Heart Failure I

Howard J. Eisen
Editor

Heart Failure I

A Comprehensive Guide to Pathophysiology and Clinical Care

Second Edition

Springer

Editor
Howard J. Eisen
Division of Cardiology
Thomas Jefferson University
Philadelphia, PA, USA

ISBN 978-3-032-12625-2 ISBN 978-3-032-12626-9 (eBook)
https://doi.org/10.1007/978-3-032-12626-9

This Springer imprint is published by the registered company Springer Nature Switzerland AG
The registered company address is: Gewerbestrasse 11, 6330 Cham, Switzerland

Contents

Molecular Changes in Heart Failure

1

Raymond C. Givens and P. Christian Schulze

Abbreviations

AKAP	A-kinase anchoring protein
ANF	Atrial natriuretic factor
AT	Angiotensin
BAD	Bcl-2-antagonist of cell death
BNP	Brain-type natriuretic peptide
cGMP	Cyclic guanine monophosphate
CHF	Congestive heart failure
CRP	C-reactive protein
DAG	Diacylglycerol
DISC	Death-induced signaling complex
ECM	Extracellular matrix
ERAD	Endoplasmic reticulum-associated degradation
ERK	Extracellular-signal-related kinase
FAK	Focal adhesion kinase
Gab	Grb2-associated binder
GSK3β	Glycogen synthase kinase 3β
HSP	Heat shock protein
ILK	Integrin-linked kinase
IP_3	Inositol triphosphate
LCAD	Long-chain acyl-CoA dehydrogenase
LTCC	L-type calcium channel
LVAD	Left ventricular assist device
MAPK	Mitogen-activated protein kinases
MCAD	Medium-chain acyl-CoA dehydrogenase
miR	Micro-RNA
MI	Myocardial infarction
MLP	Muscle LIM protein
MMP	Matrix metalloproteinase
mTOR	Molecular target of rapamycin
NF-κB	Nuclear factor kappa-light-chain-enhancer of activated B cells
NFAT	Nuclear factor of activated T cells
NOS	Nitric oxide synthase
NOX	NADPH oxidase
PI3K	Phosphoinositide-3-kinase
PKA	Protein kinase A
PKC	Protein kinase C
PPAR	Peroxisome proliferator-activated receptor
RyR2	Ryanodine receptor type 2
SAC	Stretch-activated ion channel
SERCA	Sarcoplasmic reticulum Ca^{2+} ATPase
SOC	Store-operated Ca^{2+} channel
TAC	Transaortic constriction
TGF-β	Tissue growth factor beta
TIMP	Tissue inhibitor of metalloproteinase
TNF-α	Tumor necrosis factor alpha
TnI	Troponin I

R. C. Givens
Division of Cardiology, Department of Medicine, Columbia University Medical Center, New York, NY, USA
e-mail: rg2751@cumc.columbia.edu

P. C. Schulze (✉)
Division of Cardiology, Department of Medicine, Columbia University Medical Center, New York, NY, USA

Friedrich-Schiller University, Jena, Germany

Chair, Department of Medicine, Friedrich-Schiller University, Jena, Germany
e-mail: pcs2121@cumc.columbia.edu

H. J. Eisen (ed.), *Heart Failure I*, https://doi.org/10.1007/978-3-032-12626-9_1

TnT	Troponin T
TRP	Transient receptor potential
βMHC	β-myosin heavy chain

Introduction

Over the past three centuries, medical understanding of heart failure has evolved from a simple appreciation of biomechanical and circulatory changes accompanying heart failure to recognition of the complex multiorgan physiology of this syndrome. Within the past few decades, breakthroughs in genetics and molecular investigation have revealed a vast array of cellular and molecular changes that occur in the heart and systemically as a result of hemodynamic insult. The picture of changes occurring in cardiac hypertrophy and heart failure has become increasingly complex. The goal of this chapter is to summarize the cellular and molecular changes that occur in clinical and experimental heart failure and to highlight established and potential therapeutic targets.

Compensatory Mechanisms

A large variety of myocardial insults can lead to heart failure. In the U.S., atherosclerotic coronary artery disease resulting in myocardial infarction and chronic ischemia as well as chronic arterial hypertension appear to account for the greatest population-level risk [1, 2]. There is also a rising contribution from diabetes and its associated end-organ manifestations including coronary artery disease. In contrast, infectious and valvular heart disease have declined in their impact on heart failure incidence [3].

Regardless of the nature of the initial insult, there appear to be common pathologic responses to cardiac pressure or volume overload. A hallmark finding in the stressed myocardium is hypertrophy of viable cardiomyocytes [4, 5]. The law of LaPlace indicates that the development of cardiac wall thickening due to myocyte hypertrophy is initially protective in that it serves to normalize transmural stress [6, 7]. However, persistent hypertrophy and sustained activation of the molecular pathways responsible for the initial hypertrophic response become physiologically deleterious over time [8].

More than a century of work has clarified that striated muscles such as the myocardium and skeletal muscles respond to an increased workload, e.g. hypertension, by becoming hypertrophic [9–11]. Cardiomyocytes are classically considered to be post-mitotic and, thus, cardiac hypertrophy is thought to result solely from an increase in size of existing cells. The degree to which cardiomyocyte generation from progenitor cells contributes is unclear [12]. The proliferation of non-myocyte cell types such as fibroblasts, smooth muscle cells, mesenchymal cells and the endothelium, however, may contribute significantly to the negative consequences of pathologic hypertrophy, such as myocardial and perivascular fibrosis [13, 14].

The phrase "cardiac remodeling" was originally used to describe gross structural and functional cardiac changes occurring in response to myocardial infarction but has more recently come to describe an expanding list of molecular, cellular, matricellular, metabolic, and electrical alterations resulting from sustained stress [15]. Transaortic constriction (TAC) to produce pressure overload among mice yields significant increases in myocardial thickness and relative cardiac size as early as 2 days later, and increased myocyte size and fibrosis and decreased ejection fraction by as early as 1 week [16, 17]. A pig TAC model reveals increased sarcoplasmic reticulum (SR) Ca^{2+} ATPase (SERCA) expression and activity and increased SR Ca^{2+} uptake within 6 h of TAC [18]. Treatment of rats with the nonselective β-adrenergic receptor agonist isoproterenol increased expression of the "fetal genes" c-fos and jun-B within 1 h and provoked cardiac hypertrophy by 24 h [19]. The β-adrenergic receptor blocker propranolol prevented early increases in c-fos expression. Analysis of myocardial tissue from this model by electron microscopy revealed mitochondrial swelling and disruption, intra- and extracellular edema, and fibroblast invasion by 96 h.

Persistence of stress upon the myocardium leads to progression of cardiac remodeling associated with the initial hypertrophic responses towards a maladaptive phenotype of systolic dysfunction and cardiac dilation [15]. Neurohormones of the adrenergic and renin-angiotensin-aldosterone systems provide additional cardiac stimuli that are also initially compensatory but with time contribute to adverse cardiac remodeling and multiorgan physiologic derangement. Further progressive cardiac insufficiency results in multiorgan dysfunction and death in the absence of successful intervention.

Cardiomyocyte Changes

The cardiac response to physiologic stress entails complex remodeling of cardiomyocytes and the extracellular matrix. Cardiomyocyte hypertrophy is one of the most appreciable changes in strained and failing myocardium at a microscopic level. However, sustained activation of pro-hypertrophic pathways causes cardiac dysfunction.

The pressure or volume overload caused by a physiologic insult deforms the cardiac microarchitecture. One method by which changes in extracellular mechanical forces are conveyed to the nucleus is through stretch-activated ion channels (SACs). Alterations in mechanical plasma membrane tension are sufficient to activate SACs, which are represented in mammals by transient receptor potential channels (TRPs) that are expressed in cardiomyocytes, vascular smooth muscle cells, and endothelial cells [20, 21]. A representative member, TRPC6, is located on the t-tubule membrane and is triggered to allow the influx of calcium through mechanical stretch and through association with stretch-sensitive receptors [22, 23]. TRPC6 is also activated by diacylglycerol (DAG) independent of protein kinase C (PKC) activity, and by angiotensin II receptor type 1 (AT1R) independent of angiotensin II (AT-II) [24–26]. The SAC-mediated increase in cytoplasmic Ca^{2+} entry activates the protein phosphatase calcineurin A, which can then dephosphorylate nuclear factor of activated T cells (NFAT), allowing it to enter the nucleus and induce expression of pro-hypertrophic genes, discussed below [27, 28]. The promoters of TRPC 1, 3, and 6 display NFAT consensus binding sites and TRPC isoform expression is increased in hypertrophic animal models and failing human hearts [29].

Cellular deformation is also communicated to the nucleus through the integrin family of cell surface receptors that link cytoskeletal and contractile machinery to the extracellular matrix (ECM) through their association with focal adhesion complexes and complex multimolecular structures known as a costameres. The proteins that form the costameric complex are localized to Z-discs, which form the lateral boundaries of the sarcomere, the basic contractile unit of the cardiomyocyte [30–32]. Costameres and focal adhesion complexes are linked to multiple hypertrophic signaling pathways [33, 34]. Integrins themselves bind to a large variety of extracellular ligands such as laminin, collagen, and fibronectin [35–37]. Stretch activation of integrin-associated cytoplasmic focal adhesion kinase (FAK) and integrin-linked kinase (ILK) triggers activation of phosphoinositide-3-kinase (PI3K), resulting in downstream activation of Akt and the mitogen-activated protein kinase (MAPK) cascade [38, 39]. Grb2-associated binder (Gab) proteins participate in signaling through Ras, which also triggers MAPK activation and contributes to cardiomyocyte hypertrophy [40] (Fig. 1.1).

Mechanical stretch also activates G-protein-coupled plasma membrane receptors such as AT1R and endothelin A (ETA) in cardiomyocytes and vascular smooth muscle cells, leading to indirect activation of TRP channel opening [24, 41]. Stretching of ventricular cardiomyocytes or treatment with AT-II activates AT1R, inducing activation of extracellular signal-related kinases (ERKs) and Gαq isoforms. Pressure overload in an animal model causes AT1R–dependent cardiac hypertrophy, again even in the absence of AT-II [24]. Gαq proteins activate phospholipase C, leading to an increase in cytosolic inositol triphosphate (IP_3) and DAG [42]. IP_3 activates TRP

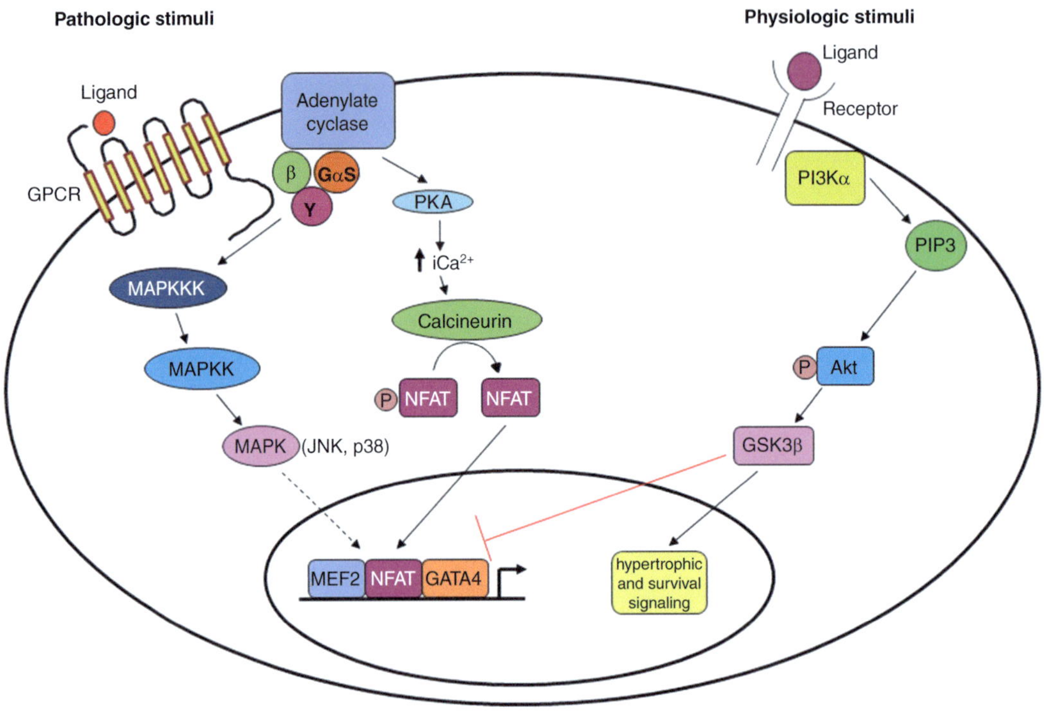

Fig. 1.1 Physiologic and pathologic hypertrophic signaling

3, 6, and 7, and also triggers an IP_3 receptor on the endoplasmic reticulum (ER), leading to Ca^{2+} release from the ER [43]. This Ca^{2+} store depletion activates plasma membrane store-operated Ca^{2+} channels (SOCs), increasing Ca^{2+} influx from extracellular sources [44] (Fig. 1.2).

Increased cytosolic concentrations of Ca^{2+} and DAG activate protein kinase C (PKC) isoforms whose signaling increases expression of early stress-response genes, such as c-fos, c-jun, jun-B, c-myc, egr-1, and heat shock protein (HSP) 70 [45]. Nkx2.5 and GATA-4, also activated by PKC signaling, may participate in PKC downregulating expression of the sarcoplasmic reticulum (SR) Ca^{2+} ATPase (SERCA), which is responsible for rapid reuptake of Ca^{2+} into the SR [46, 47]. SERCA downregulation explains much of the calcium signaling abnormalities seen in heart failure and has emerged as a potential therapeutic target [48, 49]. Changes in calcium handling associated with cardiac hypertrophy are directly involved in the cell death that characterizes the transition to systolic dysfunction and clinical heart failure [50] (Fig. 1.3).

In experimental models and in limited human data, treatment with the calcineurin inhibitors cyclosporine A or FK506 opposes the hypertrophic phenotype [51–54]. Increased cytosolic and mitochondrial Ca^{2+} concentrations provoke apoptosis [55, 56]. Calcineurin may link hypertrophy to apoptosis by dephosphorylating the pro-apoptotic protein Bcl-2-antagonist of cell death (BAD), promoting its association with Bcl-xl [57].

The actions of GATA-4 and NFAT are opposed by glycogen synthase kinase 3β (GSK3β), which inactivates these proteins through phosphorylation [58]. GSK3β is itself controlled by Akt and PKA, both of which repress GSK3β activity through phosphorylation [59, 60]. Active GSK3β is known to be a negative regulator of hypertrophy [61].

Mechanical stress upon the intact heart activates MAP kinases p38 and ERK 1/2, resulting in phosphorylation of the zinc-finger transcription factor GATA-4. As a result of phosphorylation at serine 105, GATA-4 is activated, thereby allowing its binding to DNA targets such as the BNP promoter [62–64].

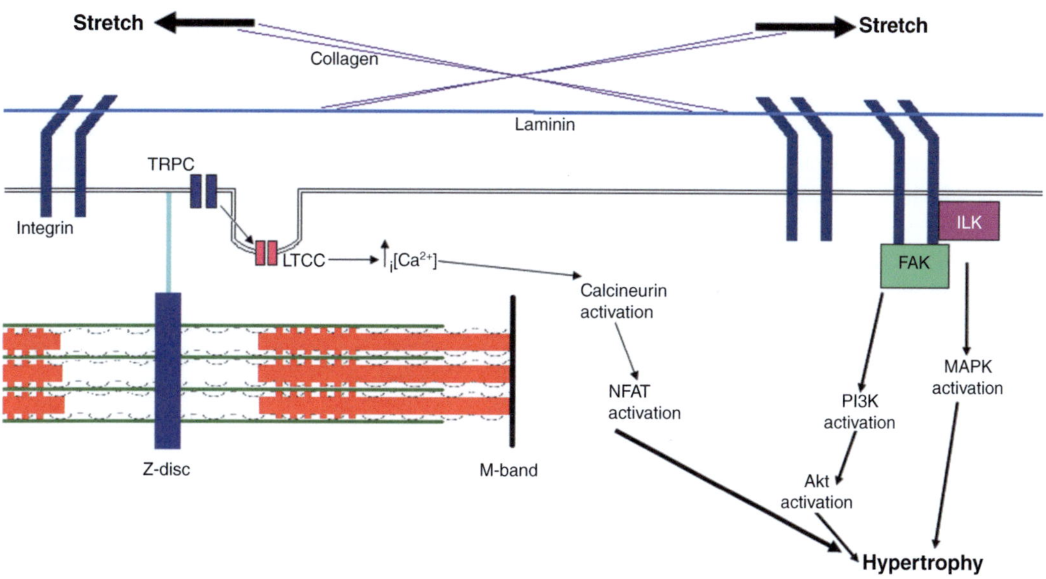

Fig. 1.2 Cardiac mechanotransduction

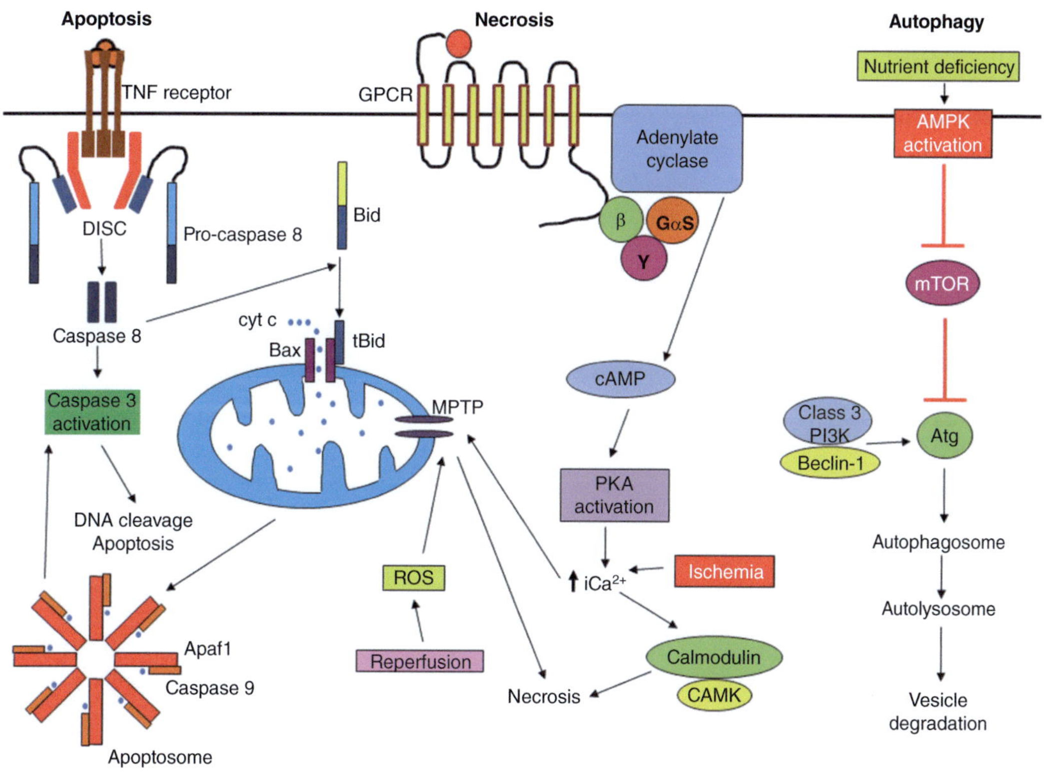

Fig. 1.3 Pathways of cellular death in heart failure

AT1R is induced by pressure overload, and the resulting increase in signaling is prohypertrophic in ways that are dependent and independent of AT-II [24]. AT1R signaling activates TRPC channels, resulting in prohypertrophic signals and derangements in calcium handling [43]. AT-II induces expression of TGF-β1 in cardiac fibroblasts, leading to increased collagen production and fibrosis [65, 66].

At a gross level, cardiac hypertrophy strongly predicts the development of clinical heart failure [67]. The pathologic hypertrophy of pressure or volume overload differs molecularly in important ways from the physiologic hypertrophy that occurs in response to exercise training or pregnancy. Re-expression of the fetal gene program appears to be absent in physiologic hypertrophy [68]. Both physiologic hypertrophy and normal cardiac growth are mediated by insulin-like growth factor 1 (IGF-1), which induces hypertrophy through an Akt pathway. Unlike pathologic hypertrophy mediators, IGF-1 activity is anti-apoptotic and IGF-1 administration in a rat model of ischemic cardiac failure leads to a preservation of systolic function and has beneficial effects on adverse cardiac remodeling [69]. Sustained experimental activation of IGF-1 pathways can, however, eventually cause a transition from physiologic hypertrophy to a more classically pathologic phenotype (Table 1.1).

While most cardiac mass is represented by the cardiomyocytes, several other cell types and extracellular structures are important in the control of cardiac function and demonstrate significant alterations in heart failure. Cardiac mast cells, fibroblasts, conductive tissue, endothelial cell, vascular smooth cells, cardiac progenitor, and resident macrophages contribute cardiac mass and biology. Fibroblasts outnumber cardiomyocytes roughly threefold in the intact heart, multiply in response to mechanical stretch, and contribute to extracellular remodeling.

Diastolic stretch activates NADPH oxidase 2 (NOX2), leading to the production of reactive oxygen species (ROS). ROS may then increase Ca2+ release from sarcoplasmic reticulum by sensitizing ryanodine receptor type 2 channels (RyR2) [70]. NOX2 activity may be critical to induction of cardiomyocyte apoptosis by hypertrophic stimuli such as AngII, as NOX2 inhibition or deletion of the NOX2 cofactor $p47^{phox}$ interferes with AngII-induced apoptosis [71].

Myocyte hypertrophy is generally characterized by the reactivation of a number of genes that

Table 1.1 Cellular and molecular changes in physiologic hypertrophy and heart failure

	Normal	Physiologic stimuli	Heart failure
Molecular changes			
"Fetal gene program"	–	–	Increased
Myosin heavy chain isoform	α-MHC	α-MHC	β-MHC
Biomarkers			
BNP	–	Unclear	Elevated
Troponin	Normal	Unknown	May be increased
Cytokine activation	Normal	Normal	Increased TNF-α, IL-6
Catecholamine levels	Normal	Normal	Increased
Cellular changes			
Cell size	Normal	Hypertrophied	Hypertrophied
Fibrosis	Normal	Normal	Increased
Cell death	Normal	Normal	Increased
Capillary density	Normal	Preserved	Decreased
Calcium cycling	Normal	Normal	Increased
Metabolism	Predominately fatty acid oxidation	Predominately fatty acid oxidation	Predominately glucose oxidation
Contractile function	Normal	Normal	Decreased
Excitation-contraction coupling	Normal	Normal	Altered

are normally expressed during fetal development but eventually become quiescent after birth [72]. This "fetal gene program" includes increased expression of GATA-4, Nkx2.5, and PTX transcription factors, is typical of cell cycle entry. These transcription factors drive the expression of classic fetal genes that are markers and essential mediators of cardiomyocyte hypertrophy, including atrial natriuretic (ANF), brain-type natriuretic peptide (BNP), α-skeletal actin, β-myosin heavy chain (βMHC), and angiotensin-II receptor type 1 (AT1R) [73, 74].

Myocardium-Vascular Mismatch

It has been observed that as cardiac hypertrophy progresses, there is relatively lower concomitant vascularization, such that the number of capillaries per area of myocardium declines [75]. Microvascular dysfunction and decreased coronary flow reserve are observed in experimental and clinic hypertrophy and heart failure even in the absence of coronary atherosclerosis [76, 77]. These changes have been linked to subendocardial ischemia in hypertrophy and may accelerate the transition to heart failure. Treatment of a rabbit TAC model with vascular endothelial growth factor (VEGF) induces MMP-2-dependent angiogenesis, delays the onset of LV dilation, and preserves LV contractility [78].

Fibroblast Proliferation and Fibrosis

The majority of cardiac cellular components are represented by cardiomyocytes, endothelial cells, vascular smooth muscle cells, and fibroblasts. But while cardiomyocytes are the necessary cells for cardiac contraction, they comprise only a third of cardiac cells. The remainder of cardiac mass is mostly comprised of fibroblasts, which are responsible for the production of the extracellular matrix (ECM) that functions as the cardiac mechanical scaffold. Additionally, ECM components contribute to the regulation of cellular growth, tissue differentiation, and angiogenesis. Cardiac fibrosis, which is characterized by the increased extracellular presence of collagens and other ECM components, is a hallmark of advanced hypertrophy and heart failure [79].

Fibroblasts can be activated by increased interstitial fluid flow to produce collagen type III and TGF-β, effects that may be opposed by blockade of the AT1 and TGF-β receptors [80]. Experimental hypertrophic stimuli such as infusion of AngII increase fibroblast production of IL-6, which leads to collagen I production from fibroblasts and may contribute to cardiomyocyte hypertrophy through paracrine signaling [81–84].

Excitation-Contraction Coupling

Cardiac contraction results from Ca^{2+}-dependent interactions of myosin and actin myofilaments. During cell membrane depolarization, Ca^{2+} enters the cardiomyocyte through L-type Ca^{2+} channels (LTCCs) located at transverse tubules, which are in proximity to the sarcoplasmic reticulum (SR) [85]. Ca^{2+} influx triggers a larger release of Ca^{2+} from the SR through ryanodine receptors (RyR2). The SR Ca^{2+}-ATPase (SERCA2A) is responsible for restoring Ca^{2+} to the SR [48]. The disappearance of SERCA2A during the progression of hypertrophy and heart failure alters the coupling of Ca^{2+} flux to the cardiomyocyte contractile apparatus [86]. In failing human hearts, there is a significant reduction in t-tubule-SR junctional dyads and thus in the co-localization of LTCCs and RyR2, indicating a degree of both physical and biochemical uncoupling of excitation from contraction [87, 88].

Sarcolemmal Proteins

Sufficient myocyte contractile force is dependent upon appropriate excitation-contraction coupling, which requires precise coordination between the entry of extracellular Ca^{2+} into the cytoplasm and the wave of Ca^{2+} release from the sarcoplasmic reticulum (SR) [89]. Transverse tubules (t-tubules) are invaginations of the surface membrane, continuous with the extracellular space, that extend into the interior of cardiac myocytes [36, 90].

T-tubules form a highly organized network that is physically coupled to the SR at Z-discs [91]. This organization is essential for coordination of excitation-contraction coupling. LTCCs are predominately localized to t-tubules and are responsible for the initial cellular Ca^{2+} influx. Ca^{2+} efflux is largely handled by the sodium-calcium exchanger (NCX), found on both tubular and non-tubular sarcolemmal [92]. The relative importance of Ca^{2+} efflux through these different domains is unclear. A population of β adrenergic receptors is localized to t-tubules, where they appear to modulate LTCC function and localize cAMP signaling [93]. In rodent heart failure models, this localization is lost, with β2 receptors redistributing from t-tubules to the cell crest, leading to diffusion of cAMP signaling [94].

Hypertrophied and failing hearts demonstrate misshapen and dilated t-tubules and tubular disorganization and disappearance, which has been called t-tubule remodeling [87]. The degree of tubular remodeling is associated with the severity of heart failure [95]. As L-type calcium channels are primarily localized to T-tubules, there is also a decline in inward calcium currents in failing myocytes [96]. In a rodent model, T-tubule disruption can be reversed after mechanical unloading with heterotopic abdominal heart transplantation [97].

Myocardial Metabolism in Heart Failure

Myocardial metabolism depends to large parts (>70% at baseline) on the utilization of fatty acids for oxidative metabolism and ATP generation. The complete oxidation of one molecule of palmitic acid as an example for the most prevalent circulating and nutritionally derived saturated fatty acid generates 129 ATP molecules. In contrast, complete oxidation of glucose results in generation of 36 ATP molecules. Therefore, oxidation of fatty acids is a more energy efficient process compared to the oxidation of glucose (Fig. 1.4).

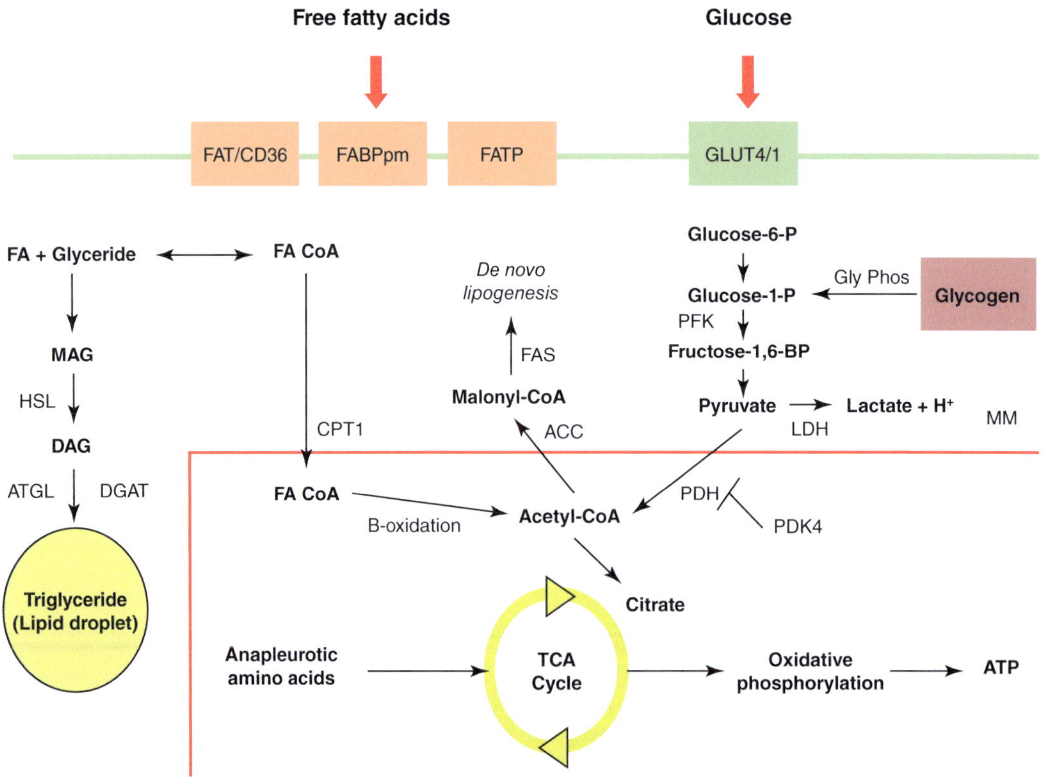

Fig. 1.4 Cardiac metabolism

The reversion to the fetal gene expression in cardiac hypertrophy and heart failure encompasses not only structural and contractile genes but also metabolic substrate utilization. During fetal development, cardiac metabolism depends primarily upon glycolysis, but the heart transitions toward fatty acid oxidation in the postnatal period [98]. While lipid metabolism may increase early in experimental hypertrophy, expression levels of fatty acid oxidation enzymes are decreased in the failing heart [99, 100]. An important determinant of fatty acid utilization and metabolism is the activity of PPARα, which targets binding sites in the promoters for the genes encoding carnitine palmitoyl transferase-I (CPT-I) and long-chain and medium-chain acyl-COA dehydrogenases (LCAD and MCAD) and activates their transcription [101]. In the hypertrophied heart, the relative shift from fatty acid to glucose utilization occurs in concert with decreased PPARα activity and expression [102]. Of note, further changes in myocardial gene expression result in a preferential generation of ATP through anaerobic metabolism, namely glycolytic breakdown of glucose to pyruvate and lactase. This is best known for myocardial metabolism in circumstances of ischemia and has been shown to produce only 8 molecules of ATP during glycolysis resulting in a severe energy (ATP)-depleted state of the failing myocardium. Reversibility of cardiac metabolism after cardiac recompensation requires up to 5 days until ATP stores reach levels known from stable heart failure patients.

Part of the repression of PPARα activity in cardiac hypertrophy may be explained by sequestration of this nuclear transcription factor in the cytoplasm by the MAP kinase kinase MEK1 [103]. The repression of PPARα expression and activity may be involved in the progression of pathological hypertrophy. Administration of PPARα ligands such as conjugated linoleic acid opposes cardiac hypertrophy in spontaneously hypertensive rat strain [104].

Ectopic accumulation of lipids in non-adipose tissues leads to lipotoxicity. In animal models and in human heart failure patients, fatty acid utilization declines and cardiac metabolism shifts back toward the fetal phenotype of glucose dependence [99, 105]. Recent work has demonstrated the myocardial accumulation of toxic lipid intermediates such as ceramide and diacylglycerol in the failing myocardium with depletion of stores of neutral lipids including triglycerides and fatty acids. Mechanical support with a left ventricular assist device (LVAD) may reverse some of the cardiac and systemic metabolic abnormalities observed in heart failure [106].

Myocardial Inflammation in Heart Failure

The progression of cardiac hypertrophy and heart failure are linked to inflammation in several ways. Elevated serum levels of TNF-α and IL-6 are seen among heart failure patients and correlate with NYHA heart failure class, the degree of cardiac cachexia, and overall prognosis [107–110]. Myocardial tissue from patients with severe heart failure obtained at the time of heart transplantation revealed an increased presence of macrophages and T lymphocytes and more endothelial activation, as indicated by the presence of intercellular adhesion molecule-1 (ICAM-1) [111].

Experimental pressure overload induces cardiac expression of proinflammatory cytokines TNF-α and IL-6, which further contribute to cardiac hypertrophy and heart failure [112–114]. TNF-α binding to its receptor TNFR1 leads to formation of the death inducing signaling complex (DISC), downstream caspase activation, and resulting apoptotic cell death. Upregulation of IL-6 expression through an α1 adrenergic receptor-A kinase anchoring protein (AKAP)-inhibitor of IκB kinase β (IKKβ) may lead to autocrine and paracrine increases in fetal and hypertrophic gene transcription through the IL-6 receptor [115]. Patients who respond clinically t o cardiac resynchronization therapy show decreased serum levels of IL-6, as well as IL-8, TNF-α, and TGF-β; among non-responders, TGF-β levels increase [116, 117].

Cell Death]

The processes outlined above contribute to apoptosis, necrosis, and autophagy, which together account for a significant increase in myocardial cell death and partly account for the transition from compensated hypertrophy to decompensated heart failure. All of the types of cell death can occur simultaneously and in close proximity to each other in failing human hearts [118]. Autophagy is the packaging of intracellular components into double-membrane autophagosomes that are then degraded by lysosomes. Autophagy can be induced by nutrient depletion, hypoxia, oxidative stress, organelle damage, and protein aggregation through pathways that are dependent upon and independent of molecular target of rapamycin (mTOR). Under conditions of ischemia, autophagy appears to be instrumental in maintaining cardiac function. With reperfusion, the continued activities of autophagic processes may lead to cell loss and resulting cardiac dysfunction. One of the pathways responsible for autophagy is AMPK. A mouse model with dominant-negative AMPK in cardiac myocytes showed decreased autophagy in response to ischemia, leading to worse cardiac function in response to myocardial infarction [119]. Some lines of evidence suggest that autophagy facilitates the development of heart failure. Mice with cardiac overexpression of beclin 1, required for autophagosome formation, have increased cardiac autophagy, ventricular dilation, cardiac fibrosis, and mortality compared to non-transgenic mice in response to transaortic constriction (TAC). Mice heterozygous for a disrupted beclin 1 gene have less cardiac autophagy and better preservation of systolic function [120]. Autophagy is repressed by mTOR, a member of the PI3K-related kinase family. Mice with a conditional cardiac knockout of raptor, an essential component of mTOR complex 1, develop severe cardiac dilation, increased autophagy, and a transition from oxidation of fatty acids to glucose utilization in response to TAC; these mice do not develop a classic initial hypertrophic response [121] (Fig. 1.3).

Increased cardiomyocyte apoptosis has been confirmed in multiple animal models of heart failure and in myocardial samples from heart failure patients [122, 123]. Important contributors to cardiomyocyte apoptosis include cytokines that are produced as part of the initial hypertrophic gene expression cascade. Serum TNF-α levels are increased among heart failure patients and are associated with worsening functional class [108, 124–126]. TNF-α expression is increased in mechanically stretched cardiomyocytes in culture and in pressure-overloaded cardiac tissue after aortic banding, correlating with apoptotic index [127, 128]. The apoptotic response is attenuated in TNF-α-knockout mice [127]. Infusion of animal models with TNF-α or cardiac-specific overexpression of TNF-α increases myocyte apoptosis and causes worsening of systolic function [129]. TNF-α binds to its receptor TNFR1, prompting formation of the death inducing signaling complex (DISC), recruitment of FADD, and activation of caspase 8, which then cleaves caspase 3, leading to activation caspase activated DNAse (CAD) and resulting DNA cleavage and apoptotic cell death [130, 131].

Cardiomyocyte necrosis due to oncotic cell death results from cellular ATP depletion, causing inactivation of ATP-dependent ion pumps and thus dissipation of energy-dependent osmotic gradients [132, 133]. Cellular swelling results and intracellular contents are released into the extracellular space. Oxygen deprivation may be a cause of ATP depletion. Decreased oxygen tension can result from coronary ischemia. Additionally, there may chronic hypoxia due to mismatch between myocyte size and vascular density in the hypertrophied heart. In advanced cardiac hypertrophy, the increased size of myocytes outpaces the production of new capillaries, leading to a relative decrease in capillary density and creating increased oxygen diffusion distance to myocytes [75]. There is also an increase in coronary vascular resistance [134].

Cellular necrosis has traditionally been considered to be an accidental and unregulated process but, in at least some cases, appears to be governed by sophisticated regulatory pathways. A plasma membrane pathway, involving some of the same molecular machinery utilized by TNF-α to promote apoptosis, has been identified [135]. The actions of TNF-α at the plasma membrane can promote either cellular survival or death, with necrosis prevailing when survival and apoptotic pathways are inhibited [136]. TNF-α binds to TNF-α receptor I (TNFRI), leading to the recruitment of a multimolecular complex that ultimately activates NF-κB, promoting cellular survival [137]. This complex can subsequently recruit Fas-associated protein with death domain (FADD), resulting in a second complex that can promote necrosis [138, 139].

The coordinated effects of metabolic derangements, cardiomyocyte death, and interstitial fibrosis cause a shift from compensated hypertrophy to decompensated heart failure. PPARγ coactivator-1 (PGC-1) isoforms α and β are both suppressed in response to experimental pressure overload, and the loss of these activities appears central to the hypertrophy-heart failure transition [140, 141]. In addition to regulating the expression of nuclear genes responsible for fatty acid import and oxidation, PGC-1 isoforms also activate the expression of transcription factors that target the mitochondrial genome, controlling the expression of oxidative phosphorylation genes and mitochondrial biogenesis [140, 142]. Cardiac PGC-1α overexpression causes unchecked mitochondrial proliferation, disrupting normal contractile structure and leading to a dilated cardiomyopathy [143]. PGC-1β-knockout mice demonstrate more cardiac fibrosis, higher levels of reactive oxygen species, and greater reduction in ejection fraction after trans-aortic banding than do wild-type mice [141].

Extracellular Matrix Changes in Heart Failure

Extracellular matrix turnover, largely catalyzed by matrix metalloproteinases (MMPs), is central to myocardial remodeling. Myocardial levels of collagenase-3 and membrane-type MMPs are increased in heart failure. Circulating levels of MMP-2 and MMP-9 are found in heart failure patients. Peroxynitrite, formed by the reaction of superoxide anion with nitric oxide, activates MMPs. Conversely, MMP inhibition lessens to effects of peroxynitrite on contractile dysfunction in isolated cardiomyocytes [144]. Animal models demonstrate the ability of pharmacologic MMP inhibition to favorably affect post-MI remodeling. Genetic deletion of tissue inhibitors of metalloproteinases (TIMPs) causes acceleration of post-MI remodeling.

Vascular Changes and Endothelial Dysfunction

Normal endothelium functions as a structural barrier between blood and the vascular wall and as a regulator of vascular tone and coagulation by balancing opposing factors [145]. One of its most important roles is the production of nitric oxide (NO) by nitric oxide synthase (NOS) isoforms. NO produces vascular smooth muscle relaxation through stimulation of guanylate cyclase production of cyclic guanosine monophosphate (cGMP). The oxidative stress that characterizes heart failure inhibits NOS production of NO. Decreased NO availability then contributes to vasoconstriction and increased after load. Vasoconstriction as well may cause a relative hypoperfusion of the hypertrophied myocardium, further contributing to ventricular dysfunction.

Impaired Nitric Oxide Coupling

In heart failure, there appears to be increased NOS production of reactive oxygen species (ROS) such as superoxide anion instead of NO, a development that has been termed NOS uncoupling. The simultaneous decline in NO and increase in ROS lead to a decline in vasodilation and myocardial relaxation [146]. The reaction of ROS with NO leads to the formation of peroxynitrite. Infusion of peroxynitrite into intact rat hearts causes production of pro-MMP-2, a transient vasodilation that is then followed by a sustained vasoconstriction, and progressive mechanical cardiac dysfunction, changes that are prevented by treatment with an MMP inhibitor and by quenching peroxynitrite with glutathione [147].

Biomarkers of Myocardial Remodelling

As proposed by Braunwald, biomarkers of heart failure may be classified into those that reflect myocyte injury, myocardial stretch, oxidative stress, neurohormonal activation, ECM remodeling, inflammation, renal dysfunction, and others that don't fit neatly into these categories [148].

B-type natriuretic peptide (BNP), most recently more commonly used in clinical practice, and atrial natriuretic peptide (ANP) are the major examples of biomarkers reflecting myocardial stretch. The value of natriuretic peptides in guiding heart failure management has been established by clinical studies [149]. Further, plasma levels of the soluble form of ST2, which is a myocardial receptor for IL-33 in its membrane-bound form, are increased in response to myocardial stretch, and predict the occurrence of heart failure among patients with an ST-segment elevation myocardial infarction (STEMI), and death among patients with established heart failure [150, 151].

Circulating cardiac troponins (Tn) I and T are the major clinical markers of myocardial injury and necrosis. Elevated serum troponin levels can be found among individuals with essential hypertension and cardiac hypertrophy [152–155]. Conventional serum TnI levels correlate with LV wall thickness among patients with hypertrophic cardiomyopathy (HCM) [156]. In a separate study, increasing high-sensitivity TnT (hs-TnT) levels correlated with worsening functional status, outflow obstruction, and with left ventricular wall thickness among HCM patients [157]. Serum TnI predicted the development of heart failure among a community-based sample of elderly men, independently of its association with blood pressure, body mass index, smoking, and history of myocardial infarction [158]. High-sensitivity TnT level associates with risk of death among patients with nonischemic dilated cardiomyopathy [159].

The serum ratio of pro-collagen type I amino-terminal propeptide (PINP) to collagen type I cross-linked carboxyterminal telopeptide (CITP), respective markers of collagen synthesis and breakdown, may predict collagen accumulation [160]. ECM turnover depends upon the activity of matrix metalloproteinase (MMP) isoforms, which belong to a large family of zinc-dependent proteases. Their activities are inhibited by tissue inhibitors of metalloproteinases. A study of patients with heart failure with preserved ejection fraction showed significant differences in levels of MMP-2, TIMP-4, and pro-collagen type III amino-terminal propeptide (PIIINP) compared to patients with LVH but not heart failure and with controls; in levels of MMP-3 and MMP-8 compared to patients with LVH alone; and in levels of MMP-7, MMP-9, TIMP-1, TIMP-2, CITP, and osteopontin. A model consisting of PIIINP, MMP-2, MMP-8, and TIMP-4 and adjusted for clinical covariates demonstrated an improved ability to distinguish patients with heart failure with preserved ejection fraction compared to a model consisting of clinical covariates alone [161].

Serum C-reactive protein (CRP) levels are elevated among heart failure patients compared to people without heart failure. Furthermore, higher CRP levels are associated with more severe heart failure and with a higher risk of death [162]. Higher levels of CRP and IL-6 predict the onset of CHF among patients with and without metabolic syndrome [163–165]. In one study of patients with severe heart failure, serum levels of TNF-α and IL-6 and soluble receptors differed significantly between survivors and nonsurvivors, higher levels predicting lower likelihood of survival [166]. Serum levels of TNF-α and of its soluble receptors (types I and II) were elevated among heart failure compared to age-matched healthy controls, and levels of the type-II soluble receptor (sTNFRII) independently predicted death [110]. Among patients with severe heart failure in a separate study, levels of IL-6, TNF-α, and IL-1β and of the soluble receptors for TNF-α and IL-2 were associated with risk of death in univariate analyses; IL-6 levels independently predicted a combined endpoint of death, new heart failure episodes, and need for heart transplantation [167]. Galectins are a family of β-galactoside-binding proteins that regulate inflammation [168]. Higher galectin-3 levels are associated with worse heart failure functional classification and with worse outcome [169, 170].

Neuregulin-1 (NRG1) is produced by coronary endothelial cells and bind to ErbB4 receptors on cardiomyocytes, prompting its interaction with HER2/neu (ErbB2) and triggering of downstream effectors such as focal adhesion kinase (FAK) that are involved in sarcomere organization and cell survival [171]. Antagonism of HER2 with the monoclonal antibody trastuzumab in addition to chemotherapy increased the risk of cardiac fourfold compared to chemotherapy alone, despite an overall oncologic and survival benefit [172]. NRG-1β levels increase with heart failure class and predict transplant-free survival [173]. In a small clinical trial, daily infusion with a recombinant human NRG-1 for 11 days produced beneficial acute hemodynamic effects (significant reductions in pulmonary capillary wedge pressure, systemic vascular resistance, and serum levels of norepinephrine and aldosterone; and increased cardiac output) and a sustained 12% increase in LV ejection fraction at 3 months [174].

Cardiac Non-coding RNA

Micro-RNAs (miRs) are noncoding molecules, 18 to 25 nucleotides in length, that silence expression of specific genes by binding to complementary segments of messenger RNA, targeting them for degradation and/or inhibiting their translation [175]. Studies comparing human heart failure and animal models have found concordance in the upregulation of mir-24, −195, 199a, and 214 in response to cardiac stress [176].

MiRs have been found to circulate stably in blood [177]. MiR-423-5p is increased in the failing human heart; plasma levels distinguish heart failure patients from healthy controls and patients with dyspnea not due to heart failure and correlated with N-terminal-pro-BNP [178]. A small clinical study demonstrated that a combination of serum levels of miR-423-5p, −320a, −22, and -92b could differentiate between heart failure patients and controls, although the interpretation is limited by significant differences between the groups in drug treatment and the prevalences of diabetes and chronic kidney disease [179]. In a separate study, miR-423-5p showed no significant differences among patients with transposition of the great arteries and a failing systemic right ventricle after atrial repair and sex- and age-matched health controls [180]. The logarithm of plasma miR-126 concentration negatively with log[BNP], declined with worsening NYHA class, and increased with clinical improvement [181]. Plasma levels of miR-499 were elevated after acute MI and viral myocarditis and during acute heart failure [182].

Conclusion

Much progress has been made in the past half-century in the understanding of the molecular changes preceding and accompanying heart failure. Continued investigation is hoped to identify new targets for prevention, diagnosis, and therapy. Studies of in vitro systems have been invaluable in unraveling the molecular and cellular mechanisms at play in heart failure. But the major breakthroughs in this area and in biomedical science generally have issued from the creation of genetically manipulated animal models. The availability of human genome sequences and our deepening understanding of inter-individual genetic variability will illuminate new discoveries in heart failure risk and treatment. Epigenetic elements, such as microRNAs, especially those that circulate in plasma may prove to be both markers and mediators of heart failure risk, progression, and response to treatment. The explosion of data resulting from all of these efforts will require advances in bioinformatics and in systems biology.

References

1. He J, Ogden LG, Bazzano LA, Vupputuri S, Loria C, Whelton PK. Risk factors for congestive heart failure in US men and women: NHANES I epidemiologic follow-up study. Arch Intern Med. 2001;161:996–1002.
2. Rich MW. Epidemiology, pathophysiology, and etiology of congestive heart failure in older adults. J Am Geriatr Soc. 1997;45:968–74.
3. Kannel WB, Ho K, Thom T. Changing epidemiological features of cardiac failure. Br Heart J. 1994;72:S3–9.
4. Savinova OV, Gerdes AM. Myocyte changes in heart failure. Heart Fail Clin. 2012;8:1–6.
5. Ruwhof C, van der Laarse A. Mechanical stress-induced cardiac hypertrophy: mechanisms and signal transduction pathways. Cardiovasc Res. 2000;47:23–37.
6. Tallarida RJ, Rusy BF, Loughnane MH. Left ventricular wall acceleration and the law of Laplace. Cardiovasc Res. 1970;4:217–23.
7. Lorell BH, Carabello BA. Left ventricular hypertrophy: pathogenesis, detection, and prognosis. Circulation. 2000;102:470–9.
8. Packer M. Neurohormonal interactions and adaptations in congestive heart failure. Circulation. 1988;77:721–30.
9. Cotton TF. Cardiac hypertrophy. Can Med Assoc J. 1914;4:709–14.
10. Stein BR, Barnes AR. Severity and duration of hypertension in relation to amount of cardiac hypertrophy. Am J Med Sci. 1948;216:661–4.
11. Hill JA, Olson EN. Cardiac plasticity. N Engl J Med. 2008;358:1370–80.
12. Laflamme MA, Murry CE. Heart regeneration. Nature. 2011;473:326–35.
13. Adler CP, Costabel U. Cell number in human heart in atrophy, hypertrophy, and under the influence of cytostatics. Recent Adv Stud Cardiac Struct Metab. 1975;6:343–55.
14. Booz GW, Baker KM. Molecular signalling mechanisms controlling growth and function of cardiac fibroblasts. Cardiovasc Res. 1995;30:537–43.
15. McKay RG, Pfeffer MA, Pasternak RC, et al. Left ventricular remodeling after myocardial infarction: a corollary to infarct expansion. Circulation. 1986;74:693–702.
16. Souders CA, Borg TK, Banerjee I, Baudino TA. Pressure overload induces early morphological changes in the heart. Am J Pathol. 2012;181:1226–35.
17. Voelkl J, Lin Y, Alesutan I, et al. Sgk1 sensitivity of Na(+)/H(+) exchanger activity and cardiac remodeling following pressure overload. Basic Res Cardiol. 2012;107:236.
18. Nediani C, Formigli L, Perna AM, et al. Early changes induced in the left ventricle by pressure overload. An experimental study on swine heart. J Mol Cell Cardiol. 2000;32:131–42.
19. Brand T, Sharma HS, Schaper W. Expression of nuclear proto-oncogenes in isoproterenol-induced cardiac hypertrophy. J Mol Cell Cardiol. 1993;25:1325–37.
20. Sharif-Naeini R, Folgering JH, Bichet D, et al. Sensing pressure in the cardiovascular system: Gq-coupled mechanoreceptors and TRP channels. J Mol Cell Cardiol. 2010;48:83–9.
21. Inoue R, Jian Z, Kawarabayashi Y. Mechanosensitive TRP channels in cardiovascular pathophysiology. Pharmacol Ther. 2009;123:371–85.
22. Dyachenko V, Husse B, Rueckschloss U, Isenberg G. Mechanical deformation of ventricular myocytes modulates both TRPC6 and Kir2.3 channels. Cell Calcium. 2009;45:38–54.
23. Spassova MA, Hewavitharana T, Xu W, Soboloff J, Gill DL. A common mechanism underlies stretch activation and receptor activation of TRPC6 channels. Proc Natl Acad Sci USA. 2006;103:16586–91.
24. Zou Y, Akazawa H, Qin Y, et al. Mechanical stress activates angiotensin II type 1 receptor without the involvement of angiotensin II. Nat Cell Biol. 2004;6:499–506.
25. Hofmann T, Obukhov AG, Schaefer M, Harteneck C, Gudermann T, Schultz G. Direct activation of human TRPC6 and TRPC3 channels by diacylglycerol. Nature. 1999;397:259–63.
26. Lemonnier L, Trebak M, Putney JW Jr. Complex regulation of the TRPC3, 6 and 7 channel subfamily by diacylglycerol and phosphatidylinositol-4,5-bisphosphate. Cell Calcium. 2008;43:506–14.
27. Molkentin JD, Lu JR, Antos CL, et al. A calcineurin-dependent transcriptional pathway for cardiac hypertrophy. Cell. 1998;93:215–28.
28. Bush EW, Hood DB, Papst PJ, et al. Canonical transient receptor potential channels promote cardiomyocyte hypertrophy through activation of calcineurin signaling. J Biol Chem. 2006;281:33487–96.
29. Kuwahara K, Wang Y, McAnally J, et al. TRPC6 fulfills a calcineurin signaling circuit during pathologic cardiac remodeling. J Clin Invest. 2006;116:3114–26.
30. Srivastava D, Yu S. Stretching to meet needs: integrin-linked kinase and the cardiac pump. Genes Dev. 2006;20:2327–31.
31. Frank D, Frey N. Cardiac Z-disc signaling network. J Biol Chem. 2011;286:9897–904.
32. Pyle WG, Solaro RJ. At the crossroads of myocardial signaling: the role of Z-discs in intracellular signaling and cardiac function. Circ Res. 2004;94:296–305.
33. Torsoni AS, Constancio SS, Nadruz W Jr, Hanks SK, Franchini KG. Focal adhesion kinase is activated and mediates the early hypertrophic response to stretch in cardiac myocytes. Circ Res. 2003;93:140–7.
34. Hoshijima M. Mechanical stress-strain sensors embedded in cardiac cytoskeleton: Z disk, titin, and associated structures. Am J Physiol Heart Circ Physiol. 2006;290:H1313–25.

35. Laser M, Willey CD, Jiang W, et al. Integrin activation and focal complex formation in cardiac hypertrophy. J Biol Chem. 2000;275:35624–30.
36. Kostin S, Scholz D, Shimada T, et al. The internal and external protein scaffold of the T-tubular system in cardiomyocytes. Cell Tissue Res. 1998;294:449–60.
37. Ahmed N, Riley C, Rice G, Quinn M. Role of integrin receptors for fibronectin, collagen and laminin in the regulation of ovarian carcinoma functions in response to a matrix microenvironment. Clin Exp Metastasis. 2005;22:391–402.
38. Taylor JM, Rovin JD, Parsons JT. A role for focal adhesion kinase in phenylephrine-induced hypertrophy of rat ventricular cardiomyocytes. J Biol Chem. 2000;275:19250–7.
39. Hauselmann SP, Rosc-Schluter BI, Lorenz V, et al. beta1-integrin is up-regulated via Rac1-dependent reactive oxygen species as part of the hypertrophic cardiomyocyte response. Free Radic Biol Med. 2011;51:609–18.
40. Wei BR, Martin PL, Hoover SB, et al. Capacity for resolution of Ras-MAPK-initiated early pathogenic myocardial hypertrophy modeled in mice. Comp Med. 2011;61:109–18.
41. Mederos Y, Schnitzler M, Storch U, Meibers S, et al. Gq-coupled receptors as mechanosensors mediating myogenic vasoconstriction. EMBO J. 2008;27:3092–103.
42. Gresset A, Sondek J, Harden TK. The phospholipase C isozymes and their regulation. Subcell Biochem 2012;58:61–94.
43. Seth M, Zhang ZS, Mao L, et al. TRPC1 channels are critical for hypertrophic signaling in the heart. Circ Res. 2009;105:1023–30.
44. Freichel M, Schweig U, Stauffenberger S, Freise D, Schorb W, Flockerzi V. Store-operated cation channels in the heart and cells of the cardiovascular system. Cell Physiol Biochem. 1999;9:270–83.
45. Rockman HA, Ross RS, Harris AN, et al. Segregation of atrial-specific and inducible expression of an atrial natriuretic factor transgene in an in vivo murine model of cardiac hypertrophy. Proc Natl Acad Sci USA. 1991;88:8277–81.
46. Wang J, Paradis P, Aries A, et al. Convergence of protein kinase C and JAK-STAT signaling on transcription factor GATA-4. Mol Cell Biol. 2005;25:9829–44.
47. Prasad AM, Inesi G. Regulation and rate limiting mechanisms of Ca2+ ATPase (SERCA2) expression in cardiac myocytes. Mol Cell Biochem. 2012;361:85–96.
48. Zarain-Herzberg A, Fragoso-Medina J, Estrada-Aviles R. Calcium-regulated transcriptional pathways in the normal and pathologic heart. IUBMB Life. 2011;63:847–55.
49. Jessup M, Greenberg B, Mancini D, et al. Calcium upregulation by percutaneous Administration of Gene Therapy in cardiac disease (CUPID): a phase 2 trial of intracoronary gene therapy of sarcoplasmic reticulum Ca2+−ATPase in patients with advanced heart failure. Circulation. 2011;124:304–13.
50. Ling H, Zhang T, Pereira L, et al. Requirement for Ca2+/calmodulin-dependent kinase II in the transition from pressure overload-induced cardiac hypertrophy to heart failure in mice. J Clin Invest. 2009;119:1230–40.
51. Dhandapany PS, Fabris F, Tonk R, et al. Cyclosporine attenuates cardiomyocyte hypertrophy induced by RAF1 mutants in Noonan and LEOPARD syndromes. J Mol Cell Cardiol. 2011;51:4–15.
52. Paoletti E, Marsano L, Bellino D, Cassottana P, Cannella G. Effect of everolimus on left ventricular hypertrophy of de novo kidney transplant recipients: a 1 year, randomized, controlled trial. Transplantation. 2012;93:503–8.
53. Di Marco GS, Reuter S, Kentrup D, et al. Cardioprotective effect of calcineurin inhibition in an animal model of renal disease. Eur Heart J. 2011;32:1935–45.
54. Hisamitsu T, Nakamura TY, Wakabayashi S. Na(+)/H(+) exchanger 1 directly binds to calcineurin A and activates downstream NFAT signaling, leading to cardiomyocyte hypertrophy. Mol Cell Biol. 2012;32:3265–80.
55. Joiner ML, Koval OM, Li J, et al. CaMKII determines mitochondrial stress responses in heart. Nature. 2012;491:269–73.
56. Yang Y, Zhu WZ, Joiner ML, et al. Calmodulin kinase II inhibition protects against myocardial cell apoptosis in vivo. Am J Physiol Heart Circ Physiol. 2006;291:H3065–75.
57. Wang HG, Pathan N, Ethell IM, et al. Ca2+−induced apoptosis through calcineurin dephosphorylation of BAD. Science. 1999;284:339–43.
58. Antos CL, TA MK, Frey N, et al. Activated glycogen synthase-3 beta suppresses cardiac hypertrophy in vivo. Proc Natl Acad Sci USA. 2002;99:907–12.
59. Stuenaes JT, Bolling A, Ingvaldsen A, et al. Beta-adrenoceptor stimulation potentiates insulin-stimulated PKB phosphorylation in rat cardiomyocytes via cAMP and PKA. Br J Pharmacol. 2010;160:116–29.
60. Webb IG, Nishino Y, Clark JE, et al. Constitutive glycogen synthase kinase-3alpha/beta activity protects against chronic beta-adrenergic remodelling of the heart. Cardiovasc Res. 2010;87:494–503.
61. Hardt SE, Sadoshima J. Negative regulators of cardiac hypertrophy. Cardiovasc Res. 2004;63:500–9.
62. Tenhunen O, Sarman B, Kerkela R, et al. Mitogen-activated protein kinases p38 and ERK 1/2 mediate the wall stress-induced activation of GATA-4 binding in adult heart. J Biol Chem. 2004;279:24852–60.
63. Kerkela R, Pikkarainen S, Majalahti-Palviainen T, Tokola H, Ruskoaho H. Distinct roles of mitogen-activated protein kinase pathways in GATA-4 transcription factor-mediated regulation of B-type natriuretic peptide gene. J Biol Chem. 2002;277:13752–60.

64. Liang Q, Wiese RJ, Bueno OF, Dai YS, Markham BE, Molkentin JD. The transcription factor GATA4 is activated by extracellular signal-regulated kinase 1- and 2-mediated phosphorylation of serine 105 in cardiomyocytes. Mol Cell Biol. 2001;21:7460–9.
65. Gao X, He X, Luo B, Peng L, Lin J, Zuo Z. Angiotensin II increases collagen I expression via transforming growth factor-beta1 and extracellular signal-regulated kinase in cardiac fibroblasts. Eur J Pharmacol. 2009;606:115–20.
66. Shivakumar K, Dostal DE, Boheler K, Baker KM, Lakatta EG. Differential response of cardiac fibroblasts from young adult and senescent rats to ANG II. Am J Physiol Heart Circ Physiol. 2003;284:H1454–9.
67. Katz AM. The cardiomyopathy of overload: a hypothesis. J Cardiovasc Pharmacol. 1991;18(Suppl 2):S68–71.
68. Eghbali M, Deva R, Alioua A, et al. Molecular and functional signature of heart hypertrophy during pregnancy. Circ Res. 2005;96:1208–16.
69. Duerr RL, Huang S, Miraliakbar HR, Clark R, Chien KR, Ross J Jr. Insulin-like growth factor-1 enhances ventricular hypertrophy and function during the onset of experimental cardiac failure. J Clin Invest. 1995;95:619–27.
70. Prosser BL, Ward CW, Lederer WJ. X-ROS signaling: rapid mechano-chemo transduction in heart. Science. 2011;333:1440–5.
71. Maejima Y, Kuroda J, Matsushima S, Ago T, Sadoshima J. Regulation of myocardial growth and death by NADPH oxidase. J Mol Cell Cardiol. 2011;50:408–16.
72. Rajabi M, Kassiotis C, Razeghi P, Taegtmeyer H. Return to the fetal gene program protects the stressed heart: a strong hypothesis. Heart Fail Rev. 2007;12:331–43.
73. Frank D, Kuhn C, Brors B, et al. Gene expression pattern in biomechanically stretched cardiomyocytes: evidence for a stretch-specific gene program. Hypertension. 2008;51:309–18.
74. Kuwahara K, Nishikimi T, Nakao K. Transcriptional regulation of the fetal cardiac gene program. J Pharmacol Sci. 2012;119:198–203.
75. Anversa P, Capasso JM. Loss of intermediate-sized coronary arteries and capillary proliferation after left ventricular failure in rats. Am J Phys. 1991;260:H1552–60.
76. Laguens R, Alvarez P, Vigliano C, et al. Coronary microcirculation remodeling in patients with idiopathic dilated cardiomyopathy. Cardiology. 2011;119:191–6.
77. Camici PG, Olivotto I, Rimoldi OE. The coronary circulation and blood flow in left ventricular hypertrophy. J Mol Cell Cardiol. 2012;52:857–64.
78. Friehs I, Margossian RE, Moran AM, Cao-Danh H, Moses MA, del Nido PJ. Vascular endothelial growth factor delays onset of failure in pressure-overload hypertrophy through matrix metalloproteinase activation and angiogenesis. Basic Res Cardiol. 2006;101:204–13.
79. Weber KT, Janicki JS, Shroff SG, Pick R, Chen RM, Bashey RI. Collagen remodeling of the pressure-overloaded, hypertrophied nonhuman primate myocardium. Circ Res. 1988;62:757–65.
80. Galie PA, Russell MW, Westfall MV, Stegemann JP. Interstitial fluid flow and cyclic strain differentially regulate cardiac fibroblast activation via AT1R and TGF-beta1. Exp Cell Res. 2012;318:75–84.
81. Ma F, Li Y, Jia L, et al. Macrophage-stimulated cardiac fibroblast production of IL-6 is essential for TGF beta/Smad activation and cardiac fibrosis induced by angiotensin II. PLoS One. 2012;7:e35144.
82. Fredj S, Bescond J, Louault C, Delwail A, Lecron JC, Potreau D. Role of interleukin-6 in cardiomyocyte/cardiac fibroblast interactions during myocyte hypertrophy and fibroblast proliferation. J Cell Physiol. 2005;204:428–36.
83. Melendez GC, McLarty JL, Levick SP, Du Y, Janicki JS, Brower GL. Interleukin 6 mediates myocardial fibrosis, concentric hypertrophy, and diastolic dysfunction in rats. Hypertension. 2010;56:225–31.
84. Martin ML, Blaxall BC. Cardiac intercellular communication: are myocytes and fibroblasts fair-weather friends? J Cardiovasc Transl Res. 2012;5:768–82.
85. Ibrahim M, Gorelik J, Yacoub MH, Terracciano CM. The structure and function of cardiac t-tubules in health and disease. Proc R Soc Lond B Biol Sci. 2011;278:2714–23.
86. Ribadeau Dumas A, Wisnewsky C, Boheler KR, Ter Keurs H, Fiszman MY, Schwartz K. The sarco(endo) plasmic reticulum Ca(2+)-ATPase gene is regulated at the transcriptional level during compensated left ventricular hypertrophy in the rat. CR Acad Sci III. 1997;320:963–9.
87. Crossman DJ, Ruygrok PN, Soeller C, Cannell MB. Changes in the organization of excitation-contraction coupling structures in failing human heart. PLoS One. 2011;6:e17901.
88. Zhang HB, Li RC, Xu M, et al. Ultrastructural uncoupling between T-tubules and sarcoplasmic reticulum in human heart failure. Cardiovasc Res. 2013;98:269–76.
89. Guo A, Zhang C, Wei S, Chen B, Song LS. Emerging mechanisms of T-tubule remodeling in heart failure. Cardiovasc Res. 2013;98:204–15.
90. Brette F, Orchard C. T-tubule function in mammalian cardiac myocytes. Circ Res. 2003;92:1182–92.
91. Kee AJ, Gunning PW, Hardeman EC. Diverse roles of the actin cytoskeleton in striated muscle. J Muscle Res Cell Motil. 2009;30:187–97.
92. Yang Z, Pascarel C, Steele DS, Komukai K, Brette F, Orchard CH. Na+–Ca2+ exchange activity is localized in the T-tubules of rat ventricular myocytes. Circ Res. 2002;91:315–22.
93. Laflamme MA, Becker PL. G(s) and adenylyl cyclase in transverse tubules of heart: implica-

tions for cAMP-dependent signaling. Am J Phys. 1999;277:H1841–8.
94. Nikolaev VO, Moshkov A, Lyon AR, et al. Beta2-adrenergic receptor redistribution in heart failure changes cAMP compartmentation. Science. 2010;327:1653–7.
95. Wei S, Guo A, Chen B, et al. T-tubule remodeling during transition from hypertrophy to heart failure. Circ Res. 2010;107:520–31.
96. He J, Conklin MW, Foell JD, et al. Reduction in density of transverse tubules and L-type Ca(2+) channels in canine tachycardia-induced heart failure. Cardiovasc Res. 2001;49:298–307.
97. Ibrahim M, Navaratnarajah M, Siedlecka U, et al. Mechanical unloading reverses transverse tubule remodelling and normalizes local Ca(2+)-induced Ca(2+)release in a rodent model of heart failure. Eur J Heart Fail. 2012;14:571–80.
98. Jolley RL, Cheldelin VH, Newburgh RW. Glucose catabolism in fetal and adult heart. J Biol Chem. 1958;233:1289–94.
99. Sack MN, Rader TA, Park S, Bastin J, McCune SA, Kelly DP. Fatty acid oxidation enzyme gene expression is downregulated in the failing heart. Circulation. 1996;94:2837–42.
100. Abdalla S, Fu X, Elzahwy SS, Klaetschke K, Streichert T, Quitterer U. Up-regulation of the cardiac lipid metabolism at the onset of heart failure. Cardiovasc Hematol Agents Med Chem. 2011;9:190–206.
101. Meng RS, Pei ZH, Yin R, et al. Adenosine monophosphate-activated protein kinase inhibits cardiac hypertrophy through reactivating peroxisome proliferator-activated receptor-alpha signaling pathway. Eur J Pharmacol. 2009;620:63–70.
102. Karbowska J, Kochan Z, Smolenski RT. Peroxisome proliferator-activated receptor alpha is downregulated in the failing human heart. Cell Mol Biol Lett. 2003;8:49–53.
103. el Azzouzi H, Leptidis S, Bourajjaj M, van Bilsen M, da Costa Martins PA, De Windt LJ. MEK1 inhibits cardiac PPARalpha activity by direct interaction and prevents its nuclear localization. PLoS One. 2012;7:e36799.
104. Alibin CP, Kopilas MA, Anderson HD. Suppression of cardiac myocyte hypertrophy by conjugated linoleic acid: role of peroxisome proliferator-activated receptors alpha and gamma. J Biol Chem. 2008;283:10707–15.
105. Tuunanen H, Engblom E, Naum A, et al. Decreased myocardial free fatty acid uptake in patients with idiopathic dilated cardiomyopathy: evidence of relationship with insulin resistance and left ventricular dysfunction. J Card Fail. 2006;12:644–52.
106. Chokshi A, Drosatos K, Cheema FH, et al. Ventricular assist device implantation corrects myocardial lipotoxicity, reverses insulin resistance, and normalizes cardiac metabolism in patients with advanced heart failure. Circulation. 2012;125:2844–53.
107. Levine B, Kalman J, Mayer L, Fillit HM, Packer M. Elevated circulating levels of tumor necrosis factor in severe chronic heart failure. N Engl J Med. 1990;323:236–41.
108. Testa M, Yeh M, Lee P, et al. Circulating levels of cytokines and their endogenous modulators in patients with mild to severe congestive heart failure due to coronary artery disease or hypertension. J Am Coll Cardiol. 1996;28:964–71.
109. Kell R, Haunstetter A, Dengler TJ, Zugck C, Kubler W, Haass M. Do cytokines enable risk stratification to be improved in NYHA functional class III patients? Comparison with other potential predictors of prognosis. Eur Heart J. 2002;23:70–8.
110. Ferrari R, Bachetti T, Confortini R, et al. Tumor necrosis factor soluble receptors in patients with various degrees of congestive heart failure. Circulation. 1995;92:1479–86.
111. Devaux B, Scholz D, Hirche A, Klovekorn WP, Schaper J. Upregulation of cell adhesion molecules and the presence of low grade inflammation in human chronic heart failure. Eur Heart J. 1997;18:470–9.
112. Baumgarten G, Knuefermann P, Kalra D, et al. Load-dependent and -independent regulation of proinflammatory cytokine and cytokine receptor gene expression in the adult mammalian heart. Circulation. 2002;105:2192–7.
113. Yokoyama T, Nakano M, Bednarczyk JL, McIntyre BW, Entman M, Mann DL. Tumor necrosis factor-alpha provokes a hypertrophic growth response in adult cardiac myocytes. Circulation. 1997;95:1247–52.
114. Bozkurt B, Kribbs SB, Clubb FJ Jr, et al. Pathophysiologically relevant concentrations of tumor necrosis factor-alpha promote progressive left ventricular dysfunction and remodeling in rats. Circulation. 1998;97:1382–91.
115. del Vescovo CD, Cotecchia S, Diviani D. A-kinase-anchoring protein-Lbc anchors IkappaB kinase beta to support interleukin-6-mediated cardiomyocyte hypertrophy. Mol Cell Biol. 2013;33:14–27.
116. Stanciu AE, Vatasescu RG, Stanciu MM, Iorgulescu C, Vasile AI, Dorobantu M. Cardiac resynchronization therapy in patients with chronic heart failure is associated with anti-inflammatory and anti-remodeling effects. Clin Biochem. 2013;46:230–4.
117. Osmancik P, Herman D, Stros P, Linkova H, Vondrak K, Paskova E. Changes and prognostic impact of apoptotic and inflammatory cytokines in patients treated with cardiac resynchronization therapy. Cardiology. 2013;124:190–8.
118. Kostin S, Pool L, Elsasser A, et al. Myocytes die by multiple mechanisms in failing human hearts. Circ Res. 2003;92:715–24.
119. Russell RR 3rd, Li J, Coven DL, et al. AMP-activated protein kinase mediates ischemic glucose uptake and prevents postischemic cardiac dysfunction, apoptosis, and injury. J Clin Invest. 2004;114:495–503.

120. Zhu H, Tannous P, Johnstone JL, et al. Cardiac autophagy is a maladaptive response to hemodynamic stress. J Clin Invest. 2007;117:1782–93.
121. Shende P, Plaisance I, Morandi C, et al. Cardiac raptor ablation impairs adaptive hypertrophy, alters metabolic gene expression, and causes heart failure in mice. Circulation. 2011;123:1073–82.
122. Sharov VG, Sabbah HN, Shimoyama H, Goussev AV, Lesch M, Goldstein S. Evidence of cardiocyte apoptosis in myocardium of dogs with chronic heart failure. Am J Pathol. 1996;148:141–9.
123. Narula J, Haider N, Virmani R, et al. Apoptosis in myocytes in end-stage heart failure. N Engl J Med. 1996;335:1182–9.
124. Dutka DP, Elborn JS, Delamere F, Shale DJ, Morris GK. Tumour necrosis factor alpha in severe congestive cardiac failure. Br Heart J. 1997;58:257–61.
125. Zhao SP, Zeng LH. Elevated plasma levels of tumor necrosis factor in chronic heart failure with cachexia. Int J Cardiol. 1997;58:257–61.
126. Nozaki N, Yamaguchi S, Shirakabe M, Nakamura H, Tomoike H. Soluble tumor necrosis factor receptors are elevated in relation to severity of congestive heart failure. Jpn Circ J. 1997;61:657–64.
127. Sun M, Chen M, Dawood F, et al. Tumor necrosis factor-alpha mediates cardiac remodeling and ventricular dysfunction after pressure overload state. Circulation. 2007;115:1398–407.
128. Stamm C, Friehs I, Cowan DB, et al. Inhibition of tumor necrosis factor-alpha improves postischemic recovery of hypertrophied hearts. Circulation. 2001;104:I350–5.
129. Haudek SB, Taffet GE, Schneider MD, Mann DL. TNF provokes cardiomyocyte apoptosis and cardiac remodeling through activation of multiple cell death pathways. J Clin Invest. 2007;117:2692–701.
130. Crow MT, Mani K, Nam YJ, Kitsis RN. The mitochondrial death pathway and cardiac myocyte apoptosis. Circ Res. 2004;95:957–70.
131. Al-Lamki RS, Brookes AP, Wang J, et al. TNF receptors differentially signal and are differentially expressed and regulated in the human heart. Am J Transplant. 2009;9:2679–96.
132. Majno G, Joris I. Apoptosis, oncosis, and necrosis. An overview of cell death. Am J Pathol. 1995;146:3–15.
133. Weerasinghe P, Buja LM. Oncosis: an important non-apoptotic mode of cell death. Exp Mol Pathol. 2012;93:302–8.
134. Tomanek RJ, Palmer PJ, Peiffer GL, Schreiber KL, Eastham CL, Marcus ML. Morphometry of canine coronary arteries, arterioles, and capillaries during hypertension and left ventricular hypertrophy. Circ Res. 1986;58:38–46.
135. Micheau O, Tschopp J. Induction of TNF receptor I-mediated apoptosis via two sequential signaling complexes. Cell. 2003;114:181–90.
136. Whelan RS, Kaplinskiy V, Kitsis RN. Cell death in the pathogenesis of heart disease: mechanisms and significance. Annu Rev Physiol. 2010;72:19–44.
137. Ea CK, Deng L, Xia ZP, Pineda G, Chen ZJ. Activation of IKK by TNFalpha requires site-specific ubiquitination of RIP1 and polyubiquitin binding by NEMO. Mol Cell. 2006;22:245–57.
138. He S, Wang L, Miao L, et al. Receptor interacting protein kinase-3 determines cellular necrotic response to TNF-alpha. Cell. 2009;137:1100–11.
139. Holler N, Zaru R, Micheau O, et al. Fas triggers an alternative, caspase-8-independent cell death pathway using the kinase RIP as effector molecule. Nat Immunol. 2000;1:489–95.
140. Riehle C, Abel ED. PGC-1 proteins and heart failure. Trends Cardiovasc Med. 2012;22:98–105.
141. Riehle C, Wende AR, Zaha VG, et al. PGC-1beta deficiency accelerates the transition to heart failure in pressure overload hypertrophy. Circ Res. 2011;109:783–93.
142. Kelly DP, Scarpulla RC. Transcriptional regulatory circuits controlling mitochondrial biogenesis and function. Genes Dev. 2004;18:357–68.
143. Lehman JJ, Barger PM, Kovacs A, Saffitz JE, Medeiros DM, Kelly DP. Peroxisome proliferator-activated receptor gamma coactivator-1 promotes cardiac mitochondrial biogenesis. J Clin Invest. 2000;106:847–56.
144. Leon H, Baczko I, Sawicki G, Light PE, Schulz R. Inhibition of matrix metalloproteinases prevents peroxynitrite-induced contractile dysfunction in the isolated cardiac myocyte. Br J Pharmacol. 2008;153:676–83.
145. Marti CN, Gheorghiade M, Kalogeropoulos AP, Georgiopoulou VV, Quyyumi AA, Butler J. Endothelial dysfunction, arterial stiffness, and heart failure. J Am Coll Cardiol. 2012;60:1455–69.
146. Silberman GA, Fan TH, Liu H, et al. Uncoupled cardiac nitric oxide synthase mediates diastolic dysfunction. Circulation. 2010;121:519–28.
147. Wang W, Sawicki G, Schulz R. Peroxynitrite-induced myocardial injury is mediated through matrix metalloproteinase-2. Cardiovasc Res. 2002;53:165–74.
148. Braunwald E. Biomarkers in heart failure. Preface. Heart Fail Clin. 2009;5:xiii–xiv.
149. Maisel AS, Krishnaswamy P, Nowak RM, et al. Rapid measurement of B-type natriuretic peptide in the emergency diagnosis of heart failure. N Engl J Med. 2002;347:161–7.
150. Shimpo M, Morrow DA, Weinberg EO, et al. Serum levels of the interleukin-1 receptor family member ST2 predict mortality and clinical outcome in acute myocardial infarction. Circulation. 2004;109:2186–90.
151. Dhillon OS, Narayan HK, Khan SQ, et al. Pre-discharge risk stratification in unselected STEMI: is there a role for ST2 or its natural ligand IL-33 when compared with contemporary risk markers? Int J Cardiol. 2013;167:2182–8.
152. Mishra RK, Li Y, Defilippi C, et al. Association of cardiac troponin T with left ventricular structure and function in CKD. Am J Kidney Dis. 2013;61(5):701–9.

153. Lowbeer C, Gustafsson SA, Seeberger A, Bouvier F, Hulting J. Serum cardiac troponin T in patients hospitalized with heart failure is associated with left ventricular hypertrophy and systolic dysfunction. Scand J Clin Lab Invest. 2004;64:667–76.
154. Sato Y, Yamamoto E, Sawa T, et al. High-sensitivity cardiac troponin T in essential hypertension. J Cardiol. 2011;58:226–31.
155. Negishi K, Kobayashi M, Ochiai I, et al. Association between fibroblast growth factor 23 and left ventricular hypertrophy in maintenance hemodialysis patients. Comparison with B-type natriuretic peptide and cardiac troponin T. Circ J. 2010;74:2734–40.
156. Kubo T, Kitaoka H, Okawa M, et al. Serum cardiac troponin I is related to increased left ventricular wall thickness, left ventricular dysfunction, and male gender in hypertrophic cardiomyopathy. Clin Cardiol. 2010;33:E1–7.
157. Moreno V, Hernandez-Romero D, Vilchez JA, et al. Serum levels of high-sensitivity troponin T: a novel marker for cardiac remodeling in hypertrophic cardiomyopathy. J Card Fail. 2010;16:950–6.
158. Sundstrom J, Ingelsson E, Berglund L, et al. Cardiac troponin-I and risk of heart failure: a community-based cohort study. Eur Heart J. 2009;30:773–81.
159. Kawahara C, Tsutamoto T, Nishiyama K, et al. Prognostic role of high-sensitivity cardiac troponin T in patients with nonischemic dilated cardiomyopathy. Circ J. 2011;75:656–61.
160. Biolo A, Fisch M, Balog J, et al. Episodes of acute heart failure syndrome are associated with increased levels of troponin and extracellular matrix markers. Circ Heart Fail. 2010;3:44–50.
161. Zile MR, Desantis SM, Baicu CF, et al. Plasma biomarkers that reflect determinants of matrix composition identify the presence of left ventricular hypertrophy and diastolic heart failure. Circ Heart Fail. 2011;4:246–56.
162. Anand IS, Latini R, Florea VG, et al. C-reactive protein in heart failure: prognostic value and the effect of valsartan. Circulation 2005;112:1428–1434.
163. Suzuki T, Katz R, Jenny NS, et al. Metabolic syndrome, inflammation, and incident heart failure in the elderly: the cardiovascular health study. Circ Heart Fail. 2008;1:242–8.
164. Bahrami H, Bluemke DA, Kronmal R, et al. Novel metabolic risk factors for incident heart failure and their relationship with obesity: the MESA (multiethnic study of atherosclerosis) study. J Am Coll Cardiol. 2008;51:1775–83.
165. Barac A, Wang H, Shara NM, et al. Markers of inflammation, metabolic risk factors, and incident heart failure in American Indians: the strong heart study. J Clin Hypertens. 2012;14:13–9.
166. Deswal A, Petersen NJ, Feldman AM, Young JB, White BG, Mann DL. Cytokines and cytokine receptors in advanced heart failure: an analysis of the cytokine database from the Vesnarinone trial (VEST). Circulation. 2001;103:2055–9.
167. Orus J, Roig E, Perez-Villa F, et al. Prognostic value of serum cytokines in patients with congestive heart failure. J Heart Lung Transplant. 2000;19:419–25.
168. Liu FT, Yang RY, Hsu DK. Galectins in acute and chronic inflammation. Ann N Y Acad Sci. 2012;1253:80–91.
169. Ueland T, Aukrust P, Broch K, et al. Galectin-3 in heart failure: high levels are associated with all-cause mortality. Int J Cardiol. 2011;150:361–4.
170. Anand IS, Rector TS, Kuskowski M, Adourian A, Muntendam P, Cohn JN. Baseline and serial measurements of galectin-3 in patients with heart failure: relationship to prognosis and effect of treatment with valsartan in the Val-HeFT. Eur J Heart Fail. 2013;15:511–8.
171. Pentassuglia L, Sawyer DB. ErbB/integrin signaling interactions in regulation of myocardial cell-cell and cell-matrix interactions. Biochim Biophys Acta. 2013;1833(4):909–16.
172. Slamon DJ, Leyland-Jones B, Shak S, et al. Use of chemotherapy plus a monoclonal antibody against HER2 for metastatic breast cancer that overexpresses HER2. N Engl J Med. 2001;344:783–92.
173. Ky B, Kimmel SE, Safa RN, et al. Neuregulin-1 beta is associated with disease severity and adverse outcomes in chronic heart failure. Circulation. 2009;120:310–7.
174. Jabbour A, Hayward CS, Keogh AM, et al. Parenteral administration of recombinant human neuregulin-1 to patients with stable chronic heart failure produces favourable acute and chronic haemodynamic responses. Eur J Heart Fail. 2011;13:83–92.
175. Mann DL. MicroRNAs and the failing heart. N Engl J Med. 2007;356:2644–5.
176. van Rooij E, Sutherland LB, Liu N, et al. A signature pattern of stress-responsive microRNAs that can evoke cardiac hypertrophy and heart failure. Pro Nat Acad Sci USA 2006;103:18255–18260, Proc Natl Acad Sci U S A.
177. Mitchell PS, Parkin RK, Kroh EM, et al. Circulating microRNAs as stable blood-based markers for cancer detection. Pro Natl Acad Sci U S A 2008;105:10513–10518, Proc Natl Acad Sci U S A.
178. Tijsen AJ, Creemers EE, Moerland PD, et al. MiR423-5p as a circulating biomarker for heart failure. Circ Res. 2010;106:1035–9.
179. Goren Y, Kushnir M, Zafrir B, Tabak S, Lewis BS, Amir O. Serum levels of microRNAs in patients with heart failure. Eur J Heart Fail. 2012;14:147–54.
180. Tutarel O, Dangwal S, Bretthauer J, et al. Circulating miR-423_5p fails as a biomarker for systemic ventricular function in adults after atrial repair for transposition of the great arteries. Int J Cardiol. 2013;167:63–6.
181. Fukushima Y, Nakanishi M, Nonogi H, Goto Y, Iwai N. Assessment of plasma miRNAs in congestive heart failure. Circ J. 2011;75:336–40.
182. Corsten MF, Dennert R, Jochems S, et al. Circulating MicroRNA-208b and MicroRNA-499 reflect myocardial damage in cardiovascular disease. Circ Cardiovasc Genet. 2010;3:499–506.

Hemodynamics and Heart Failure

2

Gary S. Ledley, Shahzad Ahmed, Haile Jones, Steven J. Rough, and Peter Kurnik

Introduction

Every year in the United States, there are approximately 550,000 newly diagnosed heart failure patients. Five million patients suffer from chronic heart failure. Acute heart failure exacerbation is the leading cause for hospitalization in Medicare patients over the age of 65. A fundamental understanding in the definition, etiology, pathophysiology and hemodynamics has led to advances in treatments.

G. S. Ledley
Department of Internal Medicine, Division of Cardiology, Drexel University College of Medicine, Philadelphia, PA, USA
e-mail: gledley@drexelmed.edu

S. Ahmed
Division of Cardiology, Hahnemann University Hospital, Drexel University College of Medicine, Philadelphia, PA, USA
e-mail: shahzad.ahmed@drexelmed.edu

H. Jones
Interventional Cardiology, Halifax Regional Cardiology, Roanoke Rapids, NC, USA
e-mail: hjones@med.unc.edu

S. J. Rough
Interventional Cardiology, Sweetwater Medical & Cardiovascular Institute, National City, CA, USA
e-mail: srough@sdcardiac.com

P. Kurnik (✉)
Division of Cardiology, Diagnostic and Interventional Cardiology, Drexel University College of Medicine, Philadelphia, PA, USA
e-mail: pkurnik@drexelmed.edu

Definition

The complete definition of heart failure is not confined solely to the heart, but involves a complex interplay between the heart and other organs. Definitions in heart failure have mainly focused on impaired pump function and clinical manifestations of venous congestion. Katz [1] states "*heart failure is a clinical syndrome in which heart disease reduces cardiac output, increases venous pressures, and is accompanied by molecular and other abnormalities that cause progressive deterioration of the failing heart*".

Etiology

The end result of heart failure is caused by a multitude of disease abnormalities. Damage to the heart varies in its clinical presentation, systemic effects on the body, in treatment and prognosis. Ischemic heart disease, pulmonary hypertension, systemic hypertension, primary heart muscle abnormalities and valvular abnormalities are a few of the causes of heart failure (Table 2.1) [2].

H. J. Eisen (ed.), *Heart Failure I*, https://doi.org/10.1007/978-3-032-12626-9_2

Table 2.1 Common etiologies of heart failure

Coronary heart disease	Acute coronary syndromes
Hypertension	Often associated with left ventricular hypertrophy and preserved ejection fraction
Cardiomyopathies	Familial/genetic or non-familial/non-genetic (including acquired, e.g. myocarditis)
	Hypertrophic (HCM), dilated (DCM), restrictive (RCM), arrhythmogenic right ventricular (ARVC), unclassified
Drugs	β-Blockers, calcium antagonists, antiarrhythmics, cytotoxic agents
Toxins	Alcohol, medication, cocaine, trace elements (mercury, cobalt, arsenic)
Endocrine	Diabetes mellitus, hypo/hyperthyroidism, Cushing syndrome, adrenal insufficiency, excessive growth hormone, phaeochromocytoma
Nutritional	Deficiency of thiamine, selenium, carnitine. Obesity, cachexia
Infiltrative	Sarcoidosis, amyloidosis, haemochromatosis, connective tissue disease
Others	Chagas' disease, HIV infection, peripartum cardiomyopathy, end-stage renal failure

Reprinted from Dickstein et al. [2], © 2008, by permission of Oxford University Press

Clinical Presentation

Heart failure can be classified as acute or chronic, compensated or decompensated, and combinations of these variables. History and physical examination skills are paramount to diagnosis in patients presenting with heart failure and their correlation to invasive hemodynamic alterations. Since the results from the Evaluation Study of Congestive Heart Failure and Pulmonary Artery Catheterization Effectiveness (ESCAPE) trial, the routine use of the invasive pulmonary artery catheter has largely fallen out of favor. Although the trial demonstrated no changes in primary endpoint with the routine utilization of right heart catheterization, there were correlations in the accuracy of jugular venous pressure (JVP) and right atrial pressure. An elevation of left ventricular filling pressures was associated with the findings of orthopnea and increased JVP. Discharge assessment of fluid status via elevated JVP and orthopnea ("wet") or decreased cardiac output with reduced perfusion ("cold") correlated with a 50% increase in risk of death or re-hospitalization at 6 months [3, 4]. Invasive pulmonary artery catheter hemodynamic assessment is utilized to aid in the understanding and diagnosis of pathophysiology in patients that do not respond to typical initial treatments (Fig. 2.1) [2]. Recognition

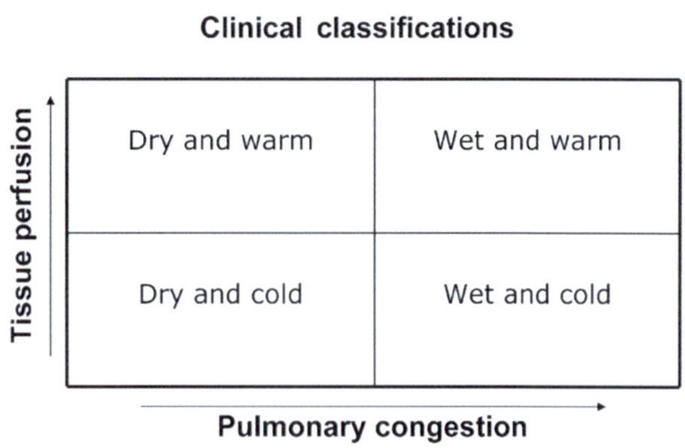

Fig. 2.1 Correlation of hemodynamic profile and invasive hemodynamic findings. (Reprinted from Dickstein et al. [2], © 2008, by permission of Oxford University Press)

of these hemodynamic characteristics can lead to alteration in therapeutic decision making.

Acute Decompensated Heart Failure

A decrease in EF due to ischemia or infarction results in primary pump failure. Acutely depressed LV function results in depressed cardiac output and venous congestion.

As the heart suffers a decrease in pump capacity there is an increase in the pressures of the venous system. The increase in venous pressure is a result of the inability of the heart to adequately accept the blood returning to the heart. Right and left atrial pressures increase. These hemodynamic alterations from a decrease in cardiac output occur within a few seconds. With the inability of a low cardiac output to provide adequate systemic perfusion, there is a response in the compensatory mechanism that results in an increase in sympathetic nervous tone.

Sympathetic stimulation results from a complex system of neurohormonal feedback. A decrease in pump function results in lower systemic arterial pressure that in turn activates the baroreceptor reflex mechanism. Ischemic heart responses, intracardiac reflexes, and other components of this feedback system contribute to sympathetic nervous system activation. Parasympathetic inhibition and sympathetic stimulation occurs within a few seconds to compensate for the acute fall in cardiac output. As sympathetic simulation occurs, the target and main effects are to the peripheral vasculature and the heart. An increase in cardiac function occurs with sympathetic stimulation to increase the recruitment of cardiac reserves within the normal and the remaining partially functional damaged myocardium. If there is diffuse damage to the ventricular myocardium during an ischemic insult, there is strengthening in the remaining functional myocytes via sympathetic stimulation. If there is no function of a portion of the ventricle, sympathetic stimulation results in the stimulation of the remaining normal myocardium. The normal myocardium attempts to compensate for the shortcomings of the damaged myocardium.

In addition to increasing myocardial muscle function, sympathetic stimulation leads to changes in the peripheral vasculature. This increase in tone in the peripheral vessels, leads to an increase in venous return. The mean systemic filling pressures are elevated increasing the flow from the venous system to the heart. The increased flow leads to increased filling of the damaged heart that in turn leads to increase in priming the heart to aid in pump function. Less than a minute in needed for the sympathetic nervous system to be completely activated (Fig. 2.2) [5, 6].

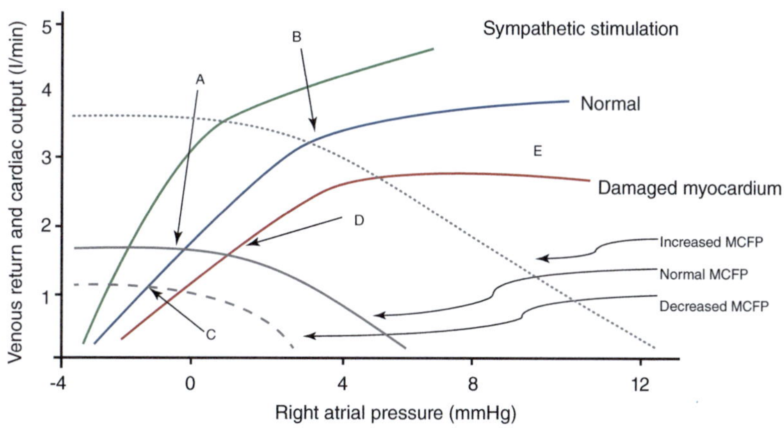

Fig. 2.2 Cardiac output and right atrial pressure relationship with varying myocardial functional states. (Reprinted from Guyton [5], © 1955, with permission from The American Physiological Society)

Chronic Heart Failure

The ischemic insult is followed by no, partial, or full recovery over weeks to months. In addition to ventricular myocardial recovery, fluid retention via renal mechanisms also occurs to compensate for this new cardiac pump status and alters the normal physiologic hemodynamics found in invasive assessments (Table 2.2) [7]. Renal function is extremely sensitive to alterations in perfusion. A low cardiac output state can lead to a decline in renal function manifested to the point of anuria. The decrease in urine output can persist until there is normalization in systemic blood pressure and cardiac output.

Blood volume is altered via renal mechanisms to affect cardiac function. Initially, moderate retention of fluid results in an increase in blood volume that is beneficial to the diminished pumping function of the heart. The increase in fluid retention increases venous return, thereby increasing blood flow to the heart.

As the damaged heart receives the increased venous return, there is a gain of cardiac function. If cardiac output becomes too low, the kidneys respond with the inability to excrete adequate amounts of sodium and water. Excess fluid retention is no longer beneficial to myocardial function, and only serves to increase cardiac workload in the damaged heart and manifests as edema.

Extravasation of fluid from the pulmonary vasculature leading to hypoxia from pulmonary edema, and systemic edema develops in various organs and contributes to their dysfunction. Myocardial functional recovery can range from full to none. After partial recovery there is fluid retention that occurs to establish a new hemodynamic state. The increase in blood volume results in an increase in venous return that provides assistance in the pumping function of the heart. The elevated venous pressure persists as the cardiac output improves. As this new steady state is established and this resting cardiac output improves, the sympathetic tone progressively abates over several weeks following an acute ischemic insult. Altered renal function that results in fluid retention persists in this new hemodynamic state. As the pumping function of the heart compensates, the sympathetic tone begins to gradually decrease transitioning from an acute phase to a chronic heart failure state.

Table 2.2 Normal hemodynamic parameters

Normal hemodynamic parameters		Pressure (mmHg)
Right atrium	*a*-wave/*v*-wave/mean	1–7/1–7/0–5
Right ventricle	Systolic/end diastolic	17–32/1–7
Pulmonary artery	Systolic/end diastolic	17–32/1–7
Left atrium	*a*-wave/*v*-wave/mean	4–12/4–15/4–15
Left ventricle	Systolic/end diastolic	90–140/5–12
Aorta	Systolic/end diastolic/mean	90–140/60–90/70–105

Reprinted with permission from Leopold and Faxon [7], © 2015, McGraw-Hill Education

Compensated and De-compensated Chronic Heart Failure

As partial recovery of the ventricular myocardial function occurs, the resting pump output from the heart normalizes with the help of an increase in atrial pressure. This increased filling pressure helps in recruitment of myocardium and improved output in the resting state. As a patient begins to exercise, the already maximized heart lacks reserve and symptoms of heart failure return. The lack of cardiac reserve is a common occurrence in heart failure patients as they achieve a resting compensated state and attempt to demand more cardiac output with exercise or systemically stressed state.

In severe cardiac failure, de-compensation occurs as a consequence of the inability of the heart to provide additional cardiac output when there are increased systemic demands. Neither sympathetic stimulation nor fluid retention can increase cardiac output to normal. Fluid retention results as the heart is unable to provide sufficient blood flow to the kidneys to excrete sodium and water.

Correlation of cardiac output on the **y** axis and the atrial filling pressures on the **x** axis is repre-

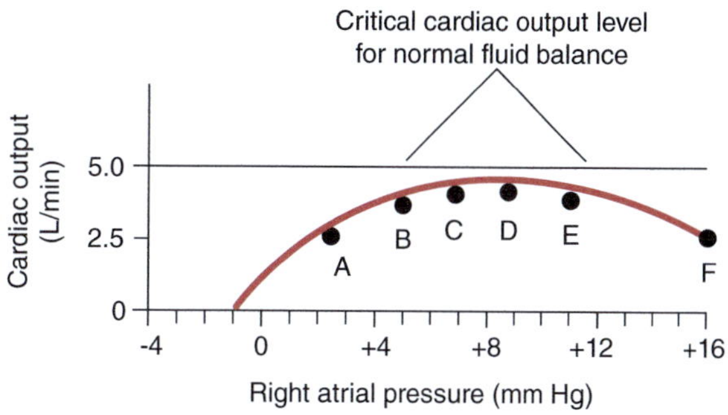

Fig. 2.3 The rise and fall of cardiac output as right atrial pressure increases. Further increase in RAP leads to a decline in cardiac output. (Reprinted from Hall [8], © 2016, with permission from Elsevier)

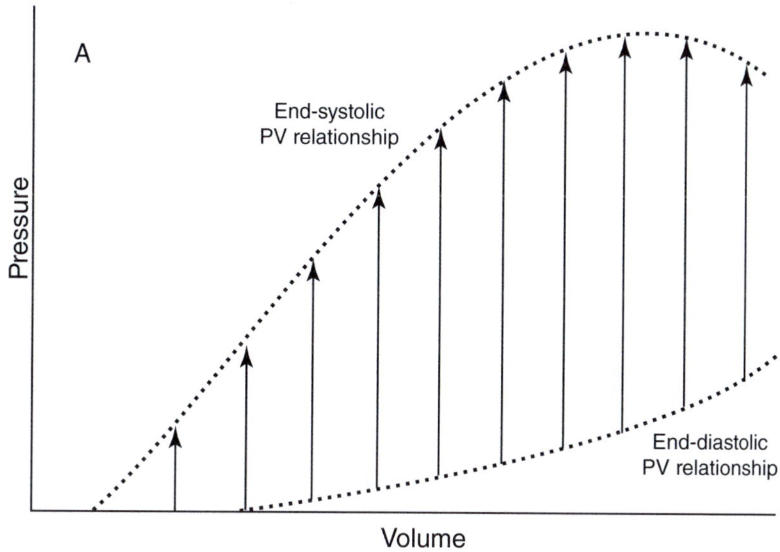

Fig. 2.4 Pressure-volume relationship within the left ventricle. As end diastolic volume increases, resulting end diastolic and systolic pressures increase. (Reprinted with permission from Katz [9], © 2011, with permission from Wolters Kluwer Health)

sented in Fig. 2.3 [8]. As a poorly functional ventricle responds to gradually increasing filling pressures, the cardiac output rises. After a certain point of maximal myocardial stretch, cardiac output falls and higher filling pressures no longer provide additional aid in cardiac function. A progressive increase in fluid retention increases filling pressures beyond the ideal ventricular size and dilatation with overstretching ensues. As progressive increases in fluid retention occur, the mean systemic filling pressures are translated to the heart, which then leads to the gradual rise and fall of cardiac output.

If the cardiac output never reaches a point of providing sufficient perfusion, specifically to the kidney, then cardiac failure is imminent, leading to systemic edema and pulmonary edema, hypoxia, pump failure and eventually death.

Pathophysiology

The Frank-Starling mechanism or Starling's Law of the heart dictates that with increasing volume in the heart there is an increase in myocardial performance that includes an increased stroke volume (Fig. 2.4) [9]. This is a manifestation of the sarcomere length-tension relationship. As the ventricle fills with blood there is distention of cardiac myocytes and less sarcomere overlap. As the myocytes are "stretched", the heart is able to increase the volume of blood it ejects. After the optimal point of overlap, the ventricle can be overstretched leading to a decrease in the amount of volume ejected from the heart. The ascending portion of the Starling curve illustrates how the increase in preload leads to the increase in cardiac output. Ventricular over filling can be detrimental. End diastolic pressures rise, and the overly "stretched" myocardium transitions to the descending portion of the Starling curve and a decrease in stroke volume and systolic pressure.

Valvular Heart Failure

Normal valvular function provides a mechanism for unidirectional flow without resistance. The limitation of blood flow during diastole or systole is cause by a stenosis in the atrio-ventricular or ventricular-arterial valves respectively.

Valvular Stenosis

Aortic stenosis and pulmonic stenosis result in a decrease in cardiac output due to increased resistance to emptying of the ventricle. This increase in resistance to cardiac output results in a measurable pressure gradient across the valve which can be measured via a dual lumen pigtail catheter, separate aortic root and left ventricular catheters, or arterial sheath and left ventricular catheter. In aortic stenosis with preserved left ventricular function, as the severity in aortic valvular stenosis increases, there is an increase in the LV chamber pressure generation. Aortic and left ventricular pressure tracings are used to measure peak to peak, maximum, and mean pressure gradients (Fig. 2.5) [10]. With the advent of increased diagnostic accuracy of echocardiography, the utilization of direct hemodynamic measurement is most strongly indicated when there is a discrepancy between clinical and echocardiographic findings.

After analysis of hemodynamic tracings, the Gorlin formula is utilized in the calculation of aortic valve area. Special circumstances with decreased systolic function, "low-output, low gradient aortic stenosis", are a subset of patients that pose diagnostic dilemmas.

Differentiation of *pseudo* aortic stenosis from true aortic stenosis in the setting of decreased cardiac output is crucial in effective management of the patient. Three particular scenarios are made apparent during dobutamine infusion with simultaneous aortic and left ventricular hemodynamic tracings obtained.

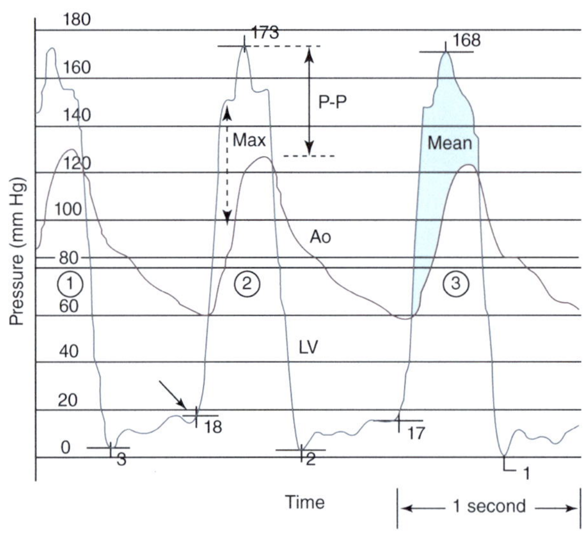

Fig. 2.5 Transaortic pressure gradient. The gradient between the left ventricle (LV) and the aorta (Ao) in aortic stenosis can be described by three invasive measures. The mean gradient (beat #3) represents the area under the left ventricular–aortic pressure curve. The peak-to-peak (P-P) gradient (beat #2) is the difference between the maximum aortic pressure and the maximum left ventricular systolic pressure. The maximum (*Max*) gradient (beat #2) is the maximum difference that can be measured between the left ventricle and aorta during systole. (Reprinted with permission from Shavelle [10], © 2014, with permission from Elsevier)

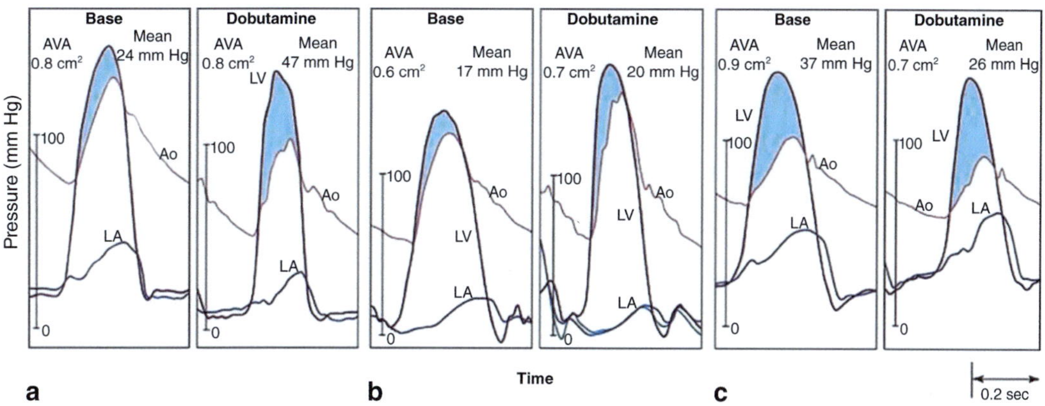

Fig. 2.6 Differentiation of three invasive measurement scenarios as a result of dobutamine infusion in "low-output, low gradient" aortic stenosis. (Reprinted with permission from Nishimura et al. [11], © 2002, with permission from Wolters Kluwer Health. And reprinted with permission from Shavelle [10], © 2014, with permission from Elsevier)

Illustrated in Fig. 2.6 is the potential findings during dobutamine challenge in patients with "low-output, low gradient" aortic stenosis [10, 11].

The far left clinical scenario both cardiac output and aortic valve mean gradient increase as a result of dobutamine infusion, thus true aortic stenosis. The middle scenario finds an increase in cardiac output with no dramatic increase in aortic valve pressure gradient, a finding of mild aortic stenosis. In the right most clinical scenario, there was no change in the aortic valve pressure gradient as a result of dobutamine infusion, truly severe aortic stenosis.

In addition to valvular stenosis that limits cardiac output, is valvular stenosis that limits cardiac filling. Mitral and tricuspid valvular stenosis affects the ability to provide adequate chamber preload. Hemodynamic findings result in an elevation in PCWP but inaccurately reflect LVEDP. PCWP in mitral stenosis is reflection of left atrial pressure but not left ventricular end diastolic pressure. Mitral stenosis results in a pressure gradient between the left atrium and the left ventricle. The classic finding on hemodynamic tracings is the elevation of pulmonary pressures, prominent "a" and "v" waves on PCWP (Fig. 2.7a, b) [12]. Simultaneous tracings within the left ventricle reveal an evident pressure gradient between PCWP and LVEDP.

One must take into account the temporal delay as the pressure of the fluid column is transmitted to the right heart catheter from the left atrium through the pulmonary vascular bed. It is therefore ideal to obtain a direct measurement of left atrial pressure via septal puncture with simultaneous left ventricular hemodynamic tracings (Fig. 2.7c) [13].

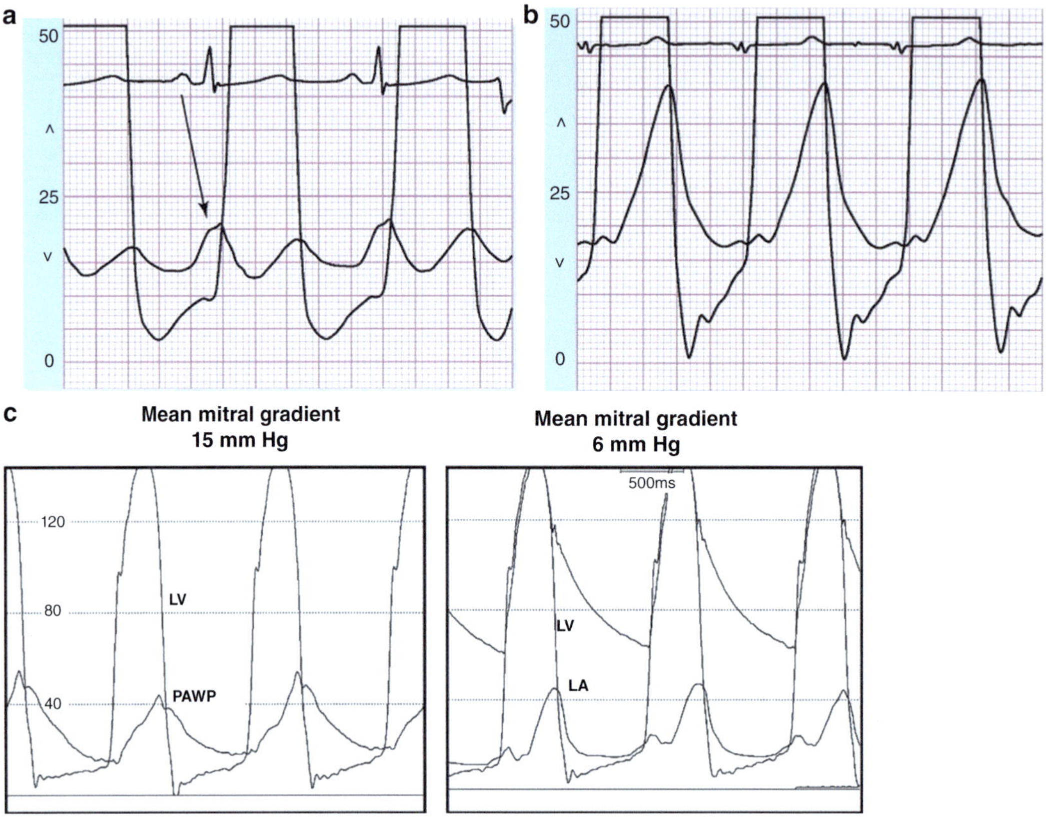

Fig. 2.7 (**a**) The "a" wave on a left atrial (shown here) or pulmonary capillary wedge pressure is accentuated in mitral stenosis (Reprinted with permission from Ragosta [12], © 2010, with permission from Elsevier) (**b**) The "v" wave may also be markedly increased in patients with mitral stenosis. This patient with mitral stenosis has no mitral regurgitation and normal systolic function. (Reprinted with permission from Ragosta [12], © 2010, with permission from Elsevier) (**c**) Measurement of the transmitral gradient by cardiac catheterization is frequently made with a simultaneous pulmonary artery wedge pressure (PAWP) and left ventricular (LV) pressure. However, as a result of the delay in transmission of the change in pressure contour and a phase shift, the gradient using a pulmonary artery wedge pressure will frequently overestimate the true transmitral gradient. *Left*, Simultaneous left ventricular and pulmonary artery wedge pressure in a patient with mitral stenosis. The measured mean gradient is 15 mmHg. *Right*, In the same patient, the transmitral gradient is measured with a left ventricular and direct left atrial (LA) pressure. The true mean transmitral gradient is only 6 mmHg (Reprinted with permission Nishimura and Carabello [13], © 2012, with permission from Wolters Kluwer Health)

Valvular Regurgitation

Aortic valvular regurgitation results in an increase in LV diastolic pressures. Acute aortic regurgitation results in the acute volume overload of the left ventricular chamber, this in turn leads to pulmonary edema, premature closure of the mitral valve and can also result in systemic shock (Fig. 2.8) [12].

Chronic aortic regurgitation results in a wide pulse pressure, high systolic and low diastolic pressures. In chronic, compensated aortic valve regurgitation, the left ventricle and systemic hemodynamics have had time to adjust, thus resulting in a normal early LVEDP. As the cardiac cycle approaches the end of the diastolic filling period, the LVEDP approaches the level of diastolic pressure. The rise of LVEDP to

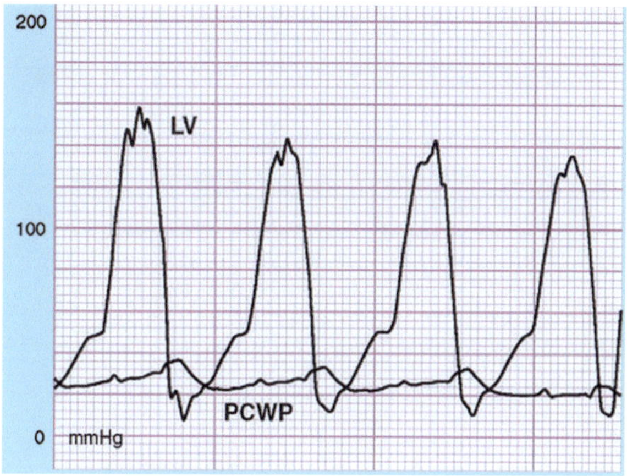

Fig. 2.8 Acute severe aortic valvular regurgitation resulting in LVEDP > PCWP. (Reprinted with permission from Ragosta [12], © 2010, with permission from Elsevier)

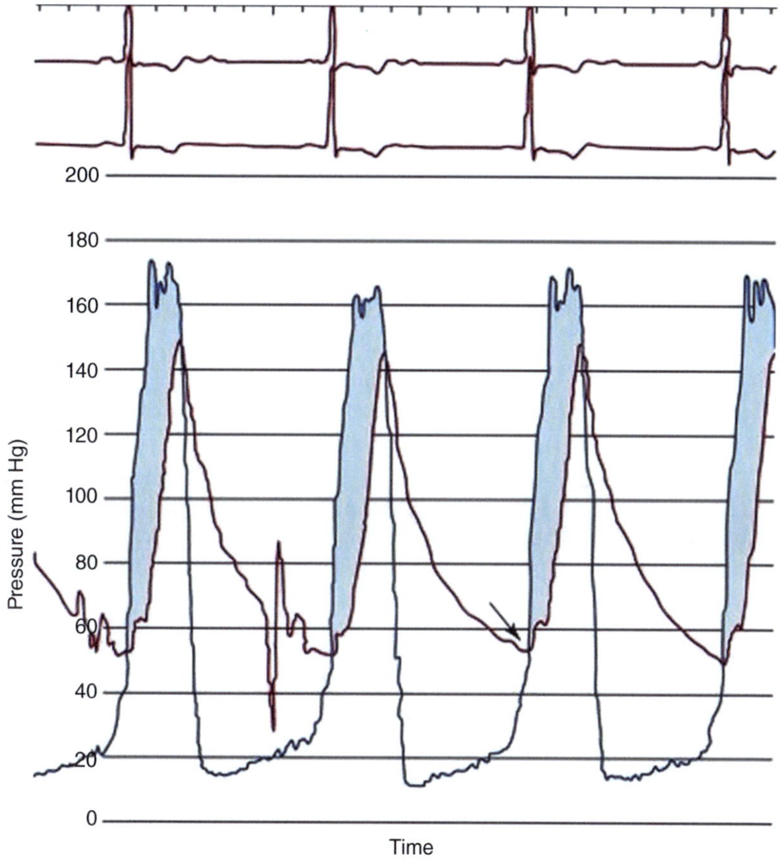

Fig. 2.9 Hemodynamics in severe aortic regurgitation. Simultaneous aortic and left ventricular pressures in a patient with mild aortic stenosis and severe aortic regurgitation. Note that the pulse pressure is wide (approximately 100 mmHg) and the aortic diastolic pressure (*arrow*) is low. (Reprinted with permission from Shavelle [10], © 2014, with permission from Elsevier)

meet diastolic pressure is known as diastasis (Fig. 2.9) [10].

Similarly, chronicity of mitral valvular regurgitation determines the findings on hemodynamic tracings. Acute mitral valvular regurgitation results in pulmonary edema and prominent "*v*" waves on PA and PCWP hemodynamic tracing illustrated with simultaneous Aortic hemodynamic tracings (Fig. 2.10) [14].

Chronic valvular regurgitation may not manifest with the classic finding of prominent "v" waves on PCWP and pulmonary artery tracings

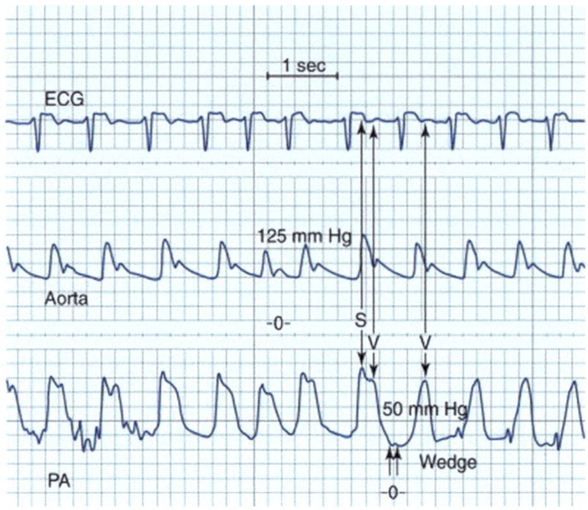

Fig. 2.10 Acute severe mitral regurgitation. Electrocardiogram (ECG), aortic (Aorta), pulmonary artery (PA) pressure (*left*), and pulmonary capillary wedge (wedge) pressure (*right*) tracings in a patient with acute severe mitral regurgitation. A prominent v wave is present in both the pulmonary artery and wedge pressure tracings. The pulmonary artery pressure is bifid because of the presence of both the pulmonary artery systolic wave (S) and the v wave. The large v wave can cause the wedge tracing to be confused with a pulmonary artery tracing. (Reprinted from Sharkey [14], © 1987, with permission from Elsevier)

as in acute mitral regurgitation. The presence of prominent of "v" waves is determined by the compliance of the left atrium in addition to its size and pressure. Given this, chronic mitral regurgitation and may manifest as normal physiologic "v" waves on hemodynamic tracings.

Unilateral Heart Failure

There are unique clinical presentations of unilateral heart failure that alter the hemodynamics related to the affected ventricle, specifically left sided heart failure in absence of right sided heart failure and vice versa.

Left sided heart failure in isolation, with normally functioning right sided ventricle leads to an increase in mean pulmonary artery pressures. In the setting of inadequate left ventricular pump function, the blood accumulates in the pulmonary vasculature and the backup in volume shifts from the systemic arterial circulation to the pulmonary vasculature. Pulmonary vasculature capillary pressures rise as a consequence of increased volume. Fluid accumulation in the pulmonary bed gradually rises to a point where the capillary network can no longer tolerate the additional fluid and begins to leak out into the interstitium. With the rise in pulmonary pressures beyond the ability of the capillary bed to hold in the fluid via osmotic mechanisms, pulmonary edema is manifested clinically as rales and dyspnea. The clinical presentation of severe pulmonary edema in the setting of acute myocardial infarction and cardiogenic shock can be dramatic resulting in profound hypoxia in less than an hour.

Isolated right ventricular failure results in a gradual increase in systemic venous pressures and a loss of preload to the left ventricular side. Right and left ventricular interdependence is a key concept in understanding the pathophysiologic alterations in hemodynamics of isolated right ventricular dysfunction. In acute right ventricular infarction, the systolic function of the pump is compromised. As right sided ventricular dysfunction occurs, right sided chamber dilatation along with a fall in systolic pressures occurs. The diastolic filling pressure of the ventricle rises and demonstrates a characteristic prominent "y" descent manifested as a dip and plateau on hemodynamic tracings (Fig. 2.11) [15].

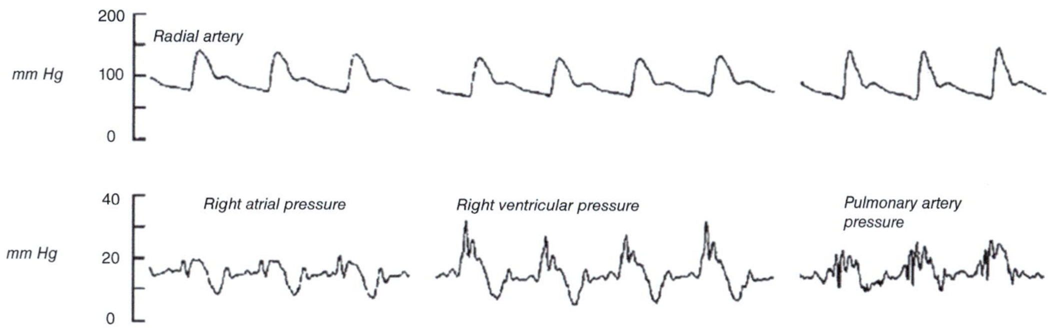

Fig. 2.11 Right ventricular infarction hemodynamic tracings. (Reprinted from Lorell et al. [15], © 1979, with permission from Elsevier)

The depressed ventricular function leads to an increase in right atrial filling pressures and a backup into venous system. Acute right ventricular chamber dilatation encroaches upon the left ventricular chamber filling. As the shared space within the pericardium is fixed, acute RV dilation results in a decrease in LV chamber filling. The enhancement of the right and left interdependence is manifested dramatically as hypotension, clear lung fields, prominent JVD all mimicking the syndrome of pericardial constriction. Experimental models of isolated RV infarct have demonstrated the inability to induce hypotension in animals where the pericardium is surgically absent. Without acute reperfusion and hemodynamic support RV infarction can be life threatening.

Constrictive Pericarditis and Restrictive Cardiomyopathy.

Restrictive cardiomyopathy is a rare form of cardiomyopathy in which the ventricle becomes abnormally rigid and lacks the flexibility to adequately expand as it fills with blood. This leads to venous congestion and heart failure.

It has distinct morphologic features allowing it to be separated from other cardiomyopathies. For example with restriction the left ventricle is usually normal in size and function unlike dilated or hypertrophic cardiomyopathies. A syndrome that poses a diagnostic dilemma with restrictive cardiomyopathy is constrictive pericarditis. They both exhibit normal ventricular size and function as well as some similar hemodynamic abnormalities.

It is extremely important for the clinician to be able to distinguish between constrictive pericarditis and restrictive cardiomyopathy since they require markedly different treatment. In some cases, invasive cardiac catheterization may be necessary to help differentiate the two. In addition the hemodynamic features of restrictive cardiomyopathy and constrictive pericarditis can be similar to tamponade and right ventricle infarction. This section will discuss the hemodynamics of these entities and how the hemodynamics can be used and differentiate between them.

Constrictive Pericarditis

Constrictive pericarditis is the end-stage of an inflammatory process affecting the pericardium, resulting in scarring and subsequent loss of the normal elasticity of the pericardial sac. In the developed world idiopathic or viral illness is the most common cause followed by post-surgical and radiation therapy (Table 2.3) [16–19].

Table 2.3 Causes of constrictive pericarditis

Idiopathic
Irradiation
Postsurgical
Infectious
Neoplastic
Autoimmune(connective tissue) disorders
Uremia
Post trauma
Sarcoid
Methylsergide therapy
Implantable defibrillator patches

Reprinted from LeWinter and Hopkins [19], © 2015, with permission from Elsevier

Pathophysiology

The pericardium is a fluid filled fibro-elastic sac that surrounds the heart. It functions to keep the heart contained in the chest cavity and stretches to accommodate physiologic changes in cardiac volume [20, 21].

In constrictive pericarditis, the total cardiac volume is fixed as a result of the non-compliant shell around the heart. The abnormal pericardium prohibits outward ventricular expansion, which is necessary to accommodate venous return. As a result, an adaptive process occurs in which the inter-ventricular septum bulges inward either into the left or right ventricle in order to accommodate myocardial blood flow into the adjacent ventricle. This maladaptive process will allow filling in one ventricle while compromising blood flow into the other. This is known as ventricular interdependence, since the amount of blood flow into one ventricle is dependent on the amount of blood flow into the other.

Ventricular interdependence is the result of the rigid pericardium, which prevents the normal reduction in intra-thoracic pressure during inspiration from being transmitted to the heart chambers. As a result during inspiration pulmonary venous pressure will decrease while left ventricular pressure remains constant. This ultimately leads to a reduction in the gradient driving filling into the LV. Reduction in LV volume allows RV filling to occur. As the RV fills, the inter-ventricular septum will shift toward the left further reducing LV filling. This septal shift occurs because outward expansion is not possible due to the constraining effects of the rigid pericardium.

During expiration the opposite sequence will occur. Pulmonary venous pressures will rise resulting in an increased trans-pulmonary gradient into the LV. As LV fillings increases the inter-ventricular septum will bulge to the right resulting in decrease flow into the RV (Fig. 2.12) [19].

With constrictive pericarditis, early diastolic filling is preserved since it is a myocardial process and not dependent upon a functioning pericardium. In fact, early filling occurs even more rapidly than normal due to elevated atrial pressures and increased suctioning form the ventricle. However; in early to mid-diastole, ventricular filling will cease abruptly due to the non-compliant pericardium. Consequently, almost all filling occurs in early diastole and systemic venous congestion results causing peripheral edema, hepatic congestion, and ascites.

Typical constrictive physiology will be evident on right atrial and left ventricle pressure recording at the time of cardiac catheterization. During early diastole the ventricular pressure initially decreases rapidly causing a steep y descent on the right atrial pressure waveform. In mid to late diastole flow abruptly ceases which is evident as a plateau after the initial downward dip (Fig. 2.13) [19, 22].

In patients with constriction right and left heart pressure recording should be performed simultaneously. Typical measurements will reveal elevated and equal RA, RV diastolic, LV diastolic, and pulmonary wedge pressures. The fillings pressures are typically elevated at approximately 20 mmHg with no more than a 3–5 mmHg difference. The RA pressure will show a preserved x descent and prominent y descent. Both RV and LV pressure tracings will show a early diastole dip followed by a plateau in mid to late diastole. Pulmonary hypertension is not usually a feature of constriction. The PA pressures are typically between 35–40 mmHg. If hypovolemia is present rapid volume challenge of 1000 cc may help to reveal typical hemodynamic features, which can be masked when fillings pressures are low [21, 23].

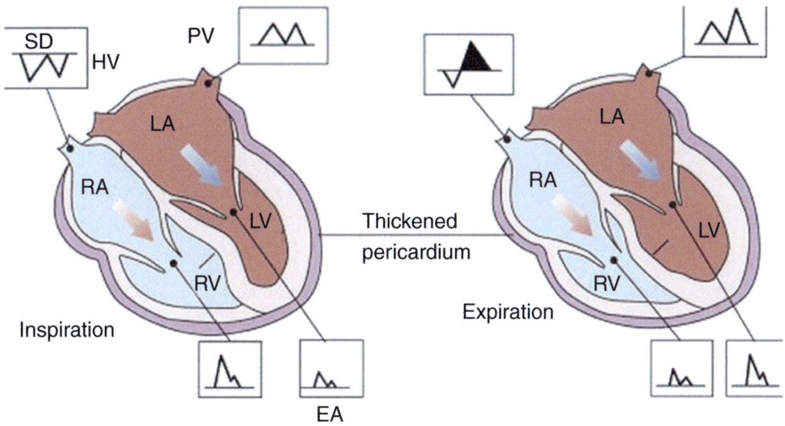

Fig. 2.12 Schematic representation of transvalvular and central venous flow velocities in constrictive pericarditis. During inspiration the decrease in LV filling results in a leftward septal shift that allows augmented flow into the right ventricle. The opposite occurs during expiration. *D* diastole, *EA* mitral inflow, *HV* hepatic vein, *LA* left atrium, *LV* left ventricle, *PV* pulmonary venous flow, *RA* right atrium, *RV* right ventricle, *S* systole. (Reprinted from LeWinter and Hopkins [19], © 2015, with permission from Elsevier)

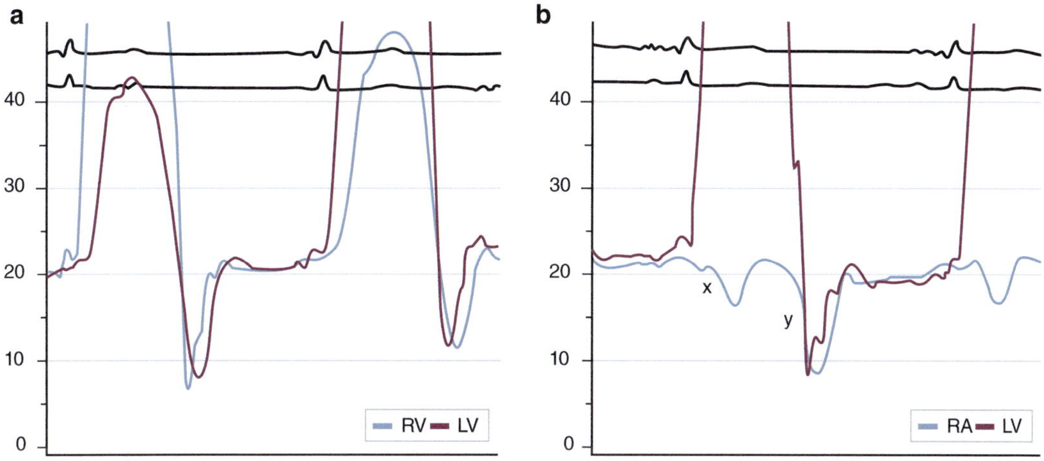

Fig. 2.13 Pressure recording in a patient with constrictive pericarditis. (**a**) Simultaneous LV and RV pressure tracing with the "dip-and-plateau waveform" or "square root sign" seen on right or left ventricular pressure waveform tracings. The black arrow represents the rapid descent, and the white arrow represents the plateau portion. (**b**) Right atrial pressure with prominent Y descent. (Reprinted from Vaitkus et al. [22], © 1996, with permission from Wolters Kluwer Health, Inc. and Reprinted from LeWinter and Hopkins [19], © 2015, with permission from Elsevier)

Clinical Presentation

Constrictive pericarditis can present with a myriad of symptoms, thus making a diagnosis solely on the basis of the clinical history is difficult. The usual presentation consists of predominantly right heart failure. Dyspnea is the most common presenting symptom and occurs in virtually all patients. Fatigue and orthopnea are common. Lower extremity edema and abdominal swelling are also common. Constrictive can mimic and be mistaken for other causes of right heart failure as well as end-stage liver disease. However it is important to note that in primary liver disease jugular venous pressures are not elevated.

Table 2.4 Causes of restrictive cardiomyopathy

Hemochromatosis
Amyloidosis (most common cause in the United States)
Sarcoidosis
Scleroderma
Carcinoid heart disease
Glycogen storage disease of the heart
Radiation
Metastatic malignancy
Anthracycline toxicity

The vast majority of patients with constriction have elevated jugular venous pressure. Elevated JVP has been reported in as many as 93% of patients with surgically confirmed constrictive pericarditis. A pericardial knock, which corresponds with the sudden cessation of ventricular filling occurs in approximately half the cases. Kussmaul's sign, which is the lack of an inspiratory decline in JVP, can be present in patients with constrictive pericarditis, however it is non-specific [17].

Restrictive Cardiomyopathy

Restrictive cardiomyopathy may be caused by various local and systemic disorders that may be categorized into 4 groups. They includes idiopathic, infiltrative, treatment-induced, and malignancy (Table 2.4) [24].

Clinical Presentation

Affected patients have signs and symptoms of pulmonary and systemic congestion resulting in dyspnea, peripheral edema, palpitations and fatigue. In advanced cases hepatosplenomegaly, ascites, and anasarca can occur from marked elevation in venous pressures.

Jugular venous pressure is generally elevated. Kussmaul's sign, which is the lack of an inspiratory decline in JVP, can be present. Also a prominent y descent may appear; however, it may not be obvious in patients with mild disease. The cardiovascular examination is often indistinguishable from that of constrictive pericarditis [25, 26].

Constrictive Pericarditis Versus Restrictive Cardiomyopathy

The history, physical examination, and radiographic findings may suggest a particular diagnosis. For example constrictive pericarditis may be suggested in patients with prior radiation or cardiothoracic surgery. Restrictive cardiomyopathy is more likely in a patient with a predisposing systemic disease such as amyloidosis. However, in many instances their clinical presentation and course overlap, making the ability to distinguish between the two syndromes difficult.

In some cases, invasive cardiac catheterization may be necessary to help differentiate (Table 2.5) [19].

In both conditions, RV and LV diastolic pressure will be elevated. However in restrictive cardiomyopathy, the difference between diastolic pressures of the LV and RV normally exceed 3–5 mmHg. In constriction those pressures usually are within 3–5 mmHg of each other. Pulmonary hypertension is rare in constriction but common in restriction. The absolute level of diastolic pressure in restriction commonly exceeds 25 mmHg whereas in constriction pressure rarely exceeds 20 mmHg. [27].

One of the most sensitive ways to differentiate constrictive pericarditis from restriction is through the respiratory effects observed between the RV and LV systolic pressures. With constriction there is discordance between RV and LV systolic pressure with respiration due to ventricular interdependence. However, with restriction ventricular interdependence does not exist because

Table 2.5 Hemodynamic features of constrictive vs restrictive cardiomyopathy

	Constriction	Restriction
Prominent Y descent	Present	Variable
Filling pressures >25 mmHg	Rare	Common
Pulmonary systolic pressure > 60 mmHg	No	Common
Square root sign	Present	Variable
Respiratory variation in LV and RV pressure	Discordant	Concordant

Reprinted from LeWinter and Hopkins [19], © 2015, with permission from Elsevier

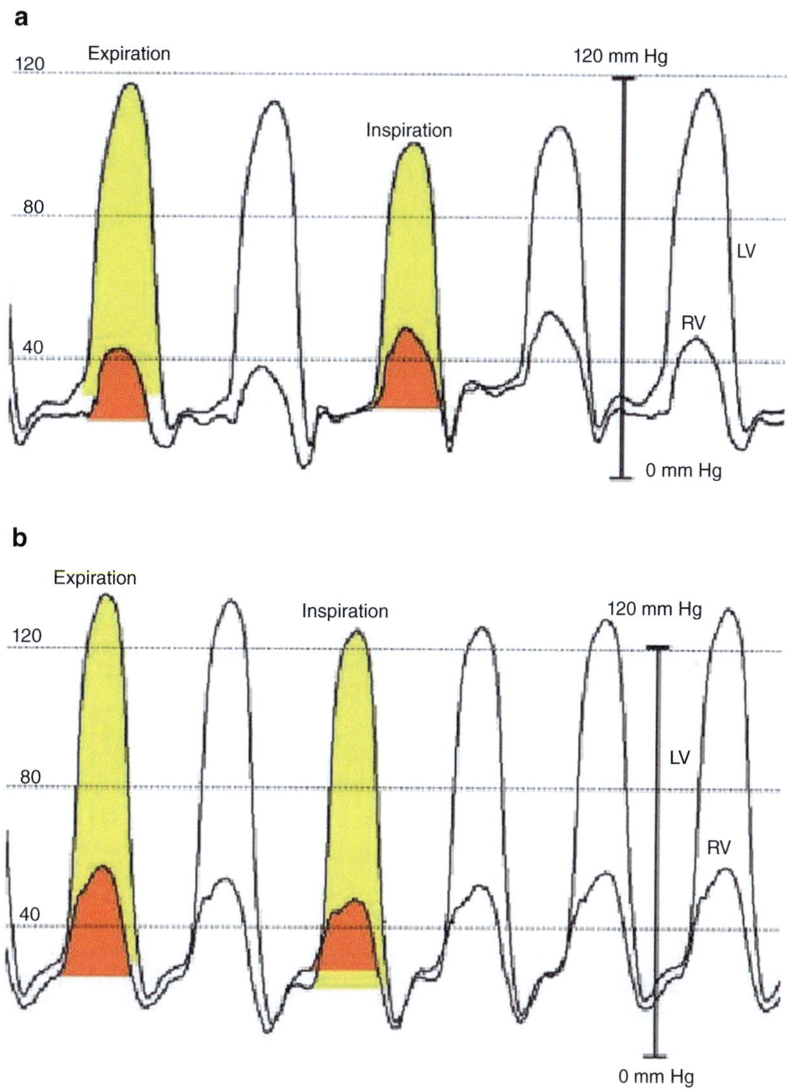

Fig. 2.14 LV and RV Pressure Recording From 2 Patients. During Expiration and Inspiration (**a**) With constrictive pericarditis LV and RV systolic pressure are discordant with respiration. During inspiration there is an increase in the RV pressure and a decrease in LV pressure. The opposite occurs during expiration (**b**) With restriction LV and RV systolic pressures are concordant during respiration. During inspiration there is a decrease in the RV pressure and a decrease in LV pressure. The opposite occurs during expiration. (Reprinted from Talreja et al. [27], © 2008, with permission from Elsevier)

the pericardium is normal. Thus in restriction RV and LV systolic pressure move concordantly with each other during the respiratory cycle (Fig. 2.14) [27].

Constriction Versus RV Infarction and Tamponade

Compressive hemodynamic effects resulting in diastolic dysfunction may be seen in other conditions besides constrictive pericarditis. In fact, any condition that causes elevated intra-pericardial pressure, i.e. from pericardial tamponade to abrupt chamber dilatation with RV infraction, will lead to increased intra-pericardial pressure and constrictive physiology. All three conditions including RV infarction may show elevation and equalization of diastolic filling pressures in the RA, RV, and PCW, as well as the LV [14, 15].

However, only constriction will exhibit dissociation between intra-thoracic and intra-cardiac pressures during the respiratory cycle (Fig. 2.15) [28]. Normally with inspiration the negative pressure created within the intra-thoracic cavity results in a simultaneous decrease in pulmonary and ventricular pressures. In constriction the rigid pericardium acts to isolate the heart leaving

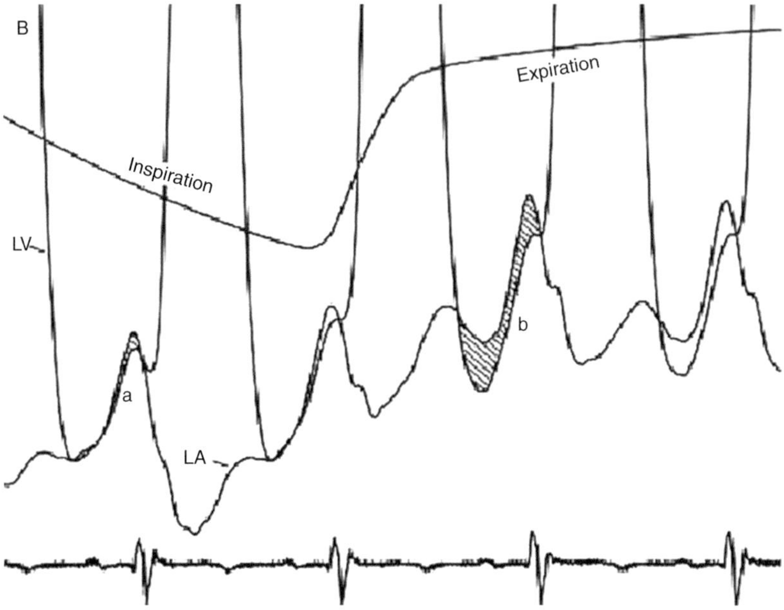

Fig. 2.15 Simultaneous pressure recording of LV and PCWP. There is significant respiratory change suggesting dissociation of intra-thoracic and intra-cardiac pressures. (Reprinted from Doshi et al. [28], © 2015, with permission from Elsevier)

it unaffected from these physiologic changes. As a result only patients with constriction will exhibit dissociation between intra-thoracic and intra-cardiac pressures, which distinguishes it from RV infarction and tamponade where the LV and wedge pressures will rise and fall concordantly.

References

1. Katz AM. Heart failure: pathophysiology, molecular biology, and clinical management. 2nd ed. Philadelphia: Lippincott Williams & Wilkins; 2009.
2. Dickstein K, Cohen-Solal A, Filippatos G, McMurray JJV, Ponikowski P, Poole-Wilson PA, ESC Committee for Practice Guidelines, et al. ESC guidelines for the diagnosis and treatment of acute and chronic heart failure 2008: the Task Force for the diagnosis and treatment of acute and chronic heart failure 2008 of the European Society of Cardiology. Developed in collaboration with the Heart Failure Association of the ESC (HFA) and endorsed by the European Society of Intensive Care Medicine (ESICM). Eur Heart J. 2008;29(19):2388–442.
3. Drazner MH, Hellkamp AS, Leier CV, Shah MR, Miller LW, Russell SD, et al. Value of clinician assessment of hemodynamics in advanced heart failure: the ESCAPE trial. Circ Heart Fail. 2008;1(3):170–7.
4. Mehra MR. Optimizing outcomes in the patient with acute decompensated heart failure. Am Heart J. 2006;151(3):571–9.
5. Guyton AC. Determination of cardiac output by equating venous return curves with cardiac response curves. Physiol Rev. 1955;35(1):123–9.
6. Henderson WR, Griesdale DEG, Walley KR, Sheel AW. Clinical review: guyton—the role of mean circulatory filling pressure and right atrial pressure in controlling cardiac output. Crit Care. 2010;14(6):243.
7. Leopold JA, Faxon DP. Diagnostic cardiac catheterization and coronary angiography. In: Kasper D, Fauci A, Hauser S, Longo D, Jameson J, Loscalzo J, editors. Harrison's principles of internal medicine. 18th ed. New York: McGraw-Hill; 2015.
8. Hall JE. Chapter 22. In: Guyton and hall textbook of medical Physiology. Published December 31, 2015.13th Edition. Philadelphia: Elsevier; 2016. p. 271–81.
9. Katz AM. Physiology of the heart. 5th ed. Philadelphia: Lippincott Williams & Wilkins; Chapter 11; 2011. p. 307–10.
10. Shavelle DM. Evaluation of valvular heart disease by cardiac catheterization and angiocardiography. In: Otto CM, Bonow RO, editors. Valvular heart disease: a companion to Braunwald's heart disease. Philadelphia: Saunders Elsevier; Chapter 7; 2014. p. 91–106.
11. Nishimura RA, Grantham JA, Connolly HM, Schaff HV, Higano ST, Holmes DR. Lowoutput, lowgradient aortic stenosis in patients with depressed left ventricular systolic function: the clinical utility of the dobu tamine challenge in the catheterization laboratory. Circulation. 2002;106(7):809–13.
12. Ragosta M. Cardiac catheterization: an atlas and DVD. 1st ed. Philadelphia: Saunders Elsevier; 2010. p. 58–74.

13. Nishimura RA, Carabello BA. Hemodynamics in the cardiac catheterization laboratory of the 21st century. Circulation. 2012;125(17):2138–50.
14. Sharkey SW. Beyond the wedge: clinical physiology and the Swan-Ganz catheter. Am J Med. 1987;83(1):111–22.
15. Lorell B, Leinbach RC, Pohost GM, Gold HK, Dinsmore RE, Hutter AM, et al. Right ventricular infarction clinical diagnosis and differentiation from cardiac tamponade and pericardial constriction. Am J Cardiol. 1979;43(3):465–71.
16. Cameron J, Oesterle SN, Baldwin JC, Hancock EW. The etiologic spectrum of constrictive pericarditis. Am Heart J. 1987;113(2 Pt 1):354–60.
17. Ling LH, Oh JK, Schaff HV, et al. Constrictive pericarditis in the modern era: evolving clinical spectrum and impact on outcome after pericardiectomy. Circulation. 1999;100(13):1380–6.
18. Bertog SC, Thambidorai SK, Parakh K, et al. Constrictive pericarditis: etiology and cause-specific survival after pericardiectomy. J Am Coll Cardiol. 2004;43(8):1445–52.
19. LeWinter MM, Hopkins WE. Pericardial diseases Chapter 71. In: Mann DL, Zipes DP, Libby P, Bonow RO, editors. Braunwald's heart disease: a textbook of cardiovascular medicine, 2-volume set. 10th ed. Philadelphia: Elsevier; 2015. p. 1636–557.
20. LeWinter MM, Myhre EESP, Slinker BK. Influence of the pericardium and ventricular interaction on diastolic function. In: Gaasch WH, LeWinter MM, editors. Heart failure and left ventricular diastolic function. Philadelphia: Lea & Febiger; 1993. p. 103–17.
21. Talreja DR, Edwards WD, Danielson GK, et al. Constrictive pericarditis in 26 patients with histologically normal pericardial thickness. Circulation. 2003;108(15):1852–7. Epub 2003 Sep 29
22. Vaitkus PT, Cooper KA, Shuman WP, Hardin NJ. Images in cardiovascular medicine constrictive pericarditis. Circulation. 1996;93(4):834–5.
23. Bush CA, Stang JM, Wooley CF, Kilman JW. Occult constrictive pericardial disease. Diagnosis by rapid volume expansion and correction by pericardiectomy. Circulation. 1977;56(6):924–30.
24. Davies MJ, Mann JM. Systemic pathology. In: The cardiovascular system. Vol 10. 1995:1409; Wald DS, Gray HH. Restrictive cardiomyopathy in systemic amyloidosis. QJM. 2003;96(5):380–2.
25. Kushwaha SS, Fallon JT, Fuster V. Restrictive cardiomyopathy. N Engl J Med. 1997;336(4):267–76.
26. Benotti JR, Grossman W, Cohn PF. Clinical profile of restrictive cardiomyopathy. Circulation. 1980;61(6):1206–12.
27. Talreja DR, Nishimura RA, Oh JK, Holmes DR. Constrictive pericarditis in the modern era: novel criteria for diagnosis in the cardiac catheterization laboratory. J Am Coll Cardiol. 2008;51(3):315–9.
28. Doshi S, Ramakrishnan S, Gupta SK. Invasive hemodynamics of constrictive pericarditis. Indian Heart J. 2015;67(2):175–82.

Imaging and Heart Failure

3

Gustavo Jardim Volpe, Henrique Turin Moreira, and Joao A. C. Lima

Abbreviations

CAD	Coronary artery disease
CCT	Cardiac computed tomography
CMR	Cardiac magnetic resonance
CRT	Cardiac resynchronization therapy
EF	Ejection fraction
HF	Heart Failure
LA	Left atria
LV	Left ventricle
LVEF	Left ventricular ejection fraction
MRI	Magnetic resonance imaging
PET	Positron emission tomography
RV	Right ventricle
RVG	Radionuclide ventriculography
SPECT	Single-photon emission computed tomography
STE	Speckle tracking echocardiography
TDI	Tissue Doppler Imaging
2D–Echo	Two-dimensional Echocardiography
3D–Echo	Three-dimensional Echocardiography

G. J. Volpe (✉) · H. T. Moreira
Hospital das Clínicas de Ribeirão Preto, Universidade de São Paulo, Ribeirão Preto, SP, Brazil
e-mail: gustavovolpe@usp.br; htmoreira@hcrp.usp.br

J. A. C. Lima
Department of Medicine, Division of Cardiology, The Johns Hopkins Hospital, Baltimore, MD, USA
e-mail: jlima@jhmi.edu

Introduction

Imaging techniques have a crucial role in heart failure (HF). For the correct diagnosis and clinical conduction of any patient with signals of impaired cardiac function, the heart function should be assessed at least once. Moreover, some studies are fundamental for differential diagnosis, and identifying reversible conditions, such as ischemic heart disease, can be the difference between success or failure in the treatment of HF [1, 2]. There has been a long way from the simple nineteenth-century chest X-ray to cutting-edge magnetic resonance imaging (MRI) sequences. Attempts to perform a detailed evaluation of all available modalities are beyond the scope of this chapter; the focus will instead be on clinical use and differential diagnosis of HF.

Chest Radiography

The use of chest X-rays in patients with heart disease goes back to the end of the nineteenth century. This modality is still a practical diagnostic test for evaluating a patient with dyspnea. It is low-cost, fast, and requires a minimal amount of radiation. As a first-line exam, the chest X-ray can help differentiate HF from primary pulmonary disease [2]. Cardiomegaly (cardiac-to-thoracic width ratio of more than 50%), Kerley B-lines, cephalization of the pulmonary vessels, and pleural effusion are the most suggestive find-

H. J. Eisen (ed.), *Heart Failure I*, https://doi.org/10.1007/978-3-032-12626-9_3

ings of HF. Variations in the cardiac area shape and size can also reveal signs of valvular disease or congenital abnormalities. However, none of the findings can, either alone or in association, establish or exclude the definitive diagnosis of impaired cardiac function. In a systematic review, Badget et al. concluded that blood vessel redistribution and cardiomegaly are the best radiographic findings for diagnosis or increased preload and reduced ejection fraction, respectively. Still, neither can adequately exclude or confirm left ventricular dysfunction [3]. Similarly, Knudsen et al. evaluated 880 patients from seven sites presenting with acute dyspnea to the emergency department. They found that—of all the signs in the chest X-ray abnormalities—only cardiomegaly had a sensitivity greater than 50% for the diagnosis of HF [4].

In clinical follow-up, chest radiography can be important to identify signs of decompensated HF. In this sense, pleural effusions, pulmonary congestion, and cephalization of the pulmonary vessels can be signals of volume overload—mainly if there is a previous examination without these findings. The differentiation between pneumonia and pulmonary congestion is often tricky, so the exam interpretation within the clinical context is critical.

Finally, the chest X-ray is essential in the first approach to a patient with suspected HF and through follow-up, but the findings should be interpreted carefully.

Echocardiography

Echocardiography comprehends all the cardiac ultrasound imaging techniques, including two- and three-dimensional echocardiography (2D- and 3D–Echo), color flow Doppler, pulsed and continuous wave Doppler, and tissue Doppler imaging (TDI). Regardless of the fast improvement in cardiovascular imaging and the development of new techniques such as cardiac MRI, echocardiography is still the method of choice in patients with suspected HF. It is a reliable, reproducible, and low-cost exam that allows a good evaluation of the anatomy and function of the heart. Nonetheless, in recent years echocardiography has been considered an extension of the physical exam due to the significant reduction in the unit size.

In the **initial evaluation** of a patient with suspected HF, 2D–Echo with Doppler flow study is the most beneficial complementary exam. It evaluates the ventricle volumes and function, atrial dimensions, and valve and pericardial abnormalities to answer three fundamental questions that could account for the clinical presentation: [1] Is the **left ventricular ejection fraction (LVEF)** preserved or reduced, [2] Is the structure of the left ventricle (LV) normal or abnormal, and [3] Are there other structural abnormalities such as valvular, pericardial, diastolic function, or right ventricular (RV) abnormalities? [5] All this information should be provided with numerical estimates, evaluation of the chambers' geometry, and regional LV wall motion (Table 3.1). The biplane method of discs (from modified Simpson's rule) is the method of choice to measure LV volumes and, therefore, the LVEF according to the American Society of Echocardiography (ASE) [6]. The methods based on the M-mode measurements, such as LVEF from the Theicholz method, are subject to variations and poor reproducibility when there is regional LV dysfunction; therefore, its use is discouraged in this clinical setting. Although the lack of correlation between ejection fraction (EF) and the LV dimensions to HF symptoms or myocardial capacity [7], they are closely related to morbidity and mortality [8, 9]. The **LV mass** and the **left atrial (LA) volume** are other essential parameters in evaluating the patient with HF, not only for their role in the differential diagnosis but also for their relationship with adverse events in those patients [10–12].

Evaluation of the **diastolic function** is also fundamental in phenotyping HF—especially in patients with symptoms and preserved LVEF. Various echocardiographic techniques can estimate LV end-diastolic pressure [2]. However, none of these modalities alone is sufficiently

Table 3.1 Normal ranges and severity classification cutoffs for 2D-derived LV mass, LVEF, and LA volume [6]

	Male				Female			
	Normal range	Mildly abnormal	Moderately abnormal	Severely abnormal	Normal range	Mildly abnormal	Moderately abnormal	Severely abnormal
LV mass/BSA (g/m^2)	49–115	43–95	116–131	> 148	43–95	96–108	109–121	>121
LVEF (%)	52–72	54–74	41–51	41–53	40–30		<30	
Maximum LA volume/BSA (mL/m^2)	16–34		35–41		42–48		>48	

2D: two-dimensional echocardiography; *BSA* body mass index, *LA* left atrium, *LVEF* left ventricular ejection fraction

accurate or reproducible to diagnose LV diastolic dysfunction definitively. Depending on the association of findings, the function could be graded according to severity in "abnormal relaxation," "pseudonormal," and "restrictive." Mild diastolic dysfunction—"abnormal relaxation"—can be detected via a decrease in early diastolic flow velocity and greater reliance on atrial contraction to fill the LV. Moderate diastolic dysfunction—"pseudonormal"—reflects an increasing left atrial pressure at the onset of diastole and an increase in early diastolic flow velocity to a level near normal filing. Severe diastolic dysfunction—"restrictive filling"—occurs when left atrial pressure is further elevated, with quick early diastolic flow and rapid equalization between LV and LA pressures in early diastole [13]. This characterization can be done based on the information from the mitral inflow Doppler, the Tissue Doppler of mitral annular motion, and the pulmonary venous flow [14], and is related to adverse outcomes [15].

Some new echocardiographic techniques are opening new horizons in cardiac non-invasive evaluation. Development of new matrix array transducers that acquire full-volume data in real-time allows the **3D–Echocardiography** (3D-echo) to get rid of off-line image reconstructions and therefore made this modality more suitable for clinical use (Fig. 3.1). The great advantage is the calculation of volumes and diameters of the heart without geometric assumptions, thus providing more accurate quantification of cardiac chambers. Some studies have shown that 3D–Echo is highly precise and reproducible for assessing LV volumes and mass compared to cardiac MRI [16, 17]. In addition, the 3D-transesophageal echocardiography is an additional imaging modality that can guide complex catheter-based procedures, surgical planning, and assessment of intra-operative results, therefore improving outcomes, especially in those at higher surgical risk, many of them with heart failure.

The **speckle tracking echocardiography** (STE) is also one of the most recent techniques incorporated into clinical routine, mainly because it can measure myocardial strains, which are sensitivity markers of global and regional ventricular functions. This modality relies on algorithms that can identify multiple unique patterns of echocardiographic pixel intensity and then automatically track them along the cardiac cycle, providing their movement in a plane (strain) and by the time (strain rate) (Fig. 3.2). Several small studies have shown correlations with strain parameters by STE and tissue alteration, such as fibrosis, and with markers of subtle myocardial disease [18]. The left ventricular global longitudinal strain has shown incremental prognostic value to LVEF in predicting major cardiovascular events and new-onset heart failure [19]. Clinical applications also include serial evaluation to detect cancer therapeutic-related cardiac dysfunction early [20]. Furthermore, the pattern of myocardial strain reductions may help to identify specific conditions, such as apical sparing in cardiac amyloidosis [21].

In patients with poor acoustic ultrasound windows, **contrast echocardiography** may be help-

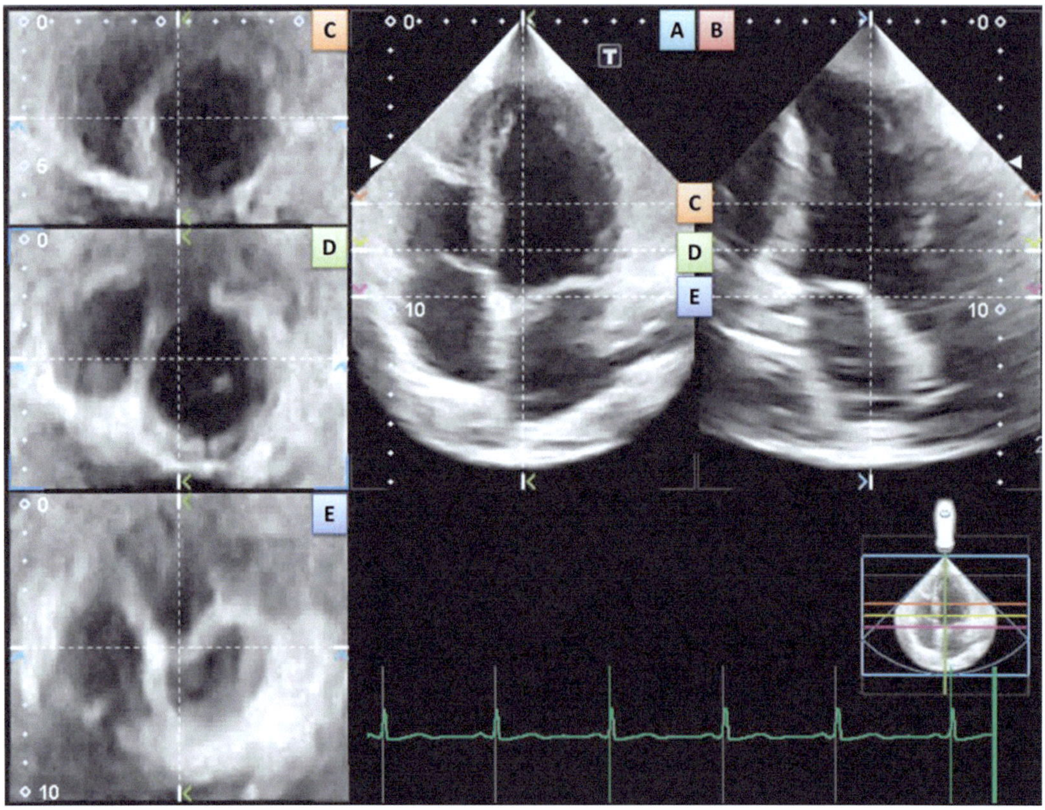

Fig. 3.1 Example of a **3D echocardiography acquisition**. The 3-dimensional full-volume data acquisition allows the imaging of multiple planes simultaneously, providing accurate measurements of chambers' volumes. (**a**) Four chamber view; (**b**) 2 chamber view; (**c–e**) short axis views

ful. This technique is based on an intravenous injection of a microbubble agent that enhances the echogenicity of blood and myocardium, thus providing better spatial resolution. Its use improves the identification of left ventricular wall motion abnormalities and provides more accurate measurements of left ventricular ejection fraction in this setting. The use of microbubble agents can also contribute to identifying small intracavitary thrombus, which may not be noticeable by conventional echocardiography. Other clinical applications include the detection of cardiac shunts, which may be the etiology of some high-output heart failure [22].

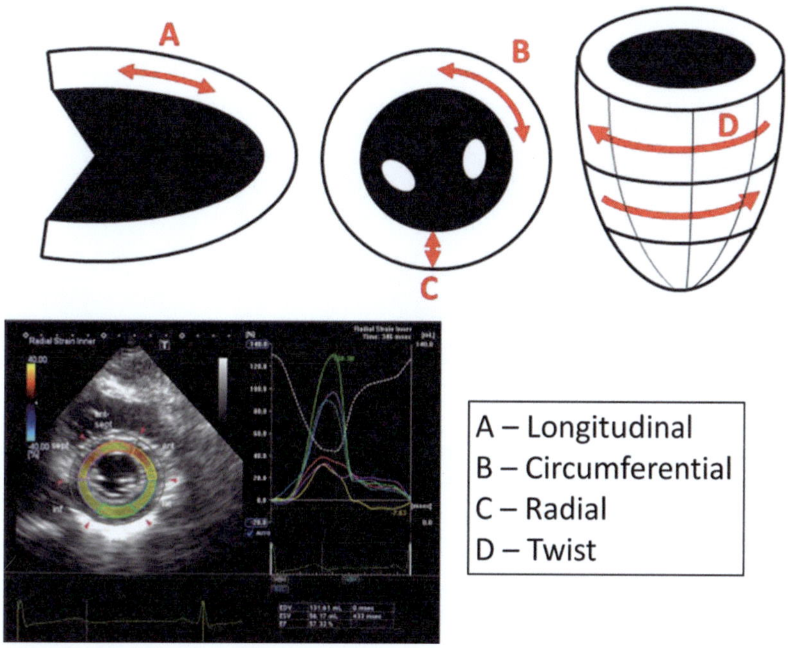

Fig. 3.2 The **strain parameters** derived from **speckle tracking echocardiography**. (**a**) Longitudinal strain demonstrates the shortening of the wall segment as the base moves towards the apex in systole; (**b**) Circumferential strain reflects the reduction in circumference of the heart in systole; (**c**) Radial strain reflects the thickening of a wall segment in systole; (**d**) Twist is the difference in degrees between apical and basal rotation. In the inferior left, there is an example of a longitudinal strain acquisition with its curves of regional systolic deformation

Cardiac Magnetic Resonance Imaging

Cardiac Magnetic Resonance (CMR) is considered one of the most valuable techniques in evaluating suspected HF. It can provide all the anatomical and functional parameters that echocardiography can provide—with additional high spatial resolution and tissue characterization. Furthermore, CMR is the gold standard for the accuracy and reproducibility of volumes, mass, and wall motion [2]. Its ability to have good image quality in most exams makes it the exam of choice for functional evaluation when 2D-Echo is non-diagnostic. A general CMR exam comprises a complete heart segmentation, with a vertical and horizontal long axis of the LV (2 and 3 chamber views), a stack of 8–12 slices in the short axis, and the left ventricle outflow tract (3 chamber view) (Fig. 3.3).

All the volumes and LV mass are usually calculated using the modified Simpson's rule in the short-axis stack, with the significant advantage of the absence of geometrical assumptions for those calculations, which is especially important given that chamber dilatation and remodeling often accompany HF (Table 3.2). Nowadays, the standard sequence for cine imaging is a balanced steady-state free precession (SSFP) with retrospective ECG gating [23], which has good spatial

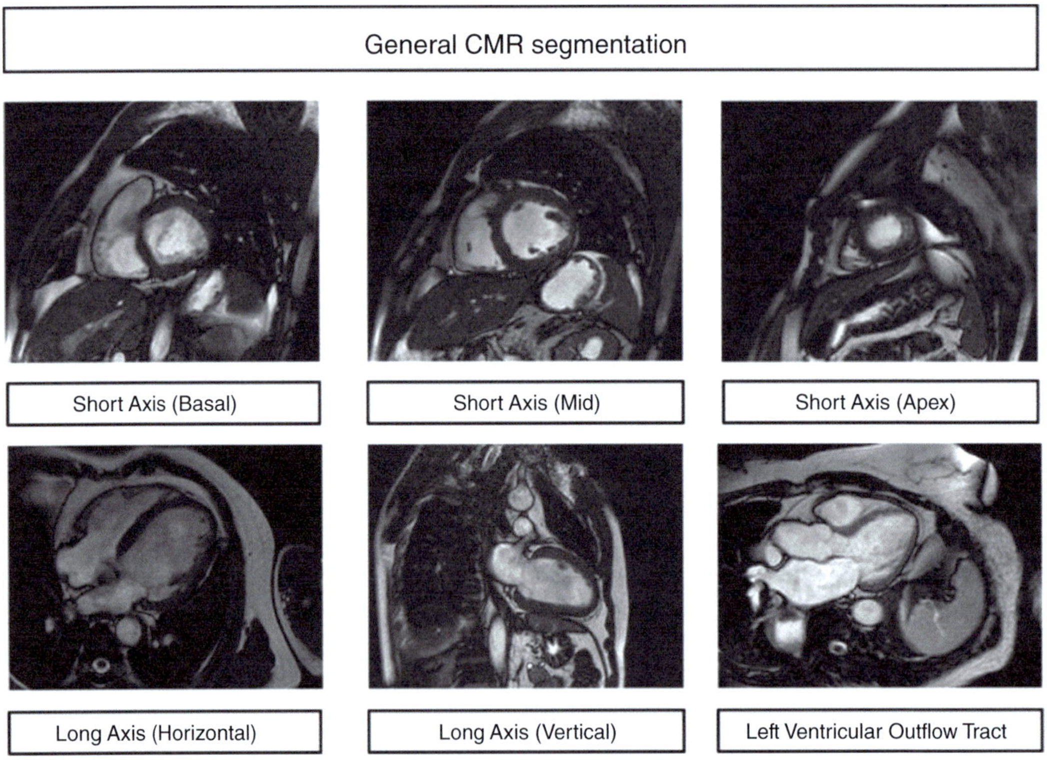

Fig. 3.3 General cardiac magnetic resonance (CMR) imaging segmentation. A CMR exam comprehends a complete segmentation of the heart, with a vertical and horizontal long axis of the LV (2 and 3 chamber views), a stack of 8–12 slices in the short axis (here with an example of basal, mid and apex) and the left ventricle outflow tract (3 chamber view)

Table 3.2 Reference values for left and right ventricular function and dimension by cardiac MRI in adults, papillary muscles included in left ventricular volume

	Women	Men
Left ventricle		
Mass (g)	43–103	57–152
Mass/BSA (g/m^2)	30–59	36–75
EDV/BSA (ml/m^2)	45–93	47–107
ESV/BSA (ml/m^2)	10–38	11–47
EF (%)	52–79	51–76
Right ventricle		
EDV/BSA (ml/m^2)	48–104	53–123
ESV/BSA (ml/m^2)	13–48	17–59
EF (%)	46–74	42–72

From the short axis, reference values based on SSFP cine images were analyzed with Argus software (Siemens, The Netherlands). These values may vary depending on image sequence, acquisition technique, and contouring. *BSA* body surface area, *EDV* end-diastolic volume, *ESV* end-systolic volume, *EF* ejection fraction.

resolution and contrast between the ventricular wall, blood, and adjacent structures. Its disadvantage is the necessity of repeated breath holds, which can be challenging for HF patients. Real-time acquisition of cine imaging could be an option for patients who cannot perform this maneuver, providing images (with lower spatial resolution than standard SSFP) acquired in 3–4 s with during free breathing [24, 25]. For a comprehensive functional assessment, phase-contrast image can be obtained for measuring valve and intra-cardiac flows. This sequence relies on phase shifting related to the motion (or flow) of the blood (or myocardium) when compared to the stationary structures, which provides a detailed pixel map where intensity is directly related to the velocity and the sign (positive or negative)

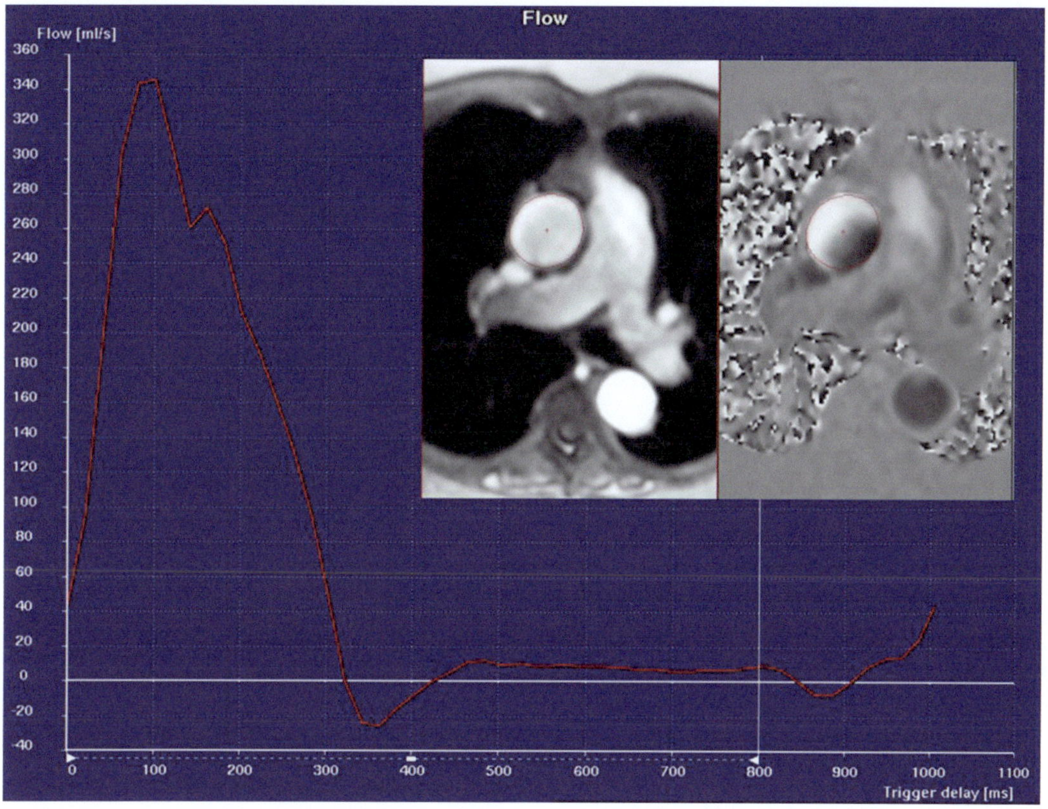

Fig. 3.4 Flow quantification of the ascending aorta with phase contrast imaging by Cardiac magnetic resonance imaging. In this example, the ROI (*red*) is placed in the ascending aorta and can be observed in the ECG-gated cine phase contrast magnitude (*left*) and phase (*right*) images during early diastole. On phase images, the bright signal intensity corresponds to cephalad flow, and the black signal to caudal flow. A plot of mean flow through the cardiac cycle in the ascending aorta can then be generated

indicates the direction (Fig. 3.4). Additionally, myocardial tagging is a powerful tool to evaluate global and regional myocardial from myocardial systolic and diastolic deformation [26].

In addition to the function analysis, **tissue characterization** is critical for HF diagnosis and provides prognostic information related to its findings. In this sense, several T1- and T2-weighted sequences, with or without gadolinium, can be performed to provide information about the composition and perfusion of the myocardium. T2- and T2*-weighted images are generally performed without contrast to bring information about the intrinsic tissue composition, such as water and iron content. When associated with other techniques, these methods can also provide information about lipid content [27–29]. T1-weighted images are generally used with contrast media to show their dynamics since gadolinium makes the T1 times shorter. Late gadolinium enhancement (LGE) and perfusion images rely on this effect to generate the images. The association of those findings makes the evaluation more powerful.

LGE techniques are a reference method for assessing myocardial replacement fibrosis [30–32]. Right after the infusion, gadolinium contrast media rapidly diffuses across the capillary membranes but not in the intracellular space. After 8–12 min, an equilibrium state is reached, and the volume of distribution of the contrast is higher in fibrotic areas, marking these areas bright white with a T1-weighted sequence. An inversion-recovery preparation pulse is set in this

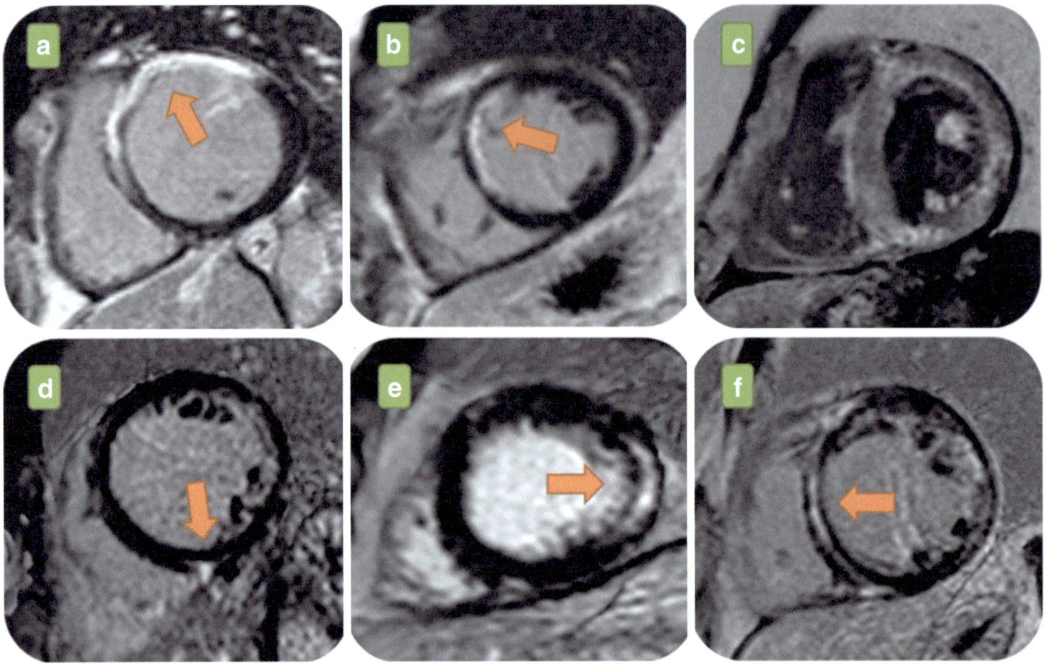

Fig. 3.5 Example of some hyperenhancement patterns in late gadolinium enhancement sequence by cardiac magnetic resonance. The orange arrows point to the main areas of the scar. Ischemic: (**a**) transmural; (**b**) subendocardial. Non-ischemic: (**c**) diffuse; (**d–f**) mid-wall. The ischemic pattern always involves the subendocardium, which is consistent with the perfusion area of an epicardial coronary artery (in these examples, the left anterior descending). The diffuse pattern is consistent with infiltrative diseases such as cardiac amyloidosis. The mid-wall patterns are less specific and can be found in idiopathic dilated cardiomyopathy, myocarditis, sarcoidosis, Chagas' heart disease, and Anderson-Fabry disease

sequence to nullify viable areas' signals to increase the image contrast. It is a valuable tool in evaluating the patient with HF because several patterns of involvement can suggest the diagnosis of some specific pathology. The hyperenhancement pattern considered "ischemic" always involves the subendocardium (or can be transmural) and should be located in a region consistent with the perfusion area of an epicardial coronary artery [33]. The ones that do not have these characteristics are considered "non-ischemic" (Fig. 3.5). For example, cardiac amyloidosis generally presents a diffuse enhancement more concentrated in the subendocardial area, while idiopathic dilated cardiomyopathy and myocarditis often show a mid-wall pattern; however, none of those patterns are pathognomonic. For CAD investigation, an ischemic LGE pattern associated with a perfusion defect can improve the accuracy of CMR to identify significant coronary obstructions. Beyond the diagnosis, the presence and the amount of scar can be related to treatment response and prognosis. The classical study from Kim et al. demonstrated poor improvement in LV function after revascularization when the transmurality of the myocardial scar assessed by LGE was more than 50% [34]. In another study, the amount of viable tissue in HF was an independent predictor of change in LVEF, mean wall motion score, and LV end-diastolic volume index in patients treated with beta-blockers [35]. Mid-wall fibrosis in non-ischemic dilated cardiomyopathy was also an independent predictor of all-cause death and hospitalization for a cardiovascular event in another subset [36]. Poor response to CRT and inducibility of ventricular tachycardia in electrophysiologic studies are also related to the presence of scars [37, 38].

CMR stress perfusion imaging is an accurate exam to investigate coronary arterial disease. It can be performed using pharmacologic or physical stress, but the first modality is far more common due to its convenience. Dipyridamole or adenosine are used to generate coronary vasodilatation; the first pass of the contrast shows areas of delayed perfusion (darker) that can be related to coronary narrowing. The dobutamine stress test relies on wall motion abnormalities like stress echocardiography. CMR stress tests are robust and highly reproducible for diagnosing coronary artery disease (CAD) [30, 39].

CMR can also provide information regarding iron overload from assessing relaxation parameter T2*. Iron overload in the myocardium produces an abnormal signal loss in T2*-weighted sequences proportional to its amount, and this effect can be used to estimate the iron content in the tissue [29]. T2* time lower than 20 ms indicates significant iron overload and is related to ventricular arrhythmias and HF [25, 40]. Moreover, the treatment with iron chelator deferoxamine—which decreases the amount of iron in the myocardium—is related to a significant increase in T2* times [40].

One of the challenges in CMR is obtaining quantitative information about myocardial tissue properties, such as relaxation times T1 and T2, which reflect the tissue's molecular environment and water content. Parametric T1 and T2 maps are images that display the pixel-wise values of these relaxation times, providing a direct and objective assessment of the myocardial tissue characteristics [41, 42]. Using T1 mapping techniques to calculate native T1 times (pre- and post-gadolinium) and the extracellular volume to assess interstitial fibrosis can potentially improve the diagnosis and treatment of HF. Parametric maps can improve MRI tissue characterization and therefore improve diagnosis due to various disturbances within the heart muscle cells (such as iron overload or glycosphingolipid accumulation in Anderson-Fabry disease), within the extracellular matrix that surrounds them (such as myocardial fibrosis or cardiac amyloidosis from excessive deposition of collagen or amyloid proteins, respectively), or both (myocardial edema with increased water content inside or outside the cells).

Cardiac Computed Tomography

Cardiac Computed Tomography (CCT) is a valuable technique for investigating obstructive CAD as a potential etiology of heart failure, especially in those with reduced LVEF. On the other hand, ruling out significant CAD is particularly important for patients with heart failure with preserved LVEF. In both clinical settings, multidetector scanners can provide high-resolution coronary angiography with excellent accuracy for detecting severe epicardial artery stenosis. Furthermore, CCT has a high negative predictive value to rule-out obstructive CAD. Detailed anatomical reconstruction imaging also offers a great advantage, with precise measurements of the chambers' diameters and volumes [43, 44].

One of the more significant CCT advantages for evaluating patients with heart failure is the possibility of maintaining medications during the patient's preparation for the exam, including beta-blockers. Images can be quickly acquired, not requesting supine positioning for long periods, which can benefit those with orthopnea. The use of prospectively ECG-triggered axial acquisition substantially reduces radiation exposure during CCT. For retrospectively ECG-gated reconstruction, tube current modulation is an alternative for this purpose. A low volume of contrast agents is required for coronary angiography and can be safely used for patients with no advanced kidney dysfunction [45].

CCT techniques continue to evolve, and some advanced image acquisition, reconstruction, and analysis can provide a combined anatomical and functional assessment of CAD. Calculating fractional flow reserve with computed tomography (FFT-CT) allows a non-invasive evaluation of functionally significant coronary lesions. This technique may identify lesion-specific ischemia and guide clinical decisions of coronary revascularization, particularly for plaques related to intermediate stenosis at anatomical evaluation [46].

Cardiac Nuclear Medicine

Nuclear medicine comprises any technique using radioactive tracers to generate images. Positron emission tomography (PET) [alone or in association with computed tomography], single-photon emission computed tomography (SPECT), and radionucleotide ventriculography (RVG) are the ones that have applications in cardiology.

The RVG was first introduced in the early 1970s and had an excellent agreement with invasive techniques to measure LVEF. [47] RVG and CMR are the most accurate and reproducible modalities for assessing ventricular function. RVG is performed by labeling the blood pool with a radioactive tracer (technetium 99 m–Tc99m) and measuring radioactivity over the anterior chest with a gamma camera. The number of counts recorded at any time is proportional to the amount of blood radioactivity, which is linearly related to the blood volumes over the cardiac cycle. One of the great advantages of this modality is not to rely on any geometric assumptions, so it is accurate regardless of the shape of the ventricle (right or left). Due to the use of ionizing radiation, however, RVG should be performed only in selected cases—when echocardiography and cardiac MRI are not possible or have low quality.

Unlike the RVG, the primary use of SPECT and PET are ischemia and viability assessment. The left ventricular function analysis can also be performed (Gated SPECT and PET-CT), but these should not be the main reason for the exam acquisition. Both modalities use radioactive flow tracers to generate the images, generally associated with pharmacologic or exercise cardiovascular stress. Although PET-CT has a higher spatial resolution, sensibility, and specificity, gated SPECT has been used as a non-invasive tool to investigate ischemia for a long time, with a good literature background of diagnostic and prognostic evaluations. Lower cost and extensive availability are other advantages of gated SPECT (Table 3.3).

Table 3.3 Clinical applications of non-invasive imaging techniques in the assessment of patients with heart failure

		Echo	CMR	SPECT	MDCT	PET
Functional evaluation						
Left ventricle	Volumes	++	+++	+	+	+
	EF	++	+++	++	+	++
	Mass	++	+++	–	+	–
Right ventricle	Volumes	++	+++	–	+	–
	EF	++	+++	–	+	–
Diastolic function		+++	+	–	–	–
Etiology						
Coronary artery disease	Ischemia	+++[a]	+++[a]	+++	+[b]	+++
	Myocardial fibrosis	–	+++	++	–	++
	Coronary anatomy	–	+	–	+++	–
Valvular	Stenosis	+++	+	–	+[c]	–
	Regurgitation	+++	++	–	–	–
Inflammatory	Myocarditis	+	+++	+	–	+
	Sarcoidosis	+	+++	+	–	+++
Hypertrophic CMP	HCM	+++	+++	–	–	–
Dilated CMP	Eosinophilic	+	+++	–	–	–
	Iron overload	+	+++	–	–	–
ARVC		++	+++	–	+	–
Restrictive CMP	Amyloidosis	++	+++	+++	–	–
	Endomyocardial fibrosis	++	+++	–	–	–
	Anderson-Fabry	+	+++	–	–	–
Unclassified CMP	Takotsubo	++	++	–	–	–
Pericardial diseases		++[d]	+++[e]	+	++[f]	–

Selection of a test in daily practice should consider availability, local expertise, costs, advantages/disadvantages, and, in the case of several questions to address, which test could best answer several of them

ARVC arrhythmogenic right ventricular cardiomyopathy, *CAD* coronary artery disease, *CMP* cardiomyopathy, *CMR* cardiac magnetic resonance, *EF* ejection fraction, *HCM* hypertrophic cardiomyopathy, *LV* left ventricle, *MDCT* multidetector computed tomography, *PET* positron emission tomography, *RV* right ventricle, *SPECT* single photon emission computed tomography

[a] Stress (dobutamine/adenosine) imaging

[b] Fractional flow reserve and stress perfusion CT imaging

[c] Including measurements of aortic valve calcium score

[d] Hemodynamic evaluation (constriction)

[e] Describes disease activity by contrast-enhanced CMR

[f] Analysis of pericardial calcification

Conclusion

Imaging exams are essential in HF patient evaluation, not only for the proper diagnosis but also for correct treatment and follow-up. Different techniques can provide different amounts of information, from the simple and limited chest X-ray to the complex and complete CMR. Today we have many modalities available, so choosing the one that will provide the desired answers with the least harm to the patient and at a lower cost is essential.

References

1. Jessup M, Abraham WT, Casey DE, Feldman AM, Francis GS, Ganiats TG, et al. 2009 focused update: ACCF/AHA Guidelines for the Diagnosis and Management of Heart Failure in Adults: a report of the American College of Cardiology Foundation/American Heart Association Task Force on Practice Guidelines: developed in collaboration with the International Society for Heart and Lung Transplantation. Circulation. 2009;119(14):1977–2016.
2. McMurray JJ, Adamopoulos S, Anker SD, Auricchio A, Bohm M, Dickstein K, et al. ESC Guidelines for

the diagnosis and treatment of acute and chronic heart failure 2012: The Task Force for the Diagnosis and Treatment of Acute and Chronic Heart Failure 2012 of the European Society of Cardiology. Developed in collaboration with the Heart Failure Association (HFA) of the ESC. Eur Heart J. 2012;33(14):1787–847.
3. Badgett RG, Mulrow CD, Otto PM, Ramirez G. How well can the chest radiograph diagnose left ventricular dysfunction? J Gen Intern Med. 1996;11(10):625–34.
4. Knudsen CW, Omland T, Clopton P, Westheim A, Abraham WT, Storrow AB, et al. Diagnostic value of B-type natriuretic peptide and chest radiographic findings in patients with acute dyspnea. Am J Med. 2004;116(6):363–8.
5. Hunt SA, Abraham WT, Chin MH, Feldman AM, Francis GS, Ganiats TG, et al. ACC/AHA 2005 Guideline Update for the Diagnosis and Management of Chronic Heart Failure in the Adult: a report of the American College of Cardiology/American Heart Association Task Force on Practice Guidelines (Writing Committee to Update the 2001 Guidelines for the Evaluation and Management of Heart Failure): developed in collaboration with the American College of Chest Physicians and the International Society for Heart and Lung Transplantation: endorsed by the Heart Rhythm Society. Circulation. 2005;112(12):e154–235.
6. Lang RM, Badano LP, Mor-Avi V, Afilalo J, Armstrong A, Ernande L, et al. Recommendations for cardiac chamber quantification by echocardiography in adults: an update from the american society of echocardiography and the European association of cardiovascular imaging. J Am Soc Echocardiogr 2015;28(1):1–39 e14.
7. Smart N, Haluska B, Leano R, Case C, Mottram PM, Marwick TH. Determinants of functional capacity in patients with chronic heart failure: role of filling pressure and systolic and diastolic function. Am Heart J. 2005;149(1):152–8.
8. Vasan RS, Larson MG, Benjamin EJ, Evans JC, Reiss CK, Levy D. Congestive heart failure in subjects with normal versus reduced left ventricular ejection fraction: prevalence and mortality in a population-based cohort. J Am Coll Cardiol. 1999;33(7):1948–55.
9. Grayburn PA, Appleton CP, DeMaria AN, Greenberg B, Lowes B, Oh J, et al. Echocardiographic predictors of morbidity and mortality in patients with advanced heart failure: the Beta-blocker Evaluation of Survival Trial (BEST). J Am Coll Cardiol. 2005;45(7):1064–71.
10. Armstrong AC, Gidding S, Gjesdal O, Wu C, Bluemke DA, Lima JA. LV mass assessed by echocardiography and CMR, cardiovascular outcomes, and medical practice. JACC Cardiovasc Imaging. 2012;5(8):837–48.
11. Quinones MA, Greenberg BH, Kopelen HA, Koilpillai C, Limacher MC, Shindler DM, et al. Echocardiographic predictors of clinical outcome in patients with left ventricular dysfunction enrolled in the SOLVD registry and trials: significance of left ventricular hypertrophy. Studies of Left Ventricular Dysfunction. J Am Coll Cardiol. 2000;35(5):1237–44.
12. Ristow B, Ali S, Whooley MA, Schiller NB. Usefulness of left atrial volume index to predict heart failure hospitalization and mortality in ambulatory patients with coronary heart disease and comparison to left ventricular ejection fraction (from the Heart and Soul Study). Am J Cardiol. 2008;102(1):70–6.
13. Kirkpatrick JN, Vannan MA, Narula J, Lang RM. Echocardiography in heart failure: applications, utility, and new horizons. J Am Coll Cardiol. 2007;50(5):381–96.
14. Redfield MM, Jacobsen SJ, Burnett JC Jr, Mahoney DW, Bailey KR, Rodeheffer RJ. Burden of systolic and diastolic ventricular dysfunction in the community: appreciating the scope of the heart failure epidemic. JAMA. 2003;289(2):194–202.
15. Tsang TS, Barnes ME, Gersh BJ, Bailey KR, Seward JB. Risks for atrial fibrillation and congestive heart failure in patients >/=65 years of age with abnormal left ventricular diastolic relaxation. Am J Cardiol. 2004;93(1):54–8.
16. Corsi C, Lang RM, Veronesi F, Weinert L, Caiani EG, MacEneaney P, et al. Volumetric quantification of global and regional left ventricular function from real-time three-dimensional echocardiographic images. Circulation. 2005;112(8):1161–70.
17. Mor-Avi V, Sugeng L, Weinert L, MacEneaney P, Caiani EG, Koch R, et al. Fast measurement of left ventricular mass with real-time three-dimensional echocardiography: comparison with magnetic resonance imaging. Circulation. 2004;110(13):1814–8.
18. Gorcsan J 3rd, Tanaka H. Echocardiographic assessment of myocardial strain. J Am Coll Cardiol. 2011;58(14):1401–13.
19. Sengelov M, Jorgensen PG, Jensen JS, Bruun NE, Olsen FJ, Fritz-Hansen T, et al. Global longitudinal strain is a superior predictor of all-cause mortality in heart failure with reduced ejection fraction. JACC Cardiovasc Imaging. 2015;8(12):1351–9.
20. Lyon AR, Lopez-Fernandez T, Couch LS, Asteggiano R, Aznar MC, Bergler-Klein J, et al. 2022 ESC Guidelines on cardio-oncology developed in collaboration with the European Hematology Association (EHA), the European Society for Therapeutic Radiology and Oncology (ESTRO) and the International Cardio-Oncology Society (IC-OS). Eur Heart J. 2022;43(41):4229–361.
21. Cohen OC, Ismael A, Pawarova B, Manwani R, Ravichandran S, Law S, et al. Longitudinal strain is an independent predictor of survival and response to therapy in patients with systemic AL amyloidosis. Eur Heart J. 2022;43(4):333–41.
22. Alherbish A, Becher H, Alemayehu W, Paterson DI, Butler CR, Anderson TJ, et al. Impact of contrast echocardiography on accurate discrimination of specific degree of left ventricular systolic dysfunction and comparison with cardiac magnetic resonance imaging. Echocardiography. 2018;35(11):1746–54.

23. Carr JC, Simonetti O, Bundy J, Li D, Pereles S, Finn JP. Cine MR angiography of the heart with segmented true fast imaging with steady-state precession. Radiology. 2001;219(3):828–34.
24. Lee VS, Resnick D, Bundy JM, Simonetti OP, Lee P, Weinreb JC. Cardiac function: MR evaluation in one breath hold with real-time true fast imaging with steady-state precession. Radiology. 2002;222(3):835–42.
25. Raman SV, Simonetti OP. The CMR examination in heart failure. Heart Fail Clin. 2009;5(3):283–300. v
26. Shehata ML, Cheng S, Osman NF, Bluemke DA, Lima JA. Myocardial tissue tagging with cardiovascular magnetic resonance. J Cardiovasc Magn Reson. 2009;11(1):55.
27. Abdel-Aty H, Simonetti O, Friedrich MG. T2-weighted cardiovascular magnetic resonance imaging. J Magn Reson Imaging. 2007;26(3):452–9.
28. Kellman P, Hernando D, Arai AE. Myocardial fat imaging. Curr Cardiovasc Imaging Rep. 2010;3(2):83–91.
29. Carpenter JP, He T, Kirk P, Roughton M, Anderson LJ, de Noronha SV, et al. On T2* magnetic resonance and cardiac iron. Circulation. 2011;123(14):1519–28.
30. Schwitter J, Arai AE. Assessment of cardiac ischaemia and viability: role of cardiovascular magnetic resonance. Eur Heart J. 2011;32(7):799–809.
31. Simonetti OP, Kim RJ, Fieno DS, Hillenbrand HB, Wu E, Bundy JM, et al. An improved MR imaging technique for the visualization of myocardial infarction. Radiology. 2001;218(1):215–23.
32. Gerber BL, Lima JA, Garot J, Bluemke DA. Magnetic resonance imaging of myocardial infarct. Top Magn Reson Imaging. 2000;11(6):372–82.
33. Mahrholdt H, Wagner A, Judd RM, Sechtem U, Kim RJ. Delayed enhancement cardiovascular magnetic resonance assessment of non-ischaemic cardiomyopathies. Eur Heart J. 2005;26(15):1461–74.
34. Kim RJ, Wu E, Rafael A, Chen EL, Parker MA, Simonetti O, et al. The use of contrast-enhanced magnetic resonance imaging to identify reversible myocardial dysfunction. N Engl J Med. 2000;343(20):1445–53.
35. Bello D, Shah DJ, Farah GM, Di Luzio S, Parker M, Johnson MR, et al. Gadolinium cardiovascular magnetic resonance predicts reversible myocardial dysfunction and remodeling in patients with heart failure undergoing beta-blocker therapy. Circulation. 2003;108(16):1945–53.
36. Assomull RG, Prasad SK, Lyne J, Smith G, Burman ED, Khan M, et al. Cardiovascular magnetic resonance, fibrosis, and prognosis in dilated cardiomyopathy. J Am Coll Cardiol. 2006;48(10):1977–85.
37. Bleeker GB, Kaandorp TA, Lamb HJ, Boersma E, Steendijk P, de Roos A, et al. Effect of posterolateral scar tissue on clinical and echocardiographic improvement after cardiac resynchronization therapy. Circulation. 2006;113(7):969–76.
38. Schmidt A, Azevedo CF, Cheng A, Gupta SN, Bluemke DA, Foo TK, et al. Infarct tissue heterogeneity by magnetic resonance imaging identifies enhanced cardiac arrhythmia susceptibility in patients with left ventricular dysfunction. Circulation. 2007;115(15):2006–14.
39. Greenwood JP, Maredia N, Younger JF, Brown JM, Nixon J, Everett CC, et al. Cardiovascular magnetic resonance and single-photon emission computed tomography for diagnosis of coronary heart disease (CE-MARC): a prospective trial. Lancet. 2012;379(9814):453–60.
40. Tanner MA, Galanello R, Dessi C, Smith GC, Westwood MA, Agus A, et al. A randomized, placebo-controlled, double-blind trial of the effect of combined therapy with deferoxamine and deferiprone on myocardial iron in thalassemia major using cardiovascular magnetic resonance. Circulation. 2007;115(14):1876–84.
41. Ugander M, Oki AJ, Hsu LY, Kellman P, Greiser A, Aletras AH, et al. Extracellular volume imaging by magnetic resonance imaging provides insights into overt and sub-clinical myocardial pathology. Eur Heart J. 2012;33(10):1268–78.
42. Bull S, White SK, Piechnik SK, Flett AS, Ferreira VM, Loudon M, et al. Human non-contrast T1 values and correlation with histology in diffuse fibrosis. Heart. 2013;99(13):932–7.
43. Miller JM, Rochitte CE, Dewey M, Arbab-Zadeh A, Niinuma H, Gottlieb I, et al. Diagnostic performance of coronary angiography by 64-row CT. N Engl J Med. 2008;359(22):2324–36.
44. Meijboom WB, Meijs MF, Schuijf JD, Cramer MJ, Mollet NR, van Mieghem CA, et al. Diagnostic accuracy of 64-slice computed tomography coronary angiography: a prospective, multicenter, multivendor study. J Am Coll Cardiol. 2008;52(25):2135–44.
45. Abbara S, Blanke P, Maroules CD, Cheezum M, Choi AD, Han BK, et al. SCCT guidelines for the performance and acquisition of coronary computed tomographic angiography: a report of the society of Cardiovascular Computed Tomography Guidelines Committee: Endorsed by the North American Society for Cardiovascular Imaging (NASCI). J Cardiovasc Comput Tomogr. 2016;10(6):435–49.
46. Abdelrahman KM, Chen MY, Dey AK, Virmani R, Finn AV, Khamis RY, et al. Coronary computed tomography angiography from clinical uses to emerging technologies: JACC state-of-the-art review. J Am Coll Cardiol. 2020;76(10):1226–43.
47. Burow RD, Strauss HW, Singleton R, Pond M, Rehn T, Bailey IK, et al. Analysis of left ventricular function from multiple gated acquisition cardiac blood pool imaging. Comparison to contrast angiography. Circulation. 1977;56(6):1024–8.

4 Acute and Chronic Right Ventricular Failure

Gabriel Sayer and Marc J. Semigran

Abbreviations

2D	Two-Dimensional
ARVC	Arrhythmogenic Right Ventricular Cardiomyopathy
CMRI	Cardiac Magnetic Resonance Imaging
CVP	Central Venous Pressure
ERA	Endothelin Receptor Antagonist
HF	Heart Failure
iNO	Inhaled Nitric Oxide
LV	Left Ventricle
LVAD	Left Ventricular Assist Device
PA	Pulmonary Artery
PAH	Pulmonary Arterial Hypertension
PCWP	Pulmonary Capillary Wedge Pressure
PDE-5I	Phosphodiesterase-5 Inhibitor
PE	Pulmonary Embolism
PH	Pulmonary Hypertension
PVR	Pulmonary Vascular Resistance
RAP	Right Atrial Pressure
RHC	Right Heart Catheterization
RIMP	Right Ventricular Index of Myocardial Performance
RV	Right Ventricle
RVAD	Right Ventricular Assist Device
RVEF	Right Ventricular Ejection Fraction
RVFAC	Right Ventricular Fractional Area Change
RVI	Right Ventricular Infarction
TAPSE	Tricuspid Annular Plane Systolic Excursion
TPG	Transpulmonary Gradient

G. Sayer
Advanced Heart Failure, Section of Cardiology, Columbia University, New York, NY, USA
e-mail: gsayer@medicine.bsd.uchicago.edu

M. J. Semigran (✉)
Cardiology Division, Massachusetts General Hospital, Boston, MA, USA
e-mail: msemigran@partners.org

Introduction

Recent research has shed new light on the importance of the right ventricle (RV) in normal cardiac physiology and its prominent role in the pathophysiology of heart failure (HF). The RV was previously overshadowed by the left ventricle (LV), whose simpler anatomy conforms better to geometric models and is more accessible to non-invasive imaging. Furthermore, early experiments falsely suggested that the RV did not contribute significantly to the generation of cardiac output [1]. However, a series of investigations over the past 25 years have provided greater insight into the RV's distinct anatomy, its performance under normal physiological conditions, and its adaptations to specific disease states. Advanced imaging, including cardiac magnetic resonance imaging (CMRI), has provided critical assistance in the study of the RV, allowing for non-invasive characterization of the RV's response to stressors, as well as a tool for measuring the success of therapies. As a result, a detailed

H. J. Eisen (ed.), *Heart Failure I*, https://doi.org/10.1007/978-3-032-12626-9_4

understanding now exists of the role of the RV in ischemic heart disease, congenital heart disease, pulmonary arterial hypertension (PAH) and chronic left-sided HF. Most importantly, studies have shown that RV failure is a crucial prognostic factor in all of these disease states. In particular, the importance of RV function in left-sided HF may outweigh the importance of LV function in terms of both morbidity and mortality.

Anatomy and Physiology of the Right Ventricle

The RV can be divided into three anatomical units: the inlet from the right atrium (including the tricuspid, the apex, and the outflow tract (infundibulum). The apex contains prominent trabeculations, in contrast to the smooth, muscular infundibulum. Viewed in cross-section, the RV resembles a crescent that lies over the anterior aspect of the LV. The free wall is thin and the overall mass of the RV is a fraction of the LV mass, despite a larger volume. The deep muscle fibers of the RV have a longitudinal orientation, resulting in a primarily vertical direction of contractile forces. The superficial muscle fibers of the RV are oriented in a more concentric direction and are intertwined with the superficial muscle fibers of the LV. This anatomical interaction between the muscular fibers of the two chambers is also present in the interventricular septum, which is typically displaced into the RV throughout the cardiac cycle. Direct muscular continuity between the LV and RV plays a significant role in ventricular interdependence, which will be discussed in further detail below.

RV contraction proceeds sequentially, initiating in the inlet, continuing through the apex and concluding in the infundibulum. The longitudinal fibers draw the apex towards the tricuspid valve, while the free wall also moves inward toward the septum. Traction on the free wall is applied by LV contraction at attachment points in the superficial muscle layer. The RV is coupled with the high compliance of the pulmonary vasculature, leading to a pressure-volume relationship that is distinct from the relationship seen in the LV. Whereas the LV continues to generate pressure until the closure of the aortic valve, RV pressure falls prior to the closure of the pulmonic valve. Ejection continues however due to the low resistance within the pulmonary circuit (Fig. 4.1) [2]. The RV takes advantage of this physiology

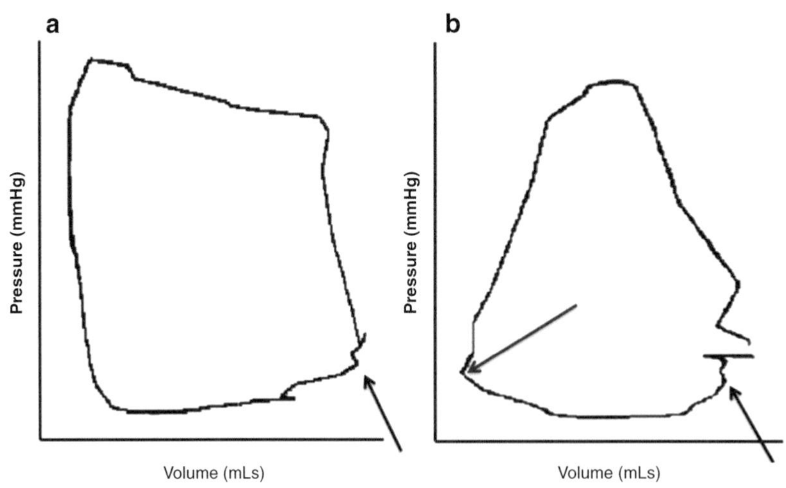

Fig. 4.1 A comparison of typical pressure-volume loops for a single cardiac cycle of the left ventricle (**a**) and right ventricle (**b**). In the left ventricle, pressure continues to increase slightly throughout the entire duration of ventricular ejection. In the right ventricle, intracardiac pressure falls prior to closure of the pulmonic valve (*red arrow*), resulting in less myocardial work. End-diastole is indicated by the black arrows (Adapted with permission from Redington [2], with permission from Elsevier)

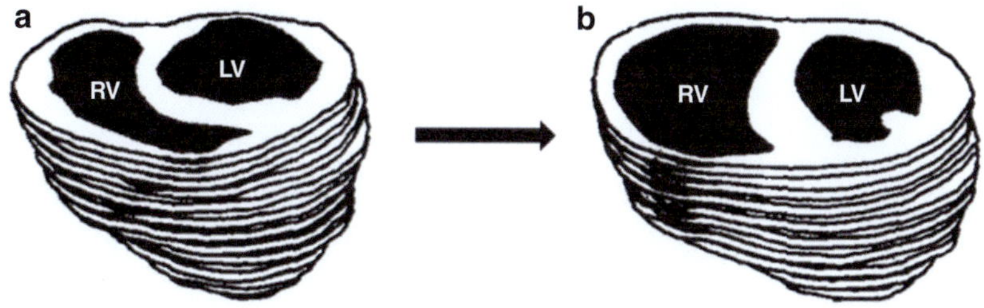

Fig. 4.2 Ventricular interdependence. During normal loading conditions (*left side of diagram*), the intraventricular septum bulges into the right ventricle (*RV*). In the context of right ventricular volume overload, the septum becomes flattened, with an increase in RV volume and a decrease in left ventricular (*LV*) volume. (Reprinted with permission from Greyson [3], © 2008, with permission from Lippincott Williams & Wilkins/Wolters Kluwer/ Society of Critical Care Medicine)

by producing an identical cardiac output to the LV with markedly reduced work and myocardial oxygen demand. However, one consequence of this interaction is the RV's heightened sensitivity to afterload, which can be deleterious in acute pressure overload states.

Ventricular interdependence occurs in both systole and diastole. Systolic interdependence is mediated by the shared musculature between the LV and the RV, which means that the contractile state of one ventricle can influence the performance of the other ventricle. Diastolic interdependence is a result of the common pericardial sac. The pericardium is unable to stretch acutely in response to ventricular dilatation, and is limited in its ability to accommodate chronic ventricular dilatation. Therefore, a volume load in either chamber will cause displacement of the septum into the other chamber, resulting in a decreased diastolic volume and an impairment of ventricular output (Fig. 4.2) [3]. As the RV is the more compliant chamber, this diastolic interaction most commonly occurs in volume overload states of the RV, such as an atrial septal defect.

Right Ventricular Adaptations to Disease States

RV pathophysiology can be broadly categorized by the mechanism of the insult and its rapidity of onset. Acute events, such as a pulmonary embolism, lead to maladaptive compensatory responses, and quickly progress to RV failure. Chronic disease processes, such as congenital heart defects, often present a gradual stress on the RV, allowing it to develop adaptive mechanisms to preserve cardiac output for a prolonged period of time prior to decompensation. Conditions characterized by volume overload are generally well tolerated by the RV due to its compliant nature. On the other hand, the RV has difficulty adapting to pressure overload due to its afterload-sensitivity (Fig. 4.3) [4]. Interestingly, the timing of onset of pressure overload is a crucial determinant of the RV response. In Eisenmenger syndrome, the RV is able to remain compensated much longer than in adult patients with acquired pulmonary hypertension (PH). This finding has been attributed to the preservation of the fetal phenotype, which is accustomed to systemic levels of vascular resistance [5]. Intrinsic myocardial diseases, such as various forms of nonischemic cardiomyopathies, may impair RV contractility, but rarely affect the RV in isolation. However, RV involvement in a cardiomyopathy can play a significant role in morbidity and mortality, particularly in the setting of pulmonary hypertension (PH). A list of diseases that cause RV dysfunction and RV failure can be found in Table 4.1.

Acute Pressure Overload

Following a submassive or massive pulmonary embolism (PE), there is a rapid rise in pulmonary vascular resistance (PVR) due to both obstructed blood flow and the release of vasoconstrictors

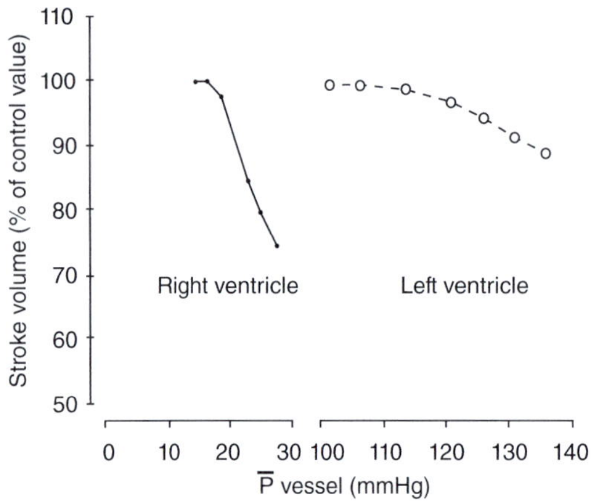

Fig. 4.3 Response of canine right ventricular and left ventricular stroke volume to acute changes in afterload. The steep slope in the right ventricle indicates enhanced sensitivity to afterload (Reprinted with permission from Abel and Waldhausen [4], © 1967, with permission from Elsevier)

[6]. Vasoconstriction may be further exacerbated by hypoxemia. The rapid rise in afterload increases RV wall tension, which quickly leads to RV dilatation and RV systolic dysfunction. As the RV pressure rises acutely, the interventricular septum shifts into the LV, reducing LV preload and further compromising cardiac output. Finally, coronary perfusion is impaired by both the compression of the right coronary artery by elevated RV wall stress and the reduction in cardiac output. In the setting of the increased myocardial oxygen demand in the failing RV, the reduction in coronary blood flow leads to a significant supply-demand imbalance. The final consequence of this sequence of events is worsening cardiac output, systemic hypotension and cardiac arrest.

Table 4.1 Causes of right ventricular failure

Acute causes	Intrinsic myocardial disease
Pulmonary embolism	Cardiomyopathy
Right ventricular infarction	Idiopathic
Sepsis	Viral
Acute lung injury	Familial
ARDS	Ischemic
TRALI	Infiltrative
Acute chest syndrome	Restrictive
Post-cardiotomy	Arrhythmogenic RV dysplasia
Pulmonary hypertensive crisis	
Cardiac tamponade	*Pericardial disease*
	Constrictive pericarditis
Chronic volume overload	*Chronic pressure overload*
Tricuspid valve regurgitation	Pulmonary arterial hypertension
Infective endocarditis	Pulmonary venous hypertension
Rheumatic disease	Left heart failure
Carcinoid	Pulmonary veno-occlusive disease
Traumatic	Hypoxia-associated PH
Pulmonic valve regurgitation	Chronic thromboembolic PH
Congenital heart disease	Congenital heart disease
Atrial septal defect	Tetralogy of Fallot
Ebstein's anomaly	Pulmonic stenosis
Coronary artery fistula	L-transposition of the great arteries
Anomalous pulmonary venous return	Pulmonary artery stenosis
	Eisenmenger's syndrome

ARDS acute respiratory distress syndrome, *PH* pulmonary hypertension, *RV* right ventricle, *TRALI* transfusion associated lung injury

Ischemia

Right ventricular infarction (RVI) occurs after occlusion of the right coronary artery in a sufficiently proximal portion to prevent perfusion of the RV branches. The immediate result of an RVI is RV free wall dyskinesis due to ischemia, although this alone may not be sufficient to produce clinical RV failure. Secondary effects include stiffening of the myocardium and dilation of the RV. Similar to the consequences of an acute PE, the acute pressure changes within the RV, in this case provoked by diastolic dysfunction, cause septal shifting and impaired LV-RV interaction. In addition septal ischemia further compromises LV performance, and diminishes the LV's ability to compensate for RV dysfunction [7].

Chronic Pressure Overload

PH is the end-product of many cardiovascular and pulmonary diseases and is the most common cause of a chronic pressure overload on the RV. As the pulmonary artery (PA) pressure gradually increases over time, the RV adapts to the increase in afterload through multiple compensatory mechanisms. Myocyte hypertrophy and the expansion of the extracellular matrix result in increased chamber thickness. At the same time, the RV remodels into a more spherical shape with a smaller radius [8]. Through the application of LaPlace's law, which states that wall stress is proportional to chamber radius and inversely proportional to chamber thickness, it is evident that the primary result of these initial adaptations is to reduce wall stress, countering the effect of the rise in afterload. In addition, central venous pressure (CVP) is allowed to rise, taking advantage of the Frank-Starling mechanism to maintain a normal stroke volume.

Several mechanisms have counterproductive effects, including reversion to a fetal gene pattern and upregulation of neurohormonal systems [8]. The result is a decrement in contractility, followed by progressive ventricular dilatation. As with acute RV pressure overload, dilatation increases myocardial oxygen demand while simultaneously reducing coronary perfusion and oxygen delivery. This supply-demand mismatch further compromises RV performance and ultimately leads to RV failure if the PH remains untreated. Both cardiac output and PA pressure fall when RV contractile reserve is no longer sufficient to maintain an adequate stroke volume (Fig. 4.4) [9].

Chronic Volume Overload

The thin, distensible wall of the RV permits it to accommodate large changes in preload without incurring significant changes in pressure. States of chronic volume overload, such as an atrial septal defect, can persist for decades prior to the development of RV dysfunction. Two consequences of persistent RV dilatation are distortion

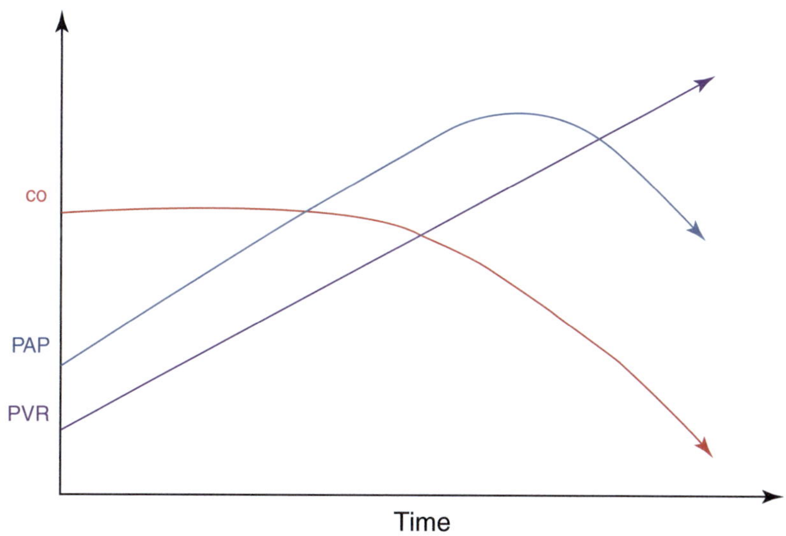

Fig. 4.4 The natural history of persistent pulmonary hypertension. As pulmonary artery pressure (*PAP*) and pulmonary vascular resistance (*PVR*) climb, cardiac output (*CO*) is initially maintained, but eventually begins to fall. When CO falls sufficiently to cause advanced RV failure, PAP fells as well due to insufficient pressure generation by the weak RV. PVR continues to rise despite falling PAP due to the concomitant fall in CO. *MPAP* mean pulmonary artery pressure, *PCWP* pulmonary capillary wedge pressure (Reprinted, with permission, from Haddad et al. [9], © 2008, with permission from Lippincott Williams & Wilkins/American Heart Association/Wolters Kluwer)

of the tricuspid annulus and septal shift. The dilated tricuspid annulus permits tricuspid regurgitation, which can further exacerbate the volume load on the RV. Septal shift occurs when the pericardium is unable to distend any further to accommodate the dilation of the RV. As noted above, septal shift can subsequently impair LV filling and adversely affect LV performance. Finally, prolonged volume overload may cause PA pressures to rise due to increased flow through the pulmonary circuit. The development of PH is often the trigger for decompensation of the chronic volume overloaded state, as the dilated RV lacks the compensatory mechanisms to augment its contractility in the setting of increased afterload [10].

Intrinsic Myocardial Disease

Arrhythmogenic right ventricular cardiomyopathy (ARVC) is a cardiomyopathy characterized by fibro-fatty replacement of myocardium, with a predilection for RV involvement. It may present with focal RV dysfunction at the sites of involvement, and may ultimately progress to RV dilatation and global RV dysfunction. The typical clinical presentation is ventricular arrhythmias, with symptoms of RV failure affecting less than 10% of ARVC patients [11]. In most patients, RV dysfunction can be present for decades without significant symptomatology. A similar observation has been made in animal experiments, in which an isolated reduction in RV contractility does not impair cardiac output in the setting of a normal PVR. In these animals, central filling pressures rise to permit sufficient flow through the pulmonary circuit. However, when PVR is raised, there is rapid cardiac decompensation, suggesting that the progression of RV dysfunction to RV failure may require the presence of an additional stressor, such as PH [12]. The Fontan operation, in which a passive conduit is created between systemic venous return and the pulmonary arteries, takes advantage of this physiology to maintain adequate flow to the LV despite the absence of RV contractility.

Diagnosis and Assessment of Right Ventricular Dysfunction and Failure

A thorough history and physical examination can provide important clues to the presence of RV failure, including the presence of a right-sided third heart sound, elevated jugular venous pressure, ascites and peripheral edema. A prominent pulmonic component of the second heart sound (P2) indicates the presence of PH. Patients may report early satiety, abdominal fullness and fatigue. Hepatic function and renal function are often compromised, and should be followed regularly in a patient with RV failure. Imaging studies play a crucial role in the initial assessment and serial monitoring of RV function. Echocardiography is the most frequently used imaging modality for RV assessment due to its ease of use, low cost and accessibility. However, CMRI has become the gold standard for evaluation of the RV because of its ability to overcome some of the anatomic limitations of two-dimensional (2D) echocardiography. While both echocardiography and CMRI can provide some assessment of RV hemodynamics, invasive measurement of intracardiac pressures by right heart catheterization is often required to diagnose the etiology of RV failure and determine the appropriate therapeutic approach.

Non-invasive Imaging Studies

RV size and function can be assessed with radionuclide ventriculography, using either first-pass or gated equilibrium techniques. While accurate measurements of volume and RV ejection fraction (RVEF) can be derived, this modality does not provide additional anatomic information, and exposes patients to radioisotopes. With the widespread availability of echocardiography, radionuclide ventriculography is rarely indicated as the primary method for RV functional assessment in the current era.

2D echocardiography has excellent spatial and temporal resolution, enabling precise evaluation of RV anatomy and valvular function. RV dimensions can be obtained through multiple views, providing an estimate of RV size. However, due to the RV's anatomic configuration, the calculation of accurate RV volumes with 2D echocardiography is not possible. Qualitatively comparing RV size to LV size in the apical view can provide a reasonable assessment of RV dilatation. Additional anatomic information that can be easily obtained is the appearance of the tricuspid and pulmonary valves, and the presence of valvular stenosis or regurgitation. Doppler evaluation of the tricuspid regurgitant jet allows the estimation of the systolic pulmonary artery pressure through the use of the modified Bernoulli equation. Important information is also provided by the appearance of the interventricular septum in the short-axis views. Pressure overload states cause flattening of the septum, particularly during systole, which volume overload states cause flattening during diastole (Fig. 4.5). With increasing pressure or volume overload, the septum is further shifted into the LV, leading to the hemodynamic effects of ventricular interdependence discussed previously.

RV function is challenging to determine with 2D echocardiography due to the lack of accurate ventricular volumes and the sensitivity of the RVEF to loading conditions. Visual assessment is the most commonly used technique but may be limited due to the complex shape of the RV. Multiple techniques are available for quantitative measurement of RV function. RV fractional area change (RVFAC) measures the change in area of the RV between diastole and systole from the apical 4-chamber view. The tricuspid annular plane systolic excursion (TAPSE) measures the vertical motion of the tricuspid valve annulus, with a value of less than 1.6 cm indicating RV dysfunction. RVFAC and TAPSE are both load-independent, and may provide varying information under different hemodynamic conditions. The RV index of myocardial performance (RIMP), also known as the Tei index, is less influenced by loading conditions, and may be a more accurate measure of underlying RV contractility [13]. This index is measured with Doppler of flow through the RV outflow tract, and is calculated as the sum of RV isovolumic contraction time and RV isovolumic relaxation time divided by ventricular ejection time.

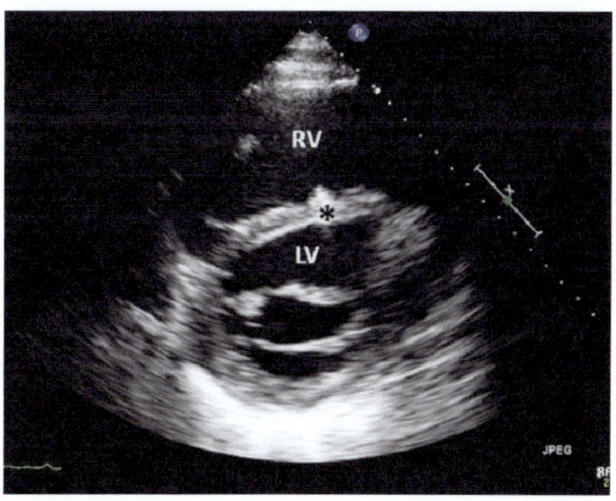

Fig. 4.5 A 2-dimensional echocardiogram image showing dilation of the right ventricle (*RV*) and flattening of the intraventricular septum (*) due to right ventricular pressure and volume overload. *LV* left ventricle

Recent advances in CMRI have established it as the best modality for obtaining accurate information about RV size and function. CMRI is not affected by the anatomic limitations that prevent 2D echocardiography from obtaining a complete picture of the RV. CMRI has excellent spatial and temporal resolution, permitting accurate assessment of RV volumes throughout the cardiac cycle. Additionally, CMRI provides information on ventricular hypertrophy, the presence of infiltrative diseases and the presence of fibrosis. For complex congenital heart disease, CMRI offers substantial advantages over 2D echocardiography for assessment of RV anatomy and function prior to and following surgical interventions. Barriers to more widespread application of CMRI in evaluation of the RV include the time required for testing, the cost of CMRI technology, and the need for technical expertise. Most importantly, CMRI is not compatible with most implantable cardiac devices, such as pacemakers, although the ongoing development of devices compatible with the magnetic field will allow for a broader application of CMRI in the assessment of RV failure [14].

Invasive Hemodynamic Assessment

Right heart catheterization (RHC) is a critical component of RV assessment, particularly in patients with PH. Measurement of the right atrial pressure (RAP), PA pressure and pulmonary capillary wedge pressure (PCWP) can distinguish the etiology of RV failure and help determine the therapeutic approach (Table 4.2). The most important information provided by RHC is about PH, which has been classified into groups by the World Health Organization:

- Group I incorporates PAH, which may be idiopathic, familial or associated with specific entities such as congenital heart disease, collagen vascular disease, HIV infection or toxins
- Group II includes PH that is found in conjunction with left heart disease and is the most common form of PH
- Group III includes PH associated with lung disease or hypoxemia
- Group IV is PH due to chronic thromboembolic disease
- Group V is a miscellaneous category

A RHC can assist in the diagnosis of PAH, by identifying PH in the presence of normal left-sided filling pressures. While left heart disease is often manifested on imaging studies by a reduced LV ejection fraction or mitral valve disease, RHC can identify elevated PCWP in the absence of valvular disease or LV dysfunction (heart failure with preserved ejection fraction). Distinguishing the underlying etiology of PH will direct the choice of therapy, as therapies that have proven benefit in some forms of PH have been shown to be harmful in PH related to left heart disease [15]. Beyond anatomy, RHC provides information about the severity of RV failure. For example, the RAP is typically about 50% of the PCWP [16]. As RV failure progresses, the RAP will approach or exceed the PCWP. Another sign of worsening RV failure is a decrease in the PA pressure despite a rising RAP due to insufficient power generation by the RV.

Another key variable obtained during right heart catheterization is the transpulmonary gradient (TPG), which is the difference between the PCWP and the mean PA pressure. This takes on importance in the assessment of PH due to left heart failure (i.e. patients with a PCWP >15 mmHg). When the PCWP is elevated, but the TPG is less than 10–12 mmHg, PH is termed "passive" or "post-capillary", indicating that the elevation in PA pressures can be solely attributed to the elevated left-sided filling pressures. When

Table 4.2 Hemodynamic profiles of different mechanisms of right ventricular failure

Cause of RV failure	RAP	PAP	PCWP	TPG	PVR	Clinical examples
Volume overload without PH	↑	↓	↓	↓	↓	ASD Isolated TV disease
Precapillary PH	↑	↑	↓	↓	↓	Idiopathic PAH CTEPH Hypoxia-associated PH Congenital Heart Disease
Postcapillary PH						
Passive	↑	↑	↑	↓	↓	Left-sided Heart Failure MV Disease
Mixed	↑	↑	↑	↑	↑	
Reactive (after vasodilator challenge)	↑	↑	↓	↓	↓	
Nonreactive (after vasodilator challenge)	↑	↑	↓	↑	↑	

ASD atrial septal defect, *CTEPH* chronic thromboembolic pulmonary hypertension, *MV* mitral valve, *PAH* pulmonary arterial hypertension, *PAP* pulmonary artery pressure, *PCWP* pulmonary capillary wedge pressure, *PH* pulmonary hypertension, *PVR* pulmonary vascular resistance, *RAP* right atrial pressure, *TPG* transpulmonary gradient, *TV* tricuspid valve the TPG is greater than 15 mmHg, the PH is termed "mixed" indicating that there is both a pre-capillary and post-capillary component of the PH. This may be secondary to vasoconstriction and pulmonary arterial remodeling as a response to chronically increased pulmonary venous pressures. Mixed PH can be further stratified into "reactive" and "nonreactive" forms through administration of a vasodilator, such as sodium nitroprusside or milrinone, to reduce the PCWP. In non-reactive PH, the TPG will remain elevated despite a lower PCWP, whereas patients with reactive PH will have concurrent decreases in the PCWP and TPG. The presence of reactive PH may indicate a more favorable prognosis, particularly when considering a patient for advanced therapies such as cardiac transplantation [17]. Whether patients with either reactive PH or non-reactive PH will benefit from selective pulmonary vasodilators is a subject of ongoing investigation.

When World Health Organization Group I PAH is present, the administration of selective pulmonary vasodilators, such as nitric oxide or epoprostenol, provides both prognostic and therapeutic information. Patients in whom the mean PA pressure drops by more than 10 mmHg to a value less than 40 mmHg without a reduction in cardiac output have an excellent prognosis, and typically respond well to calcium-channel blockers [18]. Non-responders have a worse prognosis, but still get a therapeutic benefit from selective pulmonary vasodilators.

Finally, RHC enables the calculation of the PVR, which provides a good estimate of RV afterload. PVR is both a prognostic factor, as well as a therapeutic target, that takes on considerable importance in the assessment of a patient's appropriateness for cardiac transplantation. A PVR >5 Woods Units is considered a relative contraindication to transplantation unless it can be lowered with medical therapy or mechanical circulatory support [19]. Frequency-domain analysis is an investigational method that accounts for the pressure wave reflected backwards into the main PA during late systole, and may provide a more accurate assessment of RV afterload [20].

Prognosis of Right Ventricular Failure

RV dysfunction plays a defining role in the pathogenesis of multiple diseases, ranging from left-sided HF to congenital heart disease to PH. In each of these entities, RV failure is the culmination of chronic pathophysiological disturbances, and often marks the transition to an advanced disease state. Numerous investigations have connected markers of RV dysfunction to adverse outcomes (Table 4.3). In chronic HF with LV dysfunction, RVEF, as measured by radionuclide ventriculography, invasive hemodynamics or CMRI, has been correlated with exercise capacity [21, 22], ventilatory efficiency [23], and survival [24–29]. This association has been demonstrated in both ischemic and nonischemic cardiomyopathies [24, 25, 29]. Importantly, there appears to be an additive effect of PH and RV dysfunction, leading to worse outcomes than the presence of either PH or RV dysfunction alone (Fig. 4.6) [30]. Other imaging parameters that have been associated with outcomes in chronic HF include CMRI-derived RV volumes [31], TAPSE [32–34] and RIMP [35]. Similar findings have been demonstrated in RV dysfunction due to PAH [36–40] and congenital heart disease [41, 42].

Table 4.3 Selected studies of the association of right ventricular dysfunction with adverse outcomes [21–23, 27, 29–32, 35, 36, 38–42]

	Population	Findings
Studies using radionuclide ventriculography		
Baker et al. [22]	25 pts. with symptomatic LV failure	RVEF associated with peak VO_2 LVEF not associated with peak VO_2
Lewis et al. [23]	30 pts. with symptomatic LV failure	Exercise RVEF and PVR associated with V_E/V_{CO2} slope
Di Salvo et al. [21]	67 pts. referred for OHT evaluation	RVEF >35% predictor of survival
Studies using RHC/thermodilution		
Gavazzi et al. [27]	142 pts. referred for OHT evaluation	RVEF lower in pts. who died or had OHT
Ghio et al. [30]	377 pts. with LVEF <35 % and NYHA Class III-IV	RVEF and PAP predictors of survival.
Studies using echocardiography		
Damy et al. [32]	1547 pts. referred for HF	Low TAPSE predictor of mortality
Harjai et al. [35]	60 pts. with LVEF<30%	RIMP >1.14 predictive of death
Forfia et al. [36]	63 pts. with idiopathic PAH	TAPSE <18 mm associated with mortality
Ghio et al. [38]	72 inpatients with idiopathic PAH	RV diameter > 36.5 mm associated with mortality
Yeo et al. [39]	53 pts. with idiopathic PAH	RIMP independent predictor of death
Moceri et al. [41]	181 pts. with Eisenmenger syndrome	TAPSE, RIMP and elevated CVP strongest predictors of mortality
Studies using CMRI		
Larose et al. [29]	147 pts. post-MI	RVEF <40% independent predictor of mortality
Bourantas et al. [31]	380 pts. with LVEF <45%	RVESV predicts mortality; LVESV does not predict mortality
van Wolferen et al. [40]	64 pts. with idiopathic PAH	RV dilation, low RV stroke volume and decreased LV filling predict mortality
Knauth et al. [42]	88 pts. followed up at mean of 20.7 years after TOF repair	Severe RV dilation predictor of death, VT, advanced NYHA class

CMRI cardiac magnetic resonance imaging, *HF* heart failure, *LV* left ventricle, *LVEF* left ventricular ejection fraction, *LVESV* left ventricular end systolic volume, *MI* myocardial infarction, *NYHA* New York Heart Association, *OHT* orthotopic heart transplantation, *PAH* pulmonary arterial hypertension, *PAP* pulmonary artery pressure, *PVR* pulmonary vascular resistance, *RIMP* right ventricular index of myocardial performance, *RV* right ventricle, *RVEF* right ventricular ejection fraction, *RVESV* right ventricular end systolic volume, *TAPSE* tricuspid annular plane systolic excursion, *TOF* tetralogy of Fallot, *V E/V CO2* ratio of minute ventilation to production of carbon dioxide, *VT* ventricular tachycardia

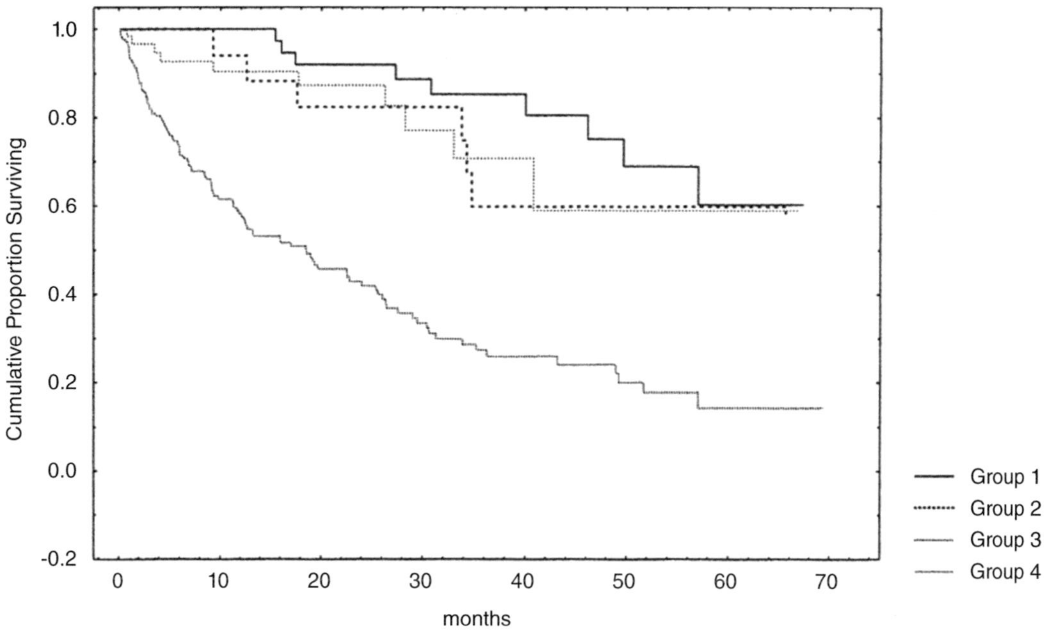

Fig. 4.6 Survival curves for heart failure patients grouped by presence or absence of pulmonary hypertension (PH) and presence or absence of an abnormal right ventricular ejection fraction (RVEF). Group 1 patients have normal RVEF and no PH. Group 2 patients have a low RVEF without PH. Group 3 patients have a normal RVEF with PH. Group 4 patients have both an abnormal RVEF and PH. The presence of both factors leads to significantly worse outcomes than any of the other three scenarios (Reprinted, with permission, from Ghio et al. [30], © 2001, with permission from Elsevier)

Management of Right Ventricular Failure

The initial approach to RV failure relies on identifying and correcting the underlying etiology. As opposed to the LV, in which dysfunction is often irreversible, the RV is highly pliable, and typically regains function after the causative factors of RV dysfunction are addressed. This is especially important in acute RV failure, where reversing the underlying disease state may drastically alter a patient's outcome. For example, coronary revascularization for an RVI reduces RV dysfunction, hemodynamic compromise and increased mortality [43]. Likewise, for an acute PE, rapid relief of the thrombotic burden through medical or surgical intervention produces a substantial survival benefit [44]. Causes of chronic RV failure are not as easily corrected, although RV function improves over time with therapy that is appropriately targeted at the underlying pathophysiology. Ultimately, managing both acute and chronic RV failure requires an understanding of the roles played by preload, afterload and contractility. A management algorithm is shown in Fig. 4.7.

Preload

Optimizing RV performance requires adequate preload to generate a sufficient stroke volume without causing a degree of RV distention that impairs LV performance through ventricular interdependence. The ideal preload required may differ between patients and will rely on both the degree of RV contractility and the severity of RV afterload. In patients with acute RV failure, central venous monitoring can guide decision-making about the volume status. Patients with

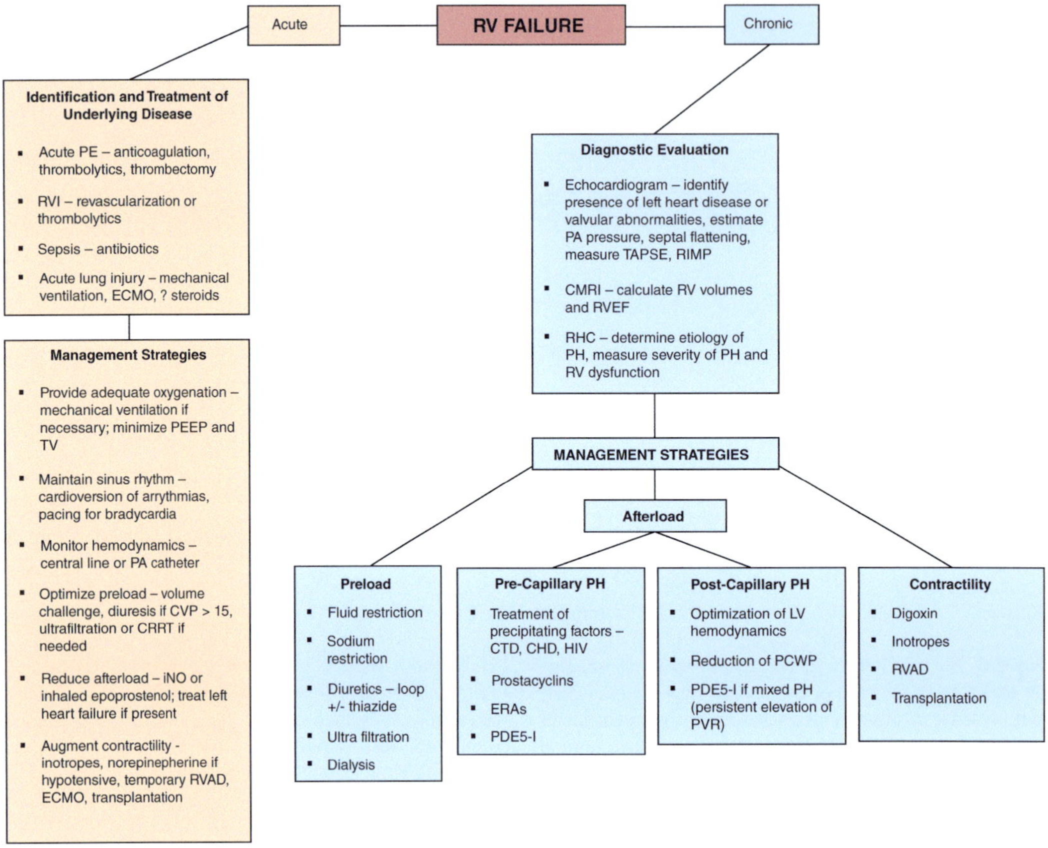

Fig. 4.7 Management algorithm for acute and chronic RV failure. Abbreviations: *CHD* congenital heart disease, *CMRI* cardiac magnetic resonance imaging, *CRRT* continuous renal replacement therapy, *CTD* connective tissue disease, *CVP* central venous pressure, *ECMO* extracorporeal membrane oxygenation, *ERA* endothelin receptor antagonist, *HIV* human immunodeficiency virus, *iNO* inhaled nitric oxide, *PA* pulmonary artery, *PDE5-I* phosphodiesterase-5 inhibitor, *PE* pulmonary embolism, *PEEP* positive end-expiratory pressure, *PH* pulmonary hypertension, *RHC* right heart catheterization, *RIMP* right ventricular index of myocardial performance, *RV* right ventricular, *RVAD* right ventricular assist device, *RVI* right ventricular infarction, *TAPSE* tricuspid annular plane systolic excursion, *TV* tidal volume

RVI are often described as “volume-sensitive”, and may require higher preloads to maintain cardiac output. However, too much volume may have deleterious consequences because RV dilation will increase wall stretch, worsen ischemia and cause septal shifting. Although mechanical ventilation is sometimes necessary in the management of patients with acute RV failure, its use should be minimized due to the adverse effects of positive end-expiratory pressure on preload.

In chronic RV failure, the focus is typically on volume removal, which is primarily achieved with loop diuretics. Selecting an agent with better oral bioavailability, such as torsemide, may be preferred in the setting of RV failure due to the possibility of intestinal edema and poor absorption. Thiazide diuretics can be added as needed to enhance diuresis. As with LV dysfunction, sodium and fluid restriction are essential to maintaining euvolemia. In extreme circumstances, ultrafiltration or hemodialysis may be required in diuretic-resistant patients, although these strategies have not been well studied in this population.

Afterload

Afterload reduction is a critical component of the management of most causes of RV failure. Addressing afterload is of particular urgency in acute RV failure due to the inability of the RV to compensate for acute changes in afterload. Persistently low oxygen saturations should be addressed with supplemental oxygen to alleviate hypoxia-induced vasoconstriction. If mechanical ventilation is required, tidal volumes should be minimized to prevent further augmentation of PA pressures.

Pulmonary vasodilators relax pulmonary vascular smooth muscle, lowering PA pressures and PVR. Inhaled nitric oxide (iNO) has the advantages of pulmonary selectivity, avoiding the hypotension associated with systemic vasodilators. It is also only active in ventilated areas of the lung, reducing the potential for V/Q mismatching. iNO is most commonly used in acute RV failure due to difficulty in administration to non-ventilated patients. Short-term hemodynamic improvements have been demonstrated with the use of iNO in the treatment of RVI [45] and in a study of intensive care patients with mixed causes of RV failure [46], but outcomes data are limited. Transitioning from iNO to oral vasodilators may prevent rapid rebound of PA pressures on discontinuation. Inhaled prostacyclins may be used as an alternative to iNO, although they have been less extensively studied.

In chronic RV failure, therapy depends on the underlying mechanism of the elevated PA pressures. In PAH, there are three classes of vasodilators that have shown clinical benefit: prostacyclins, endothelin receptor antagonists (ERAs) and phosphodiesterase-5 inhibitors (PDE-5Is). As mentioned previously, a small subset of PAH patients will respond to calcium-channel blockers, and may not require any further treatment. Outside of this subset, most PAH patients will be started on oral therapy with an ERA or PDE-5I. As the disease progresses, these patients may need to be transitioned to intravenous prostacyclin therapy. Patients who present with severe symptoms, such as syncope, often require intravenous prostacyclin therapy from the outset.

When RV failure is due to post-capillary PH (i.e. LV dysfunction or valvular disease), the initial therapeutic target is the PCWP, which should be lowered into the normal range if possible. If the PH is reactive, lowering the PCWP should also reduce PA pressures and PVR. However, if PVR remains elevated, consideration should be given to pulmonary vasodilator therapy. Sildenafil citrate, a PDE-5I, has shown benefits on hemodynamics and functional status in patients with left-sided heart failure [47–49]. A large trial to assess outcomes of patients with PH related to LV dysfunction is underway. Neither ERAs nor prostacyclins should be used for post-capillary PH due to adverse outcomes in clinical trials [15, 50].

Contractility

In acute RV failure, inotropes are often required to support the RV until the etiology can be treated. Milrinone may be the preferred agent due to its vasodilatory properties in the pulmonary vasculature, but its use is limited in patients with significant hypotension. Dobutamine and dopamine are more likely to cause tachycardia, which may exacerbate ischemia in the setting of an RVI. In some cases of RVI, mechanical support with an intraaortic balloon pump or a temporary right ventricular assist device (RVAD) has been used, although neither of these approaches has been well studied. Temporary RVADs have also been used to treat RV failure that occurs following cardiovascular surgery or cardiac transplantation.

For chronic RV failure, choices for augmenting contractility are limited. Digoxin is often used as an inotrope in the management of RV failure, based on its short-term hemodynamic benefits in patients with PAH [51]. The use of intravenous inotropes for chronic left heart failure has been associated with worse outcomes. Intravenous inotropes may be used for management of exacerbations of chronic RV failure, but the chronic administration of these agents has been associated with worse outcomes. When biventricular heart failure is refractory, a RVAD may be placed in conjunction with a left ventricular assist device (LVAD) as a means of bridging a patient to transplantation. The devices that are approved for RV support are extracorporeal (i.e. non-implantable) and are not meant for long-term support, although the development of more durable RVADs is ongoing. In some cases, these devices can be explanted once stable LVAD support has been established. Cardiac transplantation is a definitive treatment for patients with advanced RV failure that is associated with LV failure, but this therapy is limited in use due to a shortage of donor organs. Cardiac transplantation should not be attempted in patients with high PVR (>6 Woods Units) due to high risk for RV failure and graft loss postoperatively.

Summary

The onset of RV failure carries a poor prognosis in multiple diseases and is often a marker of a progression to an advanced disease state. RV failure is the end result of a series of pathophysiological adaptations that are distinct from the pathogenesis of LV failure. A detailed understanding of the RV's response to specific disease states informs the clinical management of those diseases. Imaging plays a critical role in the assessment of RV dysfunction, and can provide information about the severity of RV failure. Hemodynamic assessment with cardiac catheterization complements the findings from imaging, directing the appropriate therapeutic approach. The treatment of RV failure due is highly dependent on the underlying etiology. Acute causes respond best to removal of the offending pathophysiology. Chronic RV failure requires a targeted approach, as has been applied in the setting of PAH. Research continues into the optimal treatment strategy for PH that is secondary to left heart failure.

References

1. Starr I, Jeffers WA, Meade RH. The absence of conspicuous increments of venous pressure after severe damage to the right ventricle of the dog, with a discussion of the relation between clinical congestive failure and heart disease. Am Heart J. 1943;26(3):291–301.
2. Redington AN. Right ventricular function. Cardiol Clin. 2002;20(3):341–9.
3. Greyson CR. Pathophysiology of right ventricular failure. Crit Care Med. 2008;36(1 Suppl):S57–65.
4. Abel FL, Waldhausen JA. Effects of alterations in pulmonary vascular resistance on right ventricular function. J Thorac Cardiovasc Surg. 1967;54:886–94.
5. Hopkins WE, Waggoner AD. Severe pulmonary hypertension without right ventricular failure: the unique hearts of patients with Eisenmenger syndrome. Am J Cardiol. 2002;89(1):34–8.
6. Lualdi JC, Goldhaber SZ. Right ventricular dysfunction after acute pulmonary embolism: pathophysiologic factors, detection, and therapeutic implications. Am Heart J. 1995;130(6):1276–82.
7. Goldstein JA, Tweddell JS, Barzilai B, Yagi Y, Jaffe AS, Cox JL. Importance of left ventricular function and systolic ventricular interaction to right ventricular performance during acute right heart ischemia. J Am Coll Cardiol. 1992;19(3):704–11.
8. Bogaard HJ, Abe K, Vonk Noordegraaf A, Voelkel NF. The right ventricle under pressure: cellular and molecular mechanisms of right-heart failure in pulmonary hypertension. Chest. 2009;135(3):794–804.
9. Haddad F, Doyle R, Murphy DJ, Hunt SA. Right ventricular function in cardiovascular disease, part II: pathophysiology, clinical importance, and management of right ventricular failure. Circulation. 2008;117(13):1717–31.
10. Szabo G, Soos P, Bahrle S, Radovits T, Weigang E, Kekesi V, et al. Adaptation of the right ventricle to an increased afterload in the chronically volume overloaded heart. Ann Thorac Surg. 2006;82(3):989–95.
11. Hulot JS, Jouven X, Empana JP, Frank R, Fontaine G. Natural history and risk stratification of arrhythmogenic right ventricular dysplasia/cardiomyopathy. Circulation. 2004;110(14):1879–84.
12. Brooks H, Kirk ES, Vokonas PS, Urschel CW, Sonnenblick EH. Performance of the right ventricle under stress: relation to right coronary flow. J Clin Invest. 1971;50(10):2176–83.
13. Tei C, Dujardin KS, Hodge DO, Bailey KR, McGoon MD, Tajik AJ, et al. Doppler echocardiographic index for assessment of global right ventricular function. J Am Soc Echocardiogr. 1996;9(6):838–47.
14. Wilkoff BL, Bello D, Taborsky M, Vymazal J, Kanal E, Heuer H, et al. Magnetic resonance imaging in patients with a pacemaker system designed for the magnetic resonance environment. Heart Rhythm. 2011;8(1):65–73.
15. Califf RM, Adams KF, McKenna WJ, Gheorghiade M, Uretsky BF, McNulty SE, et al. A randomized controlled trial of epoprostenol therapy for severe congestive heart failure: The Flolan International Randomized Survival Trial (FIRST). Am Heart J. 1997;134(1):44–54.
16. Drazner MH, Hamilton MA, Fonarow G, Creaser J, Flavell C, Stevenson LW. Relationship between right and left-sided filling pressures in 1000 patients with advanced heart failure. J Heart Lung Transplant. 1999;18(11):1126–32.

17. Costard-Jackle A, Fowler MB. Influence of preoperative pulmonary artery pressure on mortality after heart transplantation: testing of potential reversibility of pulmonary hypertension with nitroprusside is useful in defining a high risk group. J Am Coll Cardiol. 1992;19(1):48–54.
18. Sitbon O, Humbert M, Jagot JL, Taravella O, Fartoukh M, Parent F, et al. Inhaled nitric oxide as a screening agent for safely identifying responders to oral calcium-channel blockers in primary pulmonary hypertension. Eur Respir J. 1998;12(2):265–70.
19. Mehra MR, Kobashigawa J, Starling R, Russell S, Uber PA, Parameshwar J, et al. Listing criteria for heart transplantation: International Society for Heart and Lung Transplantation guidelines for the care of cardiac transplant candidates--2006. J Heart Lung Transplant. 2006;25(9):1024–42.
20. Champion HC, Michelakis ED, Hassoun PM. Comprehensive invasive and noninvasive approach to the right ventricle-pulmonary circulation unit: state of the art and clinical and research implications. Circulation. 2009;120(11):992–1007.
21. Di Salvo TG, Mathier M, Semigran MJ, Dec GW. Preserved right ventricular ejection fraction predicts exercise capacity and survival in advanced heart failure. J Am Coll Cardiol. 1995;25(5):1143–53.
22. Baker BJ, Wilen MM, Boyd CM, Dinh H, Franciosa JA. Relation of right ventricular ejection fraction to exercise capacity in chronic left ventricular failure. Am J Cardiol. 1984;54(6):596–9.
23. Lewis GD, Shah RV, Pappagianopolas PP, Systrom DM, Semigran MJ. Determinants of ventilatory efficiency in heart failure: the role of right ventricular performance and pulmonary vascular tone. Circ Heart Fail. 2008;1(4):227–33.
24. Juilliere Y, Barbier G, Feldmann L, Grentzinger A, Danchin N, Cherrier F. Additional predictive value of both left and right ventricular ejection fractions on long-term survival in idiopathic dilated cardiomyopathy. Eur Heart J. 1997;18(2):276–80.
25. Polak JF, Holman BL, Wynne J, Colucci WS. Right ventricular ejection fraction: an indicator of increased mortality in patients with congestive heart failure associated with coronary artery disease. J Am Coll Cardiol. 1983;2(2):217–24.
26. de Groote P, Millaire A, Foucher-Hossein C, Nugue O, Marchandise X, Ducloux G, et al. Right ventricular ejection fraction is an independent predictor of survival in patients with moderate heart failure. J Am Coll Cardiol. 1998;32(4):948–54.
27. Gavazzi A, Berzuini C, Campana C, Inserra C, Ponzetta M, Sebastiani R, et al. Value of right ventricular ejection fraction in predicting short-term prognosis of patients with severe chronic heart failure. J Heart Lung Transplant. 1997;16(7):774–85.
28. Miszalski-Jamka T, Klimeczek P, Tomala M, Krupinski M, Zawadowski G, Noelting J, et al. Extent of RV dysfunction and myocardial infarction assessed by CMR are independent outcome predictors early after STEMI treated with primary angioplasty. JACC Cardiovasc Imaging. 2010;3(12):1237–46.
29. Larose E, Ganz P, Reynolds HG, Dorbala S, Di Carli MF, Brown KA, et al. Right ventricular dysfunction assessed by cardiovascular magnetic resonance imaging predicts poor prognosis late after myocardial infarction. J Am Coll Cardiol. 2007;49(8):855–62.
30. Ghio S, Gavazzi A, Campana C, Inserra C, Klersy C, Sebastiani R, et al. Independent and additive prognostic value of right ventricular systolic function and pulmonary artery pressure in patients with chronic heart failure. J Am Coll Cardiol. 2001;37(1):183–8.
31. Bourantas CV, Loh HP, Bragadeesh T, Rigby AS, Lukaschuk EI, Garg S, et al. Relationship between right ventricular volumes measured by cardiac magnetic resonance imaging and prognosis in patients with chronic heart failure. Eur J Heart Fail. 2011;13(1):52–60.
32. Damy T, Kallvikbacka-Bennett A, Goode K, Khaleva O, Lewinter C, Hobkirk J, et al. Prevalence of, associations with, and prognostic value of tricuspid annular plane systolic excursion (TAPSE) among out-patients referred for the evaluation of heart failure. J Card Fail. 2012;18(3):216–25.
33. Dini FL, Fontanive P, Panicucci E, Andreini D, Chella P, De Tommasi SM. Prognostic significance of tricuspid annular motion and plasma NT-proBNP in patients with heart failure and moderate-to-severe functional mitral regurgitation. Eur J Heart Fail. 2008;10(6):573–80.
34. Kjaergaard J, Akkan D, Iversen KK, Kober L, Torp-Pedersen C, Hassager C. Right ventricular dysfunction as an independent predictor of short- and long-term mortality in patients with heart failure. Eur J Heart Fail. 2007;9(6–7):610–6.
35. Harjai KJ, Scott L, Vivekananthan K, Nunez E, Edupuganti R. The Tei index: a new prognostic index for patients with symptomatic heart failure. J Am Soc Echocardiogr. 2002;15(9):864–8.
36. Forfia PR, Fisher MR, Mathai SC, Housten-Harris T, Hemnes AR, Borlaug BA, et al. Tricuspid annular displacement predicts survival in pulmonary hypertension. Am J Respir Crit Care Med. 2006;174(9):1034–41.
37. Mathai SC, Sibley CT, Forfia PR, Mudd JO, Fisher MR, Tedford RJ, et al. Tricuspid annular plane systolic excursion is a robust outcome measure in systemic sclerosis-associated pulmonary arterial hypertension. J Rheumatol. 2011;38(11):2410–8.
38. Ghio S, Pazzano AS, Klersy C, Scelsi L, Raineri C, Camporotondo R, et al. Clinical and prognostic relevance of echocardiographic evaluation of right ventricular geometry in patients with idiopathic pulmonary arterial hypertension. Am J Cardiol. 2011;107(4):628–32.
39. Yeo TC, Dujardin KS, Tei C, Mahoney DW, McGoon MD, Seward JB. Value of a Doppler-derived index combining systolic and diastolic time intervals in predicting outcome in primary pulmonary hypertension. Am J Cardiol. 1998;81(9):1157–61.

40. van Wolferen SA, Marcus JT, Boonstra A, Marques KM, Bronzwaer JG, Spreeuwenberg MD, et al. Prognostic value of right ventricular mass, volume, and function in idiopathic pulmonary arterial hypertension. Eur Heart J. 2007;28(10):1250–7.
41. Moceri P, Dimopoulos K, Liodakis E, Germanakis I, Kempny A, Diller GP, et al. Echocardiographic predictors of outcome in eisenmenger syndrome. Circulation. 2012;126(12):1461–8.
42. Knauth AL, Gauvreau K, Powell AJ, Landzberg MJ, Walsh EP, Lock JE, et al. Ventricular size and function assessed by cardiac MRI predict major adverse clinical outcomes late after tetralogy of Fallot repair. Heart. 2008;94(2):211–6.
43. Bowers TR, O'Neill WW, Grines C, Pica MC, Safian RD, Goldstein JA. Effect of reperfusion on biventricular function and survival after right ventricular infarction. N Engl J Med. 1998;338(14):933–40.
44. Kucher N, Goldhaber SZ. Management of massive pulmonary embolism. Circulation. 2005;112(2):e28–32.
45. Inglessis I, Shin JT, Lepore JJ, Palacios IF, Zapol WM, Bloch KD, et al. Hemodynamic effects of inhaled nitric oxide in right ventricular myocardial infarction and cardiogenic shock. J Am Coll Cardiol. 2004;44(4):793–8.
46. Bhorade S, Christenson J, O'Connor M, Lavoie A, Pohlman A, Hall JB. Response to inhaled nitric oxide in patients with acute right heart syndrome. Am J Respir Crit Care Med. 1999;159(2):571–9.
47. Lewis GD, Lachmann J, Camuso J, Lepore JJ, Shin J, Martinovic ME, et al. Sildenafil improves exercise hemodynamics and oxygen uptake in patients with systolic heart failure. Circulation. 2007;115(1):59–66.
48. Lewis GD, Shah R, Shahzad K, Camuso JM, Pappagianopoulos PP, Hung J, et al. Sildenafil improves exercise capacity and quality of life in patients with systolic heart failure and secondary pulmonary hypertension. Circulation. 2007;116(14):1555–62.
49. Guazzi M, Vicenzi M, Arena R, Guazzi MD. Pulmonary hypertension in heart failure with preserved ejection fraction: a target of phosphodiesterase-5 inhibition in a 1-year study. Circulation. 2011;124(2):164–74.
50. Kaluski E, Cotter G, Leitman M, Milo-Cotter O, Krakover R, Kobrin I, et al. Clinical and hemodynamic effects of bosentan dose optimization in symptomatic heart failure patients with severe systolic dysfunction, associated with secondary pulmonary hypertension--a multi-center randomized study. Cardiology. 2008;109(4):273–80.
51. Rich S, Seidlitz M, Dodin E, Osimani D, Judd D, Genthner D, et al. The short-term effects of digoxin in patients with right ventricular dysfunction from pulmonary hypertension. Chest. 1998;114(3):787–92.

Inhibition of the Renin-Angiotensin-Aldosterone System

5

Erika D. Feller

Introduction

In mild to severe heart failure, activation of the renin-angiotensin-aldosterone system is the primary abnormality. Increasing plasma levels of renin, angiotensin and aldosterone have direct effects on myocardium but also sodium and water handling, vascular contractility and reverse remodeling. Medical therapy to inhibit the renin-angiotensin-aldosterone system is the cornerstone of treatment for cardiomyopathy and heart failure.

This chapter will examine this neurohormonal pathway and discuss the deleterious effects when these pathways are activated. Current medical therapy, aimed to block activation points along the pathway, will be reviewed.

The Renin-Angiotensin-Aldosterone System

The renin-angiotensin-aldosterone system (RAAS) describes a cellular, enzymatic pathway involving primarily the heart, kidney, adrenal gland and vasculature that has various functions.

E. D. Feller (✉)
Division of Cardiology, Med-Star Health, Baltimore, MD, USA
e-mail: efeller@medicine.umaryland.edu

Perhaps, most importantly, the RAAS regulates body-fluid volume. It does so by activating a series of reactions that then affect the absorption or secretion of sodium from the kidney. Congestive heart failure describes the state when intravascular fluid becomes extravascular secondary to a poor and/or decreased cardiac output [1]. During this disturbance in fluid balance, RAAS is activated, exacerbating the problem. Thus, inhibition of RAAS is a major target for therapeutic intervention.

The RAAS is first activated when renin blood levels increase. Increased renin levels are due to multiple factors. In particular, decreased blood flow to kidneys from decreased cardiac output, as well as hypotension, can increase renin secretion. A decrease in plasma sodium levels as a result of dilution from water retention in heart failure can have a similar result. Renin is secreted by the kidney's juxtaglomerular cells into the lumen of the afferent arterioles. Angiotensinogen is released from the liver, interacts with renin to form inactive angiotensin I. Angiotensin converting enzyme (ACE) degrades angiotensin I further to form angiotensin II [2].

Most angiotensin II effects are mediated by the two receptors; angiotensin 1 receptor (AT1) and angiotensin 2 receptor (AT2). The AT1 mediates vasoconstriction and is widely expressed. The AT2 mediates vasodilation. This process happens primarily in the lungs on the endothelial

H. J. Eisen (ed.), *Heart Failure I*, https://doi.org/10.1007/978-3-032-12626-9_5

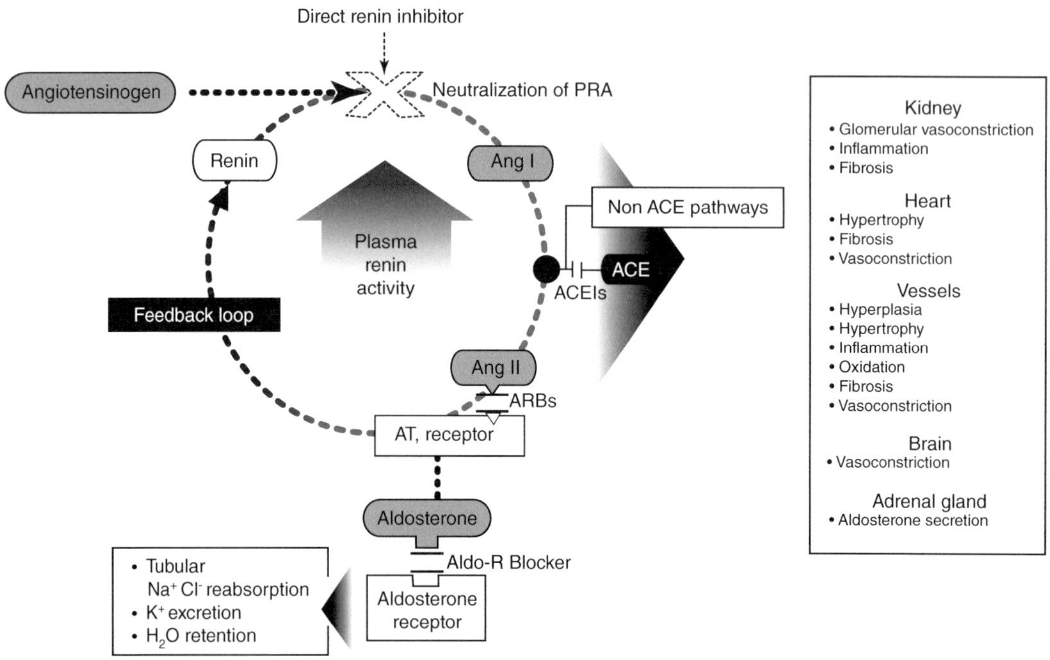

Fig. 5.1 The Renin-Angiotensin-Aldosterone System. The major components of RAAS are shown in the above figure. As depicted, an increase in plasma renin levels initiates the cascade. Multiple organ systems are involved (Reproduced with permission of Informa Healthcare, Haroonur [4], © 2008, Informa Healthcare. Reproduced with permission of Informa Healthcare)

surface of blood vessels. Angiotensin II is the main effector chemical of the RAAS.

Renin-dependent elevations in angiotensin II are associated with increases in circulating aldosterone. Aldosterone is a neurohormone and is secreted by the adrenal glands in response to angiotensin II, catecholamines, endothelins and potassium. Aldosterone works to maintain salt, water and potassium hemostasis, by binding to mineralocorticoid receptors in the kidney. Elevated levels of aldosterone add to the volume expansion seen in acute and chronic heart failure. Aldosterone has also been implicated in contributing to myocardial fibrosis [3]. Abundant myocardial fibrosis leads to cardiomyopathy and decreased myocardial systolic and diastolic function.

The major hormone of the RAAS is angiotensin II. When angiotensin II, a strong vasoconstrictor is reduced, bradykinin, a strong vasodilator is increased. In addition to its vasodilatory properties, bradykinin can release tissue plasminogen activator (tPA). tPA has anti-ischemic properties.

The RAAS system is a complex interaction between multiple organ systems to regulate body-fluid volume in hemostasis as well as disease states, namely congestive heart failure. In the initial stages of developing left ventricular systolic dysfunction, if cardiac output declines or if peripheral arterial pressure decreases RAAS is activated in order to maintain and/or increase cardiac filling pressures, cardiac output and systemic blood pressure. Figure 5.1 shows the Renin-Angiotensin-Aldosterone System [4].

Activation of the Renin-Angiotensin-Aldosterone System

The RAAS is activated in heart failure. The exact mechanisms by which activation occur are yet to be fully elucidated. Most likely, though, the combination of decreased perfusion to the kidney, decreased cardiac output, and low arterial pressure activate RAAS.

As a compensatory mechanism to decreased cardiac output, renin is released from the kidneys and is responsible for converting angiotensinogen to angiotensin I. Angiotensin I is then converted to angiotensin II by angiotensin-converting enzyme (ace). Angiotensin II stimulates the receptors AT1 and AT2.

Heart failure is defined as the pathological state in which the heart is unable to pump blood to adequately supply tissues to affect metabolism, or can do that but only with an increase in filling pressures. In the presence of an acute or subacute insult to the myocardium, which effects contractility, the heart depends on adaptive strategies to maintain pumping ability and cardiac output. Among the most important mechanism is activation of neurohormonal systems, including the sympathetic nervous system and the RAAS. The activation of RAAS can occur rapidly, over minutes to hours, to maintain cardiac function. The RAAS does this acutely by retaining salt and water to augment preload or cardiac filling. Additionally, RAAS activation can cause vasoconstriction, to help perfuse organs and tissues. Although, these mechanisms are adaptive in the short term, they are maladaptive in the long term.

As a result of activation of the RAAS, sympathetic nervous system and release of norepinephrine, myocardial hypertrophy and remodeling develop over weeks, months and years. With chronic activation of these pathways, these mechanisms become maladaptive. Although able to sustain cardiac function for some time, high filling pressures over time will ultimately cause worsening cardiac performance effecting organ perfusion and circulation. Many of the symptoms of heart failure, lower extremity swelling, dyspnea, orthopnea, paroxysmal nocturnal dyspnea, abdominal bloating are a consequence of the retention of fluid causing high filling pressures.

When the RAAS is activated in low cardiac output states, it is closely associated with the adrenergic system to maintain arterial pressure. Stimulation of beta1 adrenoceptors in the juxtaglomerular apparatus of the kidneys is a principle activator of renin release in acute heart failure. Figure 5.2 shows the activation of the Renin-Angiotensin-Aldosterone System [5].

Aldosterone is predominantly produced by the adrenal glands and, to a lesser degree, the endothelial and vascular smooth muscle cells in the heart and blood vessels. Aldosterone is regulated by the RAAS as well as potassium levels. Angiotensin II is the principal stimulator of aldosterone in the adrenal cortex [6]. Plasma levels of aldosterone can increase dramatically in patients with heart failure. This increase is attributed mainly to increased synthesis of aldosterone in response to activation of RAAS.

Aldosterone has been implicated in several harmful effects contributing to heart failure. Aldosterone vasoconstricts and also potentiates catecholamines. It upregulates inflammatory mediators such as macrophages, cytokines and chemokines. Aldosterone also plays a role in myocyte necrosis and scarring. Chronically elevated aldosterone levels contribute to myocardial fibrosis and deleterious remodeling. More recent studies have shown that aldosterone promotes platelet aggregation and activation [7, 8]. For these reasons, decreasing aldosterone levels with aldosterone inhibitors remain a therapeutic target and goal of modern heart failure therapy.

Treatment with ace-inhibitors results in an acute reduction in aldosterone levels. In chronic ace-inhibition, the reduction in aldosterone levels is weaker and more variable. This finding is referred to as aldosterone “escape” [9].

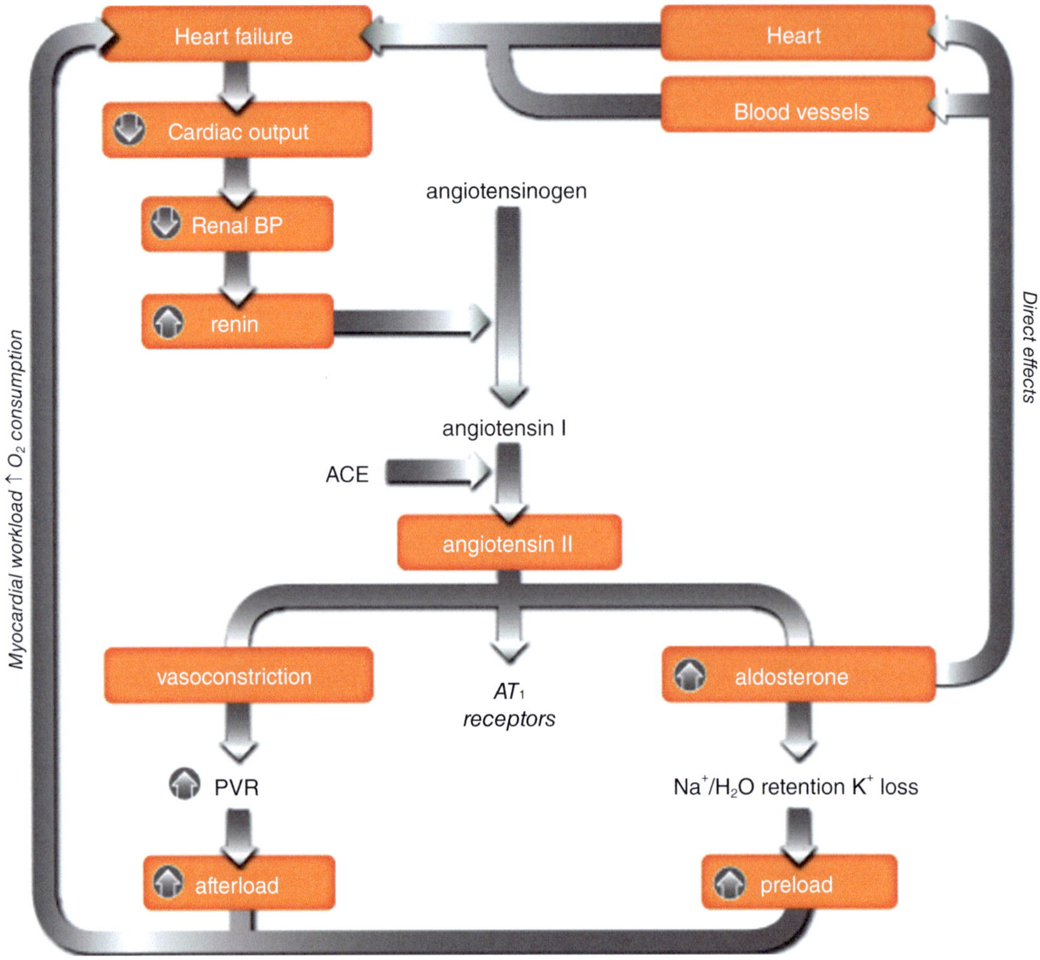

Fig. 5.2 Activation of the Renin-Angiotensin-Aldosterone System. Scheme picturing the primary hemodynamic mechanisms by which the RAAS is activated (Reproduced from Jackson et al. [5], © 2000, with permission from BMJ Publishing Group Ltd)

Effects of RAAS Activation

The actions of RAAS are beneficial in some circumstances. In heart failure, though, RAAS is chronically activated and results in deleterious effects. Chronic activation and up regulation of RAAS causes increased circulating angiotensin I, angiotensin II and aldosterone. Acute activation of RAAS maintains vascular tone or vasoconstriction. As a result, renal function is also maintained in the short term. In addition, cardiac output is preserved and left ventricular filling pressures are reduced.

Chronic activation of RAAS results in maladaptive remodeling of the myocardium. This includes fibrosis formation and myocyte hypertrophy.

Angiotensin II has several effects that contribute to the syndrome of heart failure and the progressive nature of left ventricular dysfunction. In particular, angiotensin II promotes hypertension, atherosclerosis and hypertrophic changes in the walls of arteries as well as the left ventricle [10].

Aldosterone promotes the retention of sodium and the loss of magnesium and potassium. Aldosterone also promotes sympathetic activa-

Table 5.1 Major actions of RAAS components

Chemical	Actions
Aldosterone	Cardiac fibrosis, sodium and water retention, magnesium and potassium loss, vasoconstriction, sympathetic activation, parasympathetic inhibition, impairs arterial compliance, platelet activation and aggregation, activates macrophages, stimulates growth of fibroblasts and synthesis of collagen
Angiotensin converting enzyme	Proliferative and proinflammatory signaling
Angiotensinogen	Releases angiotensin II, substrate for renin
Angiotensin I	Largely inactive precursor to angiotensin II, weak vasoconstrictor
Angiotensin II	Arterial vasoconstriction, pro-inflammatory, salt and water retention by the kidneys, stimulation of thirst, release of anti-diuretic hormone, augments norepinephrine release, remodels heart and blood vessels, induce cardiac myocyte hypertrophy, stimulates aldosterone, vasopressin, catecholamines and endothelin
Renin	Activates RAAS by cleaving angiotensinogen
Bradykinin	Vasodilator, anti-proliferative, cough, angioedema

tion, parasympathetic inhibition myocardial and vascular fibrosis. Table 5.1.

Inhibition of Raas

Earlier segments of this chapter described activation of RAAS and the detrimental effects that activation of RAAS has on the ailing and/or failing heart. The rationale for combination therapy is to inhibit the production of angiotensin II, the major hormone involved in RAAS, at every step. Angiotensin II has several harmful effects. The reduction of angiotensin II by inhibiting RAAS activation is responsible for the many positive effects of ace-inhibition, angiotensin receptor blockade and aldosterone inhibition.

The current standard therapy for heart failure and cardiomyopathy is designed to interrupt the RAAS and the sympathetic nervous system (SNS) by using a combination of medications. Multiple trials have demonstrated the beneficial effects of using medications that target different hormones. Pharmacologic approaches to blocking the effects of angiotensin II, have been aimed at decreasing its production by inhibiting angiotensin converting enzyme or by direct inhibition at the level of the angiotensin receptor 1.

Ace-Inhibition

An angiotensin-converting-enzyme inhibitor (ace-inhibitor) is considered the first line therapy in treating patients with heart failure and left ventricular dysfunction. Ace-inhibitors have shown improved survival in patients with mild to severe chronic heart failure.

Ace-inhibitors block the conversion of angiotensin I to angiotensin II and prevent the degradation of bradykinin. The efficacy of ace-inhibition is due not only to blocking the harmful effects of angiotensin II, but also due to the promotion of bradykinin, a vasodilator. It is the bradykinin that causes some of the side effects of ace inhibitors (angioedema and cough). Ace-inhibitors also block the negative feedback in renin release by decreasing renin release and the rate of angiotensin I formation. Studies have shown multiple (pleiotropic) effects of ace-inhibition.

Ace-inhibitors have been shown to decrease left ventricular hypertrophy and smooth muscle proliferation. They decrease coronary vasoconstriction and have anti-macrophage effects. Ace-inhibitors also have been shown to stabilize arterial plaque. In addition, ace-inhibitors also prevent ventricular remodeling. This has been shown clinically in patients with hypertension, symptomatic heart failure, elderly patients with heart failure and patients status-post myocardial infarction [11, 12].

Angiotensin Receptor Blockade

Angiotensin Receptor Blockers or ARBs have their effect further down the RAAS cascade. Unlike ace-inhibitors, ARBs have little effect on bradykinin, therefore no cough or angioedema. ARBs block angiotensin II at the receptor site.

While initiation of ace-inhibitors lead to a rapid decline in circulating angiotensin II, chronic use of ace-inhibitors can lead to an increase in angiotensin II, from initial decline. This increase in angiotensin II or "ACE escape" is thought to be due to conversion of angiotensin I to angiotensin II by means other than ACE. ARBs would avoid this phenomenon, based on their mechanism of action. In theory, ARBs would have a more complete blockade of angiotensin II [13].

ARBs have shown benefit in patients that are intolerant to ace-inhibitors or as an alternative to ace-inhibitors. The addition of ARBs to ace-inhibitors has shown benefit in decreasing hospital admissions, their benefit may be attenuated by increased risk of hyperkalemia. In patients intolerant to ace-inhibitors, valsartan, losartan and candesartan have shown benefits in mortality reduction [14–16].

Aldosterone Inhibition

Since the RALES trial was published in 1999, aldosterone inhibitors have been used for patients with heart failure. In the RALES trial, patients were assigned to receive aldosterone inhibitor (spironolactone) 25 mg daily or placebo. To enter the trial, patients had to have ejection fraction <35% and NYHA III–IV heart failure symptoms. The trial was stopped early due to significant benefits in the spironolactone arm. There was a 30% reduction in deaths in the spironolactone group. This was due largely to a decreased risk of progressive heart failure and a decrease in sudden cardiac death [17].

Aldosterone inhibitors block the effect of aldosterone by binding to mineralocorticoid receptors. The two major aldosterone inhibitors are spironolactone and eplerenone. Spironolactone is a non-selective mineralocorticoid receptor antagonist. It also up-regulates progesterone receptors and down-regulates androgen receptors. Some of the side effects of spironolactone-gynecomastia, changes in libido and menses-are due to this effect. Spironolactone also causes hyperkalemia, which needs to be monitored closely.

Eplerenone is a selective mineralocorticoid receptor antagonist. It has fewer side effects than Spironolactone. Importantly, it can cause hyperkalemia as well, and must be also monitored closely.

Aldosterone can stimulate angiotensin II production, leading to fibrosis. The myocardium has mineralocorticoid receptors. The amount of aldosterone produced is proportional to the degree of heart failure.

Blockade of aldosterone can also help prevent hypokalemia caused by diuretics. This strategy may help prevent arrhythmogenic deaths attributed to hypokalemia.

Aliskiren is the first direct renin inhibitor that has been trialed in a hypertensive population. It has not been fully studies in heart failure, so its properties and effects in heart failure patients is unknown.

Data Supporting Inhibition of Raas

Ace inhibitors have been shown to reduce the risk of death and hospitalization. They have also been shown to alleviate symptoms of heart failure and improve quality of life. Clinical status, as measured by New York Heart Association class (NYHA), also improves when treated with ace inhibitors.

Ace inhibitors and ARBs have been extensively studied in clinical trials in patients with congestive heart failure. The first major trial showing benefit of ace inhibitors was the CONSENSUS trial, which compared enalapril with placebo in patients with NYHA IV heart failure. The enalapril group had a 40% reduction in mortality ($p = 0.002$) and their symptoms significantly improved as measured by NYHA classification [18]. Soon after CONSENSUS, the SOLVD Treatment trial studied enalapril vs. placebo in a less ill patient population (NYHA II-IV). In SOLVD Treatment, the enalapril-treated group had a significant decrease in mortality and enjoyed fewer hospitalizations related to heart failure. In summary, this translated into a 16% relative risk reduction in death and a 26% reduction in hospitalization [19]. In SOLVD prevention trial, enalapril was studied in asymptomatic patients with ejection fraction <35%. Although in the enalapril group, there was not shown a significant reduction in mortality, there was a significant reduction in the combined endpoint of death or worsening heart failure [20].

The V-Heft II trial compared enalapril to the combination of hydralazine and isosorbide dinitrate in patients with mild-moderate heart failure and ejection fraction of <45%. Enalapril reduced mortality by 34% after 1 year and 28% at 2 years compared to the hydralazine isosorbide group [21].

More recently, trials have been designed to specifically answer the lingering question as to how to best utilize ARBs; either added to ace-inhibitors or as an alternative. In the ELITE study, patients over the age of 65 with chronic heart failure were randomized to Losartan or Captopril. The primary endpoint was worsening renal function. Although the primary endpoint showed no statistical significance, there was a decrease in mortality among the Losartan treated patients [14]. Because of this finding, ELITE II was initiated which was powered to detect a mortality benefit between ace-inhibitors and ARBs. Patients were randomized to Losartan or Captopril. They were age greater than 60 and were NYHA II-IV. There was found to be no difference in all cause mortality (primary endpoint) or cardiac arrest (secondary endpoint) between the two groups [22].

The Val-HeFT trial was undertaken to assess the utility of the ARB Valsartan in heart failure patients already receiving an ace-inhibitor and/or beta-blocker. Val-HeFT had two end points, all cause mortality and a combined end point of mortality and morbidity. There was found to be no significant difference between the two groups in terms of all cause mortality (primary endpoint). In the Losartan group, there was a risk reduction in mortality and morbidity (secondary endpoint). This was felt to be largely due to the decrease in hospital admissions for heart failure in the Valsartan group [15].

In the CHARM-Alternative trial, patients were randomized to the ARB Candesartan or placebo. Criteria for entry into the trial were NYHA II–IV, EF of 40% or less and intolerant to ace-inhibitors. The primary outcome was all cause mortality or hospital admission for heart failure. There was a 23% risk reduction of cardiovascular death or heart failure admission in those taking Candesartan [16]. This finding confirmed the VAL-HeFT subgroup analysis that ARBs had a mortality benefit in those patients intolerant to ace-inhibitors. In the CHARM-Added trial, a similar patient demographic group was studied. Patients were already taking an ace-inhibitor and were randomized to Candesartan or placebo. Cardiovascular mortality and hospitalization for heart failure were reduced in the Candesartan group [23]. This trial, as well as VAL-Heft, suggests that an ARB, when added to ace-inhibitors and beta-blockers, confer benefit. In the CHARM-Preserved study, patients with preserved ejection fractions were studied. They were randomized to Candesartan or placebo. There was no significance between the groups in terms of mortality or heart failure hospitalizations.

The RALES trial (Randomized Aldactone Evaluation Study) enrolled patients with symptomatic heart failure and ejection fractions <35%. Patients were randomized to get spironolactone or placebo. Patients enrolled were receiving ace-inhibitors, diuretics and many times, digoxin. The primary end-point was death from all causes. The trial was stopped early after an interim analysis showed that spironolactone was significantly efficacious compared to placebo. The 30% decrease in the risk of death in the spironolactone group was primarily attributed to a lower risk of death from progressive heart failure and sudden death from cardiac causes [17]. Additionally, the spironolactone group enjoyed a significant improvement in symptoms based on the New York Heart Association scale and had fewer hospital admissions for decompensated heart failure.

The RALES trial was undertaken after data emerged revealing that ace-inhibitors transiently, and not fully, suppress aldosterone.

The Eplerenone Post-Acute Myocardial Infarction Heart Failure Efficacy and Survival Study (EPHESUS) was designed to test the hypothesis that eplerenone, a selective aldosterone blocker would reduce overall mortality and cardiovascular mortality or hospitalization for cardiovascular events among patients with acute myocardial infarction complicated by diminished ejection fraction and heart failure. Patients with acute myocardial infarction, left ventricular dysfunction and heart failure were randomized to eplerenone or placebo. The primary end points were death from any cause and death from cardiovascular causes or hospitalization for heart failure, acute myocardial infarction, stroke or ventricular arrhythmia. The rate of death, cardiovascular deaths and hospitalizations and sudden death were all reduced by eplerenone [24].

Congestive heart failure is a complex syndrome. When an insult to the heart results in a change in hemodynamics and a perturbation in homeostasis, the RAAS is activated to ensure that vital organs maintain adequate perfusion. In so doing, mechanisms that improve perfusion in the short term, cause congestive symptoms and abnormal cardiac preload and afterload in the acute and chronic periods. These changes, if not checked, may result in chronic progressive damage and worsening heart failure and cardiomyopathy. The therapies that control the increase activity of the RAAS, ace-inhibitors, ARBs and aldosterone inhibitors, have been studied in multiple large scale trials, and have been shown to decrease mortality, morbidity and RAAS activation. It has yet to be shown, if other targets of the RAAS will yield similar results.

Angiotensin Receptor-Neprilysin Inhibition

In late 2014, The Paradigm-HF study was published. This double-blind trial of NYHA class II-IV heart failure patients with ejection fraction <40% were randomized to either an ace-inhibitor (enalapril) or a novel agent, neprilysin-inhibitor (sacubitril)-angiotensin receptor inhibitor (valsartan) combination.

Neprilysin is an enzyme that degrades natriuretic peptides, bradykinin and adrenomedullin [25]. Degradation of these neurohormones can result in vasoconstriction, sodium retention and myocardial remodeling; all maladaptive actions. Inhibition of neprilysin can increase the levels of these peptides countering these maladaptive actions.

The combination of inhibition of RAAS and inhibition of neprilysin had effects that were superior to inhibition of either alone, in smaller trials. In the Paradigm-HF trial, approximately 4200 patient received enalapril 10 mg twice daily and 4200 patients received combination valsartan and sacubitril, the neprilysin inhibitor. Patients in each cohort had similar baseline characteristics. The primary outcome was a composite of death from cardiovascular causes or hospitalization for heart failure. The trial was designed to detect a difference in rates of death from cardiovascular causes. The primary end point was reached in 914 patients in the valsartan/sacubitril group and 1117 patients in the enalapril group ($p < 0.001$). There were 558 cardiovascular deaths in the valsartan/sacubitril cohort and 693 cardiovascular deaths in the enalapril group ($p < 0.001$) [25]. As compared with enalapril, valsartan/sacubitril also reduced the risk of hospitalizations for heart failure, and decreased the symptoms and physical limitations associated with heart failure. The angiotensin receptor-neprilysin inhibitor significantly reduced the rates of death from any cause and from cardiovascular causes and the rates of hospitalizations for worsening heart failure as compared to enalapril [25].

The Paradigm-HF trial introduced the first new successful agent in the treatment of chronic, symptomatic heart failure in the last decade. The combination angotensin II receptor antagonist and neprilysin-inhibitor, known as Entresto, work in synergy to inhibit RAAS and increase the beneficial effects of neuropetide activity.

Due to the strength of the Paradigm-HF data for sacubitril-valsartan, the American College of

Table 5.2 RAAS inhibition

Agent	Level of evidence	Strength of recommendation	Use
Angiotensin converting enzyme ace-i	High quality research in support	Strong	Heart failure with reduced ejection fraction and prior or current symptoms
Angiotensin receptor blocker arb	High quality research in support	Strong	Intolerant to ace-i Heart failure with reduced ejection fraction and prior or current symptoms
Angiotensin receptor/ neprilysin inhibitor arb	Moderate quality research in support	Strong	Tolerating adequate doses of ace-i or arb with continued class II-III symptoms Replace to further reduce morbidity and mortality
Aldosterone receptor antagonist	High quality research in support	Strong	Add to ace-i or arb Prior or current symptoms

ACC/AHA/AHFS summary recommendations for treatment of heart failure with reduced ejection fraction

Cardiology the American Heart Association and Heart Failure Society recommended Entresto as class 1 for patients with chronic congestive heart failure, reduced ejection fraction and NYHA class II-III symptoms to replace an ace-I or ARB, in their 2016 practice guidelines [26]. (Table 5.2).

References

1. Schrier RW. Pathogenesis of sodium and water retention in high-output and low-output cardiac failure, nephrotic syndrome cirrhosis, and pregnancy. N Engl J Med. 1988;319:1065–72. 1127–1134
2. Jackson EK. Goodman and Gilman's the pharmacological basis of therapeutics. 10th ed. New York: McGraw Hill; 2001. p. 809–21.
3. Hensen J, Abraham WT, Durr J, Shrier RW. Aldosterone in congestive heart failure: analysis of determinants and role in sodium retention. Am J Nephrol. 1991;11:441–6.
4. Rashid H. Direct renin inhibition: an evaluation of the safety and tolerability of aliskiren. Curr Med Res Opin. 2008;24:2627–37.
5. Jackson G, Gibbs CR, Davies MK, Lip GYH. Pathophysiology. Br Med J. 2000;320:1676.
6. Dluhy RG, Williams GH. Aldosterone-villain or bystander? N Engl J Med. 2004;351:8–10.
7. Weber KT. Aldosterone in congestive heart failure. N Engl J Med. 2001;345:1689–97.
8. Mizuno Y, Yoshimura M, Yasue H, Sakamoto T, Ogawa H, Kugiyama K, et al. Aldosterone production is activated in failing ventricle in humans. Circulation. 2001;103:72–7.
9. Pitt B, Reichek N, Willenbrock R, Zannad F, Phillips RA, Roniker B, et al. Effects of eplerenone, enalapril, and eplerenone/enalapril in patients with essential hypertension and left ventricular hypertrophy: the 4E-left ventricular hypertrophy study. Circulation. 2003;108:1831–8.
10. McEwan PE, Gray GA, Sherry L, Webb DJ, Kenyon CJ. Differential effects of angiotensin II on cardiac cell proliferation and intramyocardial perivascular fibrosis in vivo. Circulation. 1998;98:2765–73.
11. Captopril Multicenter Trial (Captopril Multicenter Research Group). A placebo controlled trial: captopril in refractory chronic congestive heart failure. J Am Coll Cardiol. 1983;2:755–63.
12. Pilote L, Abrahamowicz M, Rodriguez E, Eisenberg MJ, Rahme E. Mortality rates in elderly patients who take different angiotensin-converting enzyme inhibitors after acute myocardial infarction: a class effect? Ann Intern Med. 2004;141:102–12.
13. Jorde UP, Ennezat PV, Lisker J, Suryadevara V, Infeld J, Cukon S, et al. Maximally recommended doses of angiotensin-converting enzyme (ACE) inhibitors do not completely prevent ACE-mediated formation of angiotensin II in chronic heart failure. Circulation. 2000;101:844–6.
14. Pitt B, Segal R, Martinez FA, Meurers G, Cowley AJ, Thomas I, et al. Randomized trial of losartan versus captopril in patients over 65 with heart failure (Evaluation of Losartan in the Elderly Study, ELITE). Lancet. 1997;349:747–52.
15. Cohn JN, Tognoni G, for the Valsartan Heart Failure Trial Investigators. A randomized trial of the angiotensin receptor blocker valsartan in chronic heart failure. N Engl J Med. 2001;341:1675.
16. Granger CB, McMurray JJ, Yusuf S, Held P, Michelson EL, Olofsson B, Ostergren J, et al. CHARM Investigators and Committees. Effects of candesartan in patients with chronic heart failure and reduced left-ventricular systolic function intolerant to angiotensin-converting-enzyme inhibitors: the CHARM-alternative trial. Lancet. 2003;362:772–6.
17. Pitt B, Zannad F, Remme WJ, Cody R, Castaigne A, Perez A, et al. The effect of spironolactone on morbid-

ity and mortality in patients with severe heart failure. Randomized aldactone evaluation study investigators. N Engl J Med. 1999;341:709–17.
18. The Consensus Trial Study Group. Effects of enalapril on mortality in severe congestive heart failure. Results of the cooperative North Scandinavian Enalapril Survival Study (Consensus). N Engl J Med. 1987;316:1429–35.
19. The SOLVD Investigators. Effect of enalapril on survival in patients with reduced left ventricular ejection fractions and congestive heart failure. N Engl J Med. 1991;325:293–302.
20. The SOLVD Investigators. Effect of enalapril on mortality and the development of heart failure in asymptomatic patients with reduced left ventricular ejection fractions. N Engl J Med. 1992;327:685–91.
21. Carson P, Ziesche S, Johnson G, Cohn JN. Racial differences in response to therapy for heart failure: analysis of the vasodilator-heart failure trials. J Card Fail. 1999;5:178–87.
22. Pitt B, Poole-Wilson PA, Segal R, Martinez FA, Dickstein K, Camm AJ, et al. Effect of losartan compared with captopril on mortality in patients with symptomatic heart failure: randomized trial—the Losartan Heart Failure Survival Study, ELITE II. Lancet. 2000;355:1582–7.
23. McMurray JJ, Ostergren J, Swedberg K, Granger CB, Held P, Michelson EL, et al. CHARM Investigators and Committees. Effects of candesartan in patients with chronic heart failure and reduced left-ventricular systolic dysfunction taking angiotensin-converting-enzyme inhibitors: the CHARM-added trial. Lancet. 2003;362:767–71.
24. Pitt B, Remme W, Zannad F, Neaton J, Martinez F, Roniker B, et al. Eperenone, a selective aldosterone blocker, in patients with left ventricular dysfunction after myocardial infarction. N Engl J Med. 2003;348:1309–21.
25. McMurray JJ, Packer M, Desai A, et al. Angiotensin-Neprilysin inhibition versus Enalapril in heart failure. N Engl J Med. 2014;371:993–1004.
26. Yancy C, et al. 2016 ACC/AHA?HFSA focused update on new pharmacological therapy for hearty failure: an update on new pharmacological therapy for heart failure: an update of the 2013 ACCF/AHA/guideline for the management of heart failure. Circulation. 2016;134

Angiotensin Receptor Neprilysin Inhibitor

6

Erika D. Feller and Omar Almaadawy

Introduction

Heart failure (HF) is a complex diagnosis that includes either a reduced ability of the heart to pump or fill with blood, leading to an inability to maintain cardiac output that matches the body's metabolic needs. Furthermore, it can be classified according to the ejection fraction (EF) into HF with reduced ejection fraction (HFrEF) with EF <40%, mildly reduced ejection fraction (HFmrEF) with EF 41–49% and preserved ejection fraction (HFpEF) with EF >50% [1]. Additionally, there are various classifications such as the New York Heart Association (NYHA) and the American College of Cardiology (ACC)/American Heart Association (AHA) [1]. HF is considered a global pandemic, affecting nearly 64 million people in 2017, and the prevalence is expected to continue to rise given the advances in treatment. In fact, there is a trend of increase in HFpEF while HFrEF has been stable [1, 2].

During the initial/acute phase of HF, a neurohormonal cascade begins with the aim of maintaining adequate cardiac output [3]. Notably, it can start as early as when left ventricular dysfunction occurs, even before the appearance of HF symptoms [3]. These include the sympathetic nervous system, renin-angiotensin-aldosterone system (RAAS), and arginine vasopressin (AVP) system [3]. These lead to an increase in heart rate, blood pressure, and fluid and sodium retention, thereby maintaining cardiac output [3]. This neurohormonal activation may be beneficial initially; however, in the long term, it leads to deleterious and maladaptive remodeling of the heart muscles along with increasing arrhythmogenicity [3]. For instance, continuous increases in blood pressure/afterload leads to hypertrophy of the cardiac muscle. Moreover, aldosterone (an end product of RAAS system activation), not only enhances sodium and fluid retention, thereby increasing the afterload on the failing heart, but it also causes myocardial and vascular fibrosis [3].

Natriuretic Peptides

ANP and BNP are peptides secreted in response to stress/stretching of heart cells, hence, increasing preload in the failing heart. This leads to an increase in the amount of circulating ANP, BNP, and N-terminal proBNP in heart failure patients. This reflex mechanism, interestingly, is helpful for the heart in the short and long term as explained, later, by the physiological effects of these hormones/enzymes [4].

Natriuretic peptides have been known since 1956, when an atrial extract was identified by Kishi et al. Later, in the 1980s, atrial (type-A)

E. D. Feller (✉)
Division of Cardiology, Med-Star Health, Baltimore, MD, USA
e-mail: efeller@medicine.umaryland.edu

O. Almaadawy
Medstar, Baltimore, MD, USA
e-mail: omar.a.almaadawy@medstar.net

H. J. Eisen (ed.), *Heart Failure I*, https://doi.org/10.1007/978-3-032-12626-9_6

natriuretic peptide (ANP), Brain (B-type) natriuretic peptide (BNP), and C-type natriuretic peptide (CNP) were discovered [5]. ANP and BNP are primarily secreted by cardiomyocytes, however, BNP is called "brain" natriuretic peptide as it was initially discovered in the porcine brain [5, 6]. At the cellular level, mRNA expression initially yields preproANP, which is later cleaved to proANP, this can further transform into B-ANP (via an unclear mechanism) or be proteolytically cleaved into ANP via the enzyme corin [4]. Regarding BNP, it is also initially made as preproBNP, which is cleaved to proBNP and further cleaved via the enzyme furin to form BNP (the active component) and N-terminal proBNP [4]. Furthermore, ANP is found in increased concentration in the atrial cells compared to ventricles, which may be as high as 1000% [4]. BNP is also found in higher concentration in atria but not to the same extent as ANP. Nevertheless, BNP is primarily secreted from the ventricular cells as they constitute up to 70% of the heart muscle [4].

ANP and BNP both activate the natriuretic peptide receptor-A (NPR-A), which in turn activates guanylyl cyclase, hence increasing the amount of cyclic guanosine monophosphate (cGMP) in the target tissues, triggering a cascade of further phosphorylation and dephosphorylation [4, 7]. This translates into different actions in different organ systems in the body, such as the cardiovascular, renal, and nervous systems, as well as other organs.

The cardiovascular and renal system is our major topic. The cGMP, via a cascade of actions, reduces cytosolic calcium leading to smooth muscle relaxation and vasodilation [7], which in turn clinically translates into afterload reduction for the failing heart. Moreover, it leads to relaxation of the mesangial cells and afferent arterioles, while constricting the efferent arterioles, leading to an increase in the glomerular filtration rate (GFR) along with suppression of sodium reabsorption in the inner medullary collecting ducts, leading to natriuresis [7, 8], furthermore reduces preload, which again helps the failing heart. Additionally, at the kidney level, BNP and ANP can directly inhibit the RAAS system. Moreover, in mice it was proven that they inhibit the expression of aldosterone synthase, hence decreasing aldosterone level and function along with ATII, which has a detrimental effect on myocardial fibrosis [8]. This is further shown in mice, in which NPR-A was knocked out causing more pronounced cardiac fibrosis exerted by ATII [4].

There are two major pathways to clear natriuretic peptides from the circulation. The first one is via binding to NPR-C, leading to a cascade of internalization and degradation of the natriuretic peptides, while the second pathway is via extracellular proteases, mainly called neprilysin [9]. This is especially important, as targeting the clearance pathways is one of the approaches used in the management of heart failure, as will be discussed below. Another minor pathway, which contributes less, is excretion in body fluids via the kidney and liver [9]. Hence, in patients with chronic kidney failure, the BNP levels may be elevated due to impaired water excretion, which leads to hypervolemia, which leads to atrial stretching and BNP secretion. Additionally, impaired secretion by the failing kidney also contributes to increased BNP [8].

Clinical Use of Natriuretic Peptides

Natriuretic peptides are utilized clinically in various ways. The AHA/ACC/HFSA guidelines recommend measuring natriuretic peptides, especially BNP and NT-proBNP, for establishing diagnosis, prognosis, and risk stratification as a class 1 recommendation [1]. ANP is not preferred as a marker due to its short half-life of 2–4 minutes, whereas NT-proBNP has a half-life of about 90 minutes and BNP has a half-life of 20 minutes [7]. According to the European Society of Cardiology (ESC), values for NT-proBNP and BNP are important in ruling in or out the diagnosis of acute heart failure. A BNP level of <100 pg/ml makes the diagnosis of HF unlikely (sensitivity of 90%, specificity of 76%, and accuracy of 83% for differentiating congestive heart failure from other causes of dyspnea), while levels >400 pg/ml are suggested to rule in the disease (I could not find sensitivity and it seems to be more arbitrary). Additionally, levels in the 100–400 pg/ml range are considered a gray zone, and if other clinical examination findings suggest HF, the diagnosis becomes more likely [10].

Moreover, natriuretic peptides are not the only diagnostic tools for HF. High levels of natriuretic peptides are risk markers for acute coronary syndrome, atrial fibrillation, myocarditis, sepsis, and rejection after heart transplantation [7]. They also have prognostic value; a study found that every 100 pg/ml increase in BNP increases the relative risk of mortality by 35% [11]. Additionally, patients presenting with shortness of breath and high troponin levels are at increased risk of HF [11]. It was found that if the BNP was >480 pg/ml, the probability of having HF within 6 months is 51% compared to 2.5% in patients with a BNP <230 pg/mL [11]. Furthermore, patients with BNP >840 pg/ml on presentation were more likely to require mechanical ventilation [11].

However, BNP levels may be low in certain conditions such as obesity [11]. Hence, in these populations, BNP should be interpreted with caution and other clinical symptoms and signs should be taken into consideration.

Angiotensin Receptor Blockers

Angiotensin receptor blockers (ARBs) act at the end of the renin-angiotensin-aldosterone system (RAAS) chain. Renin initiates the conversion of angiotensinogen, produced in the liver, into angiotensin I, which is then catalyzed in the lung endothelium into angiotensin II (ATII) via the enzyme angiotensin-converting enzyme (ACE) [3]. ATII acts on two receptors: angiotensin II type 1 receptor (AT1-R) and angiotensin II type 2 receptor (AT2-R), the latter mainly expressed in fetal tissue. Both receptors are G-protein coupled, but they exert opposing actions. For instance, AT1-R is responsible for vasoconstriction, sodium, and water retention, and in pathological states it mediates inflammation, oxidation, and fibrosis. Conversely, AT2-R stimulation by ATII leads to vasodilation, sodium excretion, and inflammation suppression, please refer to the [12]. ARBs work via blocking the AT1-R, hence leads to less vasodilation and salt and fluid retention. Valsartan, which is an essential part of ARNI (sacubitril/valsartan) has been extensively studied, especially in the Val-Heft trial which showed benefits in both mortality and morbidity over placebo in patients with HF and NYHA class II-IV [13]. The role of ACEi and ARBs was discussed extensively in the previous chapter.

Neprilysin Inhibitor

Neprilysin inhibitors represent another therapeutic strategy. ARNi, a combination medication of a Neprilysin inhibitor and an angiotensin receptor blocker (ARB). Initially, Neprilysin inhibitors alone like candoxatril failed to show benefits and were harmful, leading to vasoconstriction and hypertension [14]. This was partly because Neprilysin degrades not only natriuretic peptides but also endothelin, bradykinin, substance P, vasoactive intestinal peptide (VIP), glucagon, neurotensin, adrenomedullin, and amyloid β peptide [14]. Inhibition of Neprilysin led to increased endothelin levels, causing vasoconstriction [14]. Moreover, candoxatril potentiated the vasoconstriction of ATII, counteracting the vasodilation induced by increased BNP levels [14]. This led to the combination of Neprilysin inhibitors with RAAS inhibitors [14]. However, combining ACE inhibitors with Neprilysin inhibitors increased the risk of angioedema due to elevated bradykinin and substance-P levels, prompting the shift towards ARB and Neprilysin inhibitor combinations, resulting in the development of LCZ696 (sacubitril-valsartan) [14, 15].

ENTRESTO, the most common drug in the ARNi group, was approved by the FDA in July 2015. It has been proven to reduce mortality and hospitalization in adults with heart failure (NYHA class II-IV) with reduced ejection fraction. ENTRESTO contains two main components: valsartan and sacubitril. Valsartan blocks the AT1 receptor, leading to reduced salt and water retention, reduced sympathetic tone, vasodilation, and halted cardiac fibrosis. Sacubitril, a neprilysin inhibitor, primarily increases BNP levels, leading to natriuresis, vasodilation, and reduced sympathetic tone (FDA) [3, 15]). It is noteworthy that this combination drug tends to decrease levels of NT-proBNP, indicating a reduction in cardiac wall stress [16].

Data Supporting the Use of ARNi in Heart Failure

ARNi therapy has been well studied and has consistently shown that its use improves mortality and reduces hospitalization for HF patients, leading to FDA approval for patients with NYHA class II-IV with reduced ejection fraction. However, the ACC/AHA/HFSA guidelines recommend it for patients with NYHA class II-III, as will be explained below [1].

The PARADIGM-HF (Prospective Comparison of ARNi with ACEi to Determine Impact on Global Mortality and Morbidity in Heart Failure) trial, one of the landmark trials in heart failure research, randomly assigned 4187 individuals to valsartan/sacubitril with a dose uptitrated to 200 mg twice daily versus 4212 individuals to enalapril (an ACE inhibitor) with a dose of 10 mg twice daily in patients with HF NYHA class II-IV [17] (Figs. 6.1 and 6.2). The trial had to be discontinued earlier due to the obvious benefit of sacubitril-valsartan [17]. At a median follow-up of 27 months, death from cardiovascular disease or hospitalization for HF occurred in 21.8% of the sacubitril-valsartan group versus 26.5% of the enalapril group, with HR 0.80 (0.73–0.87, $P < 0.001$), which translates into 20% mortality and HF hospitalization reduction in the sacubitril-valsartan group [17]. Additionally, the number needed to treat to prevent one death from cardiovascular disease was 21 for sacubitril-valsartan and 32 for enalapril [17]. Regarding safety outcomes, individuals receiving sacubitril-valsartan were more likely to have hypotension episodes compared to those on enalapril, but this did not result in medication discontinuation, and furthermore, hyperkalemia >6 mmol/dl was less reported in the sacubitril-valsartan group. After this trial, the medication ENTRESTO (a combination of sacubitril and valsartan) was successfully approved by the FDA in 2015 for HF treatment as mentioned above.

However, the PARADIGM-HF trial included only a low percentage of patients with HF NYHA Class IV, around 0.6–0.8% in both groups, meaning there is no robust data for the usage of sacubitril-valsartan in patients with advanced HF, one reason why the ACC/AHA/HFSA 2022

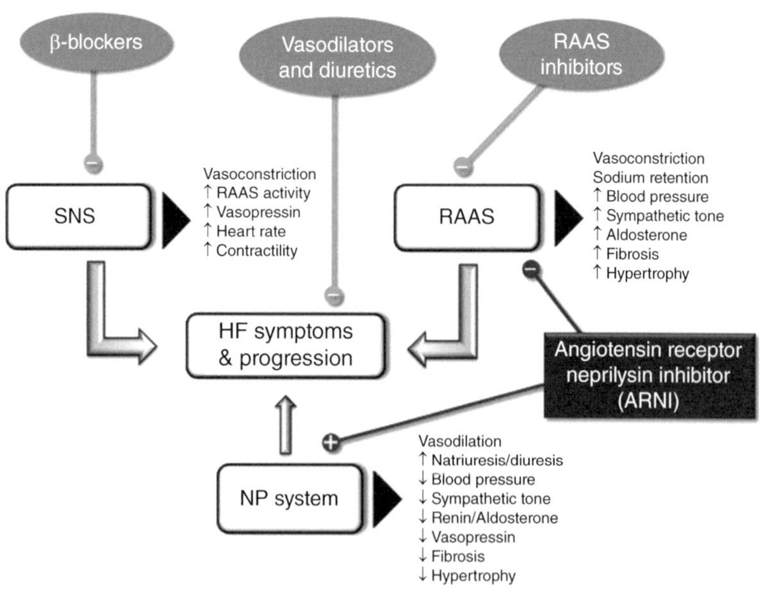

Fig. 6.1 Pathophysiology of the natriuretic peptide system and the ompact of Angiotensin Receptor-Neprilysin Inhibitors (ARNIs) on its management. (Reference Volpe et al. [27]. Under CC BY 3.0 License)

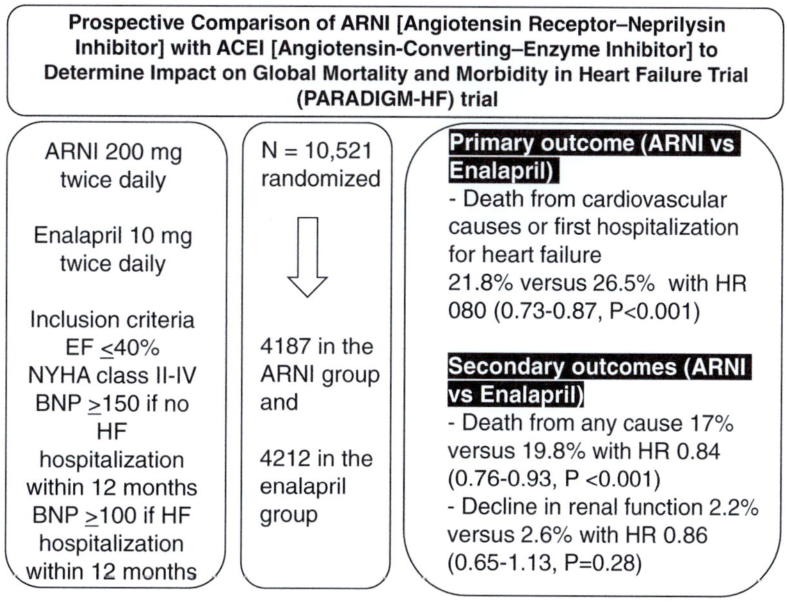

Fig. 6.2 Illustrating the main inclusion criteri and outcomes of the PARADIGM-HF trial

guidelines recommend its use only in class II-III HF [1, 18]. To test sacubitril/valsartan in NYHA class IV patients, the LIFE trial (LCZ696 in Hospitalized Advanced Heart Failure) investigators randomized patients with advanced HF (NYHA class IV) to either sacubitril/valsartan uptitrated to 97/103 mg (200-mg) twice daily or valsartan 160 mg twice daily [18]. Interestingly, the LIFE trial did not find a statistically significant difference between both groups regarding NT-proBNP level change from baseline, days alive, and heart failure events. However, it is important to note that this trial was underpowered as it only included 335 patients [18]. The insignificant difference in NT-proBNP and clinical outcomes between sacubitril/valsartan and valsartan monotherapy may be attributed to the overstimulation of RAAS in advanced HF, which reduces the effect of natriuretic peptides; moreover, the amount of BNP (active form of natriuretic peptides) decreases [18, 19].

Later, the PIONEER-HF trial assessed the safety and efficacy of starting sacubitril-valsartan with a target dose of 97/103 mg twice daily for patients with acute decompensated HF and an ejection fraction of less than 40% and NT-proBNP of >1600 pg/ml or BNP >400 pg/ml. Interestingly, most of the patients included were NYHA Class III, 61–64.3%. They randomized patients to sacubitril-valsartan versus enalapril 10 mg twice daily, with the primary outcome being the reduction in NT-proBNP and the safety outcomes including hyperkalemia, symptomatic hypotension, deteriorating kidney function, and angioedema [20]. The percent change of NT-proBNP from baseline was −46.7% vs. −25.3% with sacubitril-valsartan vs. enalapril, respectively (0.71; 95% CI, 0.63–0.81, $P < 0.001$) [20] this shows that the sacubitril/valsartan group has more NT-proBNP reduction and hence may indicate less heart wall stress. There was no significant statistical difference in the safety outcomes between the two groups [20].

Sacubitril/valsartan is safe to start for patients with acute HF hospitalization before discharge. The TRANSITION [Comparison of Pre- and Post-discharge Initiation of Sacubitril/Valsartan Therapy in HFrEF Patients After an Acute Decompensation Event] trial, which randomized patients to pre-discharge (not less than 12 h before discharge) versus post-discharge initiation of sacubitril/valsartan, did not show any significant difference in safety outcomes [21]. Hence, it is recommended to start ARNi in patients with HF before discharge, even if they are ARNi naive.

The PARADISE-MI trial (Prospective ARNI versus ACE Inhibitor Trial to Determine Superiority in Reducing Heart Failure Events after Myocardial Infarction) assessed the efficacy of ARNI versus ramipril in patients who had HF with reduced ejection fraction <40% or pulmonary congestion following myocardial infarction. A total of 5661 patients were randomized to either sacubitril/valsartan 97/103 mg twice daily or ramipril 5 mg twice daily. The data did not show any superiority of ARNI; death from cardiovascular etiologies or heart failure (either outpatient or during inpatient hospitalization), occurred in 11.9% of the sacubitril/valsartan group and in 13.2% of the ramipril group, though the HR was 0.9 in favor of sacubitril/valsartan; however, it was statistically insignificant (*P*-value = 0.17) [22].

Most of the above data is true for HFrEF, while for HFpEF, there are a few trials that assessed the efficacy of sacubitril/valsartan in HFpEF. The PARAGON-HF (Prospective Comparison of ARNI with ARB Global Outcomes in HF with Preserved Ejection Fraction) trial randomized patients with HF and ejection fraction >45% to sacubitril/valsartan 97/103 mg twice daily versus valsartan 160 mg twice daily [23]. The study found that there was no statistically significant difference in cardiovascular death, hospitalization for heart failure, or NYHA class improvement [23]. However, patients with EF <60% benefited more than those with EF >60% [23]. This was also confirmed by the PARAGLIDE-HF trial, in which patients with HF and EF >40% enrolled after an episode of HF decompensation were randomized to sacubitril/valsartan versus valsartan, it showed that the sacubitril/valsartan group showed a greater reduction in NT-proBNP, especially in the subgroup with EF <60%; otherwise, regarding the clinical outcomes as the number and times of HF hospitalization, the time to cardiovascular death was overall in favor of the sacubitril/valsartan group, but did not reach statistical significance [24]. The same pattern of results was shown in the PARALLAX (Prospective Comparison of ARNI vs. Comorbidity-Associated Conventional Therapy on Quality of Life and Exercise Capacity) trial, which randomized patients with HF with ejection fraction >40% and elevated NT-proBNP to either sacubitril/valsartan 97/103 mg twice daily or enalapril 10 mg, valsartan 160 mg, or placebo [25]. The PARALLAX trial showed that there was a greater reduction in NT-proBNP; however, there was no statistically significant difference in outcomes such as NYHA class improvement or 6-minute walk distance [25].

According to ACC/AHA/HFSA 2022 guidelines, ARNi use is well established. In stage C HF, ARNI is recommended as a class 1A for the management of patients with HFrEF with NYHA class II-III, and it is recommended over the use of ACEi and ARBs whenever feasible. Patients tolerating ACEi and ARBs should be transitioned to ARNi as it further reduces mortality and morbidity. However, a washout period of 36 hours from the last dose of ACEi should be used to prevent side effects such as angioedema [1]. Additionally, ARNi should not be used in any patients with a history of angioedema. Regarding patients with HFmrEF (EF 41–49%) and HFpEF (EF >50%), ARNI is considered a class 2b recommendation, with more benefit in patients with lower EF (i.e., on the lower side of the spectrum) [1]. In special conditions such as cardiac amyloidosis (CM), especially the transthyretin cardiomyopathy (ATTR-CM), the use of ARNi may be poorly tolerated due to vasodilation and hypotension exacerbation [1]. Moreover, in female patients who are pregnant or planning to become pregnant, the use of ARNi is contraindicated due to the risk of harmful effects on the fetus [1]. In patients with advanced kidney disease, the data about safety and tolerability are scarce, as most clinical trials included patients with an estimated glomerular filtration rate (eGFR) >30; hence, patients with eGFR <30 should be started on a lower dose of 24–26 mg twice daily and uptitrated as tolerated to reach a target of 97–103 mg twice daily [26].

Overall, the use of ARNi therapy has been extensively studied in certain classes of heart failure patients (NYHA class II-III), but some work remains to be done in patients with NYHA class IV HFrEF and in patients with HFpEF. In the future, the role of these drugs will be further defined in these patients, to maximize the effects of this powerful medication.

References

1. Heidenreich PA, Bozkurt B, Aguilar D, Allen LA, Byun JJ, Colvin MM, Deswal A, Drazner MH, Dunlay SM, Evers LR, Fang JC, Fedson SE, Fonarow GC, Hayek SS, Hernandez AF, Khazanie P, Kittleson MM, Lee CS, Link MS, Milano CA, et al. 2022 AHA/ACC/HFSA guideline for the management of heart failure: executive summary: a report of the American College of Cardiology/American Heart Association Joint Committee on Clinical Practice Guidelines. Circulation. 2022;145(18):e876–94. https://doi.org/10.1161/CIR.0000000000001062.
2. Savarese G, Becher PM, Lund LH, Seferovic P, Rosano GMC, Coats AJS. Global burden of heart failure: a comprehensive and updated review of epidemiology. Cardiovasc Res. 2023;118(17):3272–87. https://doi.org/10.1093/cvr/cvac013.
3. Manolis AA, Manolis TA, Manolis AS. Neurohumoral activation in heart failure. Int J Mol Sci. 2023;24(20):15472. https://doi.org/10.3390/ijms242015472.
4. Nakagawa Y, Nishikimi T, Kuwahara K. Atrial and brain natriuretic peptides: hormones secreted from the heart. Peptides. 2019;111:18–25. https://doi.org/10.1016/j.peptides.2018.05.012.
5. Barbieri K, Potter LR. Natriuretic peptides, their receptors and therapeutic applications. In: Encyclopedia of biological chemistry. 2nd ed; 2013.
6. Sandefur CC, Jialal I. Atrial natriuretic peptide. [Updated 2023 Aug 14]. In: StatPearls [Internet]. Treasure Island (FL): StatPearls Publishing; 2024. Available from: https://www.ncbi.nlm.nih.gov/books/NBK562257/.
7. Goetze JP, Bruneau BG, Ramos HR, Ogawa T, de Bold MK, de Bold AJ. Cardiac natriuretic peptides. Nat Rev Cardiol. 2020;17(11):698–717. https://doi.org/10.1038/s41569-020-0381-0.
8. Okamoto R, Ali Y, Hashizume R, Suzuki N, Ito M. BNP as a major player in the heart-kidney connection. Int J Mol Sci. 2019;20(14):3581. https://doi.org/10.3390/ijms20143581.
9. Potter LR. Natriuretic peptide metabolism, clearance and degradation. FEBS J. 2011;278(11):1808–17. https://doi.org/10.1111/j.1742-4658.2011.08082.x.
10. Mueller C, McDonald K, de Boer RA, Maisel A, Cleland JGF, Kozhuharov N, Coats AJS, Metra M, Mebazaa A, Ruschitzka F, Lainscak M, Filippatos G, Seferovic PM, Meijers WC, Bayes-Genis A, Mueller T, Richards M, Januzzi JL Jr, Heart Failure Association of the European Society of Cardiology. Heart Failure Association of the European Society of Cardiology practical guidance on the use of natriuretic peptide concentrations. Eur J Heart Fail. 2019;21(6):715–31. https://doi.org/10.1002/ejhf.1494.
11. Chow SL, Maisel AS, Anand I, Bozkurt B, de Boer RA, Felker GM, Fonarow GC, Greenberg B, Januzzi JL Jr, Kiernan MS, Liu PP, Wang TJ, Yancy CW, Zile MR, American Heart Association Clinical Pharmacology Committee of the Council on Clinical Cardiology; Council on Basic Cardiovascular Sciences; Council on Cardiovascular Disease in the Young; Council on Cardiovascular and Stroke Nursing; Council on Cardiopulmonary, Critical Care, Perioperative and Resuscitation; Council on Epidemiology and Prevention; Council on Functional Genomics and Translational Biology; and Council on Quality of Care and Outcomes Research. Role of biomarkers for the prevention, assessment, and management of heart failure: a scientific statement from the American Heart Association. Circulation. 2017;135(22):e1054–91. https://doi.org/10.1161/CIR.0000000000000490.
12. Fountain JH, Kaur J, Lappin SL. Physiology, renin angiotensin system. [Updated 2023 Mar 12]. In: StatPearls [Internet]. Treasure Island (FL): StatPearls Publishing; 2024. Available from: https://www.ncbi.nlm.nih.gov/books/NBK470410/.
13. Cohn JN, Tognoni G, Valsartan Heart Failure Trial Investigators. A randomized trial of the angiotensin-receptor blocker valsartan in chronic heart failure. N Engl J Med. 2001;345(23):1667–75. https://doi.org/10.1056/NEJMoa010713.
14. Hubers SA, Brown NJ. Combined angiotensin receptor antagonism and Neprilysin inhibition. Circulation. 2016;133(11):1115–24. https://doi.org/10.1161/CIRCULATIONAHA.115.018622.
15. Romero CA, Orias M, Weir MR. Novel RAAS agonists and antagonists: clinical applications and controversies. Nat Rev Endocrinol. 2015;11(4):242–52. https://doi.org/10.1038/nrendo.2015.6.
16. Docherty KF, Vaduganathan M, Solomon SD, McMurray JJV. Sacubitril/valsartan: Neprilysin inhibition 5 years after PARADIGM-HF. JACC Heart Fail. 2020;8(10):800–10. https://doi.org/10.1016/j.jchf.2020.06.020.
17. McMurray JJ, Packer M, Desai AS, Gong J, Lefkowitz MP, Rizkala AR, Rouleau JL, Shi VC, Solomon SD, Swedberg K, Zile MR, PARADIGM-HF Investigators and Committees. Angiotensin-neprilysin inhibition versus enalapril in heart failure. N Engl J Med. 2014;371(11):993–1004. https://doi.org/10.1056/NEJMoa1409077.
18. Mann DL, Givertz MM, Vader JM, et al. Effect of treatment with sacubitril/valsartan in patients with advanced heart failure and reduced ejection fraction: a randomized clinical trial. JAMA Cardiol. 2022;7(1):17–25. https://doi.org/10.1001/jamacardio.2021.4567.

19. Díez J. Chronic heart failure as a state of reduced effectiveness of the natriuretic peptide system: implications for therapy. Eur J Heart Fail. 2017;19(2):167–76. https://doi.org/10.1002/ejhf.656.
20. Velazquez EJ, Morrow DA, DeVore AD, Duffy CI, Ambrosy AP, McCague K, Rocha R, Braunwald E, PIONEER-HF Investigators. Angiotensin-Neprilysin inhibition in acute decompensated heart failure. N Engl J Med. 2019;380(6):539–48. https://doi.org/10.1056/NEJMoa1812851.
21. Wachter R, Senni M, Belohlavek J, Straburzynska-Migaj E, Witte KK, Kobalava Z, Fonseca C, Goncalvesova E, Cavusoglu Y, Fernandez A, Chaaban S, Bøhmer E, Pouleur AC, Mueller C, Tribouilloy C, Lonn E, A L Buraiki J, Gniot J, Mozheiko M, Lelonek M, et al. Initiation of sacubitril/valsartan in haemodynamically stabilised heart failure patients in hospital or early after discharge: primary results of the randomised TRANSITION study. Eur J Heart Fail. 2019;21(8):998–1007. https://doi.org/10.1002/ejhf.1498.
22. Pfeffer MA, Claggett B, Lewis EF, Granger CB, Køber L, Maggioni AP, Mann DL, McMurray JJV, Rouleau JL, Solomon SD, Steg PG, Berwanger O, Cikes M, De Pasquale CG, East C, Fernandez A, Jering K, Landmesser U, Mehran R, Merkely B, et al. Angiotensin receptor-Neprilysin inhibition in acute myocardial infarction. N Engl J Med. 2021;385(20):1845–55. https://doi.org/10.1056/NEJMoa2104508.
23. Solomon SD, McMurray JJV, Anand IS, Ge J, Lam CSP, Maggioni AP, Martinez F, Packer M, Pfeffer MA, Pieske B, Redfield MM, Rouleau JL, van Veldhuisen DJ, Zannad F, Zile MR, Desai AS, Claggett B, Jhund PS, Boytsov SA, Comin-Colet J, et al. Angiotensin-Neprilysin inhibition in heart failure with preserved ejection fraction. N Engl J Med. 2019;381(17):1609–20. https://doi.org/10.1056/NEJMoa1908655.
24. Mentz RJ, Ward JH, Hernandez AF, Lepage S, Morrow DA, Sarwat S, Sharma K, Starling RC, Velazquez EJ, Williamson KM, Desai AS, Zieroth S, Solomon SD, Braunwald E, PARAGLIDE-HF Investigators. Angiotensin-Neprilysin inhibition in patients with mildly reduced or preserved ejection fraction and worsening heart failure. J Am Coll Cardiol. 2023;82(1):1–12. https://doi.org/10.1016/j.jacc.2023.04.019.
25. Pieske B, Wachter R, Shah SJ, Baldridge A, Szeczoedy P, Ibram G, Shi V, Zhao Z, Cowie MR, PARALLAX Investigators and Committee members. Effect of sacubitril/valsartan vs standard medical therapies on plasma NT-proBNP concentration and submaximal exercise capacity in patients with heart failure and preserved ejection fraction: the PARALLAX randomized clinical trial. JAMA. 2021;326(19):1919–29. https://doi.org/10.1001/jama.2021.18463.
26. Hein AM, Scialla JJ, Edmonston D, Cooper LB, DeVore AD, Mentz RJ. Medical management of heart failure with reduced ejection fraction in patients with advanced renal disease. JACC Heart Fail. 2019;7(5):371–82. https://doi.org/10.1016/j.jchf.2019.02.009.
27. Volpe M, Carnovali M, Mastromarino V. The natriuretic peptides system in the pathophysiology of heart failure: from molecular basis to treatment. Clin Sci (Lond). 2016;130(2):57–77. https://doi.org/10.1042/CS20150469.

Inhibition of the Sympathetic Nervous System

7

Beani J. Forst and D. Eric Steidley

Introduction

Activation of the sympathetic nervous system (SNS) is a fundamental component of the pathophysiology of the development and progression of heart failure. Prolonged SNS activation contributes to several sequelae of heart failure. Over the past decades, extensive clinical research has shown that inhibition of the SNS in patients with heart failure improves outcomes, including mortality, hospitalization for heart failure, progression of symptoms, and even sudden cardiac death. The cornerstone therapy for inhibiting the SNS is the administration of drugs that antagonize the β-adrenergic receptor (β-blockers). A robust body of evidence supports the role of β-blockers in treating HFREF. Understanding the practical aspects of B-Blocker administration is essential for the practicing heart failure clinician. The role of non-pharmacologic therapies, including both device and non-device-based treatments, has also been found to deliver improved outcomes. Many of their beneficial effects arise from the inhibition of the SNS. Here, we review the literature that supports the treatment of heart failure through the direct inhibition of the SNS and offers practical advice regarding their application in clinical care.

B. J. Forst · D. E. Steidley (✉)
Mayo Clinic Arizona, Department of Cardiovascular Diseases, Phoenix, AZ, USA
e-mail: forstb@mayo.edu; steidley.d@mayo.edu

Rationale for the Inhibition of the SNS in Heart Failure

In the early twentieth century, W. B. Cannon described the sympathetic nervous system (SNS) as the regulator of "fight or flight" responses [1]. In 1948, Raymond Ahlquist, from the Department of Pharmacology at the Medical College of Georgia, published the theory that adrenaline has distinct actions on both alpha and beta receptors [2]. Strong sympathetic stimuli cause several directly measurable cardiac and peripheral vascular actions, including increased heart rate and cardiac contractility, as well as venous and arterial vasoconstriction [3]. The net effect of these changes is an increase in cardiac output, systemic blood pressure (BP), and effective circulating blood volume, which acutely support the organism's response to exogenous threats. Over the last 100 years, research into the pathophysiology of several common cardiovascular diseases, such as heart failure and hypertension, has uncovered that the SNS is not only the mediator of the "fight or flight" responses but is one of the mechanisms responsible for the continuous maintenance of cardiovascular homeostasis [4–6].

The SNS maintains cardiovascular homeostasis via a complex system of nerve relays. It generally contains two neurons extending from the central nervous system to the target organs [7]. The preganglionic neuron has its cell body in the spinal cord and projects its axon to a collection of neurons, known as a ganglion, distant from the target

H. J. Eisen (ed.), *Heart Failure I*, https://doi.org/10.1007/978-3-032-12626-9_7

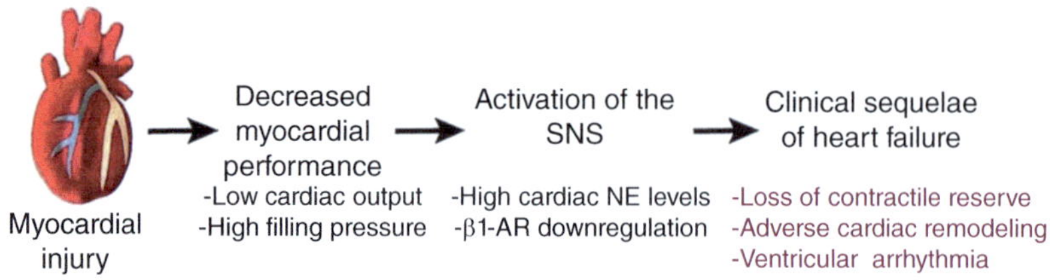

Fig. 7.1 The relationship of myocardial injury to Sympathetic Nervous Activation and progression of heart failure

organ. For the heart, the sympathetic ganglion is named the stellate ganglion, located between the subclavian artery and the first rib [8]. The axons of the postganglionic neurons project to the ventricular myocardium [9], where they release the neurotransmitter norepinephrine (NE). NE binds to specific β_1- and β_2-adrenergic receptors (AR) on the cardiac myocytes. Through G-protein coupling, internal cell signaling leads to the phosphorylation of multiple intracellular proteins, such as L-type calcium channels and the ryanodine receptor [10, 11]. These phosphorylated proteins mediate heart rate and increase contractility, primarily by elevating intracellular calcium levels.

In a simplified sense, heart failure, especially HFPEF, is decreased myocardial performance [12]. Failing cardiac muscle demonstrates decreased responsiveness to beta-receptor-mediated stimulation [13]. This suboptimal performance increases the frequency of sympathetic nerve activation via the physiologic cardiovascular reflexes of the SNS that maintain homeostasis of systemic pressure (the so-called "baroreflex"), blood volume (the "cardiopulmonary" reflex), and oxygenation (the "chemoreceptor" reflex) [14]. Activation of the SNS leads to increased NE levels in the myocardium [15], which, despite favorable acute effects, act through both direct and indirect mechanisms to enhance cardiac pathology. Bristow and colleagues were the first to show that hearts from patients with advanced cardiomyopathy had a 50% lower density of beta-1 adrenergic receptor (β_1-AR) than controls [16]. It was also shown that the degree of β_1-AR downregulation was proportional to the severity of clinical heart failure and left ventricular systolic dysfunction [17]. Elevated NE levels cause myocyte apoptosis by a direct effect [18], which worsens myocardial performance via subsequent adverse cardiac remodeling [19]. Activation of the SNS also causes alterations in the distribution of sympathetic neurons in the left ventricle [20]. These data connect the activation of SNS with the clinical sequelae of heart failure: loss of contractile reserve, progressive ventricular remodeling, and ventricular arrhythmias.

Figure 7.1 summarizes the known role of the SNS in the pathophysiology of HFREF.

Monitoring the SNS

In some future era of heart failure care, precision medicine will necessitate understanding the exact state of sympathetic nervous system activation for individual patients. We will briefly review the methods for monitoring the SNS. None of these methods have found widespread clinical application, and guideline therapy directs clinicians to initiate therapies in all eligible patients.

In patients with heart failure, SNS activation leads to high levels of NE at the synaptic cleft, which overwhelms the presynaptic transporter responsible for moving NE back into the cell [21]. These elevated norepinephrine levels result in spillover into the plasma. Plasma norepinephrine levels have been associated with worsening mortality and morbidity in heart failure [22]. However, practical and analytical challenges in measuring NE are difficult to overcome in a clinical laboratory [23]. Further, distinguishing abnormal plasma norepinephrine levels from localized, organ-specific sympathetic hyperactivity is not straightforward [24]. Consequently, plasma NE determinations have not become helpful for individual prognostication or measuring the responses to HF-directed therapy [25].

Noninvasive nuclear medicine techniques for quantifying cardiac sympathetic activity have been developed using several radiotracer agents with SPECT and PET imaging. They share the common traits of being inert to enzymatic degradation and are avidly taken up by the pre-synaptic norepinephrine transmitter. Image intensity is correlated to selective cardiac sympathetic activation. Iodine-123 Metaiodobenzylguanidine (MIBG), an analog of norepinephrine, has favorable radiopharmaceutical properties, which allow it to be centrally manufactured and distributed, and is the most widely used technique. Patients are pretreated with oral potassium to avoid uptake in the thyroid. Imaging time under the gamma camera is as little as 15 minutes. It is a helpful tool in assessing heart failure patients and prognostication for arrhythmia risk [26].

See Fig. 7.2 for an example of MIBG imaging in heart failure [27].

Decreased myocardial uptake of iodine-123 labeled MIBG was shown to be associated with adverse outcomes in heart failure patients as early as 1992 [28], but the first prospective validation of MIBG imaging was the AdreView Myocardial Imaging for Risk Evaluation in Heart Failure (ADMIRE-HF), published in 2010 [29]. In this study, 961 subjects underwent MIBG imaging and were followed for a median of 17 months. A low heart-to-mediastinum ratio of MIBG uptake predicted the risk of individual outcomes, including death, heart failure progression, arrhythmic events, and cardiac death. Treatment with carvedilol has been shown to improve MIBG uptake and suggests that monitoring SNS activation serially could allow for individualized and targeted neurohormonal therapies for heart failure [30, 31].

The sympathetic and parasympathetic nervous systems innervate the sinoatrial node, leading to heart rate fluctuations via the activation of their corresponding receptors [32]. Measurements of these normally occurring variations in the R-R interval due to autonomic tone are collectively termed heart rate variability (HRV) [33]. HRV can be measured by several parameters, the most popular of which is the standard deviation of all R-R intervals in 24 hours (SDNN) [34]. Sympathetic nervous system activation in heart failure reduces HRV [35]. Reduction in HRV is not uniform in patients with advanced cardiomyopathy [36], with several different HRV parameters having been shown to predict outcomes. Bilchik and colleagues showed that SDNN <65.3 milliseconds was associated with a 3.7-fold higher risk of mortality and a 2.4-fold higher risk of sudden cardiac death [37]. Figure 7.3 presents an example of abnormal HRV in heart failure. Carvedilol therapy improves HRV in HFREF patients [38, 39].

While these methods are not routinely used in clinical practice, they hold promise [40]. Improvements in SNS activation, as assessed by

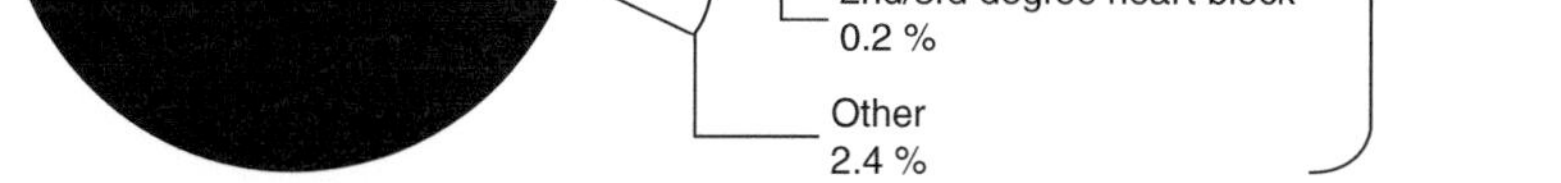

Fig. 7.2 Quantification of sympathetic nervous system activation with metaiodobenzylguanidine (MIBG) imaging. (**a**) Method for calculation of the heart-to-mediastinum ratio on MIBG imaging of the chest. Regions of interest (ROI) are drawn over the heart and mediastinum. (**b**) Normal SNS activation level and MIBG activity in a patient with a heart-to-mediastinum ratio of 1.8. (**c**) Abnormal SNS activation level and low MIBG activity in a patient with a heart-to-mediastinum ratio of 1.1 (Figure reproduced with modification from Carrió et al. [27] © 2010, with permission from Elsevier)

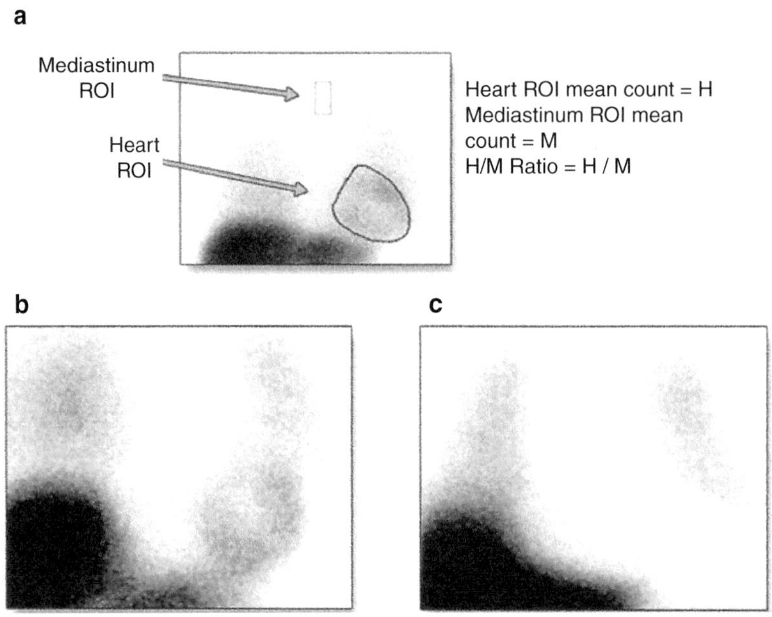

Fig. 7.3 Poincaré plots of heart rate variability from a patient with no cardiac disease and a patient with advanced cardiomyopathy. In the Poincaré plot, each R-R interval (R_nR_{n+1}) is plotted on the *x*-axis against the succeeding R-R interval ($R_{n+1}R_{n+2}$) on the *y*-axis. (**a**) Poincaré plot in a 77-year-old man without heart disease. SDNN was normal at 225.0. (**b**) Poincaré plot in a 61-year-old woman with advanced cardiomyopathy (EF 15%). SDNN was abnormal at 58.4, consistent with low heart rate variability. The patient underwent heart transplantation 3 months after this study

these methods, maybe a reasonable surrogate endpoint to clinical outcomes in trials investigating the effects of heart failure therapies.

Pharmacologic Agents: Beta-Blockers

Sir James Black, a Scottish physician and pharmacologist, is credited with developing propranolol, the first clinically useful β-adrenergic receptor antagonist (β-blocker) [41, 42]. His goal had been to find a new drug for the treatment of angina. Contrary to other research at the time, which attempted to increase the supply of oxygen to the ischemic myocardium, he reasoned that a drug that could block α- and β-AR would decrease myocardial oxygen demand and relieve cardiac symptoms. With his understanding of the effects of adrenaline on the heart, he designed a specific drug to block those receptors. He shared the 1988 Nobel Prize for Physiology or Medicine for his pioneering work in pharmacology for rational drug design. Propranolol became one of the most successful drugs of all time [42].

More than a dozen β-blockers have been developed [43]; however, only carvedilol, bisoprolol, and metoprolol succinate are approved by the U.S. Food and Drug Administration (FDA) to treat heart failure and specifically only heart failure with reduced ejection fraction. Both bisoprolol and metoprolol are "cardioselective" β-blockers, as they preferentially antagonize the β_1-AR. [44] Carvedilol is "nonselective" and antagonizes β_1-, β_2-, and α_1-AR [45] but exhibits its most prolonged-lasting effects on β_1-AR signaling [46]. Carvedilol was granted FDA in 1995 and was approved for mild to severe chronic heart failure as well as for left ventricular systolic dysfunction after myocardial infarction (regardless of the presence of heart failure) and systemic hypertension.

The pharmacology of these agents is reviewed in Table 7.1.

Table 7.1 Pharmacological properties of β-blockers approved for use in HFREF [45]

Drug	Receptor activity α	β$_1$	β$_2$	Plasma half-life (hours)	Starting dose (mg)	Target dose (mg)
Carvedilol	+	++	+	7–10	3.125 mg twice daily[a]	25 mg twice daily[b]
Bisoprolol	–	++	–	9–12	1.25 mg daily	10 mg daily
Metoprolol succinate	–	+	–	3–7	25 mg daily[a]	200 mg daily

[a]The starting dose can be halved for patients with severe heart failure, relative hypotension, or bradycardia.
[b]The maximum target dose is patients with mild to moderate heart failure weighing more than 85 kg is 50 mg twice daily.

The Evidence Basis for β-Blocker Therapy in Heart Failure with Reduced Ejection Fraction

Propranolol entered clinical use for angina and myocardial infarction in the 1960s [47]. At that time, the existing therapies for chronic heart failure were digitalis, diuretics, and bed rest [48]. Early work into the pathophysiology of heart failure suggested that the heart was functionally deinnervated in states of heart failure [49] and that an elevated heart rate seen in patients with cardiomyopathy was essential to maintain cardiac output [50]. Based on this incorrectly understood pathophysiology, it is not unsurprising that there was a decade of delay before β-blockers were applied in the treatment of heart failure.

In 1975, Waagstein and colleagues observed that treatment with propranolol improved pulmonary edema in patients with heart failure due to ischemia [51]. The mechanism of this benefit was thought to be the reduction of resting tachycardia and subsequent decrease in myocardial oxygen utilization [52]. Waagstein reasoned that patients with cardiomyopathy might benefit similarly from long-term treatment with β-blockers. They gave practolol (a selective β-1 blocker, no longer available, but similar in chemical structure to propranolol) at doses of 50 to 400 mg twice daily to seven patients with a resting tachycardia (98 +/− 13 beats/min) for 2–12 months. They observed that β-blocker treatment decreased heart failure symptoms, improved exercise tolerance, and increased ejection time, as measured by phonocardiogram, in all patients [51]. Swedberg and colleagues demonstrated the clinical utility of β-blocker therapy shortly after that [53]. They initiated 24 patients with a dilated cardiomyopathy, already being treated with diuretics and digoxin, on beta-blockade, and slowly increased dosage over 1–4 weeks. The treatment duration was at least 6 months. Survival was improved in the group compared to historical controls treated with diuretics and digoxin alone (survival at 2 years 66% versus 19%).

β-blocker therapy for HFREF was initially met with some skepticism [54]. Two smaller clinical trials with DCM patients, performed in the early 1980s, failed to show clinical benefit of β-blocker treatment, albeit with only a month of follow-up [55, 56].

The first randomized, placebo-controlled, multicenter clinical trial of β-blocker therapy in HFREF was the Metoprolol in Dilated Cardiomyopathy (MDC) trial [57]. In this trial, 383 patients with symptomatic dilated cardiomyopathy with a left ventricular EF less than 40%, already on background treatment with an angiotensin-converting enzyme inhibitor (ACEI), were treated with metoprolol tartrate or placebo and followed for up to 18 months. Metoprolol tartrate was initiated at 10 mg twice daily, and the dose was titrated upwards. The mean dose achieved was 108 mg daily. Metoprolol treatment was associated with a 34% reduction in the combined endpoint of death or need for heart transplantation, but this trend was not statistically significant. Treatment with metoprolol also improved exercise capacity and New York Heart Association (NYHA) class.

The Cardiac Insufficiency Bisoprolol Study (CIBIS) was initiated to determine the effect of β-blocker therapy on mortality in patients with dilated and ischemic cardiomyopathy and assess the tolerability of β-blocker therapy [58]. In the study, 641 patients with advanced heart failure (NYHA classes III and IV) with an LVEF <40% were treated with bisoprolol or placebo and followed for a mean of 1.9 years. Bisoprolol treatment was associated with a 20% reduction in all-cause mortality, but this was not statistically significant (confidence interval 0.56–1.15). However, there was a statistically significant decrease in hospitalization for heart failure and improvement in the NYHA class with bisoprolol treatment.

By the mid-1990s, β-blocker therapy had not yet been proven to affect mortality in heart failure. Several large-scale clinical trials were initiated in this era to determine if β-blocker therapy would indeed improve survival: (1) US Carvedilol Trials Program, (2) Cardiac Insufficiency Bisoprolol Study II (CIBIS-II), and (3) Metoprolol CR/XL Randomized Intervention Trial in Congestive Heart Failure (MERIT-HF). The US Carvedilol Trials Program consisted of four clinical trials performed as part of phase III evaluation of carvedilol and were analyzed together [44]. In the Trials program, 1094 patients with symptomatic heart failure were treated with carvedilol or a placebo [59]. The program was ended early due to the significantly lower number of deaths in patients receiving carvedilol. The annual mortality rate was 3.2% in the carvedilol group compared to 7.8% in the placebo group (a relative risk reduction of 65%). In 1995, carvedilol became the first β-blocker to be approved by the FDA for the treatment of HFrEF.

The US Carvedilol Trials Program was followed by the CIBIS-II and MERIT-HF trials publication. In CIBIS-II, treatment with bisoprolol as compared to placebo conveyed a substantial mortality benefit in patients with advanced heart failure (83% of patients were NYHA class III and 17% were NYHA class IV) and an LVEF <35% [60]. In MERIT-HF, 3991 patients with symptomatic heart failure (mostly NYHA class II and III) and an LVEF <40% were randomized to metoprolol succinate or placebo [61]. It showed statistical improvement in multiple outcomes: a 34% reduction in mortality, a 49% reduction in death from heart failure, and a 41% reduction in sudden cardiac death with metoprolol. Table 7.2 summarizes the five β-blocker trials that have shown statistically significant decreases in mortality.

Despite the favorable results of CIBIS-II, there was no widespread adoption of β-blocker therapy for patients with advanced heart failure

Table 7.2 Major clinical trials of β-blockers in HFREF show a statistically significant decrease in mortality and morbidity.

				Endpoints			
Trial	Year	Agent	Patient group	All-cause mortality	Death from HF	Sudden cardiac death	Admission for HF
US Carvedilol Study Group	1996	Carvedilol vs. placebo	NYHA II-IV, EF ≤ 35	⇓ 65%	⇓ NS	⇓ NS	⇓ 27%
CIBIS II	1999	Bisoprolol vs. placebo	NYHA III-IV EF < 35	⇓ 34%	⇓ NS	⇓ 44%	⇓ 20%
MERIT-HF	1999	Metoprolol succinate vs. placebo	NYHA II-IV EF < 40	⇓ 34%	⇓ 49%	⇓ 41%	⇓ 18%
COPERNICUS	2001	Carvedilol vs. placebo	NYHA III-IV EF < 25	⇓ 35%	NR	NR	⇓ 24%[a]
COMET	2003	Carvedilol vs. metoprolol tartrate	NYHA II-IV, EF ≤ 35	⇓ 17%	NR	NR	⇓ NS

NYHA New York heart association class, *EF* Ejection fraction, *HF* heart failure, *NR* not reported, *NS* not statistically significant.

[a]Combined endpoint of death or hospitalization

[62]. An additional concern is whether racial minorities and women, who had both been underrepresented in previous trials, would derive benefit from β-blocker therapy. In the Beta-Blocker Evaluation of Survival Trial (BEST) trial, 2708 patients with advanced symptomatic heart failure (NYHA classes III and IV) and an LVEF <35% were treated with bucindolol or placebo and followed for a mean of 24 months. The BEST study population was 30% minorities and 23% women. The trial was ended early due to the absence of a significant difference in mortality between the treatment and placebo groups (hazard ratio of 0.9). It is worth noting that there were statistically significant decreases in the secondary outcomes of death from cardiovascular causes and hospitalization for heart failure [63].

Subgroup analysis of the BEST study showed that patients of non-Black race did receive a mortality benefit from bucindolol, whereas Black patients did not. A subsequent study by Bristow and colleagues has suggested that the lack of efficacy in African American patients may be due to a specific deletion within the α_{2c}-AR gene [64]. Additional retrospective review and sub-study analysis of the MERIT-HF Trial has confirmed that β-blockers do improve outcomes in African-American patients with heart failure, although to a lesser extent than in white patients [65]. Beta Blockade appears to be 40–50% less effective in preventing death or hospitalization among African American patients with HF as compared with white individuals [66].

The Carvedilol Prospective Randomized Cumulative Survival Study Group trial (COPERNICUS) was launched in 1997 [59]. In this trial, 2289 patients with advanced symptomatic heart failure (NYHA classes III and IV) and an LVEF <25% were treated with carvedilol or placebo and followed for a mean duration of 10.4 months. The trial was stopped early due to a statistically significant 35% decrease in the risk of death. Importantly, therapy with carvedilol was well tolerated, with a higher withdrawal rate at 1 year in the placebo group over the treatment arm (18.5% vs. 14.8%).

Packer and colleagues published a meta-analysis in 2001 that showed that treatment with carvedilol led to a more significant increase in LVEF than metoprolol [67]. The Carvedilol Or Metoprolol European Trial (COMET) was designed in 2002. In this trial, 3029 patients with symptomatic heart failure and an admission for heart failure within the last 2 years were randomized to carvedilol or metoprolol tartrate [68]. The mean doses achieved were 41.6 mg daily for carvedilol and 85 mg daily for metoprolol. After a mean of 58 months, patients treated with carvedilol had a 17% lower risk of death, but there was no difference in the risk of hospital admission between the two groups. The results of the COMET trial are controversial because metoprolol tartrate is not FDA-approved for heart failure, and the dose achieved in the metoprolol arm was relatively low [69]. A post-hoc analysis of the data from the Multicenter Automatic Defibrillator Implantation Trial With Cardiac Resynchronization Therapy (MADIT-CRT) showed that carvedilol was superior to metoprolol. Over a follow-up of 3.4 years in 1515 patients with mild heart failure (NYHA class I and II, EF ≤ 30%), carvedilol treatment was associated with a 28% lower risk of death or hospitalization for heart failure as compared to metoprolol [70].

These five clinical trials form the evidence basis for utilizing β-blockers in HFREF (summarized in Table 7.2). The use of β-blockers has been shown to decrease mortality, hospitalization and death from heart failure, and sudden cardiac death; therefore, all patients with a left ventricular EF of 40% and below should be treated with a β-blocker in the absence of a significant contraindication. Guidelines from the American College of Cardiology and the Heart Failure Society of America [71] recommend that only three agents, carvedilol, bisoprolol, or metoprolol succinate, should be used to treat patients with HFREF.

In practice, clinicians caring for patients with diagnosed HFREF need to decide when to initiate medical therapy for heart failure and the other available medical treatments. This dilemma is especially pertinent for patients whose initial BP is insufficient for treatment with evidence-based doses of both agents. It is important to note that in the five β-blocker trials showing a decrease in mortality, nearly all patients (>90%) in each trial were already being treated with an ACEI or angiotensin receptor blocker (ARB). A body of data suggests that upfront initiation of a β-blocker is safe and effective. Sliwa and colleagues performed a single-center randomized trial of carvedilol or perindopril (an ACEI) as initial therapy for 78 patients with idiopathic dilated cardiomyopathy [72]. Treatment with the first agent was continued for 6 months, and the second agent was added. Endpoints were reviewed after 1 year. They found that patients in the carvedilol-first group experienced a greater improvement in NYHA class, LVEF, and B-type natriuretic peptide levels, with a higher carvedilol dose achieved. These positive findings led to the CIBIS-III trial, in which 1010 patients with symptomatic heart failure and an EF of less than 35% were randomized to monotherapy with bisoprolol or enalapril for 6 months [73]. After this time, the complimentary drug was initiated and maintained through the end of the trial. Treatment with bisoprolol-first was non-inferior to enalapril-first in the intention-to-treat sample with regards to the primary endpoint of mortality or hospitalization for HF. There was no statistical difference in the frequency of adverse events between the groups. Further analysis of CIBIS-III has shown that 60% of the adverse events occurred during the monotherapy period [74], suggesting that both guideline-based therapies should be implemented and uptitrated without delay.

In addition to a mortality benefit, β-blocker therapy has been shown to have other benefits in patients with HFREF. Treatment with carvedilol and metoprolol succinate has led to reverse remodeling of the left ventricle, characterized by an increase in the EF and a decrease in the end-systolic and end-diastolic volumes [75]. β-blocker therapy improves heart failure symptoms, lowering NYHA class by one grade and improving exercise time [76]. Only one meta-analysis of ten trials showed no significant improvement in quality of life with β-blocker therapy [77].

B-type natriuretic peptide (BNP) and N-terminal proBNP (NT-BNP) are used as both diagnostic and prognostic markers for heart failure [78]. Stanek and colleagues were among the first to examine the effect of β-blocker treatment on BNP and NT-BNP levels [79]. They found that treatment with atenolol for 6 months reduced NT-BNP but not BNP levels. In a substudy of the COPERNICUS trial, treatment with carvedilol did not decrease the median level of NT-BNP as compared to placebo but did decrease NT-BNP when analyzed as a change from baseline level for each patient (25% decrease with carvedilol as compared to 5% decrease with placebo at 6 months) [80]. Treatment with a β-blocker does not affect the utility of these prognostic markers, as BNP and NT-BNP levels remain strongly predictive of mortality [79, 81].

Considerations and Cautions with β-Blocker Therapy

Patients with chronic heart failure are a heterogeneous group with a broad spectrum of cardiovascular diseases and underlying comorbidities. Despite this heterogeneity, multiple subgroups of patients can be safely treated with β-blocker therapy, and their use has few absolute contraindications.

There are important considerations and cautions for the use of β-blockers. Table 7.3 lists the comorbidities and conditions in which β-blocker therapy is generally tolerated or should be used cautiously or avoided.

Concerns that treating HFREF with β-blockers would worsen heart failure symptoms and precipitate decompensation shortly after drug initiation have been prevalent in the past and may continue to influence prescribing practices today [94]. Hemodynamic data confirm that left ventricular systolic pressure and cardiac index acutely decrease [95]. β-blocker administration may decrease sodium excretion and increase volume overload [96]. Consistent with this, BNP and NT-BNP levels are increased compared to baseline when measured 6 weeks after β-blocker initiation and then decline by 3 months [80, 97]. Before each dose increase, the clinician should ensure the patient has maintained clinical stability regarding symptoms, volume status, heart rate, and BP. The frequency of dose increase in clinical trials has varied between 1 week (as in

Table 7.3 Comorbidities and conditions in which β-blocker therapy for HFREF is tolerated or in which therapy should be used with caution or avoided

Generally tolerated	Use with caution	Avoid use
Comorbidities		
Diabetes mellitus	Diabetes mellitus with recurrent hypoglycemic events	
Mild to moderate COPD	Severe COPD with frequent exacerbations	COPD with active bronchoconstriction
Stable RAD, treated with a cardioselective β-blocker	RAD with frequent exacerbations	RAD with active bronchoconstriction
Peripheral arterial disease without claudication	Peripheral arterial disease with claudication	Peripheral arterial disease with critical limb ischemia
Hemodynamic conditions		
Asymptomatic hypotension with SBP > 90 mmHg	Asymptomatic hypotension with SBP 80–90 mmHg	Symptomatic hypotension (e.g., orthostatic symptoms)
Stable advanced heart failure (left ventricular EF ≤ 25%)	Decompensated heart failure; resting sinus tachycardia >100 BPM	Acute hemodynamic instability or use of I.V. beta-agonist (e.g. dobutamine)
Heart rhythm conditions		
Sinus rhythm with heart rate 60–100 BPM	Sinus bradycardia with HR < 60 BPM	Sinus bradycardia with HR < 55 BPM
First-degree AV block; sinus bradycardia during sleep	Type I second-degree AV block (Wenckebach)	Type II second-degree AV block; third-degree AV block

COPD chronic obstructive pulmonary disease, *RAD* reactive airway disease, *SBP* systolic blood pressure, *EF* ejection fraction, *BPM* beats per minute, *HR* heart rate, *AV* atrioventricular [82–93]

CIBIS-II and BEST) and 2 weeks (as in MERIT-HF, COPERNICUS, and COMET), with current guidelines recommending dose increases at two-week intervals. Specialized programs for up-titration of β-blocker dose by nurses are helpful, as they have been shown to achieve higher rates of target β-blocker dose utilization compared to standard of care [98]. The STRONG-HF study found that an intensive treatment strategy of rapid up-titration of several agents was safe and reduced the risk of 180-day all-cause death or heart failure readmission compared with usual care [99]. Prior concerns about the slow up-titration of HF therapies were perhaps unfounded.

Analysis of data from the MERIT-HF trial showed that as early as 90 days after initiation of metoprolol succinate, there was a decrease in the risk of mortality or hospitalization, no change in symptoms, and a decrease in the daily dose of furosemide [100]. Even in patients at very high risk of decompensation, there was no increase in death or hospitalization at 8 weeks in the COPERNICUS trial [101].

Overall tolerability of β-blocker therapy in clinical trials has been excellent, with more patients discontinuing therapy in the placebo group than in the active treatment group [102]. Side effects of bradycardia, dizziness, and hypotension do occur more frequently with β-blocker treatment as compared to placebo but infrequent causes of discontinuation of therapy. Table 7.4 lists the incidence of these side effects as determined in a meta-analysis by Ko and colleagues [102]. B-blockers decrease the sinus rate and prolong conduction through the atrioventricular node, so use is contraindicated in patients with bradycardia (HR < 55 BPM) or high-degree AVB [103]. The role of pacemaker placement to facilitate β-blocker therapy without indications for an implantable cardiac defibrillator or cardiac resynchronization therapy (CRT) is unclear. The Dual Chamber and VVI Implantable Defibrillator II

Table 7.4 Frequency of side effects more commonly seen with β-blocker treatment than placebo by meta-analysis [102]

Side effect	Frequency during treatment with β-blocker	Frequency during treatment with placebo	Risk ratio
Hypotension	7.6%	6.1%	1.41
Dizziness	21.5%	16.6%	1.37
Bradycardia	5.7%	1.8%	3.62

Trial (DAVID-II) showed that atrial pacing at a rate of 70 BPM was safe, although it provided no clinical benefit over backup ventricular pacing at 40 BPM, in patients with HFREF (mean EF 26%) and an implanted defibrillator [104]. Notably, the percentage of patients receiving target dose β-blocker therapy was similar between the two groups, suggesting that pacemaker mode did not significantly affect β-blocker dose titration.

β-Blocker Therapy in Hospitalized Heart Failure Patients

Hospitalization for acute decompensated heart failure is common, with over one million hospitalizations annually [105, 106]. In 1999, due to studies indicating that antagonism of the adrenergic system could lead to volume overload [107], the Advisory Council To Improve Outcomes Nationwide in Heart Failure (ACTION HF) guidelines recommended that patients with decompensation requiring hospitalization should have their β-blocker dose reduced or discontinued [94]. Furthermore, *de novo* initiation or re-initiation of therapy was recommended exclusively in the outpatient setting [108].

Unfortunately, this perspective has persisted among many practicing clinicians despite significant data in the last decade that suggests the contrary. Outcomes are improved by continuing β-blocker therapy during hospitalizations or, when discontinued in the hospital, at least re-initiating therapy before discharge. In the Initiation Management Predischarge: Process for Assessment of Carvedilol Therapy in Heart Failure (IMPACT-HF) trial, 363 patients were randomized to initiation of carvedilol before discharge or at least 2 weeks after discharge [109]. The number of patients treated with any β-blocker 60 days after discharge was significantly higher in the before discharge group (91% vs. 73%), without a significant difference in outcome between the groups. Fonarow and colleagues extended these findings by analyzing patients with HFREF hospitalized in the OPTIMIZE-HF registry [110]. They found that patients who continued β-blocker therapy at hospital admission or started *de novo* had a lower mortality risk 60–90 days after discharge, even after adjusting for clinical variables predictive of post-discharge mortality. Thus, continuation of β-blocker therapy in patients with HFREF who are hospitalized for acute decompensation is recommended unless other contraindications to continued therapy, such as bradycardia or shock, are present. Data from OPTIMIZE-HF showed that patients who are initiated on β-blocker therapy while hospitalized for heart failure are three times more likely to be treated with a β-blocker at 60–90 day follow-up [111]. In a meta-analysis reviewing studies published from January 2002–2015, Prins and colleagues concluded that cessation of beta-blocker therapy in patients admitted with decompensated heart failure was associated significantly with increased in-hospital short-term mortality [112].

Patients hospitalized with acute decompensated heart failure and cardiogenic shock, who are placed on inotropic therapy for hemodynamic support, represent a particular category of patients with advanced cardiomyopathy [113]. The inotropes approved for use in the United States are the β_1-agonist, dobutamine, and the phosphodiesterase III inhibitor, milrinone. Inotropic therapy has long been used to improve hemodynamics in NYHA class IV patients with depressed cardiac output. However, given the improvement in clinical outcomes seen in patients with NYHA class IV heart failure in COPERNICUS, it might be beneficial to treat patients with advanced disease with both an inotrope and a β-blocker [114]. Mehtra and colleagues were the first to carefully study this issue by measuring the hemodynamic response to dobutamine and enoximone (an oral phosphodiesterase III inhibitor) before and after treatment with a β-blocker in 34 patients with HFREF [115]. They found that the hemodynamic effects of dobutamine infusion were blunted by treatment with metoprolol and carvedilol, but the effects of enoximone were not blunted by treatment with either agent. This trial showed that β-blockers should not be used in conjunction with dobutamine but can be used with phosphodiesterase III inhibitors. A review of four studies examining combination treatment with milrinone and β-blockers showed that co-treatment is well-tolerated and has a neutral or beneficial effect on mortality [116]. Combination treatment has also been investigated as a method to help improve cardiac function sufficiently to allow inotrope weaning [117]. We have concluded that β-blockers should not be used with dobutamine because of their blunting effect on the hemodynamic response, but they appear safe to be used with milrinone and may improve outcomes.

Optimization of β-Blocker Therapy

As with all medical therapies for heart failure, there are patient-related and system-based barriers to the optimal utilization of β-blocker therapy. Patient characteristics associated with the inability to tolerate the initiation of carvedilol in the outpatient setting include higher NYHA class, older age, lower diastolic blood pressure, and higher blood urea nitrogen concentration [118]. In a cohort of 340 patients with HFREF, 10% discontinued therapy over 2 years. The most common reason for discontinuation was a failure to restart a β-blocker after hospitalization [119] (Fig. 7.4).

Analysis of the clinical trial data supports this "target dose" strategy, with dose-related improvements in outcomes seen in the MOCHA [120], CIBS-II [121], and COMET trials [122]. This benefit has not been uniformly shown, however, as patients in MERIT-HF receiving low-dose metoprolol (≤ 100 mg daily) or high-dose metoprolol (> 100 mg daily) had a similar benefit of therapy [123]. Nonselective β-adrenergic receptor antagonists have been shown to have more significant effects on norepinephrine release then selective agents [124]. Clinicians should not assume that all beta blockers are interchangeable. In the Carvedilol Heart Failure Registry (COHERE), 55% of patients received less than the target dose of carvedilol [125].

Another potential strategy is to up-titrate the β-blocker dose based on the heart rate, as analyses of the CIBIS-II and COMET trials showed that the benefit of therapy was related to the magnitude of heart rate reduction [122, 126]. McAllister and colleagues performed a meta-analysis of 17 β-blocker clinical trials and found that the magnitude of survival benefit was related to the heart rate reduction, with a relative risk reduction for death of 18% for each decrease in heart rate by five beats/minute [127]. This meta-

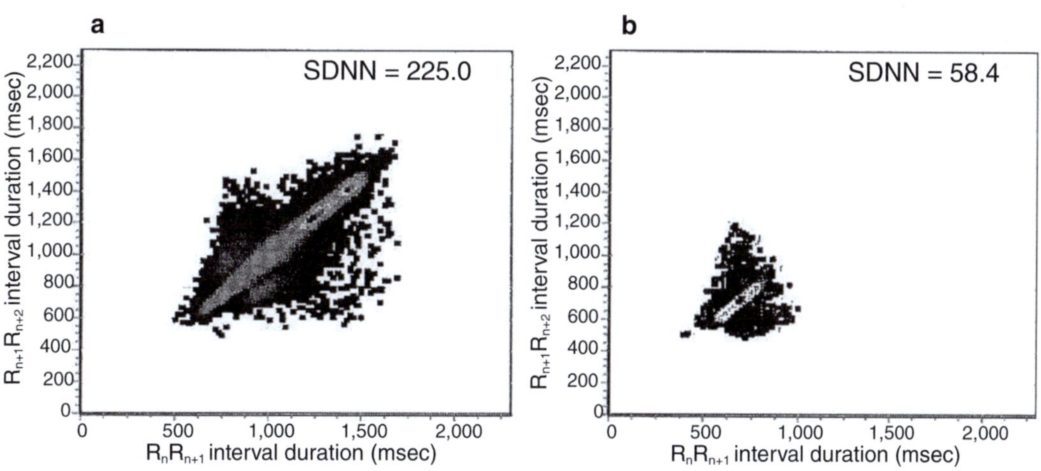

Fig. 7.4 Documented contraindications for β-blocker non-use at the time of hospital discharge in the OPTIMIZE-HF registry. In OPTIMIZE-HF, 9.4% of 18,425 patients had a documented contraindication for β-blocker treatment, as listed in the figure. (Figure reproduced with modification from Fonarow et al. [111], © 2007, with permission from Elsevier)

analysis showed no relationship between the β-blocker dose achieved and the survival benefit. The optimal dosing strategy is unclear, but guidelines recommend titration to target the doses used in the clinical trials of β-blockers [71].

β-Blocker Therapy in HF with Mid-Range or Preserved Ejection Fraction

It is well established that heart failure with preserved ejection fraction (HFpEF) is a distinct heart failure syndrome as compared to HFrEF [128]. Because of the limited understanding of the underlying myocardial biology and pathophysiology of HFpEF, it continues to present a therapeutic challenge.

When the European Society of Cardiology introduced the intermediate phenotype known as mid-range ejection fraction (HFmrEF)—defined as an EF 40–49%—guidelines suggested that HFmrEF should be managed similarly to HFpEF [129]. These guidelines were later updated to reflect a treatment strategy that better supported the shared characteristics between HFmrEF and HFrEF patients and included support for administering beta-blockers [130].

In the Study of the Effects of Nebivolol Intervention on Outcomes and Rehospitalization in Seniors with Heart Failure (SENIORS) trial, 2135 patients aged 70 or older with admission for heart failure within the last year or an EF $\leq$ 35% were randomized to treatment with nebivolol or placebo [131]. The enrolled population was a mix of patients with HFrEF (two-thirds with EF $\leq$ 35%) and mildly reduced EF (one-third with EF > 35%). After a mean of 20 months, patients treated with nebivolol had a 14% lower risk of death or hospitalization, verifying that elderly patients with heart failure benefit from β-blocker therapy. When analyzed by baseline EF, there was a similar trend toward benefit in patients with HFrEF and those with a mildly reduced EF [132].

Although no specific trials exist for beta-blockade use in HFmrEF, an individual patient data meta-analysis of 11 landmark trials showed a similar benefit of improved LVEF and prognosis in patients with a baseline EF of 40–49% and EF <40%. A 4.7% absolute reduction in cardiovascular mortality was noted in the HFmrEF population. No benefit was seen in patients with LVEF >50%; however, the randomized study group was deemed too small to draw definitive conclusions [130].

When Medicare Claims data and the OPTIMIZE-HF registry were merged, long-term outcomes of beta-blocker initiation during hospitalizations for heart failure were analyzed. HFpEF patients did not have improved survival or decreased rehospitalization for heart failure at 1 year and had worse outcomes than those with systolic dysfunction [133]. In a prospective observational cohort study using data from the Pinnacle registry, beta-blockers were administered at first encounters in outpatients older than 65 with known heart failure. Among the cohort, 400,000 patients with heart failure with ejection fraction greater than 40% used a beta-blocker at the first encounter. Their usage was associated with an increased risk for heart failure hospitalization and death in those patients with ejection fraction greater than 60% [134].

The available data suggest that the level of SNS activation is lower in HFpEF than in HFrEF [135, 136]; which may support one of the reasons behind the limited efficacy of anti-adrenergic therapies in this population. Other proposed mechanisms for the potentially harmful effects of beta-blockers may be related to the increased filling pressures associated with slowing the resting heart rate in patients with associated chronotropic incompetency, ultimately raising ventricular load and myocardial wall stress [137].

Pharmacologic Agents: Other Agents

Several non-beta-blocker pharmacologic agents also inhibit the sympathetic nervous system and have been used to treat heart failure. These agents are worth reviewing, including ACE inhibitors, Sodium Glucose Co-Transporter 2 (SGLT2) inhibitors, Angiotensin Receptor-Neprilysin Inhibitors (ARNI), and the lesser-used clonidine, moxonidine, and statins.

Ace Inhibitors

Although ACE inhibitor effects on the neuroendocrine system are a well-established mechanism of action in treating HF, sympathetic inhibition may also contribute positively as the two systems are more closely interconnected than previously realized.

The Renin Angiotensin Aldosterone System (RAAS) is a major modulator of the SNS in HF animal models, revealing that angiotensin-converting enzyme 2 (ACE2) plays a role in the upregulation of Angiotensin type 1 receptors (AT1R) in the rostral ventrolateral medulla—a receptor involved in the sympathoexcitatory pathway [138]. Additionally, angiotensin type II receptors (AT2R), which participate in sympathoinhibition, were found to be downregulated in CHF rat models [139]. Although no studies have been performed to evaluate receptor expression in the presence of ace inhibitors, one can extrapolate that should ACE2 levels decline, sympathoexcitation would also fall.

The V-HeFT II (Veterans Affairs Vasodilator-Heart Failure) trial was compared using two vasodilators in HFrEF patients: hydralazine–isosorbide dinitrate and enalapril. After 2 years of administration, the enalapril arm showed an 18% survival benefit compared to hydralazine-isosorbide dinitrate [140]. Additionally, the plasma norepinephrine increased significantly in patients assigned to hydralazine-isosorbide dinitrate than those on enalapril at both 13 weeks (p = 0.01) and 1 year (p = 0.04) (90 +/− 302 pg/mL [n = 240] versus 14 +/− 376 pg/mL [n = 265]) [140].

ARNIs

With the results of the PARADIGM-HF (Prospective Comparison of ARNI with an ACE-Inhibitor to Determine Impact on Global Mortality and Morbidity in HF) trial showing improved outcomes in patients on sacubitril-valsartan to enalapril, guidelines have shifted for the preferential use of ARNIs in HFrEF patients.

Bunsawat *et al.* showed a 17% reduction in MSNA burst frequency and a 19% reduction in MSNA burst incidence after 2 months of treatment with sacubitril-valsartan [141]. This reduction was noted in patients already on guideline-directed pharmacotherapy composed of known SNS lowering drugs (B-blockers, Aldosterone agents, and statins) [141].

Suggested mechanisms for this robust effect are related to the drug's ability to simultaneously affect both the RAAS and natriuretic peptide (NP) pathways.

Although inhibition of the SNS has been proven in both ACEI and ARNI separately, no studies currently compare the reduction of SNS activity incurred by each drug group. One could hypothesize that the SNS inhibition would be higher given the improved mortality benefits of ARNIs; however, further studies are needed.

SGLT-2 Inhibitors

In recent years, landmark clinical trials have revealed a dramatic reduction in morbidity and mortality in HF patients with the addition of SGLT-2 inhibitors (SLGT-2i). The mechanism of action of these benefits is considered multifactorial and not completely understood; however, it posits a role in inhibiting the SNS.

A study using human renal proximal tubule cells administered NE treatment, which promoted a significant translocation of SGLT2 to the cell surface. After that, dapagliflozin treatment was given in high-fat diet-fed mice, revealing a reduction of NE in the kidney and heart. Additionally, the investigators showed a reduction in the expression of tyrosine hydroxylase, an enzyme that catalyzes the rate-limiting step in catecholamine synthesis, in this model [142].

Another proposed mechanism suggests that the reduced renal stress induced by SGLT-2i inhibits renal afferent signaling to the brain [143]. This decreased sympathetic outflow enables the kidney to excrete more sodium and water, improving the overall fluid balance.

Moxonidine

Moxonidine is a centrally acting imidazoline receptor agonist, a relative of the $alpha_2$ adrenoreceptor family, and works to decrease sympathetic nervous system tone, not unlike clonidine. Although not used in the United States, it has been known as an effective anti-hypertensive agent and was considered superior to clonidine given its comparatively favorable side effect profile [144].

One of the first studies that investigated NE levels in association with moxonidine in patients with CHF showed only a Non-sustained reduction in NE, which was thought to be the result of using a standard preparation of the drug as after only one day of drug withdrawal, NE levels and heart rates began to increase [145]. This prompted the development of a sustained-release formulation of moxonidine, which was then studied in 268 patients with CHF on best standard therapy over 19 weeks [146]. Baseline norepinephrine levels were collected, and patients were randomized to placebo or 1 of 5 doses of moxonidine that were up-titrated. NE levels were collected weekly during the first 7 weeks and again at week 19 and various other time points per the study protocol. A statistically significant dose-related decrease in NE was observed, as well as reductions in heart rate and modest increases in left ventricular ejection fractions. Despite the perceived benefit, though, adverse effects were numerous, including rebound headaches and dizziness during the washout phase, but also saw an increased number of deaths in the 0.9 to 1.5 mg BID dosing regimen [146].

Occurring concurrently was a much larger randomized, double-blind, placebo-controlled trial started in 425 centers across 17 countries—The Moxonidine in Congestive Heart Failure (MOXCON) trial. The adverse effects were not dissimilar to the study above, and the trial ended early because of excess early mortality in the treatment arm [147]. Although it was unclear whether the deaths were secondary to protocol design and dosing or the mechanism of action of the drug, the study concluded that while SNS activation plays a crucial role in the pathophysiology of heart failure, its inhibition needed to be considered carefully as a treatment modality.

No further trials with moxonidine have since been pursued.

Clonidine

The harmful outcomes of the MOXCON trial caused a shift in how the central SNS was targeted, as such trials with clonidine were limited given its similar mechanism of action to moxonidine acting via $alpha_2$ adrenergic and imidazoline receptors. However, acute and chronic drug administrations have shown attenuation of the SNS without notable mortality [148–150].

Grassi *et al.* evaluated NE levels and sympathetic nerve bursts (MSNA) in 26 patients with CHF (NYHA II – III, treated with enalapril and furosemide) with a 2-month transdermal clonidine patch. They found a 46.8% ($p < 0.01$) reduction in NE without affecting exercise capacity or LVEF, as well as a 26.7% reduction in MSNA ($p < 0.01$) [149]. Although it had previously been hypothesized that the decline of NE associated with clonidine use was solely related to neurotransmitter clearance, the investigators demonstrated a true reduction in central sympathetic drive [149]. Aggarwal *et al.* revealed a similar phenomenon. However, it additionally demonstrated a concurrent reduction of the renal sympathetic tone of 32% ($p = 0.01$) [150].

Of all the previous studies, improvement in EF was either not reported or not noted. However, one prospective randomized, double-blind, placebo-controlled study of 30 chronic HF patients did establish an improvement in exercise capacity, NYHA functional class, and symptom burden as measured by the Minnesota Living with Heart Failure questionnaire (MLHFQ) [151]. The investigators urged that the harmful mortality noted with moxonidine should not be extended to clonidine and that low doses in patients who are intolerant to beta-blocker therapy may be reasonable.

Statins

Cholesterol, inflammation, and oxidative stress reduction are well-known endpoints for statin use (3-hydroxy-3-methylglutaryl-CoA reductase inhibitors), but their regulatory function on the autonomic nervous system is much less well described.

Studies performed in heart failure animal models have shown consistent reductions in renal sympathetic nerve activity (RSNA) and plasma NE concentrations [152]. When rabbits were treated with sodium nitroprusside infusion, heart rate and baroreflex response of RSNA were normalized in the group treated with simvastatin over 3 weeks. This response was documented after only 7 days of statin treatment in normolipidemic rabbits [153].

Despite these promising results, human heart failure studies have been much more variable and, subsequently, less conclusive. One prospective study evaluated eight patients with NYHA II-IV with LVEF <40% 8 weeks before and after statin discontinuation. They reported a significant increase in the incidence of MSNA upon statin discontinuation that returned to baseline 4 weeks after their re-initiation [154]. Deo *et al.* had similar findings in a small double-blinded placebo-controlled crossover study but also measured reactive oxygen species (ROS) and superoxide levels. Simvastatin use reduced resting MSNA (59 ± 5 placebo vs. 45 ± 6 statin bursts/100 heartbeats; $P < 0.05$) and significantly reduced ROS and superoxide levels, but there was no notable effect on the resting HR or systolic BP [155].

In contrast, a controlled study using 3 months of fluvastatin in ischemic cardiomyopathy patients revealed improved heart rate recovery at 1 and 3 minutes following peak exertion [156]. This finding did not correlate with statin therapy's anti-lipidemic effects, further supporting this hypothesized pleiotropic effect. A meta-analysis involving patients with heart failure and hypertension by Lewandowski *et al.* supported this sympathoinhibitory effect of statins as independent of cholesterol levels, but once again, no BP or HR changes were noted [157].

Although a sympathoinhibitory property exists within the statin drug class, the lack of consistency in dosing, timeline, and statin choice itself across study data has made its application outside of lipid-lowering therapy challenging and difficult to justify.

Non-pharmacologic Therapies for SNS Inhibition

Several non-pharmacologic therapies have been shown to reduce SNS activity in heart failure. Cardiac resynchronization therapy (CRT), continuous positive airway pressure (CPAP) for obstructive sleep apnea, and exercise training have entered standard HFREF management. Alternative therapies, such as Tai Chi and meditation, are potentially beneficial but are underutilized. Decreased SNS activity may be an early signal that a therapeutic modality could have positive clinical outcomes. While not all therapies discussed here have shown a conclusive improvement in hard clinical endpoints, many show promise in treating HF by lowering SNS activity.

CRT and Pacing

In HFREF patients with ventricular dyssynchrony, as marked by prolonged interventricular conduction, CRT is an effective procedure with both mortality and morbidity improvement [158]. CRT is discussed in further detail in Chap. 17. Three studies have shown that CRT improved HRV as measured by mean atrial cycle length [159], SDNN [160], or standard deviation of the sensed atrial-to-atrial intervals (SDAAN) [161]. Cha and colleagues also showed that CRT improves the heart-to-mediastinum ratio on MIBG imaging [160]. One aspect of CRT effectiveness derives from decreased activation of SNS in implanted patients [162].

For many years, pacemaker placement and AV Nodal ablation have been a strategy for the treatment of refractory atrial fibrillation. Earlier reports indicated a cardiac sudden death rate post-procedure of up to 7%, which was decreased to as low as 0% with the initiation of a post-procedural ventricular pacing protocol at 90 beats per minute [163]. Hamdan and colleagues attempted to determine the changes in sympathetic nerve activity due to AV junction ablation in patients with chronic atrial fibrillation [164]. They used muscle SNA, evaluated by microneurography, and measured monophasic cardiac action potential duration (APD) and effective refractory period (ERP) before and after the ablation procedure. They saw an apparent rise in sympathetic nervous system activation post-ablation, which was ameliorated by ventricular pacing at an increased rate. The exact mechanism of SNS activation in context was unclear, but the implication was significant.

Sleep Apnea

Sleep apnea comprises obstructive sleep apnea (OSA), central sleep apnea (CSA), and a mixed sleep apnea phenotype. Obstructive sleep apnea (OSA) is common in patients with HFREF, with Sin and colleagues finding a prevalence of 37% in 450 patients referred for polysomnography [165]. Muscle sympathetic nerve activity (MSNA) is the most employed technique for determining SNS activation during sleep. It can be measured directly by placing a fine needle electrode into a superficial peripheral nerve [166]. Regular sleep is associated with decreased sympathetic outflow and reduced BP and HR [167].

In contrast, patients with OSA have elevated sympathetic activation, both during episodes of apnea during sleep and even during daytime wakefulness [168]. Importantly, treatment of OSA with nocturnal CPAP has been shown to reduce sympathetic outflow, heart rate, and BP [169]. Nocturnal CPAP for even a month in a group of HF subjects (mean LVEF 25%) was associated with improved left ventricular end-systolic dimension and systolic function [170]. Patients with HFREF and OSA who are either not treated with CPAP or not fully compliant with therapy have a higher mortality [171]. As opposed to treating OSA with noninvasive positive pressure ventilation, managing CSA has been challenging. Several randomized trials show that sympathetic activity is reduced with positive airway treatment or nocturnal oxygen in patients with CSA. However, the two largest RCTs in patients with CSA and HfrEF were not only negative concerning their primary outcomes but also associated with excess mortality [172]. The pathophysiology of this finding is not fully understood [173].

Vagal Nerve Stimulation

Vagal nerve stimulation (VNS) is a potential therapy for heart failure with reduced ejection fraction (HFrEF). The rationale is that VNS can increase efferent parasympathetic input to the heart and reduce the effects of an overly active SNS, which may help halt or reverse the progression of heart failure [174]. Concurrent to the activation of the SNS that occurs in HFREF is the withdrawal of vagal activity [175]. Chronic vagal nerve electrical stimulation (VNS) improved HRV and led to reverse remodeling in a pacing-induced animal model of HFREF [176]. In the Cardiofit Multicenter trial, the safety and efficacy of the CardioFit VNS device were evaluated in an uncontrolled trial of 32 patients with HFREF [177]. After 6 months of therapy, 41% of patients experienced a severe adverse event, not unanticipated for a novel device. However, there were significant improvements in heart failure symptoms, 6-minute walk distance, and EF. If VNS therapy improves outcomes, non-invasive markers of SNS activation, such as low HRV and low heart-to-mediastinum ratio on MIBG, may identify patients who may benefit from this therapy.

However, despite promising preclinical and pilot clinical studies, the two large, controlled trials—NECTAR-HF and INOVATE-HF—failed to demonstrate benefit [178]. The clinical application of VNS in these phase III studies was believed to be performed before a sufficient degree of understanding of the complex pathophysiology of autonomic electrical modulation, leading to an underestimation of its potential benefit. The complicated issues of delivering the correct type of VNS (i.e., pulse amplitude, frequency, duration, and duty cycle) may account for the failure of these trials [179]. A more extensive randomized trial (ANTHEM-HFrEF) with an adaptive design should overcome some challenges. In the study, most patients were identified as having NYHA Class 3 symptoms with an average LVEF of approximately 26%. The subjects were well-treated, with over 80% on ACEI/ARB/ARNI and nearly all on beta-blockers. However, it failed to show a difference in the primary endpoint of CV death or HF hospitalization with over more than three years of follow-up. Perhaps disappointingly, the sponsor halted the trial, with only half the expected subjects enrolled. When the researchers analyzed the change in the Kansas City Cardiomyopathy Questionnaire (KCCQ) overall summary score from the start of the study to 9 months later, they found that Vagal Nerve Stimulation (VNS) did have a positive effect. The score improved by 13.1 points for patients with VNS, compared to an improvement of 7.5 points for those without VNS (one-sided $P < 0.001$). This indicates an advantage for VNS in improving the quality of life for these subjects [180].

Baroreflex Activation Therapy

Baroreflex activation therapy (BAT) is one such device-based approach. It involves an implanted pulse generator, an external programming system and leads near the carotid sinus to deliver electrical pulses to the carotid baroreceptors. This electrical stimulation activates the baroreflex system, increasing parasympathetic output and inhibiting sympathetic activity. In a proof-of-concept study, 11 patients with heart failure (HF), New York Heart Association (NYHA) class III, and left ventricular ejection fraction (LVEF) of less than 40% who were ineligible for cardiac resynchronization therapy (CRT) received Baroreflex Activation Therapy (BAT) with Barostim™ neo [181]. After 6 months, there was a significant improvement in baroreflex sensitivity, LVEF, NYHA class, Minnesota Living with HF (MLHFQ) score, and 6-minute walk distance, with only one complication (perioperative anemia). This was followed by the phase II HOPE4HF (Barostim® Hope of HF Study) trial, which randomized 146 patients with LVEF ≤35% and NYHA functional class III to either medical therapy alone or BAT and medical therapy. BAT with medical therapy improved NYHA functional class, MLHFQ score, and 6-minute walk distance and demonstrated an excellent safety profile with freedom from major adverse neurological and cardiovascular events of 97.2% [182].

BeAT-HF was a prospective, multicenter, randomized 2-arm, parallel-group trial designed to test the safety and effectiveness of BAT with the BAROSTIM NEO system (CVRx, Minneapolis, Minnesota) in patients with HFrEF [183]. The trial was designed under the FDA's Breakthrough Devices Program implemented after the twenty-first Century Cures Act to promote and accelerate patient access to technologies for treating life-threatening or debilitating diseases. The trial was designed to encompass a pre-market phase that examined three effectiveness endpoints (6MHW, QOL, and NT-proBNP) and one safety endpoint (major adverse neurological or cardiovascular system or procedure-related event-free rate). Subsequently, 408 patients with LVEF ≤35% and NYHA functional class II-III with an NT-proBNP <1600 pg/mL were enrolled. BAT significantly improved these outcomes at 6 months, with a low adverse event profile [184]. This led to an FDA-approved indication for BAT in 2019. The pre-market phase used an FDA-approved adaptive design and developed four study cohorts (A, B, C, and D). The post-market phase of all four cohorts was concluded and presented at ESC Congress 2023, and the primary endpoint of composite CV mortality and heart failure morbidity was not a statistically significant trend that favored BAT. Long-term safety and long-term symptom improvement continued to statistically favor BAT to a degree over other therapies for heart failure. Published results are forthcoming.

Exercise

Exercise training has been prescribed to improve the quality of life and outcomes in patients with heart failure [185]. In the Heart Failure: A Controlled Trial Investigating Outcomes of Exercise Training (HF-ACTION) trial, implementing a structured exercise program led to a statistically significant decrease in the composite endpoint of all-cause mortality or hospitalization [186]. A review of multiple studies by Gademan et al. demonstrates that exercise training improves heart rate variability in heart failure patients [187]. Furthermore, Roveda and colleagues recorded muscle sympathetic nerve activity in 16 patients with HFREF and found that it decreased significantly after exercise training in HFREF patients, even to the levels seen in normal controls [188]. Exercise intensity in earlier studies was moderate-intensity continuous training (MICT); however, more recent literature has focused on the clinical benefits of high-intensity interval training (HIIT) [189].

In a small but elegantly designed study, Sales and colleagues compared the effects of HITT on muscle sympathetic nerve activity and peripheral vascular function in patients with HFREF [190]. While cardiopulmonary exercise fitness (peak VO2) measurements, left ventricular ejection fraction, and blood pressure were unchanged between the MICT and HITT groups, high-intensity training significantly improved MSNA and brachial artery blood flow responsiveness. As expected, both types of training improved all parameters over the 12-week study compared to a no-training cohort. In a meta-analysis of training modes between traditional MICT, combined aerobic and resistance training (CT) and (HIIT) in a population of HFPEF and HFREF patients, HIIT was significantly more effective than MIT for improving peak VO2 and LVEF [191].

Meditation

Emotional stress affects the level of activation of the SNS via the hypothalamus [192]. This heart-brain connection is most clinically relevant in stress cardiomyopathy (also known as Takotsubo cardiomyopathy), in which sudden, severe, mental, or physical stress leads to acute myocardial dysfunction [193]. Stress cardiomyopathy is felt to be mediated, at least in part, by high circulating levels of catecholamines [194]. Therefore, it is not surprising that non-pharmacologic therapies aimed at decreasing mental stress have been shown to have benefits in heart failure. Tai Chi, also known as Tai Chi Chuan, is a mind–body exercise that originated in China over 1000 years ago that blends the three components of movement, meditation and deep breathing [195]. In 2004, Yeh and colleagues randomized 30 patients with HFREF to 12 weeks of Tai Chi training or no training [196]. After the study, patients in the Tai Chi group demonstrated an improved quality of life, improved six-minute walk distance, and a trend toward lower BNP levels. Meditation has also been shown to lower norepinephrine levels and increase Minnesota Living with Heart Failure Questionnaire scores [197]. These alternative therapies can potentially improve the quality of life and outcomes in patients with several cardiovascular disease states.

Renal Denervation

The relationship between the kidney and the SN is complex and likely plays a role in a variety of cardiovascular diseases, including hypertension and heart failure. Renal denervation (RDN) therapy is a minimally invasive technique that employs radiofrequency energy using a specialized catheter placed into the renal arteries. The U.S. Food and Drug Administration (FDA) has recently approved two renal denervation (RDN) systems for the treatment of refractory hypertension: the Medtronic Symplicity Spyral RDN System, which uses four RFA electrodes and the Recor Medical Paradise Ultrasound RDN System. Regardless of the device used, operators can effectively ablate afferent and efferent renal nerves, which run along the entire length of the renal vessels.

Brandt et al. first reported that RDN significantly reduced LV mass and improved diastolic function at 6 months in 46 patients with refractory hypertension, while no significant changes were observed in control patients [198]. The first randomized, open-controlled trial to evaluate the effectiveness of RDN in HFpEF patients was terminated early due to recruitment difficulties (only 25 HFpEF patients were randomized 2:1 to receive RDN or medication). The trial did not detect improved QOL (MLWHFQ score), exercise function, BNP, and cardiac remodeling at 12 months, although RDN improved VO2 peak and E/e′ at 3 months [199]. Schirmer SH et al. found that the improvement of LV hypertrophy and diastolic function by RDN after 6 months was unrelated to a reduction in systolic blood pressure and heart rate, suggesting a direct effect of RDN on changes in the cardiac phenotype [200]. The ongoing UNLOAD-HFpEF (Renal Denervation to Treat Heart Failure with Preserved Ejection Fraction) trial is the first randomized, sham-controlled, double-blind pilot trial that will further address the role of RDN in HFpEF.

Conclusions

Activation of the SNS is among the fundamental neurohormonal abnormalities in heart failure [201]. Initially, SNS activation is compensatory but subsequently contributes to disease progression and the clinical sequelae of heart failure. A few pioneering clinical studies in the 1970s showed that treatment with β-blockers dramatically improved the clinical status of heart failure patients, which critically altered the notions about the pathophysiology of the chronic heart failure state. Multicenter clinical trials subsequently enrolled many thousands of subjects and have shown unrefutably that β-blockers improve clinical outcomes in patients with HFREF [202] and that the mechanism of this improvement is the inhibition of the SNS. While a small number of patients do not tolerate β-blocker therapy due to comorbidities, the greatest challenge is the appropriate application and up-titration of this life-saving therapy. Currently, several non-beta blocker pharmacologic therapies also appear to impact the sympathetic nervous system in heart failure patients and have been shown to provide mortality and morbidity benefits. Various device therapies are reaching widespread clinical applicability, most of which rest on the foundational appreciation that inhibiting the sympathetic nervous system is central to achieving clinical effectiveness. Understanding how to measure and manipulate the SNS will allow researchers to develop future therapeutic interventions to combat the complex clinical syndrome of heart failure.

References

1. Cannon WB. Bodily changes in pain, hunger, fear and rage. New York/Littleton: D. Appleton and Co.; 1929.
2. Ahlquist RP. A study of the adrenotropic receptors. Am J Phys. 1948;153(3):586–600.
3. Malpas SC. Sympathetic nervous system overactivity and its role in the development of cardiovascular disease. Physiol Rev. 2010;90(2):513–57. PubMed CrossRef.
4. Wenger NK, Greenbaum LM. From adrenoceptor mechanisms to clinical therapeutics: Raymond Ahlquist, Ph.D., 1914–1983. J Am Coll Cardiol. 1984;3(2 Pt 1):419–21.
5. Limbird LE. Historical perspective for understanding of adrenergic receptors. Curr Top Membr. 2011;67:1–17.
6. Wachter SB, Gilbert EM. Beta-adrenergic receptors, from their discovery and characterization through their manipulation to beneficial clinical application. Cardiology. 2012;122(2):104–12.
7. Jänig W. The integrative action of the autonomic nervous system: neurobiology of homeostasis. Cambridge: Cambridge University Press; 2006. CrossRef.
8. Janes RD, Brandys JC, Hopkins DA, Johnstone DE, Murphy DA, Armour JA. Anatomy of human extrinsic cardiac nerves and ganglia. Am J Cardiol. 1986;57(4):299–309. PubMed CrossRef.
9. Randall WC, Szentivanyi M, Pace JB, Wechsler JS, Kaye MP. Patterns of sympathetic nerve projections onto the canine heart. Circ Res. 1968;22(3):315–23. PubMed CrossRef.
10. Fuller MD, Emrick MA, Sadilek M, Scheuer T, Catterall WA. Molecular mechanism of calcium channel regulation in the fight-or-flight response. Sci Signal. 2010;3(141):ra70. https://doi.org/10.1126/scisignal.2001152. PubMed PubMedCentral CrossRef.

11. Shan J, Kushnir A, Betzenhauser MJ, Reiken S, Li J, Lehnart SE, et al. Phosphorylation of the ryanodine receptor mediates the cardiac fight or flight response in mice. J Clin Invest. 2010;120(12):4388–98. PubMed PubMedCentral CrossRef.
12. Katz AM, Konstam MA. Heart failure: pathophysiology, molecular biology, and clinical management. 2nd ed. Philadelphia: Lippincott Williams & Wilkins; 2012.
13. Ginsburg R, Bristow MR, Billingham ME, Stinson EB, Schroeder JS, Harrison DC. Study of the normal and failing isolated human heart: decreased response of failing heart to isoproterenol. Am Heart J. 1983;106(3):535–40. PubMed CrossRef.
14. Floras JS. Sympathetic nervous system activation in human heart failure. J Am Coll Cardiol. 2009;54(5):375–85.
15. Swedberg K, Viquerat C, Rouleau JL, Roizen M, Atherton B, Parmley WW, et al. Comparison of myocardial catecholamine balance in chronic congestive heart failure and in angina pectoris without failure. Am J Cardiol. 1984;54(7):783–6. PubMed CrossRef.
16. Bristow MR, Ginsburg R, Minobe W, Cubicciotti RS, Sageman WS, Lurie K, et al. Decreased catecholamine sensitivity and beta-adrenergic-receptor density in failing human hearts. N Engl J Med. 1982;307(4):205–11. PubMed CrossRef.
17. Fowler MB, Laser JA, Hopkins GL, Minobe W, Bristow MR. Assessment of the beta-adrenergic receptor pathway in the intact failing human heart: progressive receptor down-regulation and subsensitivity to agonist response. Circulation. 1986;74(6):1290–302. PubMed CrossRef.
18. Communal C, Singh K, Pimentel DR, Colucci WS. Norepinephrine stimulates apoptosis in adult rat ventricular myocytes by activation of the beta-adrenergic pathway. Circulation. 1998;98(13):1329–34. PubMed CrossRef.
19. Narula J, Haider N, Virmani R, DiSalvo TG, Kolodgie FD, Hajjar RJ, et al. Apoptosis in myocytes in end-stage heart failure. N Engl J Med. 1996;335(16):1182–9. PubMed CrossRef.
20. Cao JM, Fishbein MC, Han JB, Lai WW, Lai AC, Wu TJ, et al. Relationship between regional cardiac hyperinnervation and ventricular arrhythmia. Circulation. 2000;101(16):1960–9. PubMed CrossRef.
21. Bohm M, La Rosée K, Schwinger RH, Erdmann E. Evidence for reduction of norepinephrine uptake sites in the failing human heart. J Am Coll Cardiol. 1995;25(1):146–53. PubMed CrossRef.
22. Cohn JN, Levine TB, Olivari MT, Garberg V, Lura D, Francis GS, Simon AB, Rector T. Plasma norepinephrine as a guide to prognosis in patients with chronic congestive heart failure. N Engl J Med. 1984;311:819–23.
23. Hjemdahl P. Plasma catecholamines—analytical challenges and physiological limitations. Bailliere Clin Endocrinol Metab. 1993;7(2):307–53.
24. Goldstein DS, McCarty R, Polinsky RJ, Kopin IJ. Relationship between plasma norepinephrine and sympathetic neural activity. Hypertension. 1983;5(4):552–9.
25. Verschure D, Nakajima K, Verberne H. Cardiac 123I-mIBG imaging in heart failure. Pharmaceuticals. 2022;15(6):656.
26. Thackeray JT, Bengel FM. Assessment of cardiac autonomic neuronal function using PET imaging. J Nucl Cardiol. 2013;20(1):150–65. PubMed CrossRef.
27. Carrió I, Cowie MR, Yamazaki J, Udelson J, Camici PG. Cardiac sympathetic imaging with mIBG in heart failure. JACC Cardiovasc Imaging. 2010;3(1):92–100. PubMed CrossRef.
28. Merlet P, Valette H, Dubois-Randé JL, Moyse D, Duboc D, Dove P, et al. Prognostic value of cardiac metaiodobenzylguanidine imaging in patients with heart failure. J Nucl Med. 1992;33(4):471–7. PubMed.
29. Jacobson AF, Senior R, Cerqueira MD, Wong ND, Thomas GS, Lopez VA, et al. Myocardial Iodine-123 meta-iodobenzylguanidine imaging and cardiac events in heart failure. J Am Coll Cardiol. 2010;55(20):2212–21. PubMed CrossRef.
30. Cohen-Solal A, Rouzet F, Berdeaux A, Le Guludec D, Abergel E, Syrota A, et al. Effects of carvedilol on myocardial sympathetic innervation in patients with chronic heart failure. J Nucl Med. 2005;46(11):1796–803. PubMed.
31. Kasama S, Toyama T, Hatori T, Sumino H, Kumakura H, Takayama Y, et al. Evaluation of cardiac sympathetic nerve activity and left ventricular remodeling in patients with dilated cardiomyopathy on the treatment containing carvedilol. Eur Heart J. 2007;28(8):989–95. PubMed CrossRef.
32. DiFrancesco D. The role of the funny current in pacemaker activity. Circ Res. 2010;106(3):434–46. PubMed CrossRef.
33. Frenneaux MP. Autonomic changes in patients with heart failure and in post-myocardial infarction patients. Heart. 2004;90(11):1248–55. PubMed PubMedCentral CrossRef.
34. Heart rate variability: standards of measurement, physiological interpretation and clinical use. Task force of the European Society of Cardiology and the North American Society of Pacing and Electrophysiology. Circulation. 1996;93(5):1043–65.
35. Casolo G, Balli E, Taddei T, Amuhasi J, Gori C. Decreased spontaneous heart rate variability in congestive heart failure. Am J Cardiol. 1989;64(18):1162–7. PubMed CrossRef.
36. Ponikowski P, Anker SD, Chua TP, Szelemej R, Piepoli M, Adamopoulos S, et al. Depressed heart rate variability as an independent predictor of death in chronic congestive heart failure secondary to ischemic or idiopathic dilated cardiomyopathy. Am J Cardiol. 1997;79(12):1645–50. PubMed CrossRef.

37. Bilchick KC, Fetics B, Djoukeng R, Fisher SG, Fletcher RD, Singh SN, et al. Prognostic value of heart rate variability in chronic congestive heart failure (veterans affairs' survival trial of antiarrhythmic therapy in congestive heart failure). Am J Cardiol. 2002;90(1):24–8. PubMed CrossRef.
38. Mortara A, La Rovere MT, Pinna GD, Maestri R, Capomolla S, Cobelli F. Nonselective beta-adrenergic blocking agent, carvedilol, improves arterial baroreflex gain and heart rate variability in patients with stable chronic heart failure. J Am Coll Cardiol. 2000;36(5):1612–8. PubMed CrossRef.
39. Bullinga JR, Alharethi R, Schram MS, Bristow MR, Gilbert EM. Changes in heart rate variability are correlated to hemodynamic improvement with chronic carvedilol therapy in heart failure. J Card Fail. 2005;11(9):693–9. PubMed CrossRef.
40. Strauss HW, Johnson MN, Schöder H, Tamaki N. Metaiodobenzylguanidine imaging comes of age. A new arrow in the prognostic quiver for heart failure patients. J Am Coll Cardiol. 2010;55(20):2222–4. PubMed CrossRef.
41. Black JW, Crowther AF, Shanks RG, Smith LH, Dornhorst AC. A new adrenergic beta-receptor antagonist. Lancet. 1964;1(7342):1080–1. PubMed CrossRef.
42. Stapleton MP. Sir James Black and propranolol. The role of the basic sciences in the history of cardiovascular pharmacology. Tex Heart Inst J. 1997;24(4):336–42. PubMed PubMedCentral.
43. Frishman WH, Alwarshetty M. Beta-adrenergic blockers in systemic hypertension: pharmacokinetic considerations related to the current guidelines. Clin Pharmacokinet. 2002;41(7):505–16. PubMed CrossRef.
44. Bristow MR. Treatment of chronic heart failure with beta-adrenergic receptor antagonists: a convergence of receptor pharmacology and clinical cardiology. Circ Res. 2011;109(10):1176–94. PubMed CrossRef.
45. Brunton L, Chabner B, Knollman B. Goodman and Gilman's the pharmacological basis of therapeutics. 12th ed. Columbus: McGraw-Hill Education; 2010.
46. Kindermann M. Carvedilol but not metoprolol reduces beta-adrenergic responsiveness after complete elimination from plasma in vivo. Circulation. 2004;109(25):3182–90. PubMed CrossRef.
47. Snow PJ. Effect of propranolol in myocardial infarction. Lancet. 1965;2(7412):551–3. PubMed CrossRef.
48. Burch GE, Walsh JJ, Ferrans VJ, Hibbs R. Prolonged bed rest in the treatment of the dilated heart. Circulation. 1965;32(5):852–6. PubMed CrossRef.
49. Chidsey CA, Braunwald E, Morrow AG, Mason DT. Myocardial norepinephrine concentration in man -- effects of reserpine and of congestive heart failure. N Engl J Med. 1963;269:653–8. PubMed CrossRef.
50. Gaffney TE, Braunwald E. Importance of the adrenergic nervous system in the support of circulatory function in patients with congestive heart failure. Am J Med. 1963;34:320–4. PubMed CrossRef.
51. Waagstein F, Hjalmarson A, Varnauskas E, Wallentin I. Effect of chronic beta-adrenergic receptor blockade in congestive cardiomyopathy. Br Heart J. 1975;37(10):1022–36. PubMed PubMedCentral CrossRef.
52. Gobel FL, Norstrom LA, Nelson RR, Jorgensen CR, Wang Y. The rate-pressure product as an index of myocardial oxygen consumption during exercise in patients with angina pectoris. Circulation. 1978;57(3):549–56. PubMed CrossRef.
53. Swedberg K, Hjalmarson A, Waagstein F, Wallentin I. Prolongation of survival in congestive cardiomyopathy by beta-receptor blockade. Lancet. 1979;1(8131):1374–6. PubMed CrossRef.
54. Goodwin JF. The frontiers of cardiomyopathy. Br Heart J. 1982;48(1):1–18. PubMed PubMed Central CrossRef.
55. Ikram H, Fitzpatrick D. Double-blind trial of chronic oral beta blockade in congestive cardiomyopathy. Lancet. 1981;2(8245):490–3. PubMed CrossRef.
56. Currie PJ, Kelly MJ, McKenzie A, Harper RW, Lim YL, Federman J, et al. Oral beta-adrenergic blockade with metoprolol in chronic severe dilated cardiomyopathy. J Am Coll Cardiol. 1984;3(1):203–9. PubMed CrossRef.
57. Waagstein F, Bristow MR, Swedberg K, Camerini F, Fowler MB, Silver MA, et al. Beneficial effects of metoprolol in idiopathic dilated cardiomyopathy. Metoprolol in Dilated Cardiomyopathy (MDC) trial study group. Lancet. 1993;342(8885):1441–6. PubMed CrossRef.
58. Investigators C, Committees A. Randomized trial of beta-blockade in heart failure. The Cardiac Insufficiency Bisoprolol Study (CIBIS). Circulation. 1994;90(4):1765–73. CrossRef.
59. Packer M, Coats AJ, Fowler MB, Katus HA, Krum H, Mohacsi P, et al. Effect of carvedilol on survival in severe chronic heart failure. N Engl J Med. 2001;344(22):1651–8. PubMed CrossRef.
60. The Cardiac Insufficiency Bisoprolol Study II (CIBIS-II): a randomised trial. Lancet. 1999;353(9146):9–13.
61. Group M-HS. Effect of metoprolol CR/XL in chronic heart failure: Metoprolol CR/XL Randomised Intervention Trial in Congestive Heart Failure (MERIT-HF). Lancet. 1999;353(9169):2001–7. CrossRef
62. Macdonald PS, Keogh AM, Aboyoun CL, Lund M, Amor R, McCaffrey. DJ. Tolerability and efficacy of carvedilol in patients with New York Heart Association class IV heart failure. J Am Coll Cardiol. 1999;33(4):924–31. PubMed CrossRef.
63. Beta-Blocker Evaluation of Survival Trial Investigators. A trial of the beta-blocker bucindolol in patients with advanced chronic heart failure. N Engl J Med. 2001;344(22):1659–67.

64. Bristow MR, Murphy GA, Krause-Steinrauf H, Anderson JL, Carlquist JF, Thaneemit-Chen S, et al. An alpha-2c-adrenergic receptor polymorphism alters the norepinephrine-lowering effects and therapeutic response of the beta-blocker bucindolol in chronic heart failure. Circ Heart Fail. 2010;3(1):21–8. PubMed CrossRef.
65. Goldstein S, Deedwania P, Gottlieb S, Wikstrand J. Metoprolol CR/XL in black patients with heart failure (from the metoprolol CR/XL randomized intervention trial in chronic heart failure). Am J Cardiol. 2003;92(4):478–80.
66. Lanfear DE, Hrobowski TN, Peterson EL, Wells KE, Swadia TV, Spertus JA, et al. Association of beta-blocker exposure with outcomes in heart failure differs between African American and white patients. Circ Heart Fail. 2012;5(2):202–8. PubMed PubMedCentral CrossRef.
67. Packer M, Antonopoulos GV, Berlin JA, Chittams J, Konstam MA, Udelson JE. Comparative effects of carvedilol and metoprolol on left ventricular ejection fraction in heart failure: results of a meta-analysis. Am Heart J. 2001;141(6):899–907. PubMed CrossRef.
68. Poole-Wilson PA, Swedberg K, Cleland JGF, Di Lenarda A, Hanrath P, Komajda M, et al. Comparison of carvedilol and metoprolol on clinical outcomes in patients with chronic heart failure in the Carvedilol Or Metoprolol European Trial (COMET): randomised controlled trial. Lancet. 2003;362(9377):7–13. PubMed CrossRef.
69. Bristow MR, Feldman AM, Adams KF Jr, Goldstein S. Selective versus nonselective beta-blockade for heart failure therapy: are there lessons to be learned from the COMET trial? J Card Fail. 2003;9(6):444–53. PubMed CrossRef.
70. Ruwald MH, Ruwald ACH, Jons C, Alexis J, McNitt S, Zareba W, et al. Effect of metoprolol versus carvedilol on outcomes in MADIT-CRT (Multicenter Automatic Defibrillator Implantation Trial with Cardiac Resynchronization Therapy). J Am Coll Cardiol. 2013;61(14):1518–26. PubMed CrossRef.
71. Heidenreich PA, Bozkurt B, Aguilar D, et al. 2022 AHA/ACC/HFSA guideline for the management of heart failure: a report of the American College of Cardiology/American Heart Association Joint Committee on Clinical Practice Guidelines. J Am Coll Cardiol. 2022;79:e263–421. PubMed CrossRef.
72. Sliwa K, Norton GR, Kone N, Candy G, Kachope J, Woodiwiss AJ, et al. Impact of initiating carvedilol before angiotensin-converting enzyme inhibitor therapy on cardiac function in newly diagnosed heart failure. J Am Coll Cardiol. 2004;44(9):1825–30. PubMed CrossRef.
73. Willenheimer R, van Veldhuisen DJ, Silke B, Erdmann E, Follath F, Krum H, et al. Effect on survival and hospitalization of initiating treatment for chronic heart failure with bisoprolol followed by enalapril, as compared with the opposite sequence: results of the Randomized Cardiac Insufficiency Bisoprolol Study (CIBIS) III. Circulation. 2005;112(16):2426–35. PubMed CrossRef.
74. Funck-Brentano C, van Veldhuisen DJ, van de Ven LLM, Follath F, Goulder M, Willenheimer R, et al. Influence of order and type of drug (bisoprolol vs. enalapril) on outcome and adverse events in patients with chronic heart failure: a post hoc analysis of the CIBIS-III trial. Eur J Heart Fail. 2011;13(7):765–72. PubMed CrossRef.
75. Kramer DG, Trikalinos TA, Kent DM, Antonopoulos GV, Konstam MA, Udelson JE. Quantitative evaluation of drug or device effects on ventricular remodeling as predictors of therapeutic effects on mortality in patients with heart failure and reduced ejection fraction. J Am Coll Cardiol. 2010;56(5):392–406. PubMed PubMed Central CrossRef.
76. Abdulla J, Kober L, Christensen E, Torppedersen C. Effect of beta-blocker therapy on functional status in patients with heart failure — a meta-analysis. Eur J Heart Fail. 2006;8(5):522–31. PubMed CrossRef.
77. Dobre D, van Jaarsveld CHM, deJongste MJL, Haaijer Ruskamp FM, Ranchor AV. The effect of beta-blocker therapy on quality of life in heart failure patients: a systematic review and meta-analysis. Pharmacoepidemiol Drug Saf. 2007;16(2):152–9. PubMed CrossRef.
78. Maisel A, Mueller C, Adamsjr K, Anker S, Aspromonte N, Cleland J, et al. State of the art: using natriuretic peptide levels in clinical practice. Eur J Heart Fail. 2008;10(9):824–39. PubMed CrossRef.
79. Stanek B, Frey B, Hülsmann M, Berger R, Sturm B, Strametz-Juranek J, et al. Prognostic evaluation of neurohumoral plasma levels before and during beta-blocker therapy in advanced left ventricular dysfunction. J Am Coll Cardiol. 2001;38(2):436–42. PubMed CrossRef.
80. Hartmann F, Packer M, Coats AJ, Fowler MB, Krum H, Mohacsi P, et al. NT-proBNP in severe chronic heart failure: rationale, design and preliminary results of the COPERNICUS NT-proBNP substudy. Eur J Heart Fail. 2004;6(3):343–50. PubMed CrossRef.
81. Hartmann F, Packer M, Coats AJ, Fowler MB, Krum H, Mohacsi P, Rouleau JL, Tendera M, Castaigne A, Anker SD, Amann-Zalan I, Hoersch S, Katus HA. Prognostic impact of plasma N-terminal pro-brain natriuretic peptide in severe chronic congestive heart failure: a substudy of the carvedilol prospective randomized cumulative survival (COPERNICUS). Trial Circ. 2004;110(13):1780–6. PubMed CrossRef.
82. Haas SJ, Vos T, Gilbert RE, Krum H. Are beta-blockers as efficacious in patients with diabetes mellitus as in patients without diabetes mellitus who have chronic heart failure? A meta-analysis of large-scale clinical trials. Am Heart J. 2003;146(5):848–53. PubMed CrossRef.
83. Shorr RI, Ray WA, Daugherty JR, Griffin MR. Antihypertensives and the risk of serious

hypoglycemia in older persons using insulin or sulfonylureas. JAMA. 1997;278(1):40–3. PubMed CrossRef.
84. Rodger JC, Sheldon CD, Lerski RA, Livingstone WR. Intermittent claudication complicating beta-blockade. Br Med J. 1976;1(6018):1125. PubMed PubMedCentral CrossRef.
85. Radack K, Deck C. Beta-adrenergic blocker therapy does not worsen intermittent claudication in subjects with peripheral arterial disease. A meta-analysis of randomized controlled trials. Arch Intern Med. 1991;151(9):1769–76. PubMed CrossRef.
86. Broadley KJ. Beta-adrenoceptor responses of the airways: for better or worse? Eur J Pharmacol. 2006;533(1–3):15–27. PubMed CrossRef.
87. McNeill RS. Effect of a beta-adrenergic-blocking agent, propranolol, on asthmatics. Lancet. 1964;2(7369):1101–2. PubMed CrossRef.
88. Salpeter SR, Ormiston TM, Salpeter EE. Cardioselective beta-blockers in patients with reactive airway disease: a meta-analysis. Ann Intern Med. 2002;137(9):715–25. PubMed CrossRef.
89. Kotlyar E, Keogh AM, Macdonald PS, Arnold RH, McCaffrey DJ, Glanville AR. Tolerability of carvedilol in patients with heart failure and concomitant chronic obstructive pulmonary disease or asthma. J Heart Lung Transplant. 2002;21(12):1290–5. PubMed CrossRef.
90. Rutten FH, Zuithoff NPA, Hak E, Grobbee DE, Hoes AW. Beta-blockers may reduce mortality and risk of exacerbations in patients with chronic obstructive pulmonary disease. Arch Intern Med. 2010;170(10):880–7. PubMed CrossRef.
91. Salpeter S, Ormiston T, Salpeter E. Cardioselective beta-blockers for chronic obstructive pulmonary disease. Cochrane Database Syst Rev. 2005;4:CD003566.
92. Jabbour A, Macdonald PS, Keogh AM, Kotlyar E, Mellemkjaer S, Coleman CF, et al. Differences between beta-blockers in patients with chronic heart failure and chronic obstructive pulmonary disease: a randomized crossover trial. J Am Coll Cardiol. 2010;55(17):1780–7. PubMed CrossRef.
93. Mentz RJ, Wojdyla D, Fiuzat M, Chiswell K, Fonarow GC, O'Connor CM. Association of beta-blocker use and selectivity with outcomes in patients with heart failure and chronic obstructive pulmonary disease (from OPTIMIZE-HF). Am J Cardiol. 2012;111(4):582–7. PubMed CrossRef.
94. Advisory council to improve outcomes nationwide in heart failure. Consensus recommendations for the management of chronic heart failure. Am J Cardiol. 1999;83(2A):1A–38A.
95. Haber HL, Simek CL, Gimple LW, Bergin JD, Subbiah K, Jayaweera AR, et al. Why do patients with congestive heart failure tolerate the initiation of beta-blocker therapy? Circulation. 1993;88(4):1610–9. PubMed CrossRef.
96. Epstein SE, Braunwald E. The effect of beta adrenergic blockade on patterns of urinary sodium excretion. Studies in normal subjects and in patients with heart disease. Ann Intern Med. 1966;65(1):20–7. PubMed CrossRef.
97. Davis ME, Richards AM, Nicholls MG, Yandle TG, Frampton CM, Troughton RW. Introduction of metoprolol increases plasma b-type cardiac natriuretic peptides in mild, stable heart failure. Circulation. 2006;113(7):977–85. PubMed CrossRef.
98. Driscoll A, Krum H, Wolfe R, Tonkin A, Study Group BENCH. Nurse-led titration of beta-adrenoreceptor blocking agents in chronic heart failure patients in the community. J Card Fail. 2011;17(3):224–30. PubMed CrossRef.
99. Mebazaa A, Davison B, Chioncel O, Cohen-Solal A, Diaz R, Filippatos G, et al. Safety, tolerability and efficacy of up-titration of guideline-directed medical therapies for acute heart failure (STRONG-HF): a multinational, open-label, randomised, trial. Lancet. 2022;400(10367):1938–52.
100. Gottlieb SS, Fisher ML, Kjekshus J, Deedwania P, Gullestad L, Vitovec J, et al. Tolerability of beta-blocker initiation and titration in the metoprolol CR/XL randomized intervention trial in congestive heart failure (MERIT-HF). Circulation. 2002;105(10):1182–8. PubMed CrossRef.
101. Krum H, Roecker EB, Mohacsi P, Rouleau JL, Tendera M, Coats AJS, et al. Effects of initiating carvedilol in patients with severe chronic heart failure: results from the COPERNICUS study. JAMA. 2003;289(6):712–8. PubMed CrossRef.
102. Ko DT, Hebert PR, Coffey CS, Curtis JP, Foody JM, Sedrakyan A, et al. Adverse effects of beta-blocker therapy for patients with heart failure: a quantitative overview of randomized trials. Arch Intern Med. 2004;164(13):1389–94. PubMed CrossRef.
103. Proclemer A, Gradnik R, Savonitto S, Feruglio GA. Electrophysiological effects of bisoprolol. Eur Heart J. 1987;8(Suppl M):81–5. PubMed CrossRef.
104. Wilkoff BL, Kudenchuk PJ, Buxton AE, Sharma A, Cook JR, Bhandari AK, et al. The DAVID (Dual Chamber and VVI Implantable Defibrillator) II trial. J Am Coll Cardiol. 2009;53(10):872–80. PubMed CrossRef.
105. Agarwal MA, Fonarow GC, Ziaeian B. National trends in heart failure hospitalizations and readmissions from 2010 to 2017. JAMA Cardiol. 2021;6(8):952–6. https://doi.org/10.1001/jamacardio.2020.7472.
106. Bozkurt B, Ahmad T, Alexander KM, Baker WL, Bosak K, Breathett K, et al. Heart failure epidemiology and outcomes statistics: a report of the Heart Failure Society of America. J Card Fail. 2023;29(10):1412–51.
107. Weil JV, Chidsey CA. Plasma volume expansion resulting from interference with adrenergic function in normal man. Circulation. 1968;37(1):54–61. PubMed CrossRef.
108. Heart Failure Society of America (HFSA) Practice Guidelines. HFSA guidelines for management of patients with heart failure caused by left ventricular

systolic dysfunction--pharmacological approaches. J Card Fail. 1999;5(4):357–82. CrossRef.
109. Gattis WA, O'Connor CM, Gallup DS, Hasselblad V, Gheorghiade M. IMPACT-HF investigators and coordinators. Predischarge initiation of carvedilol in patients hospitalized for decompensated heart failure: results of the initiation management predischarge: process for assessment of carvedilol therapy in heart failure (IMPACT-HF) trial. J Am Coll Cardiol. 2004;43(9):1534–41. PubMed CrossRef.
110. Fonarow GC, Abraham WT, Albert NM, Stough WG, Gheorghiade M, Greenberg BH, et al. Influence of beta-blocker continuation or withdrawal on outcomes in patients hospitalized with heart failure. J Am Coll Cardiol. 2008;52(3):190–9. PubMed CrossRef.
111. Fonarow G, Abraham W, Albert N, Stough W, Gheorghiade M, Greenberg B, O'Connor CM, et al. Prospective evaluation of beta-blocker use at the time of hospital discharge as a heart failure performance measure: results from OPTIMIZE-HF. J Card Fail. 2007;13(9):722–31. PubMed CrossRef.
112. Prins K, Neill J, Tyler J, Eckman P, Duval S. Effects of Beta-blocker withdrawal in acute decompensated heart failure. JACC: Heart Fail. 2015;3(8):647–53.
113. Gorodeski EZ, Chu EC, Reese JR, Shishehbor MH, Hsich E, Starling RC. Prognosis on chronic dobutamine or milrinone infusions for stage d heart failure. Circ Heart Fail. 2009;2(4):320–4. PubMed CrossRef.
114. De Marco T, Chatterjee K. Phosphodiesterase inhibitors in refractory heart failure: bridge to beta-blockade? J Am Coll Cardiol. 1998;31(6):1341–3. PubMed CrossRef.
115. Metra M, Nodari S, D'Aloia A, Muneretto C, Robertson AD, Bristow MR, et al. Beta-blocker therapy influences the hemodynamic response to inotropic agents in patients with heart failure: a randomized comparison of dobutamine and enoximone before and after chronic treatment with metoprolol or carvedilol. J Am Coll Cardiol. 2002;40(7):1248–58. PubMed CrossRef.
116. Jennings DL, Thompson ML. Use of combination therapy with a beta-blocker and milrinone in patients with advanced heart failure. Ann Pharmacother. 2009;43(11):1872–6. PubMed CrossRef.
117. Shakar SF, Abraham WT, Gilbert EM, Robertson AD, Lowes BD, Zisman LS, et al. Combined oral positive inotropic and beta-blocker therapy for treatment of refractory class IV heart failure. J Am Coll Cardiol. 1998;31(6):1336–40. PubMed CrossRef.
118. Krum H, Ninio D, MacDonald P. Baseline predictors of tolerability to carvedilol in patients with chronic heart failure. Heart. 2000;84(6):615–9. PubMed PubMedCentral CrossRef.
119. Parameswaran AC, Tang WHW, Francis GS, Gupta R, Young JB. Why do patients fail to receive beta-blockers for chronic heart failure over time? A "real-world" single-center, 2-year follow-up experience of beta-blocker therapy in patients with chronic heart failure. Am Heart J. 2005;149(5):921–6. PubMed CrossRef.
120. Bristow MR, Gilbert EM, Abraham WT, Adams KF, Fowler MB, Hershberger RE, et al. Carvedilol produces dose-related improvements in left ventricular function and survival in subjects with chronic heart failure. MOCHA investigators. Circulation. 1996;94(11):2807–16. PubMed CrossRef.
121. Simon T. Bisoprolol dose–response relationship in patients with congestive heart failure: a subgroup analysis in the Cardiac Insufficiency Bisoprolol Study (CIBIS II). Eur Heart J. 2003;24(6):552–9. PubMed CrossRef.
122. Metra M, Torp-Pedersen C, Swedberg K, Cleland JG, Di Lenarda A, Komajda M. Influence of heart rate, blood pressure, and beta-blocker dose on outcome and the differences in outcome between carvedilol and metoprolol tartrate in patients with chronic heart failure: results from the COMET trial. Eur Heart J. 2005;26(21):2259–68. PubMed CrossRef.
123. Wikstrand J, Hjalmarson A, Waagstein F, Fagerberg B, Goldstein S, Kjekshus J, et al. Dose of metoprolol CR/XL and clinical outcomes in patients with heart failure: analysis of the experience in metoprolol CR/XL randomized intervention trial in chronic heart failure (MERIT-HF). J Am Coll Cardiol. 2002;40(3):491–8. PubMed CrossRef.
124. Azevedo ER, Kubo T, Mak S, Al-Hesayen A, Schofield A, Allan R, et al. Nonselective versus selective β-adrenergic receptor blockade in congestive heart failure. Circulation. 2001;104(18):2194–9.
125. Fowler MB, Lottes SR, Nelson JJ, Lukas MA, Gilbert EM, Greenberg B, et al. Beta-blocker dosing in community-based treatment of heart failure. Am Heart J. 2007;153(6):1029–36. PubMed CrossRef.
126. Lechat P, Hulot JS, Escolano S, Mallet A, Leizorovicz A, Werhlen-Grandjean M, et al. Heart rate and cardiac rhythm relationships with bisoprolol benefit in chronic heart failure in CIBIS II trial. Circulation. 2001;103(10):1428–33. PubMed CrossRef.
127. McAlister FA, Wiebe N, Ezekowitz JA, Leung AA, Armstrong PW. Meta-analysis: beta-blocker dose, heart rate reduction, and death in patients with heart failure. Ann Intern Med. 2009;150(11):784–94. PubMed CrossRef.
128. Borlaug BA, Paulus WJ. Heart failure with preserved ejection fraction: pathophysiology, diagnosis, and treatment. Eur Heart J. 2010;32(6):670–9.
129. Ponikowski P, et al. 2016 ESC Guidelines for the diagnosis and treatment of acute and chronic heart failure: The Task Force for the diagnosis and treatment of acute and chronic heart failure of the European Society of Cardiology (ESC). Developed with the special contribution of the Heart Failure Association (HFA) of the ESC. Eur J Heart Fail. 2016;18(8):891–975.
130. Cleland JGF, et al. Beta-blockers for heart failure with reduced, mid-range, and preserved ejection fraction: an individual patient-level analysis

of double-blind randomized trials. Eur Heart J. 2017;39(1):26–35.
131. Flather MD, et al. Randomized trial to determine the effect of nebivolol on mortality and cardiovascular hospital admission in elderly patients with heart failure (SENIORS). Eur Heart J. 2005;26(3):215–25.
132. van Veldhuisen DJ, et al. Beta-blockade with nebivolol in elderly heart failure patients with impaired and preserved left ventricular ejection fraction: data from SENIORS (study of effects of Nebivolol intervention on outcomes and rehospitalization in seniors with heart failure). J Am Coll Cardiol. 2009;53(23):2150–8.
133. Hernandez AF, et al. Clinical effectiveness of beta-blockers in heart failure: findings from the OPTIMIZE-HF (organized program to initiate lifesaving treatment in hospitalized patients with heart failure) registry. J Am Coll Cardiol. 2009;53(2):184–92.
134. Arnold SV, et al. Beta-blocker use and heart failure outcomes in mildly reduced and preserved ejection fraction. JACC: Heart Fail. 2023;11(8, Part 1):893–900.
135. Benedict CR, et al. Comparative neurohormonal responses in patients with preserved and impaired left ventricular ejection fraction: results of the studies of left ventricular dysfunction (SOLVD) registry. The SOLVD investigators. J Am Coll Cardiol. 1993;22(4 Suppl A):146a–53a.
136. Carson P, et al. Mild systolic dysfunction in heart failure (left ventricular ejection fraction >35%): baseline characteristics, prognosis and response to therapy in the vasodilator in heart failure trials (V-HeFT). J Am Coll Cardiol. 1996;27(3):642–9.
137. Meyer M, et al. Association between β-blockers and outcomes in heart failure with preserved ejection fraction: current insights from the SwedeHF registry. J Card Fail. 2021;27(11):1165–74.
138. Zucker IH, et al. Regulation of central angiotensin type 1 receptors and sympathetic outflow in heart failure. Am J Physiol Heart Circ Physiol. 2009;297(5):H1557–66.
139. Gao L, et al. Imbalance of angiotensin type 1 receptor and angiotensin II type 2 receptor in the rostral ventrolateral medulla: potential mechanism for sympathetic overactivity in heart failure. Hypertension. 2008;52(4):708–14.
140. Cohn JN, et al. A Comparison of enalapril with hydralazine–isosorbide dinitrate in the treatment of chronic congestive heart failure. N Engl J Med. 1991;325(5):303–10.
141. Bunsawat K, et al. Sympathoinhibitory effect of sacubitril-valsartan in heart failure with reduced ejection fraction: a pilot study. Auton Neurosci. 2021;235:102834.
142. Matthews VB, et al. Role of the sympathetic nervous system in regulation of the sodium glucose cotransporter 2. J Hypertens. 2017;35(10):2059–68.
143. Sano M. A new class of drugs for heart failure: SGLT2 inhibitors reduce sympathetic overactivity. J Cardiol. 2018;71(5):471–6.
144. Ernsberger PR, et al. A second generation of centrally acting antihypertensive agents act on putative I1-Imidazoline receptors. J Cardiovasc Pharmacol. 1992;20:S1–S10.
145. Swedberg K, et al. The effects of moxonidine, a novel imidazoline, on plasma norepinephrine in patients with congestive heart failure. Moxonidine investigators. J Am Coll Cardiol. 2000;35(2):398–404.
146. Swedberg K, et al. Effects of sustained-release moxonidine, an Imidazoline agonist, on plasma norepinephrine in patients with chronic heart failure. Circulation. 2002;105(15):1797–803.
147. Cohn JN, et al. Adverse mortality effect of central sympathetic inhibition with sustained-release moxonidine in patients with heart failure (MOXCON). Eur J Heart Fail. 2003;5(5):659–67.
148. Azevedo ER, Newton GE, Parker JD. Cardiac and systemic sympathetic activity in response to clonidine in human heart failure. J Am Coll Cardiol. 1999;33(1):186–91.
149. Grassi G, et al. Effects of chronic clonidine administration on sympathetic nerve traffic and baroreflex function in heart failure. Hypertension. 2001;38(2):286–91.
150. Aggarwal A, et al. Regional sympathetic effects of low-dose clonidine in heart failure. Hypertension. 2003;41(3):553–7.
151. Moorman AJ, Stratton JR, Levy WC. Clonidine therapy in patients with heart failure improves exercise efficiency, functional class and symptoms. Int J Cardiol. 2011;150(3):372–3.
152. Pliquett RU, et al. Simvastatin normalizes autonomic neural control in experimental heart failure. Circulation. 2003;107(19):2493–8.
153. Gao L, et al. Simvastatin therapy normalizes sympathetic neural control in experimental heart failure. Circulation. 2005;112(12):1763–70.
154. Gomes ME, et al. Sympathoinhibitory effect of statins in chronic heart failure. Clin Auton Res. 2010;20(2):73–8.
155. Deo SH, et al. Statin therapy lowers muscle sympathetic nerve activity and oxidative stress in patients with heart failure. Am J Physiol Heart Circ Physiol. 2012;303(3):H377–85.
156. Katircibasi MT, et al. Decreased heart rate recovery in patients with heart failure: effect of fluvastatin therapy. Int Heart J. 2005;46(5):845–54.
157. Lewandowski J, et al. The effect of statins on sympathetic activity: a meta-analysis. Clin Auton Res. 2015;25(2):125–31.
158. Linde C, Ellenbogen K, McAlister FA. Cardiac resynchronization therapy (CRT): clinical trials, guidelines, and target populations. Heart Rhythm. 2012;9(Suppl):S3–S13. PubMed CrossRef.
159. Adamson PB, Kleckner KJ, VanHout WL, Srinivasan S, Abraham WT. Cardiac resynchronization therapy improves heart rate variability in

patients with symptomatic heart failure. Circulation. 2003;108(3):266–9. PubMed CrossRef.
160. Cha YM, Chareonthaitawee P, Dong YX, Kemp BJ, Jae KO, Miyazaki C, et al. Cardiac sympathetic reserve and response to cardiac resynchronization therapy. Circ Heart Fail. 2011;4(3):339–44. PubMed CrossRef.
161. Fantoni C, Raffa S, Regoli F, Giraldi F, La Rovere MT, Prentice J, et al. Cardiac resynchronization therapy improves heart rate profile and heart rate variability of patients with moderate to severe heart failure. J Am Coll Cardiol. 2005;46(10):1875–82. PubMed CrossRef.
162. Moreira RI, Abreu A, Portugal G, Oliveira L, Oliveira M, Rodrigues I, et al. Prognostic effect and modulation of cardiac sympathetic function in heart failure patients treated with cardiac resynchronization therapy. J Nucl Cardiol. 2020;27(1):283–90.
163. Geelen P, Brugada J, Andries E, Brugada P. Ventricular fibrillation and sudden death after radiofrequency catheter ablation of the atrioventricular junction. Pacing Clin Electrophysiol. 1997;20:343–8.
164. Hamdan MH, Page RL, Sheehan CJ, Zagrodzky JD, Wasmund SL, Ramaswamy K, Joglar JA, Smith ML. Increased sympathetic activity after atrioventricular junction ablation in patients with chronic atrial fibrillation. J Am Coll Cardiol. 2000;36:151–8.
165. Sin DD, Fitzgerald F, Parker JD, Newton G, Floras JS, Bradley TD. Risk factors for central and obstructive sleep apnea in 450 men and women with congestive heart failure. Am J Respir Crit Care Med. 1999;160(4):1101–6. PubMed CrossRef.
166. Lanfranchi PA, Pépin J-L, Somers VK. Chapter 14 - cardiovascular physiology: autonomic control in health and in sleep disorders. In: Kryger M, Roth T, Dement WC, editors. Principles and practice of sleep medicine. 6th ed. Elsevier; 2017. p. 142–54.e4.
167. Somers VK, Dyken ME, Mark AL, Abboud FM. Sympathetic-nerve activity during sleep in normal subjects. N Engl J Med. 1993;328(5):303–7. PubMed CrossRef.
168. Somers VK, Dyken ME, Clary MP, Abboud FM. Sympathetic neural mechanisms in obstructive sleep apnea. J Clin Invest. 1995;96(4):1897–904. PubMed PubMedCentral CrossRef.
169. Usui K, Bradley TD, Spaak J, Ryan CM, Kubo T, Kaneko Y, et al. Inhibition of awake sympathetic nerve activity of heart failure patients with obstructive sleep apnea by nocturnal continuous positive airway pressure. J Am Coll Cardiol. 2005;45(12):2008–11. PubMed CrossRef.
170. Kaneko Y, Floras JS, Usui K, Plante J, Tkacova R, Kubo T, et al. Cardiovascular effects of continuous positive airway pressure in patients with heart failure and obstructive sleep apnea. N Engl J Med. 2003;348(13):1233–41. PubMed CrossRef.
171. Kasai T, Narui K, Dohi T, Yanagisawa N, Ishiwata S, Ohno M, et al. Prognosis of patients with heart failure and obstructive sleep apnea treated with continuous positive airway pressure. Chest. 2008;133(3):690–6. PubMed CrossRef
172. Javaheri S, Brown LK, Khayat RN. Update on apneas of heart failure with reduced ejection fraction: emphasis on the physiology of treatment: part 2: central sleep apnea. Chest. 2020;157(6):1637–46.
173. Tamisier R, Pépin J-L, Woehrle H, Salvat M, Barone-Rochette G, Rocca C, et al. Effect of adaptive servo-ventilation for central sleep apnoea in systolic heart failure on muscle sympathetic nerve activity: a SERVE-HF randomised ancillary study. Eur Respir J. 2023;61(2):2200384.
174. Dusi V, Angelini F, Zile MR, De Ferrari GM. Neuromodulation devices for heart failure. Eur Heart J Suppl. 2022;24(Supplement_E):E12–27.
175. Olshansky B, Sabbah HN, Hauptman PJ, Colucci WS. Parasympathetic nervous system and heart failure: pathophysiology and potential implications for therapy. Circulation. 2008;118(8):863–71. PubMed CrossRef.
176. Zhang Y, Popovic ZB, Bibevski S, Fakhry I, Sica DA, Van Wagoner DR, et al. Chronic vagus nerve stimulation improves autonomic control and attenuates systemic inflammation and heart failure progression in a canine high-rate pacing model. Circ Heart Fail. 2009;2(6):692–9. PubMed CrossRef.
177. De Ferrari GM, Crijns HJGM, Borggrefe M, Milasinovic G, Smid J, Zabel M, et al. Chronic vagus nerve stimulation: a new and promising therapeutic approach for chronic heart failure. Eur Heart J. 2011;32(7):847–55. PubMed CrossRef.
178. Anand IS, Konstam MA, Klein HU, Mann DL, Ardell JL, Gregory DD, et al. Comparison of symptomatic and functional responses to vagus nerve stimulation in ANTHEM-HF, INOVATE-HF, and NECTAR-HF. ESC Heart Fail. 2020;7(1):76–84.
179. Dusi V, De Ferrari GM. Vagal stimulation in heart failure. Herz. 2021;46(6):541–9.
180. Konstam MA. ANTHEM HF-rEF pivotal study: primary and supplemental endpoint results. Presented at: HFSA 2023; 2023.
181. Gronda E, Seravalle G, Brambilla G, et al. Chronic baroreflex activation effects on sympathetic nerve traffic, baroreflex function, and cardiac haemodynamics in heart failure: a proof-of-concept study. Eur J Heart Fail. 2014;16:977–83.
182. Abraham WT, Zile MR, Weaver FA, et al. Baroreflex activation therapy treats heart failure with a reduced ejection fraction. JACC Heart Fail. 2015;3:487–96.
183. Zile MR, Abraham WT, Lindenfeld J, Weaver FA, Zannad F, Graves T, et al. First granted example of novel FDA trial design under expedited access pathway for premarket approval: BeAT-HF. Am Heart J. 2018;204:139–50.
184. Zile MR, Abraham WT, et al. Baroreflex activation therapy in patients with heart failure with reduced ejection fraction. J Am Coll Cardiol. 2020;76:1–13.
185. McKelvie RS, Teo KK, McCartney N, Humen D, Montague T, Yusuf S. Effects of exercise training in patients with congestive heart failure: a criti-

cal review. J Am Coll Cardiol. 1995;25(3):789–96. PubMed CrossRef.
186. O'Connor CM, Whellan DJ, Lee KL, Keteyian SJ, Cooper LS, Ellis SJ, et al. Efficacy and safety of exercise training in patients with chronic heart failure: HF-ACTION randomized controlled trial. JAMA. 2009;301(14):1439–50. PubMed PubMedCentral CrossRef.
187. Gademan MGJ, Swenne CA, Verwey HF, van der Laarse A, Maan AC, van de Vooren H, et al. Effect of exercise training on autonomic derangement and neurohumoral activation in chronic heart failure. J Card Fail. 2007;13(4):294–303. PubMed CrossRef.
188. Roveda F, Middlekauff HR, Rondon MUPB, Reis SF, Souza M, Nastari L, et al. The effects of exercise training on sympathetic neural activation in advanced heart failure: a randomized controlled trial. J Am Coll Cardiol. 2003;42(5):854–60. PubMed CrossRef.
189. Wisløff U, Støylen A, Loennechen JP, Bruvold M, Rognmo Ø, Haram PM, Tjønna AE, Helgerud J, Slørdahl SA, Lee SJ, et al. Superior cardiovascular effect of aerobic interval training versus moderate continuous training in heart failure patients: a randomized study. Circulation. 2007;115:3086–94.
190. Sales AK, Azevedo L, Silva TC, Rodrigues A, Oliveira P, Jordão C, et al. High-intensity interval training decreases muscle sympathetic nerve activity and improves peripheral vascular function in patients with heart failure with reduced ejection fraction. Circ: Heart Fail. 2020;13(8):e007121.
191. Edwards J, Shanmugam N, Ray R, Jouhra F, Mancio J, Wiles J, et al. Exercise mode in heart failure: a systematic review and meta-analysis. Sports Medicine - Open. 2023;9(1)
192. DiMicco JA, Samuels BC, Zaretskaia MV, Zaretsky DV. The dorsomedial hypothalamus and the response to stress: part renaissance, part revolution. Pharmacol Biochem Behav. 2002;71(3):469–80. PubMed CrossRef.
193. Akashi YJ, Goldstein DS, Barbaro G, Ueyama T. Takotsubo cardiomyopathy: a new form of acute, reversible heart failure. Circulation. 2008;118(25):2754–62. PubMed PubMedCentral CrossRef.
194. Wittstein IS, Thiemann DR, Lima JAC, Baughman KL, Schulman SP, Gerstenblith G, et al. Neurohumoral features of myocardial stunning due to sudden emotional stress. N Engl J Med. 2005;352(6):539–48. PubMed CrossRef.
195. Huston P, McFarlane B. Health benefits of tai chi. What is the evidence? Can Fam Physician. 2016;62(11):881–90.
196. Yeh GY, Wood MJ, Lorell BH, Stevenson LW, Eisenberg DM, Wayne PM, et al. Effects of tai chi mind-body movement therapy on functional status and exercise capacity in patients with chronic heart failure: a randomized controlled trial. Am J Med. 2004;117(8):541–8. PubMed CrossRef.
197. Curiati JA, Bocchi E, Freire JO, Arantes AC, Braga M, Garcia Y, et al. Meditation reduces sympathetic activation and improves the quality of life in elderly patients with optimally treated heart failure: a prospective randomized study. J Altern Complement Med. 2005;11(3):465–72. PubMed CrossRef.
198. Brandt MC, Mahfoud F, Reda S, Schirmer SH, Erdmann E, Böhm M, et al. Renal sympathetic denervation reduces left ventricular hypertrophy and improves cardiac function in patients with resistant hypertension. J Am Coll Cardiol. 2012;59:901–9.
199. Patel HC, Rosen SD, Hayward C, Vassiliou V, Smith GC, Wage RR, et al. Renal denervation in heart failure with preserved ejection fraction (RDT-PEF): a randomized controlled trial. Eur J Heart Fail. 2016;18:703–12.
200. Schirmer SH, Sayed MM, Reil JC, Ukena C, Linz D, Kindermann M, et al. Improvements in left ventricular hypertrophy and diastolic function following renal denervation: effects beyond blood pressure and heart rate reduction. J Am Coll Cardiol. 2014;63:1916–23.
201. Rundqvist B, Elam M, Bergmann-Sverrisdottir Y, Eisenhofer G, Friberg P. Increased cardiac adrenergic drive precedes generalized sympathetic activation in human heart failure. Circulation. 1997;95(1):169–75. PubMed CrossRef.
202. Chatterjee S, Biondi-Zoccai G, Abbate A, D'Ascenzo F, Castagno D, Van Tassell B, et al. Benefits of beta blockers in patients with heart failure and reduced ejection fraction: network meta-analysis. Br Med J. 2013;346:f55. https://doi.org/10.1136/bmj.f55. CrossRef.

Further Reading

Benedict CR, Weiner DH, Johnstone DE, Bourassa MG, Ghali JK, Nicklas J, et al. Comparative neurohormonal responses in patients with preserved and impaired left ventricular ejection fraction: results of the Studies of Left Ventricular Dysfunction (SOLVD) registry. J Am Coll Cardiol. 1993;22(Suppl A):146A–53A. PubMed CrossRef.
Borlaug BA, Paulus WJ. Heart failure with preserved ejection fraction: pathophysiology, diagnosis, and treatment. Eur Heart J. 2011;32(6):670–9. PubMed CrossRef.
Carson P, Johnson G, Fletcher R, Cohn J. Mild systolic dysfunction in heart failure (left ventricular ejection fraction >35%): baseline characteristics, prognosis and response to therapy in the vasodilator in heart failure trials (V-HeFT). J Am Coll Cardiol. 1996;27(3):642–9. PubMed CrossRef.
Cheng RK, Horwich TB, Fonarow GC. Relation of systolic blood pressure to survival in both ischemic and nonischemic systolic heart failure. Am J Cardiol.

2008;102(12):1698–705. PubMed PubMedCentral CrossRef.

El-Refai M, Peterson EL, Wells K, Swadia T, Sabbah HN, Spertus JA, et al. Comparison of beta-blocker effectiveness in heart failure patients with preserved ejection fraction versus those with reduced ejection fraction. J Card Fail. 2013;19(2):73–9. PubMed PubMedCentral CrossRef.

Flather MD, Shibata MC, Coats AJ, Van Veldhuisen DJ, Parkhomenko A, Borbola J, et al. Randomized trial to determine the effect of nebivolol on mortality and cardiovascular hospital admission in elderly patients with heart failure (SENIORS). Eur Heart J. 2004;26(3):215–25. CrossRef.

Hernandez AF, Hammill BG, O'Connor CM, Schulman KA, Curtis LH, Fonarow GC. Clinical effectiveness of beta-blockers in heart failure. J Am Coll Cardiol. 2009;53(2):184–92. PubMed PubMedCentral CrossRef.

Rouleau JL, Roecker EB, Tendera M, Mohacsi P, Krum H, Katus HA, et al. Influence of pretreatment systolic blood pressure on the effect of carvedilol in patients with severe chronic heart failure. J Am Coll Cardiol. 2004;43(8):1423–9. PubMed CrossRef.

Soläng L, Malmberg K, Rydén L. Diabetes mellitus and congestive heart failure. Further knowledge needed. Eur Heart J. 1999;20(11):789–95. PubMed CrossRef.

van Veldhuisen DJ, Cohen-Solal A, Bohm M, Anker SD, Babalis D, Roughton M, et al. Beta-blockade with nebivolol in elderly heart failure patients with impaired and preserved left ventricular ejection fraction. J Am Coll Cardiol. 2009;53(23):2150–8. PubMed CrossRef.

Yeh GY, McCarthy EP, Wayne PM, Stevenson LW, Wood MJ, Forman D, et al. Tai chi exercise in patients with chronic heart failure: a randomized clinical trial. Arch Intern Med. 2011;171(8):750–7. PubMed PubMedCentral CrossRef.

Sodium Glucose Transport Protein-2 (SGLT-2) Inhibitors

8

Dorothy Jung and Omaima Ali

Introduction

Sodium glucose transport 2 (SGLT2) inhibitors are the newest class of pharmacologic therapies used in managing heart failure. Initially introduced as oral anti-diabetic drugs in the 2010s, SGLT2 inhibitors were found to have unexpected beneficial effects on cardiovascular outcomes in patients with type 2 diabetes. Several large clinical trials in the last 5 years have shown that SGLT2 inhibitors reduce cardiovascular mortality and heart failure hospitalizations in patients regardless of whether they have diabetes or not. This benefit is observed in both patients with reduced ejection fraction as well as patients with preserved ejection fraction. The class of medications has since been adopted as one of four pillars of guideline-directed medical therapies in the management of heart failure with reduced ejection fraction (HFrEF) and heart failure with mildly reduced ejection fraction (HFmrEF). It is also the only medication that holds a class 2a recommendation for the management of heart failure with preserved ejection fraction (HFpEF).

D. Jung · O. Ali (✉)
Division of Cardiology, Penn State Hershey Medical Center, Hershey, PA, USA
e-mail: djung@pennstatehealth.psu.edu; oali@pennstatehealth.psu.edu

History of SGLT2 Inhibitors

Sodium-Glucose Cotransporters

In 1960, Robert Crane proposed the novel concept of coupling the active transport of a molecule across a cell membrane with an ion gradient [1]. Specifically, he demonstrated that intestinal glucose absorption occurs by the active transport of glucose into intestinal cells coupled with sodium transport down the sodium gradient that exists across the cell membrane. It was not until the 1980s that the protein responsible for this cotransport of molecules was identified in the small intestine: it was named the sodium-glucose cotransporter (SGLT1).

Discovery of the sodium-glucose cotransporter in the intestine (SGLT1) eventually led to discovery of the same sodium-glucose co-transporter in the proximal tubule of the renal nephron (It had been noted in the early 1980s that the proximal portion of the rat kidney tubule could absorb more glucose than the distal tubule.). Additional studies identified a similar co-transporter more proximal in the tubule and with a much higher capacity for glucose transport than SGLT1; this co-transporter was named sodium-glucose cotransporter 2 (SGLT2).

SGLT2 is responsible for 90% of total glucose absorption from the urine, while SGLT1 is responsible for the remaining 10%. Researchers naturally wondered whether inhibition of SGLT2 would decrease blood glucose levels

H. J. Eisen (ed.), *Heart Failure I*, https://doi.org/10.1007/978-3-032-12626-9_8

and, ultimately, have positive effects on patients with diabetes. SGLT2 inhibition had already been observed in patients with familial renal glucosuria (FRG). These patients have genetic mutations that lead to the downregulation of SGLT2 activity; patients subsequently lose significant amounts of glucose in their urine. Interestingly, patients do not become hypoglycemic or suffer from serious side effects of the disease.

Phlorizin and the Development of SGLT2 Inhibitors

Phlorizin was first isolated from the bark of an apple tree in 1835. Its bitter taste was thought similar to that of the cinchona tree extract (now known as quinine), an anti-malarial remedy dating back to the 1600s. Phlorizin was used primarily to treat malaria until the late 1800s when Joseph Von Mering observed that phlorizin produced glycosuria [2]. At the time, glycosuria was considered a marker of 'sound kidneys', so phlorizin became a tool for the study of renal function in man. In 1933, Homer Smith used phlorizin-induced glucose excretion in urine to measure renal blood flow and glomerular filtration rates [3]. His study also demonstrated that intravenous formulations of phlorizin could be used safely in humans.

After discovering sodium-glucose cotransport in the 1960s, Robert Crane went on to demonstrate that phlorizin competitively inhibits this cotransport mechanism in the small intestine. Given its known ability to inhibit SGLT1, phlorizin was thus used as the starting point for synthesizing the first SGLT2 inhibitors (Fig. 8.1). Phlorizin itself was not developed as an SGLT2 inhibitor as it is poorly absorbed orally and its non-selective inhibition of SGLT1 leads to impaired glucose absorption in the small intestine.

Dapaglifozin was the first SGLT2 inhibitor to be approved for medical use. It was approved in the European Union in 2012 after demonstrating a significant reduction in glycosylated hemoglobin levels in patients with type 2 diabetes mellitus compared to placebo. Canaglifozin and then Empaglifozin followed suit.

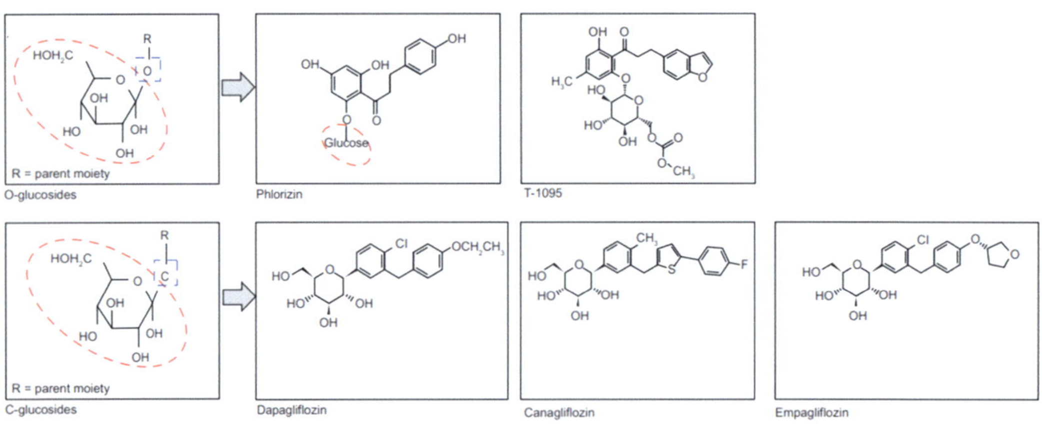

Fig. 8.1 Phlorizin is an O-glucoside derivative, which renders it unstable in the small intestine. Early SGLT2 inhibitors—dapaglifozin, canaglifozin, empaglifozin—derived from phlorizin were structurally modified to be C-glucosides and thus more stable in the small intestine. (Reproduced with permission from Nauck [31])

SGLT2 Inhibitors: Mechanism of Action in Heart Failure

Structural Mechanism of Action

Sodium-glucose cotransporters, part of the leucine-transporter (LeuT) family, work by an alternating access mechanism in which they first bind sodium (Na+) and glucose from the extracellular side and then transition to an inward-facing conformation and release the molecules into the cytoplasm. Glucose transport 'uphill' against its concentration gradient is coupled with sodium transport 'downhill' its concentration gradient (Fig. 8.2). SGLT1 is considered a high-affinity, low-capacity cotransporter: it binds glucose and galactose but not fructose and transports one glucose molecule for every two sodium ions [4]. It is expressed primarily in the small intestine and kidneys, and is also found in human salivary glands, liver, lung, skeletal muscle, heart and pancreatic alpha-cells. SGLT2 is considered a low-affinity, high-capacity transport: it binds glucose > galactose > fructose and transports one glucose molecule for one sodium ion. It is predominantly expressed in the kidneys but has also

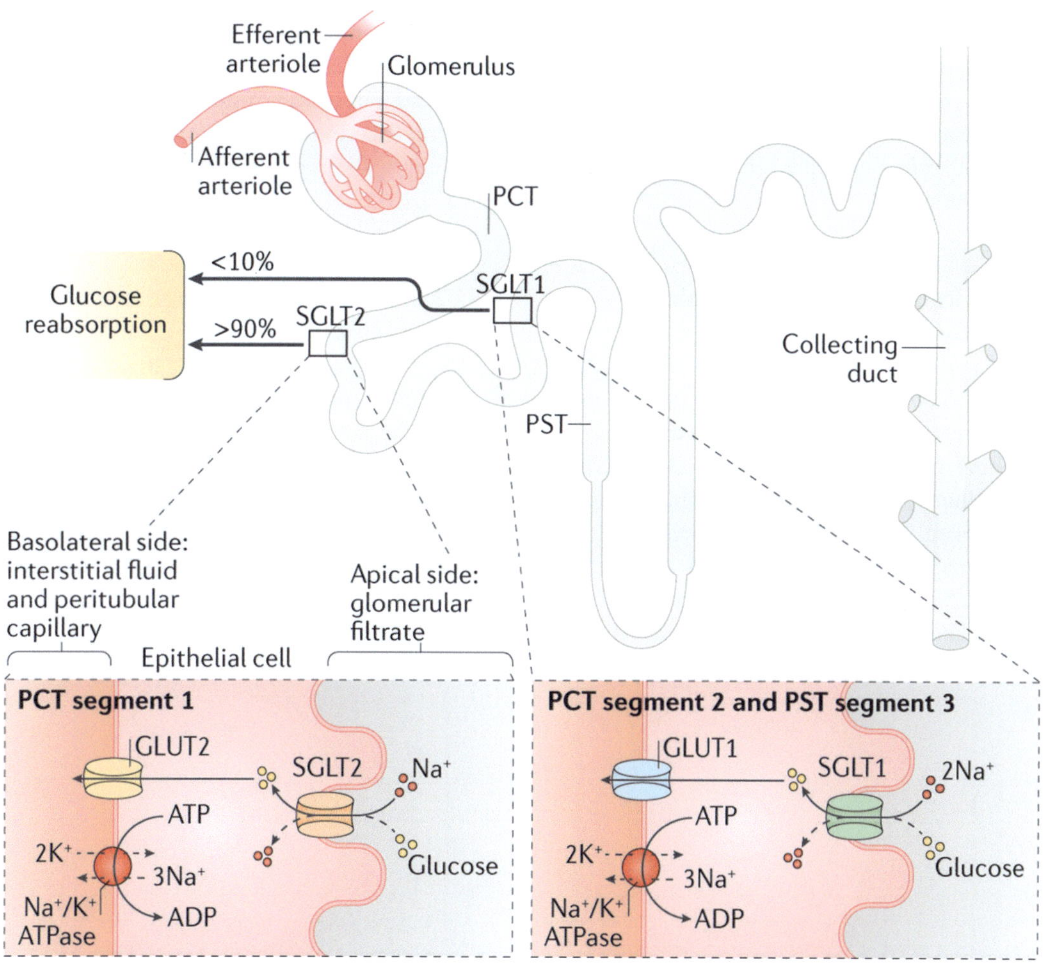

Fig. 8.2 Most (>90%) of the glucose is reabsorbed from the glomerular filtrate into the epithelial cells via sodium–glucose cotransporter 2 (SGLT2) in segment 1 of the proximal convoluted tubule (PCT); the remainder of the glucose (<10%) is reabsorbed via SGLT1 in PCT segment 2 and proximal straight tubule (PST) segment 3. (Reproduced with permission from Cowie and Fisher [32])

been found in the mammary glands, testis, liver, lung, intestine, skeletal muscle, spleen, cerebellum, and pancreatic alpha-cells. The physiologic roles of the other SGLTs—SGLT3, SGLT4, SGLT5, and SGLT6—are unknown.

SGLT2, also known as glifozins or flozins, are considered phlorizin-derivatives and are composed of a sugar moiety bound to an aromatic aglycon tail. Unlike phlorizin, glifozins are not rapidly degraded in the small intestine; this is accomplished with the addition of an anion (ie chloride in dapaglifozin and empaglifozin, fluoride in canaglifozin) in the chemical structure to stabilize the molecule. The structural basis of how inhibitors block transport is unknown [5]. SGLT2 inhibitors likely stabilize a Na-bound, outward-facing conformation of the sodium-glucose cotransporter, 'locking' it in such a way that it cannot transport glucose or sodium into the epithelial cells lining the renal proximal convoluted tubule.

SGLT2 Inhibition and Cardiac Metabolism

SGLT2 inhibition also appears to positively affect cardiac metabolism through several avenues. It causes an increase in circulating ketones, which leads to an increase in myocardial adenosine triphosphate (ATP) levels. It appears to decrease oxidative stress in cardiac myocytes as well as endothelial cells, which may directly contribute to their beneficial effects on cardiac remodeling. SGLT2 inhibitors also increase erythropoietin and, by extension, the oxygen supply to cardiac myocytes. Finally, inhibition of SGLT2 is thought to inhibit sodium-hydrogen ion exchange which causes an increase in mitochondrial calcium levels and an overall improvement in mitochondrial function that reduces oxidative stress and reduces the incidence of cardiac arrhythmias [7].

SGLT2 Inhibition and Systemic Hemodynamics

Inhibition of sodium and glucose uptake results in sodium and glucose excretion in the urine. The resulting natriuretic and osmotic effect reduces intracellular and extracellular volumes by the same token [6]. This ultimately leads to a sustained reduction in intravascular volume and blood pressure which offloads the heart by reducing cardiac preload and afterload, respectively.

SGLT2 Inhibitors and Cardiac Autonomic Activity

SGLT2 inhibitors appear to decrease cardiac sympathetic activity and increase parasympathetic nerve activity (Fig. 8.3). Offloading the heart and improving myocardial oxygen supply and demand contribute to this phenomenon. SGLT2 inhibitors may also act through increased vagal tone to decrease brainstem activity and subsequently control heart rate.

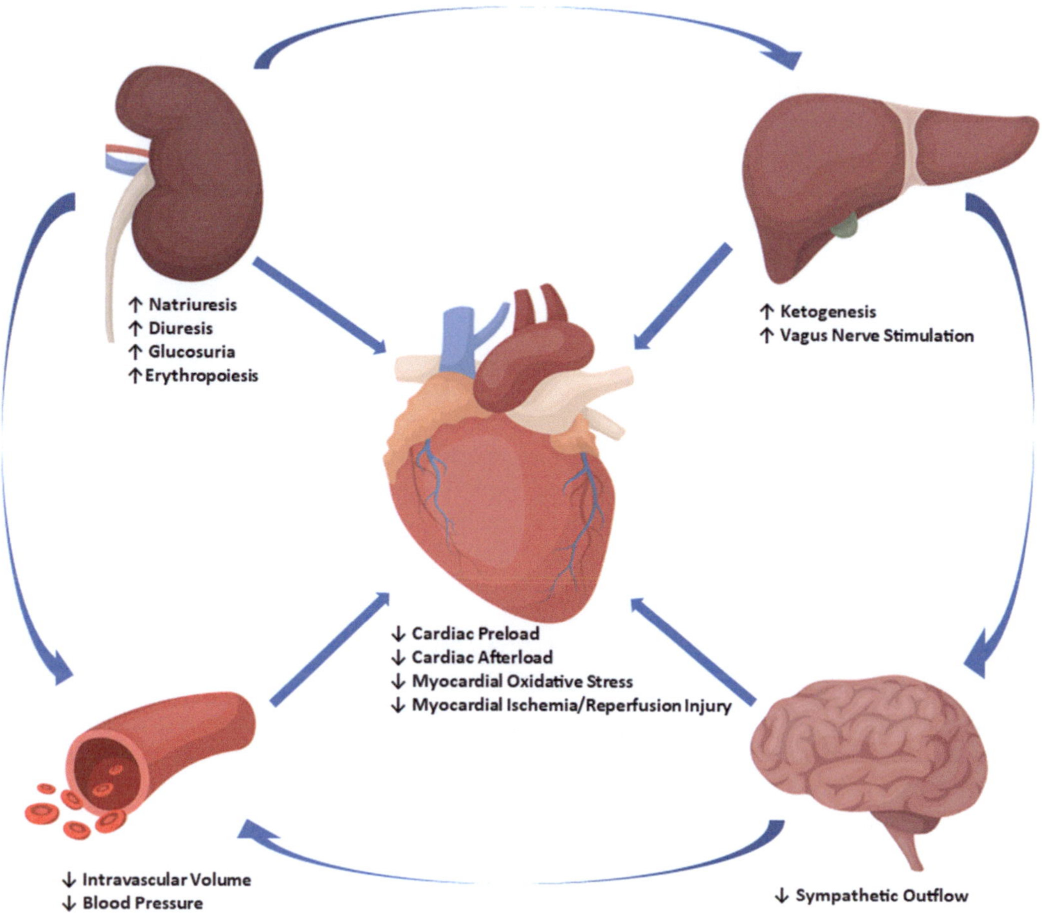

Fig. 8.3 Proposed mechanisms of action of sodium-glucose cotransporter 2 inhibitors in patients with heart failure

SGLT2 Inhibitors: Adverse Effects

Genital Mycotic Infections

The most common adverse effect of SGLT2 inhibition is genital mycotic infections, which is not unexpected given the glycosuria-inducing effect of the medication. Genital mycotic infections, which present as mycotic vulvovaginitis in women and mycotic balanitis in men, occur at an incidence of 5–15% in patients on SGLT2 inhibitors. They disproportionately affect women 4-to-1 compared to men and are more common in women who are premenopausal, obese, and/or have had prior mycotic infections [8]. Surprisingly, there does not appear to be an association between baseline HgA1c levels and incidence of genital mycotic infection. Most cases respond well to standard therapy.

Urinary Tract Infections

There is inconsistent data on the increased risk of urinary tract infections (UTI) with SGLT2 inhibitors. A pooled safety analysis of dapagliflozin showed a higher incidence of UTI in patients who received the 5 mg dose of dapagliflozin but not the 10 mg dose, which is the dose recommended for patients with heart failure [9]. A more contemporary meta-analysis showed a dose-dependent increased risk of urinary tract infections in patients taking dapagliflozin but not with other SGLT2 inhibitors [10]. There may be an increased risk of urinary tract and genital infections in women over the age of 65. However, being on an SGLT2 inhibitor does not seem to pose a greater risk of contracting a UTI when compared to other oral diabetes medications [11, 12]. Nevertheless, the Food and Drug Administration (FDA) has issued a warning regarding the risk of urinary tract infections in this class of medications.

Ketoacidosis

The increased risk of ketoacidosis in SGLT2 inhibition is attributed to decreased fasting plasma glucose concentrations, which leads to glucagon secretion and inhibition of insulin secretion. This in turn results in an increase in plasma free fatty acids and a subsequent increase in fat oxidation and ketone production. Several studies have shown, however, that patients with normal glucose tolerance (and patients with prediabetes) are not at increased risk of ketoacidosis on SGLT2 inhibitors [13–15]. This appears to be because patients without diabetes do not experience a decrease in fasting plasma glucose while on an SGLT2 inhibitor [16]. It is important to note that patients on SGLT2 inhibitors who are actively fasting for surgery are at increased risk for developing postoperative euglycemic ketoacidosis. These patients are now advised to stop taking their SGLT2-inhibitor 3–4 days prior to surgery to minimize this risk.

Bone Fragility

An increased risk of bone fractures was noted in the initial trial group studying cardiovascular outcomes in patients with diabetes who were given canaglifozin. Patients receiving canaglifozin at 100 mg and 300 mg experienced 1.4 and 1.5 bone fractures per 100 patient-years, respectively, compared to 1.1 per 100-patient-years in the placebo arm [17]. Bone density studies done at the 2-year mark for patients on canaglifozin also showed a decrease in total hip bone mineral density [18]. This information would seem to indicate that canaglifozin causes increased bone fragility leading to increased risk of fracture. It is worthwhile noting, however, that the increased incidence of bone fractures noted in the canaglifozin arm occurred after a relatively short period of time - at 12 weeks after starting the drug. Furthermore, while canaglifozin was associated with a decrease in total hip bone mineral density, it was not associated with decreased bone mineral density at other sites (ie femoral neck, lumbar spine, distal forearm) and it was associated with increased biomarkers of bone formation and resorption which may have been due at least in part to weight loss in patients studied. Neither decreased bone mineral density nor increased incidence of bone fracture has been observed in dapaglifozin or empaglifozin.

Hypotension

SGLT2 inhibitors have been associated with a decrease in blood pressure. This decrease may be associated with osmotic diuresis and natriuresis leading to plasma volume reduction, body weight loss, local RAAS inhibition, and release of nitric oxide. The data on whether SGLT2 inhibitors cause symptomatic hypotension, however, is less clear. In EMPEROR-Reduced, patients randomized to the empaglifozin arm with systolic blood pressures <110 mm Hg experienced a similar risk of hypotension when compared to placebo and an at-least similar treatment benefit when compared to patients with higher systolic blood pressures [19]. DAPA-HF similarly showed a statistically insignificant, placebo-corrected decrease in systolic blood pressure of <3 mm Hg in patients who received dapaglifozin.

Amputation

Canaglifozin was also associated with an increased risk of amputation in patients with diabetes in the CANVAS trial [20]. A subsequent analysis of case safety reports suggests that the increased risk of amputation may extend to empaglifozin and dapaglifozin; however, the absolute number of amputations reported was low (ie fewer than 100 out of over 8 million cases) [21].

Lipoproteins

Several trials have noted a small increase in LDL-c in patients initiated on an SGLT2 inhibitor with as yet undefined clinical significance [22]. There appears to be a similar favorable effect on HDL-c and triglycerides with SGLT2 inhibitor initiation. Further studies are warranted to evaluate the potential implications of SGLT2 inhibition on lipoprotein-mediated atherosclerotic cardiovascular risk.

Hypoglycemia

It is important to note that SGLT inhibitors as monotherapy add-ons to metformin have not been associated with hypoglycemia. There is, however, an increased incidence of hypoglycemia if taken with sulfonylureas and/or insulin.

SGLT2 Inhibitors and Renal Dysfunction

Post-marketing reports for canaglifozin and dapaglifozin were notable for a relatively high number of associated acute kidney injury, which appeared to improve with discontinuation of the drugs. Several trials have since shown that not only can SGLT2 inhibitors be safely used in patients with chronic kidney disease but that their use decreases the risk of adverse renal adverse events and abrupt declines in renal function [23]. The Canaglifozin and Renal Events in Diabetes with Established Nephropathy Clinical Evaluation (CREDENCE) included patients with type 2 diabetes and mean eGFR 56 ml/min/1.73 m^2 [24]. Canaglifozin reduced the risk of kidney failure, doubling of serum creatinine level or death from renal or cardiovascular causes when compared to placebo. The Dapaglifozin and Prevention of Adverse Outcomes in Chronic Kidney Disease (DAPA-CKD) trial, which included patients with slightly lower eGFR (mean 43 ml/min/1.73 m^2) compared to patients in CREDENCE, showed a statistically significant reduction in the primary composite outcome of a sustained decline in eGFR of at least 50%, kidney failure or death from renal or cardiovascular causes in those patients who received dapaglifozin compared to those who received placebo [25]. Similar renal protective effects have been observed in trials evaluating SGLT2 inhibitors in patients with heart failure (ie pooled analysis of DAPA-HF and EMPEROR-Reduced). Studies on SGTL2 inhibitor use in patients with heart failure with preserved ejection fraction (HFpEF) are limited to date. Safety data from the Dapaglifozin in Heart Failure with Mildly Reduced or Preserved Ejection Fraction (DELIVER) trial showed no difference in acute kidney injury between the dapaglifozin and placebo arms.

Empaglifozin at the 10 mg daily dose is currently indicated for patients with heart failure and estimated glomerular filtration rates (eGFR) ≥20 mL/min/1.73 m^2. This is based off pooled analysis of the EMPEROR-Reduced and EMPEROR-Preserved trials which showed potential benefit for patients with heart failure and severe, pre-dialysis, renal dysfunction. Dapaglifozin has not been studied in patients with eGFR <25 mL/min/1.73 m^2; it is thus indicated in heart failure patients with eGFR ≥25 mL/min/1.73 m^2.

SGLT2 Inhibitors: The Heart Failure Trials

Long-term cardiovascular outcomes trials on diabetes medications have been mandated by the Food and Drug Administration since 2008, ever since accumulated data on thiazolidinediones suggested an increased risk of myocardial infarction with that class of drug. Empaglifozin Cardiovascular Outcome Event Trial in Type 2 Diabetes Patients (EMPA-REG OUTCOME) was one such trial that followed adverse cardiovascular events in diabetic patients prescribed either empaglifozin or placebo. Unexpectedly,

EMPA-REG OUTCOME demonstrated a clear reduction in the composite outcome of major adverse cardiovascular events, cardiovascular mortality, any cause mortality or heart failure hospitalization in patients with type 2 diabetes and high cardiovascular risk in the empaglifozin arm when compared to placebo. These results were also observed in the cardiovascular outcomes trial for canaglifozin (CANVAS). And while The Multicenter Trial to Evaluate the Effect of Dapagliflozin on the Incidence of Cardiovascular Events (DECLARE-TIMI 58) did not show a reduction in risk of major adverse cardiovascular events in patients on dapaglifozin, it did show a lower rate of heart failure hospitalizations and cardiovascular death in those patients. These results led to studies on the effects of SGLT2 inhibitors specifically on patients with heart failure, regardless of diabetes status.

Heart Failure with Reduced Ejection Fraction

The first of these studies was in 2019, evaluating the cardiovascular effects of SGLT2 inhibitors in patients with heart failure with reduced ejection fraction (HFrEF) in 2019 (Table 8.1). Dapaglifozin in Patients with Heart Failure and Reduced Ejection fraction (DAPA-HF) was a multi-center, double-blind, randomized control trial that evaluated a composite outcome of worsening heart failure or cardiovascular death in patients receiving either dapaglifozin or placebo. The study found that those in the dapaglifozin arm were at lower risk of worsening heart failure or cardiovascular death compared to those in the placebo arm. The study also showed a statistically significant improvement in symptoms in patients receiving dapaglifozin compared to those patients getting placebo. These outcomes were replicated in the EMPEROR-Reduced trial in 2020 in patients taking empaglifozin compared to those taking placebo.

The SOLOIST-WHF trial followed patients with diabetes and heart failure on sotaglifozin. In

Table 8.1 Relevant clinical trials evaluating sodium glucose co-transporter 2 inhibitors (SGLT2i) in patients with heart failure with reduced ejection fraction (HFrEF)

Key trials examining SGLT2i in HFrEF		
Trial	Population	Primary outcomes
DAPA-HF	All patients with LVEF ≤40%, NT-ProBNP ≥600 pg/ml NYHA class II to IV symptoms 42% with diabetes	Dapaglifozin 10 mg reduced the risk of cardiovascular death, HF hospitalizations, or urgent HF visit
DEFINE-HF	All patients with LVEF ≤40%, NT-ProBNP ≥400 pg/ml or BNP ≥100 pg/ml NYHA class II to III symptoms	Dapaglifozin 10 mg improved quality of life as evaluated using the KCCQ or caused a significant decrease in NT-ProBNP at 12 weeks
EMPEROR-reduced	All patients with LVEF ≤40%, NT-ProBNP ≥600 pg/ml NYHA class II to IV symptoms	Empaglifozin 10 mg reduced cardiovascular mortality or HF hospitalization and improved quality of life as evaluated using the KCCQ
Meta-analysis of DAPA-HF and EMPEROR-reduced		SGLT2i reduced all-cause death by 13%
SOLOIST-WHF	Patients hospitalized with HF, SBP ≥100, NT-ProBNP ≥600 pg/ml 100% with type II diabetes 79% with LVEF <50%	Sotaglifozin 200–400 mg reduced the risk of death, HF hospitalizations or urgent HF visits and improved quality of life as evaluated using the KCCQ

BNP brain natriuretic peptide, *HF* heart failure, *HFrEF* heart failure with reduced ejection fraction, *KCCQ* Kansas City Cardiomyopathy Questionnaire, *LVEF* left ventricular ejection fraction, *NT-ProBNP* n-terminal pro-brain natriuretic peptide, *NYHA* New York Heart Association, *SBP* systolic blood pressure, *SGLT2i* sodium-glucose cotransporter 2 inhibitor addition to confirming a reduced risk of cardiovascular death and hospitalization in the SGLT2 inhibitor arm compared to placebo, this trial noted a time to sustained reduction of risk of 27 days. The study is also the only study to date to show a reduced risk of cardiovascular death in the SGLT2 inhibitor arm. It is worth noting, however, that this was only shown in on-treatment analysis but not in the pooled intention-to-treat analysis. The trial was also stopped prematurely due to loss of funding during COVID.

Heart Failure with Preserved Ejection Fraction

SGLT2 inhibitors have been shown to benefit patients with heart failure with preserved ejection fraction (HFpEF), which cannot be said without qualifiers about most medications shown to benefit the HFrEF patient population (ie ARNIs, MRAs) (Table 8.2). In the EMPEROR-PRESERVED trial, empagliflozin was shown to reduce the risk of cardiovascular death or heart failure hospitalization amongst patients with heart failure with preserved ejection fraction (LVEF ≥50%) [24]. It is worth noting that the benefit was driven by a reduction in heart failure hospitalization. No medication to date has been shown to reduce cardiovascular death or death from any cause in the HFpEF population. Of the four pillars of guideline-directed medical therapies in the HFrEF population, SGLT2 inhibitors are the only class of medications with a class 2a recommendation for use in HFpEF patients in the 2022 ACC/AHA/HFSA Guidelines for the Management of Heart Failure. ARB/ARNI and MRA hold a class 2b recommendation [26].

Empagliflozin was also shown to benefit renal function in patients with preserved ejection fraction in EMPEROR-PRESERVED. Patients were noted to have a slower decline in renal function on empagliflozin compared to placebo and were at lower risk of acute kidney injury.

Patients also reported overall symptom improvement on empagliflozin and were less likely to show deterioration, as assessed using the Kansas City Cardiomyopathy Questionnaire (KCCQ). This improvement in quality of life was replicated in the SGLT2 inhibitor arm of the Empagliflozin in Patients Hospitalized for Acute

Table 8.2 Relevant clinical trials evaluating sodium glucose co-transporter 2 inhibitors (SGLT2i) in patients with heart failure with preserved ejection fraction (HFpEF)

Key trials examining SGLT2i in HFpEF		
Trial	Population	Primary outcomes
CHIEF-HF	All patients with LVEF ≥40% and baseline KCCQ score ≤80	Canaglifozin 100 mg improved symptoms of HF as evaluated using KCCQ
PRESERVED-HF	All patients with LVEF >45%, NT- ProBNP ≥225 pg/ml or BNP ≥75 pg/ml NYHA class II to IV symptoms	Dapaglifozin 10 mg improved symptoms and physical limitations from HF in 12 weeks as measured by KCCQ-CS
DELIVER	All patients with LVEF >40% NYHA class II to IV symptoms 45% with diabetes	Dapaglifozin 10 mg reduced cardiovascular mortality, HF hospitalizations, or urgent HF visits by 18%
Meta-analysis including DELIVER and EMPEROR-preserved	>78% with diabetes	SGLT2i reduced cardiovascular death or first hospitalization for heart failure, driven by a reduction in heart failure hospitalizations
EMPEROR-preserved	All patients with LVEF >40% 49% with diabetes	Empaglifozin 10 mg reduced the risk of cardiovascular death or HF hospitalizations, driven by a reduction in hospitalizations

BNP brain natriuretic peptide, *HF* heart failure, *HFpEF* heart failure with preserved ejection fraction, *KCCQ* Kansas City Cardiomyopathy Questionnaire, *LVEF* left ventricular ejection fraction, *NT-ProBNP* n-terminal pro-brain natriuretic peptide, *NYHA* New York Heart Association, *SBP* systolic blood pressure, *SGLT2i* sodium-glucose co-transporter 2 inhibitor

Heart Failure (EMPULSE) trial [27]. Patients were also noted to have greater reduction in body weight on empaglifozin in this trial compared to placebo.

In the Dapaglifozin Evaluation to Improve the Lives of Patients with Preserved Ejection Fraction Hart Failure (DELIVER) trial, patients in the dapaglifozin arm were noted to have a 1.8 mm Hg reduction in systolic blood pressure (SBP) compared to placebo [28]. Notably, the beneficial effect of SGLT2 inhibitors in DELIVER was observed consistently irrespective of diabetes status and across the range of frailty, baseline SBP, NT-ProBNPs, and body mass index (BMI) studied.

Heart Failure with Mildly Reduced Ejection Fraction

There is a growing body of evidence to suggest that patients with mildly reduced ejection fraction (HFmrEF), defined as having an LVEF 40% or greater and less than 50%, may benefit from the same guideline directed medical therapies found to be beneficial for patients with LVEF less than 40%. On subgroup analysis, the EMPEROR-PRESERVED trial provided clinical evidence that SGLT2 inhibitors reduce heart failure mortality and heart failure hospitalizations not only in patients with preserved ejection fractions but also in HFmrEF patients. In fact, the largest benefit was noted among the HFmrEF patients in this study. These findings were later confirmed in the DELIVER trial. There are no prospective randomized control trials on SGLT2 inhibitors in patients specifically with HFmrEF, however. For this reason, the use of SGLT2 inhibitors in patients with mildly reduced ejection fraction is a class 2b recommendation in the 2022 AHA/ACC/HFSA Guidelines for the management of heart failure.

SGLT2 Inhibitors and Cardio-Oncology

SGLT2 inhibitors may reduce the rate of heart failure hospitalization in patients with diabetes and cancer who are treated with anthracyclines [29]. A retrospective study of diabetic patients on an SGLT2 inhibitor at the time of anthracycline treatment found that these patients were less likely to be newly diagnosed with heart failure, be admitted to the hospital for heart failure, and develop a clinically significant arrhythmia compared to diabetic patients not on an SGLT2 inhibitor while being treated with an anthracycline [30]. These patients also had lower overall mortality as well as a lower composite of sepsis and neutropenic fever. A more contemporary study with a larger patient population failed to observe this mortality benefit; however, the study did show a lower risk of hospitalization in the arm of patients on SGLT2 inhibitors. Further investigation in the form of randomized controlled trials is warranted.

SGLT2 Inhibitors: Ongoing Investigations in Heart Failure

Several trials are underway to refine our understanding of the optimal use of SGLT2 inhibitors in various patient populations. EMPACT-MI and PRESTIGE-MI will evaluate the effect of SGLT2 inhibitors on patients who have sustained acute myocardial infarctions. Other patient populations of unique interest include those with cardiac amyloidosis and those with end-stage renal disease.

Additional avenues of investigation include evaluating the combined effects of SGLT2 inhibitors with other guideline-directed medical therapies in the heart failure population as well as the optimal timing of initiating these therapies.

RECEDE-CHF will evaluate the effect of loop diuretics and SGLT2 inhibitors on major adverse cardiovascular events in heart failure patients. Another study aims to evaluate the effects of angiotensin-receptor/neprilysin-inhibitors and SGLT2 inhibitors on ventricular remodeling.

Several studies are also underway to evaluate the clinical applicability of posited mechanisms of action by which SGLT2 inhibitors achieve their favorable effects on the heart failure patient population. ERTU-SODIUM will look at ertuglifozin's effects on interstitial volume, plasma volume, subcutaneous sodium storage and the functionality of the subcutaneous glycosaminoglycan network in HFrEF patients. VERTICAL will look at its effects on cardiac fibrosis inhibition. DAPA-MEMRI will assess the effect of dapaglifozin on calcium in heart failure patients.

The last 5 years have seen tremendous pharmacologic advancement in the management of heart failure. SGLT2 inhibitors are now one of four classes of medications which clearly benefit patients with reduced ejection fraction. They are the only class of medications that have shown benefit in the management of heart failure with preserved ejection fraction. The next 5 years will hopefully add to our understanding of how SGLT2 inhibitors achieve their salubrious effects on heart failure patients and steer future pharmaceutical innovation in the field.

References

1. Crane RK, Krane SM. Studies on the mechanism of the intestinal active transport of sugars. Biochim Biophys Acta. 1959;31(2):397–401.
2. Ehrenkranz JR, Lewis NG, Kahn CR, Roth J. Phlorizin: a review. Diabetes Metab Res Rev. 2005;21(1):31–8.
3. Chasis H, Jolliffe N, Smith HW. The action of phlorizin on the excretion of glucose, xylose, sucrose, creatinine and urea by man. J Clin Invest. 1933;12(6):1083–90.
4. Sano R, Shinozaki Y, Ohta T. Sodium-glucose cotransporters: functional properties and pharmaceutical potential. J Diabetes Investig. 2020;11(4):770–82.
5. Bisignano P, Ghezzi C, Jo H, Polizzi NF, Althoff T, Kalyanaraman C, et al. Inhibitor binding mode and allosteric regulation of Na(+)-glucose symporters. Nat Commun. 2018;9(1):5245.
6. Kubota Y, Shimizu W. Clinical benefits of sodium-glucose cotransporter 2 inhibitors and the mechanisms underlying their cardiovascular effects. JACC: ASIA. 2022;2:287–93.
7. Packer M, Anker SD, Butler J, Filippatos G, Zannad F. Effects of sodium-glucose cotransporter 2 inhibitors for the treatment of patients with heart failure: proposal of a novel mechanism of action. JAMA Cardiol. 2017;2(9):1025–9.
8. Bhatt DL, Szarek M, Steg PG, Cannon CP, Leiter LA, McGuire DK, et al. Sotagliflozin in patients with diabetes and recent worsening heart failure. N Engl J Med. 2021;384(2):117–28.
9. Johnsson KM, Ptaszynska A, Schmitz B, Sugg J, Parikh SJ, List JF. Urinary tract infections in patients with diabetes treated with dapagliflozin. J Diabetes Complicat. 2013;27(5):473–8.
10. Behzadi P, Behzadi E, Pawlak-Adamska EA. Urinary tract infections (UTIs) or genital tract infections (GTIs)? It's the diagnostics that count. GMS Hyg Infect Control. 2019;14:Doc14.
11. Monzo L, Ferrari I, Cicogna F, Tota C, Cice G, Girerd N, et al. Sodium-glucose co-transporter 2 inhibitors in heart failure: an updated evidence-based practical guidance for clinicians. Eur Heart J Suppl. 2023;25(Suppl C):C309–c15.
12. Lega IC, Bronskill SE, Campitelli MA, Guan J, Stall NM, Lam K, et al. Sodium glucose cotransporter 2 inhibitors and risk of genital mycotic and urinary tract infection: a population-based study of older women and men with diabetes. Diabetes Obes Metab. 2019;21(11):2394–404.
13. Persson F, Rossing P, Vart P, Chertow GM, Hou FF, Jongs N, et al. Efficacy and safety of dapagliflozin by baseline glycemic status: a prespecified analysis from the DAPA-CKD trial. Diabetes Care. 2021;44(8):1894–7.
14. Anker SD, Butler J, Filippatos G, Khan MS, Marx N, Lam CSP, et al. Effect of empagliflozin on cardiovascular and renal outcomes in patients with heart failure by baseline diabetes status: results from the EMPEROR-reduced trial. Circulation. 2021;143(4):337–49.
15. Petrie MC, Verma S, Docherty KF, Inzucchi SE, Anand I, Belohlavek J, et al. Effect of dapagliflozin on worsening heart failure and cardiovascular death in patients with heart failure with and without diabetes. JAMA. 2020;323(14):1353–68.
16. Al Jobori H, Daniele G, Adams J, Cersosimo E, Triplitt C, DeFronzo RA, et al. Determinants of the increase in ketone concentration during SGLT2 inhibition in NGT, IFG and T2DM patients. Diabetes Obes Metab. 2017;19(6):809–13.
17. Watts NB, Bilezikian JP, Usiskin K, Edwards R, Desai M, Law G, et al. Effects of canagliflozin on fracture risk in patients with type 2 diabetes mellitus. J Clin Endocrinol Metab. 2016;101(1):157–66.
18. Bilezikian JP, Watts NB, Usiskin K, Polidori D, Fung A, Sullivan D, et al. Evaluation of bone mineral density and bone biomarkers in patients with type 2 dia-

betes treated with canagliflozin. J Clin Endocrinol Metab. 2016;101(1):44–51.
19. Girerd N. Low blood pressure and managing drugs in HF: where do SGLT2 inhibitors stand? J Am Coll Cardiol. 2021;78(13):1349–51.
20. Neal B, Perkovic V, Mahaffey KW, de Zeeuw D, Fulcher G, Erondu N, et al. Canagliflozin and cardiovascular and renal events in type 2 diabetes. N Engl J Med. 2017;377(7):644–57.
21. Khouri C, Cracowski JL, Roustit M. SGLT-2 inhibitors and the risk of lower-limb amputation: is this a class effect? Diabetes Obes Metab. 2018;20(6):1531–4.
22. Halimi S, Verges B. Adverse effects and safety of SGLT-2 inhibitors. Diabetes Metab. 2014;40(6 Suppl 1):S28–34.
23. van der Aart-van der Beek AB, de Boer RA, Heerspink HJL. Kidney and heart failure outcomes associated with SGLT2 inhibitor use. Nat Rev Nephrol. 2022;18(5):294–306.
24. Perkovic V, Jardine MJ, Neal B, Bompoint S, Heerspink HJL, Charytan DM, et al. Canagliflozin and renal outcomes in type 2 diabetes and nephropathy. N Engl J Med. 2019;380(24):2295–306.
25. Heerspink HJL, Stefánsson BV, Correa-Rotter R, Chertow GM, Greene T, Hou F-F, et al. Dapagliflozin in patients with chronic kidney disease. N Engl J Med. 2020;383(15):1436–46.
26. Heidenreich PA, Bozkurt B, Aguilar D, Allen LA, Byun JJ, Colvin MM, et al. 2022 AHA/ACC/HFSA guideline for the management of heart failure: a report of the American College of Cardiology/American Heart Association Joint Committee on Clinical Practice Guidelines. Circulation. 2022;145(18):e895–e1032.
27. Voors AA, Angermann CE, Teerlink JR, Collins SP, Kosiborod M, Biegus J, et al. The SGLT2 inhibitor empagliflozin in patients hospitalized for acute heart failure: a multinational randomized trial. Nat Med. 2022;28(3):568–74.
28. Peikert A, Goyal P, Vaduganathan M, Claggett BL, Kulac IJ, Miao ZM, et al. Dapagliflozin in heart failure with mildly reduced or preserved ejection fraction according to polypharmacy status. JACC Heart Fail. 2023;11:1380–93.
29. Abdel-Qadir H, Carrasco R, Austin PC, Chen Y, Zhou L, Fang J, et al. The association of sodium-glucose cotransporter 2 inhibitors with cardiovascular outcomes in anthracycline-treated patients with cancer. JACC CardioOncol. 2023;5(3):318–28.
30. Gongora CA, Drobni ZD, Quinaglia Araujo Costa Silva T, Zafar A, Gong J, Zlotoff DA, et al. Sodium-glucose co-transporter-2 inhibitors and cardiac outcomes among patients treated with anthracyclines. JACC Heart Fail. 2022;10(8):559–67.
31. Nauck M. Update on developments with SGLT2 inhibitors in the management of type 2 diabetes. Drug Des Devel Ther. 2014;8:1335–80. https://doi.org/10.2147/DDDT.S50773.
32. Cowie MR, Fisher M. SGLT2 inhibitors: mechanisms of cardiovascular benefit beyond glycaemic control. Nat Rev Cardiol. 2020;17(12):761–72.

Management of the Patient with Heart Failure with Preserved Ejection Fraction

9

Jeffrey D. Wessler and Mathew S. Maurer

Introduction

Since its first formal characterization three decades ago as *congestive heart failure with normal systolic function* [1] heart failure with preserved ejection fraction (HFPEF) has emerged as an increasingly common and challenging entity within the field of heart failure. Several early studies conducted on hypertrophic and infarcted hearts demonstrated diminished diastolic left ventricular (LV) filling and led to coining of the term *diastolic heart failure* [2, 3]. Yet as our understanding of heart failure has grown, the term "diastolic heart failure" was replaced by the nomenclature "heart failure with a preserved ejection fraction" by national guidelines in part because of diverse pathophysiologic mechanisms beyond diastolic dysfunction that contribute to the observed phenotype and are potential targets for therapy [4]. The following chapter will cover the management of patients with HFPEF. After presenting an overview of the scope and pathophysiology of the condition, we will detail the diagnostic approach and treatment options before concluding with a look at the future directions in HFPEF.

J. D. Wessler (✉)
Department of Medicine, Columbia University Medical Center, New York, NY, USA
e-mail: jdw2170@columbia.edu

M. S. Maurer
Department of Medicine, Columbia University Medical Center, Allen Hospital of New York Presbyterian, New York, NY, USA
e-mail: msm10@columbia.edu

Epidemiology

HFPEF is a disease primarily effecting older adults. The incidence and prevalence of heart failure are increasing and it has been projected that these rates will continue well into the twenty-first Century. More than six million Americans have been diagnosed with heart failure in the United States [5]. The total number of admissions for heart failure in the United States is greater than one million per year [5]. Readmission rates are as high as 30–60% within 3–6 months after discharge [6]. The incidence and prevalence of heart failure are strikingly age-dependent, with prevalence rates in adults over 80 years of age approaching 10% and mortality rates increasing exponentially with advancing age in all major demographic subgroups of the United States population [5]. Although several factors have contributed to the rise in heart failure, principal among them is the progressive aging of the population. The exponential increase in the prevalence of heart failure has been attributed to the increase in prevalence and cumulative duration of systemic hypertension and coronary artery disease with advancing age and age-related changes in cardiac structure and function, which occur even in the absence of overt clinically defined cardio-

H. J. Eisen (ed.), *Heart Failure I*, https://doi.org/10.1007/978-3-032-12626-9_9

vascular disease [7, 8]. Consistent with the high prevalence and substantial mortality associated with this disorder, heart failure is currently one of the most common reasons for hospital admission in adults older than 65 years of age. It is not only one of the most common diagnosis related group in the Medicare population, it is also the most costly, with estimated annual inpatient expenditures in excess of $15 billion [9].

Of all patients suffering from heart failure, the majority have preserved ejection fraction. While these changes in the heart failure phenotype are thought to be relatively new, the distribution of different ejection fraction consistent with HFREF (<40%), HFPEF (40–55%) and with HFNEF (>55%) in several large epidemiologic studies at the inception of these cohorts demonstrates that most individuals with heart failure in the community have a normal or preserved ejection fraction (see Fig. 9.1). These individuals are more likely to be elderly, female, have higher body mass index (BMI), higher blood pressure, and lower hemoglobin than those with reduced ejection fraction. The rate of hospitalization for HFPEF now exceeds that of heart failure with reduced ejection fraction (HFREF), and 6-month re-hospitalization approaches 50% [10–12]. Patients with HFPEF are characteristically affected by multiple co-morbidities that contribute to their disease—including obesity, hypertension, anemia, diabetes, coronary artery disease, and chronic kidney disease—as well as multiple non-cardiac comorbidities seen more commonly in older adults—including chronic pulmonary disease, liver disease, thyroid dysfunction, and cancer [10, 13]. Not surprisingly, therefore, though the mortality rates in HFPEF are similar to HFREF, the cause of death in HFPEF is more commonly attributed to non-cardiovascular causes [14], as is the reason for readmission after a hospitalization for acute decompensated heart failure [9].

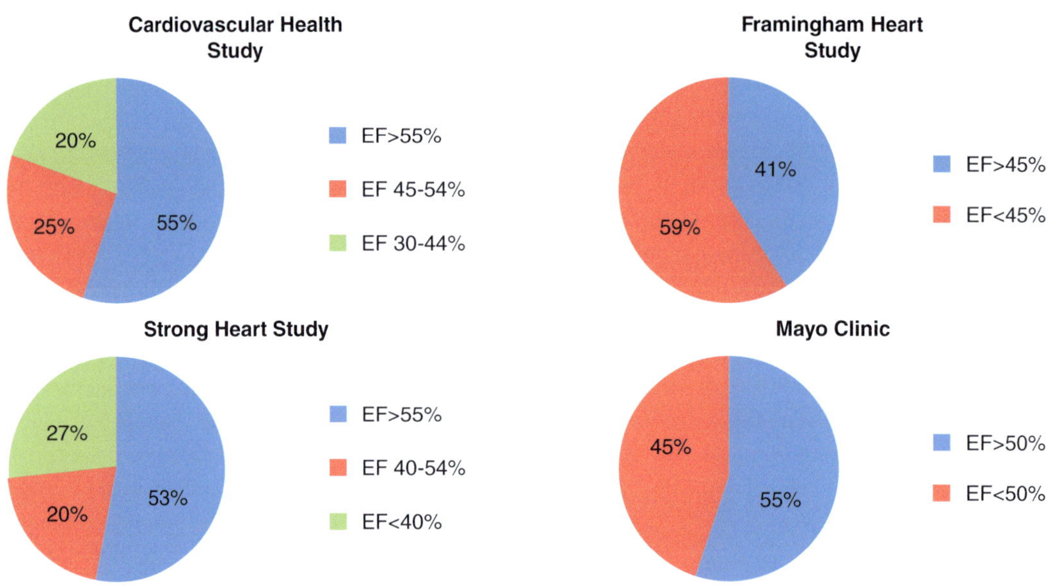

Fig. 9.1 Prevalence of HFPEF in four major epidemiologic cohorts [15–18]

Pathophysiology

The traditional classification of HFPEF as *diastolic heart failure* is based on the premise that a single pathophysiologic mechanism underlies the genesis of HFPEF. Yet as understanding progressed and recognition that HFPEF is a complex clinical syndrome with multiple operative pathophysiologic mechanisms including several different subgroups of patients, it became apparent that diastolic dysfunction was inadequate to explain all cases of HFPEF [19]. Rational sub grouping of patients into cohorts that have operational and targetable pathophysiologic mechanisms can be appreciated by assessment of the pressure-volume (PV) relations that characterize different populations with HFPEF [20, 21]. PV measurements provide a systematic means of characterizing overall, systolic and diastolic properties of the heart, as well as isovolumetric pressure volume area (PVA_{iso}), which when indexed to EDP provides an afterload independent measure of the pump function of the ventricle [22]. End-systolic PV relation (ESPVR) and end-diastolic PV relation (EDPVR) in particular reflect global ventricular chamber pump properties that effect overall cardiac function. These parameters are in turn determined by intrinsic myocardial properties (systolic and diastolic function), but also by muscle mass, chamber architecture (how myocardial fibers are assembled), chamber shape, and sequence of myocardial activation.

Data from PV analyses in both animal and human studies have revealed at least three different phenotypes of HFPEF that are depicted in Fig. 9.2. In the first, patients have a normal ESPVR and upward shifted EDPVR—(e.g. reduced chamber capacitance or diastolic dysfunction) with normal chamber contractility (e.g. preserved systolic function) (Fig. 9.2a).

Patients with this classic diastolic heart failure paradigm have intrinsic myocardial disease causing impairment in cardiac relaxation and passive ventricular filling. Such severe and isolated diastolic dysfunction is often found in hypertrophic cardiomyopathy and infiltrative diseases such as cardiac amyloidosis. These patients with isolated diastolic dysfunction can be identified clinically by the presence of heart failure and a normal ejection fraction without

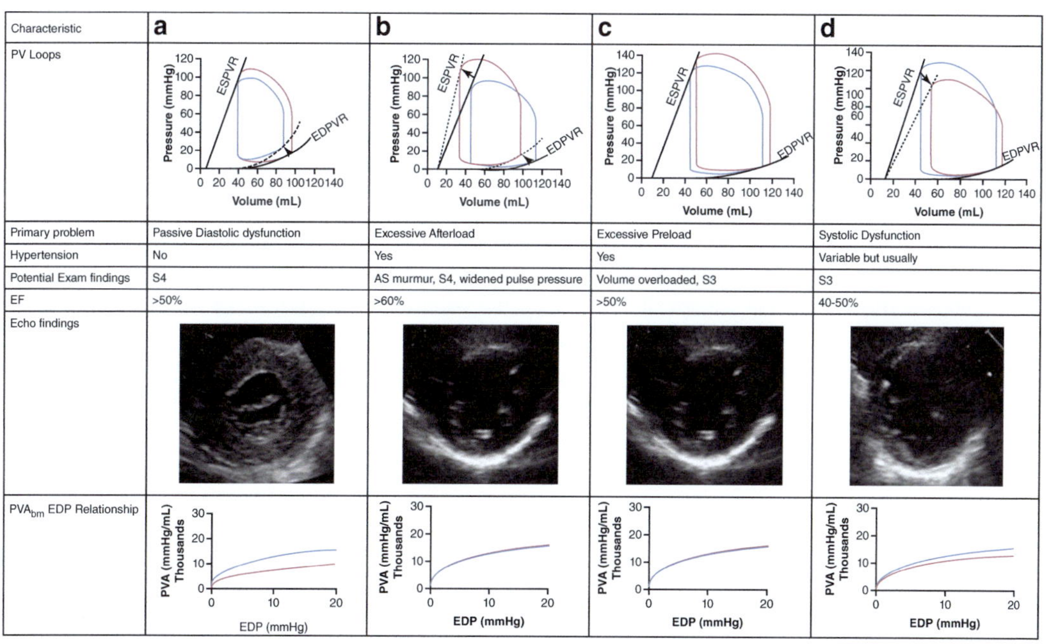

Fig. 9.2 Phenotypic characterization of HFPEF by pressure volume relations with associated clinical characteristics by primary problem. (**a**) Diastolic dysfunction. (**b**) Excessive afterload. (**c**) Excessive preload. (**d**) Systolic dysfunction

concomitant hypertension [23]. Physical exam findings are often notable for signs and symptoms of a stiff ventricle, including an S4 gallop and other classic but non-specific signs of heart failure such as pulmonary congestion and elevated jugular venous distension. In subjects with restrictive cardiomyopathies the jugular venous pressure often has a "double dip" which is indicative of the rapid "x" and "y" descent seen on the right atrial pressure tracing in patients with restriction. Ejection fraction is usually greater than 50% in the early phases of these conditions, and on echocardiogram Doppler evidence of diastolic dysfunction ranging from impaired relaxation to a restrictive filling pattern can be observed—although Doppler will be notably abnormal and indistinguishable in each of the following phenotypes of HFPEF [24]. Finally, the PVA_{iso} will be lower than normal in these subjects indicative of left ventricular pump dysfunction as a primary pathophysiologic mechanism underlying the phenotype.

In the second paradigm of HFPEF, ESPVR and EDPVR are both shifted upward and leftward, with a resulting decrease in chamber capacitance but with concomitant enhanced chamber systolic function—as evidenced by the upward shift of the ESPVR (Fig. 9.2b). In such subjects, the area between the ESPVR and EDPVR will be unchanged and the PVA_{iso} will remain normal. Examples of clinical conditions that produce this phenotype include increased afterload from chronic hypertension (usually from central conduit artery stiffening) and severe aortic stenosis. These two clinical scenarios are the most common causes of this phenotype in older adults with HFPEF. With normal physiologic aging, increasing central conduit arterial stiffness from collagen crosslinking leads to an increased arterial elastance with concomitant hypertension. Consequent concentric hypertrophy of the left ventricle yields subsequent reliance on atrial filling with corresponding left atrial (LA) enlargement [7, 8, 25, 26]. Similarly, concentric remodeling with a small ventricular chamber is seen in patients with aortic stenosis who are characterized by this phenotype according to this paradigm. Ejection fraction is often supranormal in these patients (>60%) as a result of an increase in end systolic elastance with a similar echocardiographic phenotype characterized by a normal to small LV chamber size, concentric LV hypertrophy and LA enlargement [27].

In the third subtype of HFPEF, patients can display normal ESPVR and normal or slightly rightward and downward shifted EDPVR (e.g. normal or increased capacitance) with increased end diastolic pressures. The latter results from an increased central volume that could be caused by either an expanded blood volume or a shift of the blood volume toward the central circulation from veno-constriction. Indeed, most of the blood volume in mammalian species is in the venous bed, and small changes in venous tone can result in large shift of blood volume back to the central circulation resulting in left ventricular overfilling [28]. Pathophysiologically, this phenotype is characterized by increased preload without significant alteration in LV systolic or diastolic function (e.g. the ESPVR and EDPVR are not significantly different from normal) (Fig. 9.2c) [29]. Although these patients also have hypertension, the primary operative mechanism is increased preload due conditions that expand the blood volume such as renal dysfunction, obesity, anemia and others. Indeed, age-related changes in non-cardiac systems including renal, pulmonary, endocrine, and autonomic nervous systems have been documented to produce a state of salt sensitive hypertension characterized by excessive salt and water retention [30–32]. The diminished pulmonary vascular capacitance with pulmonary arterial hypertension and endothelial dysfunction coupled with the volume redistribution that accompany advancing age (decreased beta-2 adrenergic responsiveness of the veins reduces venous capacitance) predispose the aging adult to the development of symptomatic pulmonary edema in the setting of normal LV systolic function. Patients display signs of volume overload on physical exam, and can have an S3 gallop. Ejection fraction is commonly >50% and echocardiography shows a mildly dilated LV that often is unrecognized [33]. LV pump function as indexed by the PVA_{iso} to EDP relation is supranormal in these subjects suggesting that the myocardium is performing more work at any given filling pressure.

Finally, subtle reductions in systolic function as evidenced by a reduction in LV chamber contractile function (either from a downward shifted ESPVR or increased V_0 [volume axis intercept of the ESPVR]) can cause neurohormonal activation that leads to salt and water retention (Fig. 9.2d) [34, 35]. In these subjects, the EF may be low normal or slightly reduced (e.g. ~40–50%). The primary mechanism in this underappreciated subtype is systolic dysfunction and PVA_{iso} to EDP relation that demonstrates a downward shift compared consistent with reduced chamber contractile strength. These patients are often hypertensive, and on physical exam will appear most similarly to patients with a mild form of systolic heart failure as demonstrated by non-invasive PV analysis [36].

The pathophysiology of HFPEF is heterogeneous, involving multiple physiologic domains in both cardiac and non-cardiac systems—and manifesting in patients with multiple co-morbid conditions. Despite the multifactorial etiology of the syndrome, there are several clinical signs and symptoms consistently present in patients that characterize the phenotype(s) of HFPEF: (i) Labile blood pressure with high resting LVEDP, (ii) predisposition for acute pulmonary edema, and (iii) effort intolerance with diminished exercise capacity [37–39]. Appreciating the distinct pathophysiologic mechanisms that contribute to these phenotypes is essential in guiding therapeutic interventions and in advancing the understanding and management of this condition.

Diagnosis

Diagnosing HFPEF presents a clinical challenge stemming from its diverse etiology. Making the diagnosis of HFPEF is particularly difficult because: (1) there is no specific measure (such as EF in HFREF) to define the syndrome, (2) other disorders common in older adults (such as obesity with confounding comorbidities) can mimic the clinical syndrome, and (3) precise criteria have not been widely adapted. The original criteria developed to distinguish HFPEF from HFREF called for the presence of a clinical heart failure syndrome, a normal EF, and evidence of diastolic dysfunction by either catheterization or echocardiography [40]. Since then, several guidelines have been published that broaden the requirement of diastolic dysfunction to surrogate markers of diastolic LV dysfunction such as LV hypertrophy, LA enlargement, atrial fibrillation, or elevated plasma natriuretic peptides (NP) levels (Fig. 9.3) [41–45].

In the most recent guideline published by the Heart Failure and Echocardiography Associations of the European Society of Cardiology (ESC), the diagnosis of HFPEF required signs or symptoms of heart failure, a LVEF >50%, a LVEDV Index <97 mL/m^2, and evidence of diastolic LV dysfunction as shown by LVEDP >16 mmHg, pulmonary capillary wedge pressure (PCWP) >12 mmHg or ratio of mitral peak velocity of early filling (E) to early diastolic mitral annular velocity (E/E') >15 alone. Alternatively criteria include an elevated NP with E/E'>8, a mitral flow velocity Doppler signal showing a ratio of early to late flow (E/A) <0.5 with deceleration time (DT) >280 ms, a pulmonary vein flow velocity signal showing a Ard-Ad >30 ms (Ard = duration of reverse pulmonary vein atrial systole flow; Ad = duration of mitral valve atrial wave flow), a LA size >40 mL/m^2, or a LV mass >149 g/m^2 in men or >122 g/m^2 in women [43]. These guidelines represent consensus criteria with ongoing validation studies needed to verify their utility (in particularly for those that are non-invasive). Although invasive measurements with cardiac catheterization remain the gold standard for identifying HFPEF, the invasive nature of catheterization makes it impractical to obtain during routine evaluation for all patients with the HFPEF phenotype.

The diagnostic criteria above are largely based on the premise that elevated filling pressures remain the primary hemodynamic abnormality in HFPEF. Yet in a recent study assessing the diagnostic utility of these ESC guidelines, only 25% of patients with HFPEF and unexplained dyspnea who underwent invasive diagnostic testing fulfilled ESC criteria for HFPEF with evidence of elevated filling pressures at rest [46]. Indeed, a significant proportion of the patients demonstrated left ventricular stiffness, dyssynchrony, and dynamic mitral regurgitation, confirming patients with HFPEF can experience heart failure

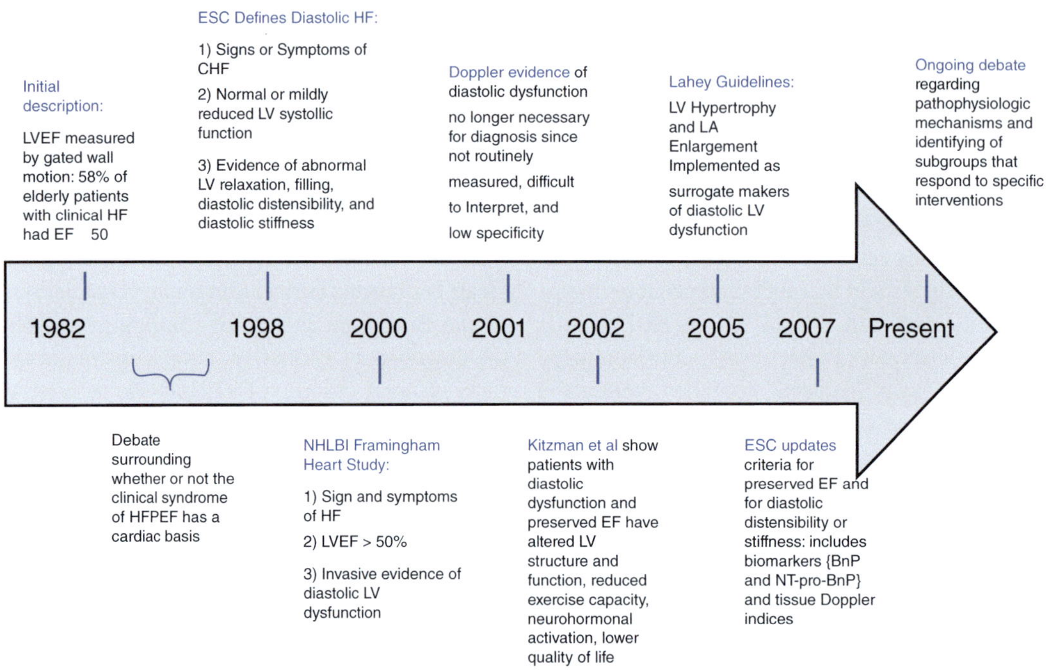

Fig. 9.3 Evolution of HFPEF from initial description to current diagnostic guidelines [41]

symptoms without demonstrating significant elevated filling pressures at rest or during hand grip exercise (increased afterload), leg lift (increased preload), nitroprusside infusion (decreased afterload), or dobutamine infusion (increased contractility). The specificity of these guidelines was also challenged, with 20–40% of health controls demonstrating borderline E/E' despite no evidence of heart failure and normal filling pressures [46]. Similarly, in a recent study assessing hemodynamic response to volume challenge in healthy young volunteers, older women, and patients with HFPEF, filling pressures (assessed by PCWP and mean pulmonary artery pressures [MPAP]) rose significantly with volume loading in all of the groups [47]. This raises additional concern for the validity of the cut points utilized to define an elevated filling pressure characteristic of HFPEF, suggesting more testing is needed to determine the threshold at which to classify HFPEF.

Despite these findings, several studies have validated the diagnostic capacity of various non-invasive estimates of elevated filling pressures. Conventional and tissue Doppler echocardiographic indices have been measured against conductance catheter PV loop analyses in patients with diastolic dysfunction (confirmed by invasively measured indices for diastolic relaxation [tau], LVEDP and LVEDV), demonstrating the LV filling index E/E' to have the highest ability to detect diastolic dysfunction (86% sensitivity) [48]. This measure (E/E') has subsequently been evaluated against LA volume index and LV mass index, demonstrating increased sensitivity of detecting HFPEF in patients with LA size >40 mL/m^2 and LV mass >149 g/m^2 in men or >122 g/m^2 in women [46]. Yet when these non-invasive indices were compared with pulmonary capillary wedge pressure (PCWP) assessed by right heart catheterizations, the non-invasive E/E' did not reliably track changes in left-sided filling pressures [49]. This disconnect between patients with HFPEF and non-elevated filling pressures at rest has been examined further by a study of euvolemic patients with exertional dyspnea, preserved EF, and normal cardiac filling pressures at rest: during exercise, patients demonstrated significantly abnormal hemodynamic responses including elevated PCWP [50]. While exercise hemodynamics may lack specificity as abnormal findings can be found in normal aging, it presents an attractive method to yield findings that may not be apparent at rest. The role of exercise hemodynamics in the diagnosis of HFPEF presents an emerging area of potentially improved diagnostic sensitivity. Although further validation of exercise hemodynamics in the diagnosis of HFPEF is necessary, it may be useful in the evaluation of patients who do not meet other established criteria for HFPEF.

Finally, the measurement of circulating natriuretic peptides (NP) has been suggested as an adjunctive diagnostic tool, but is also confounded by the influence of common co-morbidities present in patients with HFPEF on the presence of elevated NP [46]. Recent studies have demonstrated the association between NP and HFPEF, however validation of this marker in the diagnosis of HFPEF needs to be verified in ongoing clinical studies [51, 52].

Given the non-specific nature of the current non-invasive measures and their lack of correlation with invasive measures, the diagnostic utility of the ESC criteria have been called into question [35, 49]. Since many older adults have comorbid conditions that mimic the symptoms of dyspnea, fatigue, paroxysmal nocturnal dyspnea, orthopnea and leg swelling classically associated with heart failure, the specificity of the clinical diagnosis of HFPEF is reduced. Similarly, physical exam findings are both difficult to assess and notoriously non-specific for diagnostic criteria, and the diagnostic EF cutoff defining "preserved EF" has not been consistently used in diagnostic studies [3, 13, 21, 42, 52–54]. The nature of these diagnostic dilemmas has created a clinical challenge for the treating physician. Consequently, many clinicians have opted for an approach to diagnosis that employs a combination of the previous diagnostic strategies that is tailored to specific clinical settings and includes a clinical phenotype consistent with heart failure, a preserved EF, and echocardiographic evidence for LV hypertrophy and LA enlargement [51].

Treatment

Despite advances in our understanding of the causes and mechanisms driving the development of HFPEF, treatment options remain limited. Over the past two decades, clinical trials in HFPEF have primarily focused on drugs that have demonstrated mortality benefit in HFREF. Multiple drug trials have now been completed, yet no single agent has shown mortality benefit, and pharmaceutical options for HFPEF remain elusive. In contrast, lifestyle modifications have exhibited consistent benefit in patients with HFPEF, and novel therapies show promise in targeting several of the non-*diastolic dysfunction* etiologies of HFPEF.

The rationale behind many of the large pharmaceutical trials is that drugs that reduce ventricular hypertrophy or improve myocardial relaxation should benefit patients with HFPEF. This premise is primarily based on improving diastolic function, which as previously mentioned is only one of several mechanistic contributors to HFPEF. The following drug classes have been studied in large randomized placebo-controlled clinical trials (Table 9.1): beta-blockers, angiotensin-converting enzyme inhibitors (ACEi), angiotensin receptor blockers (ARB), aldosterone antagonists, and digoxin.

Each of these trials is notable for including subjects with clinical HFPEF and, with the exception of RAAM-PEF, having greater than 100 and up to 4128 patients (I-PRESERVE). The trial subjects had a mean age ranging from 63 years to 76 years, and EF cutoffs ranging from ≥35 to ≥50%. None of these trials demonstrated mortality benefit, and most failed to show benefit in the endpoint of heart failure hospitalizations; only candesartan (CHARM-P) and perindopril (PEP-CHF) exhibited decreased hospitalizations. Finally, despite a lack of placebo-controlled trials demonstrating clinical benefit of diuretic use in HFPEF, in the Hong Kong diastolic heart failure study of 150 elderly patients with HFPEF, diuretics significantly reduced heart failure symptoms and improved quality of life, and neither ramipril nor irbesartan demonstrated additional effect [66]. Diuretics remain essential therapy in the symptomatic control of volume overloaded states, although their use should be cautioned among preload dependent euvolemic patients. See Table 9.2 [67–77].

Table 9.1 Large pharmacologic trials for HFPEF [55–65]

Trial, year	DIG study (1997) [55, 56]	CHARM-P (2003) [65]	SWEDIC (2004) [57]	PEP-CHF (2006) [58]	SENIORS (2009) [64]
Drug	Digoxin	Candesartan	Carvedilol	Perindopril	Nebivolol
n	988	3023	113	850	752
Mean age (years)	63	67	67	75	76
Inclusion criteria	CHF diagnosis	NYHA II-IV, prior cardiac hospitalization	DHF by echocardiography	HF symptoms, LAE, Impaired LV filling, Cardiac hospitalization in prior 6 mo	HF symptoms, Cardiac hospitalizations in prior 12 mo
EF (%)	>45	>40	>45	≥40	≥35
Primary outcome	Composite death or HF hospitalizations	Composite CV death or HF hospitalization	Regression of diastolic LV dysfunction by Doppler	Composite all-cause mortality or HF hospitalization	Composite all-cause mortality or CV hospitalizations
Results	No mortality benefit (HR 0.82; 95% CI 0.63–1.07); ↓ 2-year HF Hospitalizations (HR 0.66; 95% CI 0.47–0.91, p = 0.012)	No mortality benefit (HR 0.89; 95% CI 0.77–1.03; p = 0.118); ↓ 3-year Hospitalizations (p = 0.017)	No significant change in composite diastolic LV function; ↑ E/A (p = <0.05)	No mortality benefit was seen over 2.1 year (HR 0.92; 95% CI 0.70–1.21, p = 0.545); ↓ 1-year hospitalizations (HR 0.628; 95% CI 0.408–0.966, p = 0.033)	No reduction (HR (0.81; 95% CI 0.63–1.04, p = 0.720)
Trial, year	I-PRESERVE (2008) [62]	RAAM-PEF (2011) [60]	ELAND (2012) [59]	Aldo-DHF (2013) [61]	TOPCAT, ongoing [63]
Drug	Irbesartan	Eplerenone	Nebivolol	Spironolactone	Spironolactone
n	4128	44	116	422	3445
Mean age (years)	72	70	66	67	69
Inclusion criteria	NYHA II–IV, Cardiac hospitalization in prior 6 months	NYHA II/III, BNP ≥100 pg/mL	NYHA II/III, ESC criteria of DHF	NYHA II/III, echocardiographic DHF	HF signs and symptoms, HF hospitalization in prior 12 months
EF (%)	≥40	≥50	>45	≥50	≥45
Primary outcome	Composite all-cause mortality or CV hospitalizations	6MWD	6MWD	E/E', peak VO2	Composite CV mortality or HF hospitalizations
Results	No reduction over 49.5 months of follow-up (HR 0.95; 95% CI 0.86–1.05; p = 0.35)	No improvement (p = 0.91)	No improvement (p = 0.094)	↓ E/E' (adj. mean difference –1.5; 95% CI –2.0–0.9; p < 0.001); No improvement peak VO2 (p = 0.81)	Reduction in HF hospitalization (HR 0.83; 95% CI 0.69–0.99; p = 0.04). No reduction in mortality (HR 0.89; 95% CI 0.77–1.04; p = 0.14)

EF ejection fraction, *NYHA* New York Heart Association, *CHF* congestive heart failure, *DHF* diastolic heart failure, *HF* heart failure, *LAE* left atrial enlargement, *LV* left ventricle, *CV* cardiovascular, *HR* hazard ratio, *CI* confidence interval, *E/E'* ratio of mitral peak velocity of early filling (E) to early diastolic mitral annular velocity (E')

Table 9.2 Lifestyle/exercise interventions in the treatment of HFPEF [67–78]

Study, year	Type of study	n	Population	Age	EF cutpoint	Intervention	Outcome	Results
Exercise								
Gary et al. (2004) [67]	RCT	32	Women, NYHA II/III DHF	68	≥45%	3 months of home-based low-to-moderate intensity exercise	6MWT, QOL, GDS	6MWT–840 ± 366 ft to 1043 ± 317 ft vs 824 ± 367 ft to 732 ± 408 ft ($P = 0.002$); ↑ QOL and ↓GDS
Smart et al. (2007) [68]	Non-randomized, non-placebo controlled	26	DHF by delayed relaxation or pseudonormal filling	65	>45%	16 weeks of supervised cycle ergometer ExT	Peak VO2, E/E', QOL	30% ↑ Peak VO2 ($p < 0.001$); No change E/E' ($p = 0.38$); ↑ QOL
Korzeniowska-Kubacka et al. (2010) [69]	RCT	48	Men, Post-MI with mild diastolic dysfunction by TDI	56	≥50%	18 weeks supervised aerobic training (3 sessions/week)	Exercise capacity, Echocardiography	↑ Peak VO2 ($p < 0.0001$); No change E/E'
Kitzman et al. (2010) [70]	Randomized, attention controlled	53	Ambulatory patients with isolated HFPEF (no coronary, pulmonary, valvular disease)	70	≥50%	16 weeks of supervised aerobic exercise training	Exercise performance, QOL, Echocardiography, Neuroendocrine function	↑ Peak VO2 ($p = 0.0002$); ↑ Physical QOL ($p = 0.03$); No change in doppler echocardiography; No change in BNP ($p = 0.06$)
Edelman et al. (2011) [71]	RCT	64	Outpatients, NYHA II/III, diastolic dysfunction by echocardiogram	65	≥50%	24 weeks of supervised aerobic cycling	Exercise capacity, Echocardiography, QOL	↑ Peak VO2 ($p < 0.001$); ↓ E/E' and LAVI ($p < 0.001$); ↑ QOL
Fujimato et al. (2012) [72]	Non-randomized, non-controlled	11	HF by Framingham criteria plus e/o pulmonary congestion	75	>45%	1 year of exercise training (3×/week for 25 min)	RHC, Doppler echocardiography, aterial stiffness, exercise testing, ventricular-arterial coupling	No change in LV compliance or volumes, arterial stiffiness, E/E', peak VO2, or ventricular-arterial coupling
Haykowsky et al. (2012) [73]	Randomized, attention-controlled	40	Ambulatory patients with isolated HFPEF (no coronary, pulmonary, valvular disease)	69	≥50%	16 weeks of supervised aerobic exercise training	Peak VO2 and echocardiography	↑ Peak VO2 ($p = 0.002$; No change in EDV, SV, CO; ↑ Peak arterial-venous oxygen difference ($p = 0.03$)

(continued)

Table 9.2 (continued)

Study, year	Type of study	n	Population	Age	EF cutpoint	Intervention	Outcome	Results
Smart et al. (2012) [74]	RCT	25	Dyspneic clinic patients with delayed relaxation or pseudonormal filling	65	>45%	16 weeks of supervised, outpatient, cycle ergometer ExT (3 × 30 min sessions/week)	Peak VO2, Echocardiography, QOL, GDS	25% ↑ Peak VO2 (p = 0.02); No change E/E' (p = 0.52); No change QOL or GDS
Kitzman et al. 2016 [75]	RCT	100	Older obese patients with chronic, stable HFPEF	67	≥ 50%	20 wks of exercise, diet or both	Peak VO2, QOL	Peak VO2 ↑ by both interventions. Exercise 1.2 mL/kg body mass/min (95% CI 0.7–1.7), p < 0.001; Diet 1.3 mL/kg body mass/min (95% CI 0.8–1.8), p < 0.001; Combination joint effect 2.5 mL/kg/min. No change QOL.
Salt-restriction								
GAP-HF (2009) [76]	Retrospective cohort	443	Discharge diagnosis of primary HF	75	≥50%	Discharge recommendation for sodium restricted diet	30-day combined death and readmission	OR 0.43 (95% CI 0.24–0.79; p = 0.007)
Hummel et al. (2012) [77]	Pilot study, non-randomized, non-controlled	13	Systemic hypertension, e/o diastolic dysfunction by catheterization or echocardiography	72	≥50%	21 days of sodium-restricted DASH diet (all food provided)	BP, Laboratory, Echocardiography, Functional testing	↓ Clinic and 24-hr BP (SBP 155–>138, p = 0.02); ↓ Urinary F2-isoprostane and urinary sodium excretion; No change in E/E' (p = 0.45); No change; ↑ 6MWT (p = 0.006)
GOURMET-HF (2014) [78]	RCT	66	Older adults after hospitalization for ADHF	≥65	≥50% (stratified, also recruiting <50%)	4 weeks of preprepared, home-delivered DASH/SRD-compliant meals	QOL, Adherence, Salt taste affinity testing, Echocardiography, Systemic inflammation and oxidative stress reduction, functional testing, adverse events	Results pending

RCT randomized-controlled trial, *NYHA* New York Heart Association, *DHF* diastolic heart failure, *6MWT* 6-min walk test, *HF* heart failure, *QOL* quality of life, *6MWD* 6-min walk distance, *GDS* geriatric depression scale, *VO2* oxygen uptake, *ExT* exercise training, *E/E'* ratio of mitral peak velocity of early filling (E) to early diastolic mitral annular velocity (E'), *TDI* tissue Doppler imaging, *BNP* brain-natriuretic peptide, *LAVI* left atrial volume index, *RHC* right heart catheterization, *EDV* end-diastolic volume, *SV* stroke volume, *CO* cardiac output, *OR* odds ratio, *DASH* dietary approaches to stop hypertension, *SBP* systolic blood pressure, *GOURMET-HF* geriatric out of hospital randomized meal trial in heart failure, *ADHF* acute decompensated heart failure, *SRD* sodium restricted diet

Owing in part to the neutral results of pharmacologic therapy but also the increased understanding of the multifactorial etiology of HFPEF, lifestyle modifications have been increasingly studied over the past decade. Evidence-supported interventions include exercise training, weight loss, smoking cessation, cardiac rehabilitation/physical therapy, and low-sodium diet (Table 9.2) [67, 68, 70, 76, 79–83]. Although many of these studies have been limited by a lack of randomization, no placebo-control, small numbers of patients, and less clinically relevant endpoints, they offer valuable insight into the utility of non-pharmacologic treatment in HFPEF. While exercise training, including weight loss and cardiac rehabilitation/physical therapy are now being integrated into clinical guidance for HFPEF [84], salt-restricted diets remain controversial. Low sodium diets have predominantly been studied in the outpatient setting and have been observed to show benefit in vital sign and laboratory measurements [77, 85, 86]. Although most studies have not focused on mortality outcomes, the GAP-HF study demonstrated reduced 30-day combined mortality and readmission with discharge recommendations for a sodium-restricted diet in 443 patients with HFPEF [76]. These findings have been tempered, however, by a recent study in patients with HFREF suggesting low salt diet may increase mortality and HF-related hospitalizations [87]. Whereas these findings raise concern that salt-restriction may be harmful in patients with systolic dysfunction, they may also be viewed as further evidence of the mechanistic and corresponding therapeutic differences between HFPEF and HFREF.

Limited data is available on the use of interventional procedures in the treatment of HFPEF—including percutaneous coronary intervention (PCI), coronary artery bypass grafting (CABG), aortic valve replacement (AVR) and cardiac resynchronization therapy (CRT). Although a study of 46 patients hospitalized with acute pulmonary edema showed that revascularization with PCI or CABG did not effect the recurrence of pulmonary edema [88]. ACC/AHA guidelines recommend revascularization if symptomatic myocardial ischemia is judged to be contributing to worsening of cardiac function [89]. Observations by Hachicha et al., in 331 patients with EF > 50% and severe aortic stenosis (AS; aortic valve area < 0.6) demonstrated that paradoxical low flow states (characteristic of patients with HFPEF) were associated with a worsened 3-year survival [90]. This has contributed to the class I recommendation for AVR in symptomatic patients with HFPEF and AS [91]. Finally, CRT (see Table 9.3) has emerged as a potential therapeutic option for HFPEF based on recent data showing decreased LV dyssynchrony, decreased LVEDP and improved LVESV, however prospective data is ongoing and necessary before clinical CRT guidelines are recommended [104, 105].

In addition to CRT, several other novel therapies have emerged as additional therapeutic possibilities for HFPEF. These include neutral endopeptidase inhibitors [96], recombinant human relaxin-2 [93], barostimulation [94, 95] and renal denervation [97]. Neutral endopeptidase inhibition is based on the hypothesis that reducing the degradation of NP will lower sympathetic drive via the inhibition of the renin-aldosterone-angiotensin (RAA) system, causing antiproliferative and antihypertrophic effects on myocardium. Serelaxin, a recombinant human relaxin-2, causes vasodilation and increased inotropy, and has demonstrated symptomatic relief of dyspnea in patients with HFPEF. Barostimulation has similarly been shown to decrease adrenergic stimulation, leading to reduced ventricular-vascular stiffening with corresponding harmful myocardial remodeling. Finally, renal denervation has demonstrated reduced sodium reabsorption with reduced blood pressure and corresponding ventricular hypertrophy. Recent and ongoing studies are examining the effects of these emerging therapies on various clinical endpoints in HFPEF (See Table 9.3).

In contrast to the above pharmaceutical, lifestyle and interventional therapies that have shown mixed promise in the treatment of HFPEF, several agents have been observed to cause harm and worsen outcomes in HFPEF. Drugs to avoid include those causing fluid retention such as the thiazolinediones (TZDs) pioglitazone or rosiglitazone, and non-steroidal anti-inflammatory

Table 9.3 Additional therapies in HFPEF [92–103]

Therapy	Neutral endopeptidase inhibitors [96]	Recombinant human relaxin-2 [93]	Cardiac resynchronization therapy [92, 98]	Barostimulation [94, 95]	Renal denervation [97, 99]
Summary	Increases plasma concentrations of natriuretic peptides, which inhibit RAA system activity, lower sympathetic drive, and have antiproliferative and antihypertrophic effects	Causes decreased systemic vascular resistance (vasodilation), increased cardiac output (inotropy), and increased renal blood flow	The prevalence of electrical and mechanical ventricular dyssynchrony in HFPEF is less than HFREF but still significant, suggesting a therapeutic role for cardiac resynchronization as a therapeutic target	Reduces the activity of the SNS, leading to diminished hypertension, renal dysfunction, vascular stiffness and myocardial ischemia. Currently being studied to determine carotid baroreceptor stimulation on outcomes in patients with HFPEF	Decreases sodium reabsorption and RAA system activity; has been show to reduce blood pressure, renal dysfunction and cardiac hypertrophy in patients with resistant hypertension
Ongoing studies	PARAMOUNT [103], a phase 2 RCT of ARNI LCZ696 in 301 patients with NYHA II/III, EF ≥ 40%, and NT-proBNP >400 pg/mL, demonstrated reduced NT-proBNP (783–605 pg/mL) compared to valsartan at 12 weeks follow-up	RELAX-AHF [93], a RCT of Serelaxin in 1161 patients with acute HF. Patients with HFPEF (26% of patients) experienced relief of dyspnea by visual analogue scale through day 5 of treatment	KaRen registry [102], a prospective observational study characterizing the prevalence of electrical or mechanical dyssynchrony in HFPEF with resulting effect on prognosis	HOPE4HF [94], a RCT of Baroreflex Activation Therapy (BAT) in ~540 patients on CV death or HF hospitalizations	SYMPLICITY-HF [100] and SWAN-HF [101], two open-label feasibility and safety/efficacy studies of renal denervation and renal sympathetic modification on patients with HF

drugs (NSAIDS). Such drugs can cause increased sodium and water retention leading to edema and hypertension with subsequent worsening of volume overloaded states. This has led to an AHA Consensus Statement about the increased risk of heart failure with the use of TZDs [106]. Similar caution should be used with drugs causing renal impairment, and in over-diuresis as above in patients with euvolemia for whom preload is essential to maintain cardiac output.

There has been much discussion and several proposed explanations for the apparent disconnect in therapeutic success between HFREF and HFPEF—including differences in myocardial structure [107, 108] flaws in diagnostic methods for inclusion criteria [109] and inappropriate trial design [13]. What is clear is that the success of future of HFPEF treatments will require a novel approach that integrates the multifaceted causes and diverse population that comprise this syndrome distinct from HFREF. In a recent study, however, examining differences in treatment strategies pursued by cardiologists for HF patients according to EF, patients with HFPEF were treated similarly as patients with HFREF, suggesting a lack of integrating known data into current practice [110].

Incorporating the above data together with an appreciation of its multifaceted etiology yields a heterogeneous approach to the management of HFPEF. Clinicians must consider a broad differential diagnosis for the patient presenting with a clinical phenotype consistent with HFPEF. Although data supporting the treatment of co-morbid conditions such as anemia, dyslipidemia, chronic renal disease, chronic pain, and diabetes are mixed (including one study showing improved survival with statin use compared to ACEi, beta-blocker, or calcium channel blockers [111] and another showing no benefit of subcutaneous epoetin alpha [ESA] administration on LVEDV or submaximal exercise but an improvement in peak VO2 in those able to exercise [112], co-morbid conditions should be embraced in the overall treatment strategy with the understanding that peripheral mechanisms of HFPEF may contribute significantly to the clinical phenotype and that non-cardiovascular causes of recurrent hospitalization are the major cause of 30–90 day readmissions [9]. Similar to the multimodal approach championed in the current practice of geriatric medicine, treatment could be aimed at multiple components, including both cardiac and non-cardiac domains.

Conclusion

As the burden of HFPEF rises with our aging population, managing this condition has become increasing complex. Clinicians must take care to understand the multifactorial pathogenesis that defines this syndrome, and the subsequent diagnostic approach used to classify patients. Treatment approaches are evolving, with an emphasis on optimizing volume status, controlling blood pressure and managing comorbid conditions which may exacerbate symptoms. Successful strategies may involve a new approach that does not rely on single interventions but is instead broadly based by addressing targeted goals rather than a single endpoint. Focusing management on improvements in several domains (i.e. vital signs, lifestyle changes, comorbidities, functional limitations and sarcopenia) would direct care at improving target blood pressure control, weight loss, exercise goals and rehabilitation, or diabetes management—based on the understanding that these incremental effects contribute to the overall HFPEF phenotype in a majority of patients. The result would be a treatment approach that addresses the complexity of HFPEF through its fundamental elements. By incorporating a multifaceted approach with our understanding of its complex etiology, further advances in HFPEF trial design will greatly benefit the future management of this condition.

References

1. Dougherty AH, Naccarelli GV, Gray EL, Hicks CH, Goldstein RA. Congestive heart failure with normal systolic function. Am J Cardiol. 1984;54(7):778–82. PubMed CrossRef.
2. Hanrath P, Mathey DG, Siegert R, Bleifeld W. Left ventricular relaxation and filling pattern in different forms of left ventricular hypertrophy: an echocardiographic study. Am J Cardiol. 1980;45(1):15–23. PubMed CrossRef.
3. Sanderson JE, Gibson DG, Brown DJ, Goodwin JF. Left ventricular filling in hypertrophic cardiomyopathy. An angiographic study. Br Heart J. 1977;39(6):661–70. CrossRef.
4. Hunt SA, Abraham WT, Chin MH, Feldman AM, Francis GS, Ganiats TG, et al. ACC/AHA 2005 guideline update for the diagnosis and management of chronic heart failure in the adult: a report of the American College of Cardiology/American Heart Association Task Force on Practice Guidelines (Writing Committee to Update the 2001 Guidelines for the Evaluation and Management of Heart Failure): developed in collaboration with the American College of Chest Physicians and the International Society for Heart and Lung Transplantation: endorsed by the Heart Rhythm Society. Circulation. 2005;112(12):e154–235. CrossRef
5. Roger VL, Go AS, Lloyd-Jones DM, Benjamin EJ, Berry JD, Borden WB, et al. Executive summary: heart disease and stroke statistics – 2012 update: a report from the American Heart Association. Circulation. 2012;125(1):188–97. PubMed CrossRef.
6. Jencks SF, Williams MV, Coleman EA. Rehospitalizations among patients in the medicare fee-for-service program. N Engl J Med. 2009;360(14):1418–28. PubMed CrossRef.
7. Lakatta EG, Levy D. Arterial and cardiac aging: major shareholders in cardiovascular disease enterprises: part I: aging arteries: a "set up" for vascular disease. Circulation. 2003;107(1):139–46. PubMed CrossRef.
8. Lakatta EG, Levy D. Arterial and cardiac aging: major shareholders in cardiovascular disease enterprises: part II: the aging heart in health: links to heart disease. Circulation. 2003;107(2):346–54. PubMed CrossRef.

9. Fida N, Pina IL. Trends in heart failure hospitalizations. Curr Heart Fail Rep. 2012;9(4):346–53. PubMed CrossRef.
10. Lam CS, Donal E, Kraigher-Krainer E, Vasan RS. Epidemiology and clinical course of heart failure with preserved ejection fraction. Eur J Heart Fail. 2011;13(1):18–28. PubMed CrossRef.
11. Owan TE, Hodge DO, Herges RM, Jacobsen SJ, Roger VL, Redfield MM. Trends in prevalence and outcome of heart failure with preserved ejection fraction. N Engl J Med. 2006;355(3):251–9. PubMed CrossRef.
12. Steinberg BA, Zhao X, Heidenreich PA, Peterson ED, Bhatt DL, Cannon CP, et al. Trends in patients hospitalized with heart failure and preserved left ventricular ejection fraction: prevalence, therapies, and outcomes. Circulation. 2012;126(1):65–75. PubMed CrossRef.
13. Bhuiyan T, Maurer MS. Heart failure with preserved ejection fraction: persistent diagnosis. Therapeutic Enigma Curr Cardiovasc Risk Rep. 2011;5(5):440–9. PubMed CrossRef.
14. Henkel DM, Redfield MM, Weston SA, Gerber Y, Roger VL. Death in heart failure: a community perspective. Circ Heart Fail. 2008;1(2):91–7. PubMed PubMedCentral CrossRef.
15. Bursi F, Weston SA, Redfield MM, Jacobsen SJ, Pakhomov S, Nkomo VT, et al. Systolic and diastolic heart failure in the community. JAMA. 2006;296(18):2209–16. PubMed CrossRef.
16. Devereux RB, Roman MJ, Liu JE, Welty TK, Lee ET, Rodeheffer R, et al. Congestive heart failure despite normal left ventricular systolic function in a population-based sample: the Strong Heart Study. Am J Cardiol. 2000;86(10):1090–6. PubMed CrossRef.
17. Kitzman DW, Gardin JM, Gottdiener JS, Arnold A, Boineau R, Aurigemma G, et al. Importance of heart failure with preserved systolic function in patients > or = 65 years of age. CHS Research Group. Cardiovascular Health Study. Am J Cardiol. 2001;87(4):413–9. PubMed CrossRef.
18. Lee DS, Gona P, Vasan RS, Larson MG, Benjamin EJ, Wang TJ, et al. Relation of disease pathogenesis and risk factors to heart failure with preserved or reduced ejection fraction: insights from the framingham heart study of the national heart, lung, and blood institute. Circulation. 2009;119(24):3070–7. PubMed PubMedCentral CrossRef.
19. Kliger C, King DL, Maurer MS. A clinical algorithm to differentiate heart failure with a normal ejection fraction by pathophysiologic mechanism. Am J Geriatr Cardiol. 2006;15(1):50–7. PubMed CrossRef.
20. Lakatta EG. Cardiovascular regulatory mechanisms in advanced age. Physiol Rev. 1993;73(2):413–67. PubMed.
21. Maurer MS, Spevack D, Burkhoff D, Kronzon I. Diastolic dysfunction: can it be diagnosed by Doppler echocardiography? J Am Coll Cardiol. 2004;44(8):1543–9. PubMed CrossRef.
22. Lakatta EG. Arterial and cardiac aging: major shareholders in cardiovascular disease enterprises: part III: cellular and molecular clues to heart and arterial aging. Circulation. 2003;107(3):490–7. PubMed CrossRef.
23. Kawaguchi M, Hay I, Fetics B, Kass DA. Combined ventricular systolic and arterial stiffening in patients with heart failure and preserved ejection fraction: implications for systolic and diastolic reserve limitations. Circulation. 2003;107(5):714–20. PubMed CrossRef.
24. Burton A. Physiology and biophysics of the circulation. 2nd ed. Chicago: Year Book Medical Publishers; 1972.
25. Duarte D, Santos-Araujo C, Leite-Moreira AF. Hypertension and angiogenesis in the aging kidney: a review. Arch Gerontol Geriatr. 2011;52(3):e93–102. PubMed CrossRef.
26. Maurer MS, Kronzon I, Burkhoff D. Ventricular pump function in heart failure with normal ejection fraction: insights from pressure-volume measurements. Prog Cardiovasc Dis. 2006;49(3):182–95. PubMed CrossRef.
27. Hotta H, Uchida S. Aging of the autonomic nervous system and possible improvements in autonomic activity using somatic afferent stimulation. Geriatr Gerontol Int. 2010;10(Suppl 1):S127–36. PubMed CrossRef
28. Miller MR. Structural and physiological age-associated changes in aging lungs. Semin Respir Crit Care Med. 2010;31(5):521–7. PubMed CrossRef.
29. Abramov D, Helmke S, Rumbarger Lel K, King DL, Maurer MS. Overestimation of left ventricular mass and misclassification of ventricular geometry in heart failure patients by two-dimensional echocardiography in comparison with three-dimensional echocardiography. Echocardiography. 2010;27(3):223–9. PubMed CrossRef.
30. He KL, Burkhoff D, Leng WX, Liang ZR, Fan L, Wang J, et al. Comparison of ventricular structure and function in Chinese patients with heart failure and ejection fractions >55% versus 40% to 55% versus <40%. Am J Cardiol. 2009;103(6):845–51. PubMed PubMedCentral CrossRef.
31. He KL, Dickstein M, Sabbah HN, Yi GH, Gu A, Maurer M, et al. Mechanisms of heart failure with well preserved ejection fraction in dogs following limited coronary microembolization. Cardiovasc Res. 2004;64(1):72–83. PubMed CrossRef.
32. Munagala VK, Hart CY, Burnett JC Jr, Meyer DM, Redfield MM. Ventricular structure and function in aged dogs with renal hypertension: a model of experimental diastolic heart failure. Circulation. 2005;111(9):1128–35. PubMed PubMedCentral CrossRef.

33. Gandhi SK, Powers JC, Nomeir AM, Fowle K, Kitzman DW, Rankin KM, et al. The pathogenesis of acute pulmonary edema associated with hypertension. N Engl J Med. 2001;344(1):17–22. PubMed CrossRef.
34. Kitzman DW, Higginbotham MB, Cobb FR, Sheikh KH, Sullivan MJ. Exercise intolerance in patients with heart failure and preserved left ventricular systolic function: failure of the Frank-Starling mechanism. J Am Coll Cardiol. 1991;17(5):1065–72. PubMed CrossRef.
35. Zile MR, Gaasch WH, Carroll JD, Feldman MD, Aurigemma GP, Schaer GL, et al. Heart failure with a normal ejection fraction: is measurement of diastolic function necessary to make the diagnosis of diastolic heart failure? Circulation. 2001;104(7):779–82. PubMed CrossRef.
36. Vasan RS, Levy D. Defining diastolic heart failure: a call for standardized diagnostic criteria. Circulation. 2000;101(17):2118–21. PubMed CrossRef.
37. Lam CS. Heart failure with preserved ejection fraction: invasive solution to diagnostic confusion? J Am Coll Cardiol. 2010;55(16):1711–2. PubMed CrossRef.
38. Paulus WJ, Tschope C, Sanderson JE, Rusconi C, Flachskampf FA, Rademakers FE, et al. How to diagnose diastolic heart failure: a consensus statement on the diagnosis of heart failure with normal left ventricular ejection fraction by the Heart Failure and Echocardiography Associations of the European Society of Cardiology. Eur Heart J. 2007;28(20):2539–50. PubMed CrossRef.
39. Yturralde RF, Gaasch WH. Diagnostic criteria for diastolic heart failure. Prog Cardiovasc Dis. 2005;47(5):314–9. PubMed CrossRef.
40. Penicka M, Bartunek J, Trakalova H, Hrabakova H, Maruskova M, Karasek J, et al. Heart failure with preserved ejection fraction in outpatients with unexplained dyspnea: a pressure-volume loop analysis. J Am Coll Cardiol. 2010;55(16):1701–10. PubMed CrossRef.
41. Luchi RJ, Snow E, Luchi JM, Nelson CL, Pircher FJ. Left ventricular function in hospitalized geriatric patients. J Am Geriatr Soc. 1982;30(11):700–5. PubMed CrossRef.
42. Bhella PS, Pacini EL, Prasad A, Hastings JL, Adams-Huet B, Thomas JD, et al. Echocardiographic indices do not reliably track changes in left-sided filling pressure in healthy subjects or patients with heart failure with preserved ejection fraction. Circ Cardiovasc Imaging. 2011;4(5):482–9. PubMed PubMedCentral CrossRef.
43. Emery WT, Jadavji I, Choy JB, Lawrance RA. Investigating the European Society of Cardiology Diastology guidelines in a practical scenario. Eur J Echocardiogr. 2008;9(5):685–91. PubMed CrossRef.
44. Fujimoto N, Borlaug BA, Lewis GD, Hastings JL, Shafer KM, Bhella PS, et al. Hemodynamic responses to rapid saline loading: the impact of age, sex, and heart failure. Circulation. 2013;127(1):55–62. PubMed CrossRef.
45. Kasner M, Westermann D, Steendijk P, Gaub R, Wilkenshoff U, Weitmann K, et al. Utility of Doppler echocardiography and tissue Doppler imaging in the estimation of diastolic function in heart failure with normal ejection fraction: a comparative Doppler-conductance catheterization study. Circulation. 2007;116(6):637–47. PubMed CrossRef.
46. Jeevanantham V, Shrivastava R, Nannapaneni S, Khan A, Sengodan M, Nautiyal A, et al. Elevated B-type natriuretic peptide level: use with caution in patients with multiple co-morbidities and presenting with dyspnea. Indian Heart J. 2007;59(1):64–8. PubMed.
47. Bishu K, Deswal A, Chen HH, LeWinter MM, Lewis GD, Semigran MJ, et al. Biomarkers in acutely decompensated heart failure with preserved or reduced ejection fraction. Am Heart J. 2012;164(5):763–70 e3. PubMed CrossRef.
48. Edelmann F, Schmidt AG, Gelbrich G, Binder L, Herrmann-Lingen C, Halle M, et al. Rationale and design of the 'aldosterone receptor blockade in diastolic heart failure' trial: a double-blind, randomized, placebo-controlled, parallel group study to determine the effects of spironolactone on exercise capacity and diastolic function in patients with symptomatic diastolic heart failure (Aldo-DHF). Eur J Heart Fail. 2010;12(8):874–82. PubMed CrossRef.
49. Zile MR, Brutsaert DL. New concepts in diastolic dysfunction and diastolic heart failure: Part I: diagnosis, prognosis, and measurements of diastolic function. Circulation. 2002;105(11):1387–93. PubMed CrossRef.
50. Borlaug BA, Nishimura RA, Sorajja P, Lam CS, Redfield MM. Exercise hemodynamics enhance diagnosis of early heart failure with preserved ejection fraction. Circ Heart Fail. 2010;3(5):588–95. PubMed PubMedCentral CrossRef.
51. Melenovsky V, Borlaug BA, Rosen B, Hay I, Ferruci L, Morell CH, et al. Cardiovascular features of heart failure with preserved ejection fraction versus nonfailing hypertensive left ventricular hypertrophy in the urban Baltimore community: the role of atrial remodeling/dysfunction. J Am Coll Cardiol. 2007;49(2):198–207. PubMed CrossRef.
52. Petrie MC, Hogg K, Caruana L, McMurray JJ. Poor concordance of commonly used echocardiographic measures of left ventricular diastolic function in patients with suspected heart failure but preserved systolic function: is there a reliable echocardiographic measure of diastolic dysfunction? Heart. 2004;90(5):511–7. PubMed PubMedCentral CrossRef.
53. Kindermann M, Reil JC, Pieske B, van Veldhuisen DJ, Bohm M. Heart failure with normal left ventricular ejection fraction: what is the evidence? Trends Cardiovasc Med. 2008;18(8):280–92. PubMed CrossRef.

54. Palmieri V, Innocenti F, Pini R, Celentano A. Reproducibility of Doppler echocardiographic assessment of left ventricular diastolic function in multicenter setting. J Am Soc Echocardiogr. 2005;18(2):99–106. PubMed CrossRef.
55. The Digitalis Investigation Group. The effect of digoxin on mortality and morbidity in patients with heart failure. N Engl J Med. 1997;336(8):525–33. CrossRef.
56. Ahmed A, Rich MW, Fleg JL, Zile MR, Young JB, Kitzman DW, et al. Effects of digoxin on morbidity and mortality in diastolic heart failure: the ancillary digitalis investigation group trial. Circulation. 2006;114(5):397–403. PubMed PubMedCentral CrossRef.
57. Bergstrom A, Andersson B, Edner M, Nylander E, Persson H, Dahlstrom U. Effect of carvedilol on diastolic function in patients with diastolic heart failure and preserved systolic function. Results of the Swedish Doppler-echocardiographic study (SWEDIC). Eur J Heart Fail. 2004;6(4):453–61. PubMed CrossRef.
58. Cleland JG, Tendera M, Adamus J, Freemantle N, Polonski L, Taylor J. The perindopril in elderly people with chronic heart failure (PEP-CHF) study. Eur Heart J. 2006;27(19):2338–45. PubMed CrossRef.
59. Conraads VM, Metra M, Kamp O, De Keulenaer GW, Pieske B, Zamorano J, et al. Effects of the long-term administration of nebivolol on the clinical symptoms, exercise capacity, and left ventricular function of patients with diastolic dysfunction: results of the ELANDD study. Eur J Heart Fail. 2012;14(2):219–25. PubMed CrossRef.
60. Deswal A, Richardson P, Bozkurt B, Mann DL. Results of the Randomized Aldosterone Antagonism in Heart Failure with Preserved Ejection Fraction trial (RAAM-PEF). J Card Fail. 2011;17(8):634–42. PubMed CrossRef.
61. Edelmann F, Wachter R, Schmidt AG, Kraigher-Krainer E, Colantonio C, Kamke W, et al. Effect of spironolactone on diastolic function and exercise capacity in patients with heart failure with preserved ejection fraction: the Aldo-DHF randomized controlled trial. JAMA. 2013;309(8):781–91. PubMed CrossRef.
62. Massie BM, Carson PE, McMurray JJ, Komajda M, McKelvie R, Zile MR, et al. Irbesartan in patients with heart failure and preserved ejection fraction. N Engl J Med. 2008;359(23):2456–67. PubMed CrossRef.
63. Shah SJ, Heitner JF, Sweitzer NK, Anand IS, Kim HY, Harty B, et al. Baseline characteristics of patients in the treatment of preserved cardiac function heart failure with an aldosterone antagonist (TOPCAT). Trial Circ Heart Fail. 2013;6:184–92. PubMed CrossRef.
64. van Veldhuisen DJ, Cohen-Solal A, Bohm M, Anker SD, Babalis D, Roughton M, et al. Beta-blockade with nebivolol in elderly heart failure patients with impaired and preserved left ventricular ejection fraction: data from SENIORS (Study of Effects of Nebivolol Intervention on Outcomes and Rehospitalization in Seniors With Heart Failure). J Am Coll Cardiol. 2009;53(23):2150–8. PubMed CrossRef.
65. Yusuf S, Pfeffer MA, Swedberg K, Granger CB, Held P, McMurray JJ, et al. Effects of candesartan in patients with chronic heart failure and preserved left-ventricular ejection fraction: the CHARM-Preserved Trial. Lancet. 2003;362(9386):777–81. PubMed CrossRef.
66. Yip GW, Wang M, Wang T, Chan S, Fung JW, Yeung L, et al. The Hong Kong diastolic heart failure study: a randomised controlled trial of diuretics, irbesartan and ramipril on quality of life, exercise capacity, left ventricular global and regional function in heart failure with a normal ejection fraction. Heart. 2008;94(5):573–80. PubMed CrossRef.
67. Gary RA, Sueta CA, Dougherty M, Rosenberg B, Cheek D, Preisser J, et al. Home-based exercise improves functional performance and quality of life in women with diastolic heart failure. Heart Lung. 2004;33(4):210–8. PubMed CrossRef.
68. Smart N, Haluska B, Jeffriess L, Marwick TH. Exercise training in systolic and diastolic dysfunction: effects on cardiac function, functional capacity, and quality of life. Am Heart J. 2007;153(4):530–6. PubMed CrossRef.
69. Korzeniowska-Kubacka I, Bilinska M, Michalak E, Kusmierczyk-Droszcz B, Dobraszkiewicz-Wasilewska B, Piotrowicz R. Influence of exercise training on left ventricular diastolic function and its relationship to exercise capacity in patients after myocardial infarction. Cardiol J. 2010;17(2):136–42. PubMed.
70. Kitzman DW, Brubaker PH, Morgan TM, Stewart KP, Little WC. Exercise training in older patients with heart failure and preserved ejection fraction: a randomized, controlled, single-blind trial. Circ Heart Fail. 2010;3(6):659–67. PubMed PubMedCentral CrossRef.
71. Edelmann F, Gelbrich G, Dungen HD, Frohling S, Wachter R, Stahrenberg R, et al. Exercise training improves exercise capacity and diastolic function in patients with heart failure with preserved ejection fraction: results of the Ex-DHF (Exercise training in Diastolic Heart Failure) pilot study. J Am Coll Cardiol. 2011;58(17):1780–91. PubMed CrossRef.
72. Fujimoto N, Prasad A, Hastings JL, Bhella PS, Shibata S, Palmer D, et al. Cardiovascular effects of 1 year of progressive endurance exercise training in patients with heart failure with preserved ejection fraction. Am Heart J. 2012;164(6):869–77. PubMed CrossRef.
73. Haykowsky MJ, Brubaker PH, Stewart KP, Morgan TM, Eggebeen J, Kitzman DW. Effect of endurance training on the determinants of peak exercise oxygen consumption in elderly patients with stable compensated heart failure and preserved ejection fraction.

J Am Coll Cardiol. 2012;60(2):120–8. PubMed PubMedCentral CrossRef.
74. Smart NA, Haluska B, Jeffriess L, Leung D. Exercise training in heart failure with preserved systolic function: a randomized controlled trial of the effects on cardiac function and functional capacity. Congest Heart Fail. 2012;18(6):295–301. PubMed CrossRef.
75. Kitzman DW, Brubaker P, Morgan T, Haykowsky M, Hundley G, Kraus WE, et al. Effect of caloric restriction or aerobic exercise training on peak oxygen consumption and quality of life in obese older patients with heart failure with preserved ejection fraction: a randomized clinical trial. JAMA. 2016;315(1):36–46. PubMed PubMedCentral CrossRef.
76. Hummel SL, DeFranco AC, Skorcz S, Montoye CK, Koelling TM. Recommendation of low-salt diet and short-term outcomes in heart failure with preserved systolic function. Am J Med. 2009;122(11):1029–36. PubMed PubMedCentral CrossRef.
77. Hummel SL, Seymour EM, Brook RD, Kolias TJ, Sheth SS, Rosenblum HR, et al. Low-sodium dietary approaches to stop hypertension diet reduces blood pressure, arterial stiffness, and oxidative stress in hypertensive heart failure with preserved ejection fraction. Hypertension. 2012;60(5):1200–6. PubMed PubMedCentral CrossRef.
78. Wessler JD, Maurer MS, Hummel SL. Evaluating the safety and efficacy of sodium-restricted/dietary approaches to stop hypertension diet after acute decompensated heart failure hospitalization: design and rationale for the Geriatric OUt of hospital Randomized MEal Trial in Heart Failure (GOURMET-HF). Am Heart J. 2015;169(3):342–8 e4. PubMed PubMedCentral CrossRef.
79. Bibbins-Domingo K, Chertow GM, Coxson PG, Moran A, Lightwood JM, Pletcher MJ, et al. Projected effect of dietary salt reductions on future cardiovascular disease. N Engl J Med. 2010;362(7):590–9. PubMed PubMedCentral CrossRef.
80. Conard MW, Haddock CK, Poston WS, Spertus JA. The impact of smoking status on the health status of heart failure patients. Congest Heart Fail. 2009;15(2):82–6. PubMed CrossRef.
81. Hinderliter AL, Babyak MA, Sherwood A, Blumenthal JA. The DASH diet and insulin sensitivity. Curr Hypertens Rep. 2011;13(1):67–73. PubMed PubMedCentral CrossRef.
82. Meurrens K, Ruf S, Ross G, Schleef R, von Holt K, Schluter KD. Smoking accelerates the progression of hypertension-induced myocardial hypertrophy to heart failure in spontaneously hypertensive rats. Cardiovasc Res. 2007;76(2):311–22. PubMed CrossRef.
83. Sacks FM, Svetkey LP, Vollmer WM, Appel LJ, Bray GA, Harsha D, et al. Effects on blood pressure of reduced dietary sodium and the Dietary Approaches to Stop Hypertension (DASH) diet. DASH-Sodium Collaborative Research Group. N Engl J Med. 2001;344(1):3–10. PubMed CrossRef.
84. Hunt SA. ACC/AHA 2005 guideline update for the diagnosis and management of chronic heart failure in the adult: a report of the American College of Cardiology/American Heart Association Task Force on Practice Guidelines (Writing Committee to Update the 2001 Guidelines for the Evaluation and Management of Heart Failure). J Am Coll Cardiol. 2005;46(6):e1–82. PubMed CrossRef.
85. Hirota S, Sadanaga T, Mitamura H, Fukuda K. Spot urine-guided salt reduction is effective in Japanese cardiology outpatients. Hypertens Res. 2012;35(11):1069–71. PubMed CrossRef.
86. Sadanaga T, Ando K, Hirota S, Mitamura H, Tsuchihashi T, Kohsaka S, et al. B-type natriuretic peptide levels are decreased by reducing dietary salt intake in patients with compensated heart failure with preserved ejection fraction. Intern Med J. 2013;43:663–7. PubMed CrossRef.
87. Dinicolantonio JJ, Pasquale PD, Taylor RS, Hackam DG. Low sodium versus normal sodium diets in systolic heart failure: systematic review and meta-analysis. Heart. 2013; Epub 2013 March 12.
88. Kramer K, Kirkman P, Kitzman D, Little WC. Flash pulmonary edema: association with hypertension and reoccurrence despite coronary revascularization. Am Heart J. 2000;140(3):451–5. PubMed CrossRef.
89. Hunt SA, Abraham WT, Chin MH, Feldman AM, Francis GS, Ganiats TG, et al. 2009 focused update incorporated into the ACC/AHA 2005 Guidelines for the Diagnosis and Management of Heart Failure in Adults: a report of the American College of Cardiology Foundation/American Heart Association Task Force on Practice Guidelines: developed in collaboration with the International Society for Heart and Lung Transplantation. Circulation. 2009;119(14):e391–479. PubMed CrossRef.
90. Hachicha Z, Dumesnil JG, Bogaty P, Pibarot P. Paradoxical low-flow, low-gradient severe aortic stenosis despite preserved ejection fraction is associated with higher afterload and reduced survival. Circulation. 2007;115(22):2856–64. PubMed CrossRef.
91. Bonow RO, Carabello BA, Chatterjee K, de Leon AC Jr, Faxon DP, Freed MD, et al. 2008 focused update incorporated into the ACC/AHA 2006 guidelines for the management of patients with valvular heart disease: a report of the American College of Cardiology/American Heart Association Task Force on Practice Guidelines (Writing Committee to revise the 1998 guidelines for the management of patients with valvular heart disease). Endorsed by the Society of Cardiovascular Anesthesiologists, Society for Cardiovascular Angiography and Interventions, and Society of Thoracic Surgeons. J Am Coll Cardiol. 2008;52(13):e1–142. PubMed CrossRef.

92. De Sutter J, Van de Veire NR, Muyldermans L, De Backer T, Hoffer E, Vaerenberg M, et al. Prevalence of mechanical dyssynchrony in patients with heart failure and preserved left ventricular function (a report from the Belgian Multicenter Registry on dyssynchrony). Am J Cardiol. 2005;96(11):1543–8. PubMed CrossRef.
93. Filippatos G, Teerlink JR, Farmakis D, Cotter G, Davison BA, Felker GM, et al. Serelaxin in acute heart failure patients with preserved left ventricular ejection fraction: results from the RELAX-AHF trial. Eur Heart J. 2014;35(16):1041–50. PubMed CrossRef.
94. Georgakopoulos D, Little WC, Abraham WT, Weaver FA, Zile MR. Chronic baroreflex activation: a potential therapeutic approach to heart failure with preserved ejection fraction. J Card Fail. 2011;17(2):167–78. PubMed CrossRef.
95. Lovett EG, Schafer J, Kaufman CL. Chronic baroreflex activation by the Rheos system: an overview of results from European and North American feasibility studies. Conf Proc IEEE Eng Med Biol Soc. 2009;2009:4626–30. PubMed.
96. Mangiafico S, Costello-Boerrigter LC, Andersen IA, Cataliotti A, Burnett JC Jr. Neutral endopeptidase inhibition and the natriuretic peptide system: an evolving strategy in cardiovascular therapeutics. Eur Heart J. 2013;34:886–893c. PubMed CrossRef.
97. Schlaich MP, Krum H, Sobotka PA, Esler MD. Renal denervation and hypertension. Am J Hypertens. 2011;24(6):635–42. PubMed CrossRef.
98. Yu CM, Zhang Q, Yip GW, Lee PW, Kum LC, Lam YY, et al. Diastolic and systolic asynchrony in patients with diastolic heart failure: a common but ignored condition. J Am Coll Cardiol. 2007;49(1):97–105. PubMed CrossRef.
99. Zile MR, Little WC. Effects of autonomic modulation: more than just blood pressure. J Am Coll Cardiol. 2012;59(10):910–2. PubMed CrossRef.
100. ClinicalTrials.gov ID: NCT01392196.
101. ClinicalTrials.gov ID: NCT01402726.
102. Donal E, Lund L, Linde C, Daubert JC. Is cardiac resynchronization therapy an option in heart failure patients with preserved ejection fraction? Justification for the ongoing KaRen project. Arch Cardiovasc Dis. 2010;103(6–7):404–10. PubMed CrossRef.
103. Solomon SD, Zile M, Pieske B, Voors A, Shah A, Kraigher-Krainer E, et al. The angiotensin receptor neprilysin inhibitor LCZ696 in heart failure with preserved ejection fraction: a phase 2 double-blind randomised controlled trial. Lancet. 2012;380(9851):1387–95. PubMed CrossRef.
104. Chung ES, Katra RP, Ghio S, Bax J, Gerritse B, Hilpisch K, et al. Cardiac resynchronization therapy may benefit patients with left ventricular ejection fraction >35%: a PROSPECT trial substudy. Eur J Heart Fail. 2010;12(6):581–7. CrossRef.
105. Penicka M, Kocka V, Herman D, Trakalova H, Herold M. Cardiac resynchronization therapy for the causal treatment of heart failure with preserved ejection fraction: insight from a pressure-volume loop analysis. Eur J Heart Fail. 2010;12(6):634–6. PubMed CrossRef.
106. Nesto RW, Bell D, Bonow RO, Fonseca V, Grundy SM, Horton ES, et al. Thiazolidinedione use, fluid retention, and congestive heart failure: a consensus statement from the American Heart Association and American Diabetes Association. Circulation. 2003;108(23):2941–8. PubMed CrossRef.
107. van Heerebeek L, Borbely A, Niessen HW, Bronzwaer JG, van der Velden J, Stienen GJ, et al. Myocardial structure and function differ in systolic and diastolic heart failure. Circulation. 2006;113(16):1966–73. PubMed CrossRef.
108. Kitzman DW, Little WC, Brubaker PH, Anderson RT, Hundley WG, Marburger CT, et al. Pathophysiological characterization of isolated diastolic heart failure in comparison to systolic heart failure. JAMA. 2002;288(17):2144–50. PubMed CrossRef.
109. Paulus WJ, van Ballegoij JJ. Treatment of heart failure with normal ejection fraction: an inconvenient truth! J Am Coll Cardiol. 2010;55(6):526–37. PubMed CrossRef.
110. Cohen Solal A, Leurs I, Assyag P, Beauvais F, Clerson P, Contre C, et al. Optimization of heart FailUre medical treatment after hospital discharge according to left ventricUlaR Ejection fraction: the FUTURE survey. Arch Cardiovasc Dis. 2012;105(6–7):355–65. PubMed CrossRef.
111. Fukuta H, Sane DC, Brucks S, Little WC. Statin therapy may be associated with lower mortality in patients with diastolic heart failure: a preliminary report. Circulation. 2005;112(3):357–63. PubMed CrossRef.
112. Maurer MS, Teruya S, Chakraborty B, Helmke S, Mancini D. Treating anemia in older adults with Heart Failure with a Preserved Ejection Fraction (HFPEF) with epoetin alfa: single blind randomized clinical trial of safety and efficacy. Circ Heart Fail. 2013;6:254–63. PubMed CrossRef.

Acute Decompensated Heart Failure: Classification, Epidemiology and Pathophysiology

10

Daniel Fishbein

Introduction

Hospitalization for heart failure (HF) has emerged as major worldwide public health problem over the last three decades. Heart failure is the most common cause for hospitalization in patients over the age of 65 years in the United States. There are an estimated one million hospitalizations annually in the US with a primary diagnosis of heart failure accounting for 5–10% of all hospitalizations. Three million patients are hospitalized annually with a primary or secondary diagnosis of heart failure. Approximately 5.1–5.8 million Americans have HF and it is estimated that the prevalence of heart failure will increase by 46% from 2012 to 2030 [1–4]. The European Society of Cardiology represents 51 countries with a population of >900 million people. At least 15 million Europeans have heart failure and an equal number have asymptomatic left ventricular dysfunction [2].

The direct and indirect costs associated with HF in the US in 2009 are estimated to exceed $37 billion. Most of these costs are attributable to hospitalization for HF. The number of hospitalizations for HF has triple in the last three decades. The increase in the prevalence of heart failure appears to be due to a number of factors including: the aging of the U.S. population in association with the increased incidence of heart failure with advancing age; improved survival after myocardial infarction resulting in more patients living with left ventricular dysfunction; and better prevention of arrhythmia-related death in patients with chronic left ventricular systolic dysfunction [5].

D. Fishbein (✉)
Department of Medicine, Division of Cardiology, University of Washington Medical Cente, Seattle, WA, USA
e-mail: dfish@uw.edu

Definition

Acutely Decompensated Heart Failure (ADHF) can be defined as the new onset or recurrence of heart failure signs and symptoms that require urgent or emergent treatment and that result in hospitalization. A number of other terms have been used in the literature including: Acute Heart Failure Syndromes (AHFS), Acute Heart Failure (AHF) and Acute Decompensation of Chronic Heart Failure (ADCHF). The number of terms used in the literature reflects that ADHF is not a single diagnosis but rather, a group of related syndromes caused by a number of different primary underlying cardiovascular diseases that may be made worse by a variety of cardiac and non-cardiac conditions.

In patients with ADHF, there is significant heterogeneity in the underlying pathophysiology, precipitants, time course, clinical presentation and underlying cause of heart disease. However, pulmonary congestion due to elevated left atrial pressure with associated symptoms of dyspnea

H. J. Eisen (ed.), *Heart Failure I*, https://doi.org/10.1007/978-3-032-12626-9_10

with or without clinical evidence of low cardiac output is a consistent finding in patients with this syndrome.

Approximately 80% of patients hospitalized with ADHF have a previous diagnosis of heart failure, 15% have new onset heart failure, and 5% have advanced or refractory heart failure. Underlying cardiovascular diseases including coronary artery disease, hypertension, valvular heart disease and cardiomyopathy are often present. Non-cardiac conditions including kidney dysfunction, pulmonary disease, diabetes, thyroid disease, anemia, substance abuse, obesity, sleep apnea, and infection are often present and may contribute to heart failure decompensation [6].

Epidemiology

The number of hospitalizations with heart failure as a primary or secondary diagnosis tripled from 1979 to 2004, increasing from 1,274,000 in 1974 to 3,860,000 in 2004. Heart failure was the primary diagnosis in 30–35% of these admissions. Age-adjusted hospitalization rates also increased during this period. More than 80% of these hospitalizations were in patients age 65 years or older and were paid by Medicare or Medicaid [7].

There has, however, been a recent decline noted in hospitalization rates for ADHF. In an analysis of inpatient National Claims History files from the Centers for Medicare & Medicaid Services (CMS) which identified all fee-for-service Medicare beneficiaries who were hospitalized for HF from 1998 to 2008, the heart failure hospitalization rates adjusted for age, gender and race declined from 2845 per 100,000 person-years in 1998 to 2007 per 100,000 person-years in 2008 (a decline of 29.5%; $p < 0.001$). Black men had the lowest rate of age-adjusted decline for all race-gender categories. Importantly, risk-adjusted 1-year mortality after hospitalization decreased from 31.7% in 1999 to 29.6% in 2008 (a decline of 6.6%; $p < 0.001$) [8].

Several large multicenter observational registries in the United States and Europe have significantly improved our understanding of the demographics, clinical characteristics, comorbidities, management patterns and outcomes of patients admitted with ADHF. Prior to these registries, our understanding of ADHF came largely from studies of younger patients with moderate to severe systolic dysfunction that were enrolled in single-center or multicenter randomized controlled clinical trials conducted predominantly at academic heart failure centers. The observational registries were designed to enroll a more representative sample of patients with ADHF that included all patients admitted with heart failure at geographically diverse academic and non-academic medical centers.

The Organized Program to Initiate Lifesaving Treatment in Hospitalized Patients with Heart Failure (OPTIMIZE-HF) used HF case ascertainment methods to identify 48,612 patients hospitalized at 259 centers in the United States for new or worsening HF as the primary cause of admission or who developed significant HF symptoms during hospitalization for a different diagnosis. Using a web-based registry, detailed data were collected including demographics, medical history, signs and symptoms, medications, laboratories, diagnostic testing procedures, discharge status, outcomes and adherence to performance indicators. A pre-specified subgroup that was $\geq$10% of the total number of patients was followed for 60–90 days after discharge for the collection of outcomes data [9].

The Acute Decompensated Heart Failure National Data Registry (ADHERE) database was a prospective observational registry that was developed to provide a large national database to describe clinical characteristics, management and outcomes of patients hospitalized with heart failure at 285 hospitals in the United States. Thirty one percent of the participating institutions were academic hospitals. From 2002 to 2004, data were collected from 159,168 hospitalizations beginning with the point of initial care and ending with the patients' discharge or in-hospital death [10–12].

The EuroHeart Failure Survey I (EHFS I) was a retrospective registry in which deaths or discharges from 115 hospitals (50% university hospitals) from 24 European countries were screened to identify patients with known or suspected heart failure. Demographics, clinical characteristics, evaluation, treatment and outcomes were assessed [13–15]. The EuroHeart Failure Survey II (EHFS II) was a prospective observational registry that recruited 3580 patients hospitalized for HF at 133 centers (47% university hospitals) in 30 European countries. Using a web based registry, detailed data were collected including demographics, clinical characteristics, etiology, treatment and outcome [16].

The findings from the U.S. and European trials are largely concordant. ADHF disproportionately affects the elderly; the mean age in the registries was 73 years. One quarter of the patients in OPTIMIZE-HF were more than 83 years old [17]. Men and women were equally represented in the U.S. registries while men represented two thirds of the hospitalized patients in EHFS II [16]. Women with ADHF tend to be older, are less likely to have coronary artery disease and are more likely to have hypertension and preserved systolic function [17].

Over 70% of patients with ADHF in the U.S. registries had a history of hypertension. A history of hypertension was reported in 63% of patients in EHFS II [16]. Elevation of systolic blood pressure is common at the time of presentation to the emergency department (ED). Mean initial systolic blood pressure on presentation to the emergency department (ED) was 143 mmHg in OPTIMIZE-HF and 144 mmHg in ADHERE. Half of the patients in ADHERE and OPTIMIZE-HF had an initial systolic pressure of greater than 140 mmHg [10, 18]. Renal dysfunction is common. The mean serum creatinine was 1.8 mg/dL in both ADHERE and OPTIMIZE; 20% of patients in ADHERE had a serum creatinine of greater than 2.0 mg/dL [10, 18].

Approximately half of patients in ADHERE and OPTIMIZE had normal or near normal systolic function defined as a left ventricular ejection fraction (LVEF) ≥40% [19, 20]. Patients with heart failure with preserved ejection fraction (HFpEF) were more likely to be older, female, Caucasian, and have a higher systolic blood pressure on admission and less likely to have had a prior myocardial infarction when compared with patients with heart failure with reduced ejection fraction (HFrEF). In-hospital mortality was lower in patients with HFpEF compared to patients with HFrEF in both ADHERE (2.8% vs. 3.9%) and OPTIMIZE-HF (2.9% vs. 3.9%). In ADHERE, patients with HFpEF had a similar length of stay and duration of intensive care unit stay when compared with patients with HFrEF [19]. In OPTIMIZE-HF, patients with HFpEF and HFrEF had similar 60–90 day post-discharge mortality (9.5% vs. 9.8%, respectively) and rehospitalization rates (29.2% vs. 29.9%, respectively). Findings were similar when patients with an LVEF between 40% and 50% were compared with patients with an LVEF ≥50% [20]. In an analysis of the data from EHFS I, mortality during the 12-week post-discharge follow-up period was higher in patients with HFrEF compared to patients with HFpEF (12% vs 10%). There were no differences in readmission rates during the 12 week follow up period [21].

Eighteen percent of patients in OPTIMIZE-HF and 20% of patients in ADHERE were African American. African American patients in OPTIMIZE-HF were younger (mean age 63.6 years compared with 75.2 years for non-African American patients), were more likely to have systolic dysfunction and a hypertensive etiology of heart failure and significantly less likely to have ischemic heart disease than non- African American patients. African American patients were more likely to receive evidence-based medications but less likely to receive discharge instructions and smoking cessation counseling. African American race was an independent predictor of lower in-hospital mortality but not of hospital length of stay or multivariable adjusted post-discharge outcomes [22].

In ADHERE, 75% of patients had a prior history of HF and 33% had a HF admission within the prior 6 months. Eighty eight percent of patients in OPTIMIZE-HF had a prior history of heart failure. Thirty seven percent of patients in EHFS II had new onset HF; 42% of these patients presented with an acute coronary syndrome [10, 16, 17].

Comorbid conditions are common in patients admitted with ADHF. A history of hypertension was present in over 70% of patients in the U.S. registries and 53% and 62.5% in EHFS I and II, respectively. Over 40% of patients had diabetes in the U.S. registries (27% and 32.8% in EHFS I and II, respectively). Renal insufficiency was present in 30% of patients and chronic lung disease was present in 30% of patients in the U.S. registries.

Outcomes

There are significant differences in length of stay, in-hospital mortality, rehospitalization rates and post-discharge mortality when registry data from the US and Europe are compared. Median length of stay is 4 days in the U.S [10, 17] compared with 9–11 days in Europe [13, 16]. In-hospital mortality is approximately 4% in the U.S [10, 17]. and 6.7% in Europe [16].

The 60–90 day post-discharge mortality reported in OPTIMIZE-HF was 10.4% [17]. In EHFS I, 13% of patients died between admission and the 12-week follow-up visit. 6.9% of patients died during the index hospitalization [13]. Readmission rate 60–90 days after discharge was approximately 30% in OPTIMIZE and 24% in EHFS I. An analysis of Medicare claims data found that 26.9% of Medicare beneficiaries who were hospitalized for heart failure were rehospitalized within 30 days. However, only 37% of patients who were rehospitalized were rehospitalized for heart failure [23].

Two large, retrospective observational studies have demonstrated reductions in hospital length of stay, in-hospital mortality, and 30-day mortality and an increase in 30 day readmission rates. An analysis from the Veterans Affairs Health Care System of 50,125 patients with a first hospitalization for HF from 2002 to 2006 showed a decrease in in-hospital, 30 day and 1 year mortality from 4.7, 7.1, and 27.7% in 2002 to 2.8, 5.0, and 24.3% in 2006, respectively ($p < 0.0001$). Thirty-day readmission rate for heart failure increased from 5.6 in 2002 to 6.1% in 2006 ($p = 0.11$) [24]. Another analysis of 6,955,461 Medicare fee-for-service hospitalizations for heart failure between 1993 and 2006 demonstrated a decrease in in-hospital mortality from 8.5% in 1993 to 4.3% in 2006 and a decrease in 30-day mortality from 12.8% to 10.7% over the same time period. Thirty-day readmission rates increased from 17.2% to 20.1% over the same time period. The risk adjusted 30-day mortality risk ratio was 0.92 and the 30-day readmission risk ratio was 1.11 in 2005–2006 compared with 1993–1994 [25].

A large prospective observational study reported outcomes in 69,958 beneficiaries of the French national health insurance general scheme who were hospitalized with heart failure in 2009 [26]. Patients who were hospitalized for heart failure and did not have a previous diagnosis of HF or prior HF hospitalization were included in the analysis. The in-hospital mortality was 6.4%. The 1-month, 1-year and 2-year survival rates were 89%, 71%, and 60%, respectively. Heart failure and all-cause readmission free rates were 55% and 43% at 1 year and 27% and 17% at 2 years, respectively. Factors associated with a better 2 year survival rate in patients less than 70 years who survived 1 month after discharge were: female gender, age <55 years, absence of comorbidities, and use of an angiotensin converting enzyme inhibitor or angiotensin receptor blocker, beta-blocker, lipid-lowering agent or oral anticoagulant during the month following discharge.

Classification of ADHF

Heart failure is the final common pathway for a broad range of cardiovascular disorders. Patients with ADHF have diverse underlying causes of cardiac dysfunction, time course of symptom development, co-morbid conditions and precipitants, and underlying pathophysiology. A number of attempts have been made to classify ADHF based on onset, underlying heart disease, underlying hemodynamic abnormalities and clinical profiles.

The International Working Group on Acute Heart Failure Syndromes [6] emphasized the time course of development of HF and the American College of Cardiology/American

Heart Association (ACC/AHA) stage in their classification of ADHF:

1. Worsening chronic heart failure: with reduced or preserved LVEF. ACC/AHA Stage C heart failure. Seventy percent of all admissions.
2. De novo heart failure: most commonly caused by acute coronary syndrome (ACS); also, acute myocarditis or sudden increase in blood pressure in a patient with a non-compliant left ventricle. Many with either ACC/AHA Stage A (risk factors but no structural heart disease) or Stage B (pre-existing structural heart disease but without signs or symptoms of heart failure). Twenty five percent of all admissions.
3. Advanced heart failure: severe LV systolic dysfunction, associated with progressively worsening low output state, refractory to conventional heart failure therapy and requiring specialized therapies (LVAD, heart transplant, hospice). ACC/AHA Stage D 5% of all admissions.

The 2009 ACCF/AHA Guidelines for the Diagnosis and Management of Heart Failure in Adults [27] have described three clinical profiles of patients with ADHF that focus on clinical manifestations of congestion and systemic perfusion:

1. The patient with volume overload, manifested by pulmonary and/or systemic congestion, frequently precipitated by an acute increase in chronic hypertension.
2. The patient with profound depression of cardiac output manifested by hypotension, renal insufficiency, and/or shock syndrome.
3. The patient with signs and symptoms of both fluid overload and shock.

The European Society of Cardiology (ESC) has described six clinical scenarios for patients presenting with ADHF in their 2008 Guidelines for the Diagnosis and Treatment of Acute and Chronic Heart Failure [2]. EHFS II used a modification of the ESC scenarios to characterize patients included in the registry [16]:

1. Worsening or decompensated chronic heart failure: history of progressive worsening of known chronic heart failure. Signs and symptoms of worsening heart failure with evidence of pulmonary and systemic venous congestion. Patients can have either reduced or preserved ejection fraction. (65% of patients in EHFS II).
2. Pulmonary edema: Patients who present with severe respiratory distress, tachypnea with diffuse pulmonary rales, hypoxia with oxygen saturation <90% (without supplemental oxygen) with alveolar edema on chest X-ray. (16% of patients in EHFS II).
3. Hypertensive heart failure: Patients have signs and symptoms of heart failure with high blood pressure (generally ≥180/100 mmHg). There is commonly evidence of high sympathetic tone with tachycardia and signs of vasoconstriction. Patients are more likely to have preserved systolic function. Frequently, these patients present with evidence of pulmonary congestion without signs of systemic congestion. The response to HF therapy is generally rapid and the in-hospital mortality is low (1.5% in EHFS II). (11% of patients in EHFS II).
4. Cardiogenic shock: Patients with evidence of end-organ hypoperfusion due to heart failure with adequate or elevated LV end-diastolic pressure. Typically, these patients have a reduced systolic blood pressure (<90 mmHg), oliguria, and low cardiac index (<2.2 L/min/m^2). Many patients will also have severe pulmonary congestion. Mortality in this population is high. (4% of patients in EHFS II).
5. Isolated right heart failure: evidence of systemic venous congestion, elevated jugular venous pressure and low cardiac output without evidence of pulmonary congestion.
6. Acute coronary syndrome complicated by heart failure: (This was not included as a separate classification in EHFS II) heart failure with a clinical picture and laboratory evidence of an acute coronary syndrome. Approximately 13.6% of patients with ACS have associated signs and symptoms of heart

failure [28, 29]. In EHFS II, ACS was the precipitating factor in 42% of patients who presented with new onset or de novo heart failure and 23% of patients who had preexisting heart failure.

A recent American Heart Association Scientific Statement on Acute Heart Failure Syndromes has also emphasized the concept of clinical profiles of patients presenting with ADHF [30].

ADHF has also been characterized by the presence or absence of systolic dysfunction. Patients with heart failure with normal or near normal left ventricular ejection fraction are described as having heart failure with preserved ejection fraction (HFpEF). Patients with heart failure with significant reduction in LVEF (and generally with left ventricular dilation) are characterized as having heart failure with reduced ejection fraction (HFrEF). Patients with HFpEF are more likely to be female, older, Caucasian, have hypertension and atrial fibrillation and less likely to have coronary artery disease. Length of stay for patients with HFpEF is similar to patients with HFrEF but in-hospital mortality is lower. Long-term survival is somewhat better in patients with HFpEF but readmission rates and functional class are similar in patients with HFpEF compared with patients with HFrEF [20, 21, 31].

Pathophysiology

ADHF is a syndrome due to a broad range of cardiovascular disorders. The underlying pathophysiology is heterogeneous and depends on the nature, time course and severity of the underlying cardiac disease and the presence and severity of non-cardiac precipitating factors. The heterogeneity of patients with ADHF makes it difficult to develop a single pathophysiologic model. Despite this heterogeneity, there are some important themes in patients with ADHF that guide the approach to patient management.

Neurohormonal Activation and Salt and Water Retention

In heart failure, there is a decrease in cardiac output that results in activation of baroreceptors in the central circulation in response to "vascular under-filling". This causes activation of the sympathetic nervous system resulting in an increase in sympathetic outflow to the kidney and systemic vasoconstriction.

Decreased renal blood flow and sympathetic stimulation of the kidney cause release of renin from the juxtaglomerular apparatus which, in turn, results in conversion of angiotensinogen to angiotensin I which is converted to angiotensin II by angiotensin converting enzyme (ACE) and other tissue proteases. Angiotensin II is a potent vasoconstrictor that causes systemic vasoconstriction, renal arterial efferent > afferent vasoconstriction, activation of the sympathetic nervous system, stimulation of sodium retention in the proximal tubule of the kidney, release of aldosterone, release of arginine vasopressin, and stimulation of thirst centers in the brain.

Aldosterone increases sodium and water reabsorption in the distal tubule and collecting duct contributing to extracellular fluid expansion and systemic congestion. Aldosterone also increases sodium and water absorption in the colon. Hepatic congestion in the setting of elevated right atrial pressure decreases aldosterone metabolism leading to higher aldosterone levels. In heart failure, patients do not have "aldosterone escape" so that, unlike patients with isolated hyperaldosteronism, the distal tubule continues to reabsorb sodium in response to elevated aldosterone levels.

Stimulation of central baroreceptors and increased angiotensin II levels stimulate the non-osmotic release of arginine vasopressin from the posterior pituitary gland. This leads to increased free water reabsorption in the collecting ducts which worsens volume overload and leads to the development of hyponatremia.

In heart failure, retention of sodium and water is mediated by decreased systemic and renal perfusion, activation of the sympathetic nervous system and activation of the renin angiotensin aldosterone system (RAAS). In many patients, salt and water retention cannot be reversed by pharmacologic blockade of the RAAS and sympathetic nervous system suggesting that neurohormonal activation is not the only mechanism responsible for salt and water retention [32–34]. Increases in sodium and water intake are mediated by an increase in thirst caused by stimulation of central thirst centers mediated by activation of baroreceptors in the central circulation and excessive production angiotensin II. Systemic congestion is a result of an increase in total body salt and water mediated by a decrease in sodium and water excretion and an increase in intake.

Activation of the sympathetic nervous system and RAAS cause systemic vasoconstriction and an increase in systemic vascular resistance (SVR). Increases in SVR result in a decrease in stroke volume and cardiac output in patients with systolic dysfunction and an increase in functional mitral regurgitation in patients with ventricular dilation.

Pulmonary Congestion

Most patients with ADHF present with the primary symptom of dyspnea either at rest or with activity. This is true for patients with new-onset or chronic heart failure and for patients with and without systolic dysfunction. Many patients have evidence on physical exam of pulmonary and systemic venous congestion [10, 17].

Dyspnea in patients with ADHF is caused by an elevation in left atrial and pulmonary capillary pressure. The movement of fluid from the pulmonary capillary space to the pulmonary interstitium is determined by a balance between hydrostatic and oncotic pressures in the pulmonary capillary and the pulmonary interstitial space. The major factor that causes fluid to move out of the capillary is a difference between the higher hydrostatic pressure within the pulmonary capillary and the lower hydrostatic pressure in the surrounding interstitium. This movement of fluid is opposed by the difference between the colloid osmotic pressure (which is mainly provided by the concentration of albumin) in the capillary space and the interstitium, which reduces the transudation of fluid out of the capillary. In normal physiology, lymphatic washout of albumin that enters the interstitium results in an increase in the osmotic gradient between the interstitium and pulmonary capillary which reduces transudation of fluid. In normal physiology, fluid continuously moves from the capillary space into the interstitium and is then removed by the lymphatic system. When hydrostatic pressure in the pulmonary capillary significantly increases, transudation of fluid into the interstitium increases with potential for "spillover" into the alveolar space [35].

There are several protective mechanisms that prevent the development of pulmonary edema (fluid entering the alveolar space). First, the alveolar-capillary unit is composed of a thin and thick side. The thin side is made up of a capillary closely opposed to the alveolar air space. The capillary endothelium and alveolar epithelium are attenuated, the basal laminae of the alveolar epithelium and capillary endothelium are fused and the permeability to salt and water is low. The thick portion of the alveolar capillary unit contains an interstitial matrix with a gel-like protein component that separates the alveolar epithelium from the capillary endothelium. With a rise in capillary hydrostatic pressure, edema first forms in the interstitial compartment away from areas of gas exchange. Second, as fluid enters the interstitial compartment, hydrostatic pressure rises and oncotic pressure falls, which serves to oppose further movement into the interstitial space. Third, fluid that forms in the interstitium travels along a negative pressure gradient to the interlobular septae, the bronchovascular space and the hila. Edema fluid also collects in the pleural space. Lymphatic vessels in the interlobular septae, peribronchovascular sheath and pleura facilitate clearance of lung water. Pulmonary lymphatics are highly recruitable and, over time, are able to increase clearance of lung water by more than tenfold. Fourth, active Na + transport across the alveolar-capillary barrier by type II alveolar epithelial cells lining the alveoli is responsible for clearance of alveolar edema. Na+ enters the alveolar epithelial cells through apical amiloride sensitive Na+ channels and other Na+ channels and, by a process that consumes energy, is pumped out of the cell by the Na+,K + -ATPase located in the basolateral membrane [35–40].

In patients with HFpEF or HFrEF, the LV filling pressure required to support a given amount of left ventricular work is increased. As left ventricular end-diastolic pressure (LVEDP) rises, so do left atrial and pulmonary capillary pressures. As pulmonary capillary pressure increases, there is an increase in the transmural filtration of fluid into the pulmonary interstitium. There is a point at which the capacity of the lymphatic system to remove fluid from the interstitium is exceeded and fluid begins to accumulate in the alveoli. Animal data suggest that there is a threshold beyond which interstitial fluid begins to accumulate and that the rate of fluid accumulation is linearly related to pulmonary capillary wedge pressure.

The accumulation of extravascular fluid in the pulmonary interstitium and alveoli is associated with symptoms of dyspnea, orthopnea, paroxysmal dyspnea, and impaired gas exchange. Symptoms and pulmonary function are influenced by water content of the lungs. The underlying pathophysiology of dyspnea in ADHF is multifactorial and complex with contributions from: decreased lung volume; airflow obstruction from reflex bronchoconstriction; geometric decrease in airway size from decreased lung volumes, intraluminal edema fluid and mucosal swelling; decreased lung compliance; decreased alveolar-capillary membrane conductance with acute and chronic decreases in DLCO; impaired gas exchange due to alveolar edema; arterial hypoxemia; increased work of breathing; respiratory muscle weakness in the chronically ill patient; activation of chest wall sensors, an increase in the elastic work of breathing due to vascular engorgement and cardiac enlargement with chest wall expansion past the usual or physiologic position; and stimulation of nerve endings in response to vascular distention and interstitial edema [35].

Transition from Compensated to Decompensated Heart Failure

A traditional understanding of why patients with chronic heart failure develope ADHF suggests that patients with chronic heart failure commonly experience a gradual increase in total body salt and water reflected by gradual weight gain and the gradual development of signs and symptoms of pulmonary and systemic venous congestion. While this paradigm occurs in some patients with chronic heart failure, it may not be applicable to the majority of patients with ADHF. A nested case-control study of patients referred to a home monitoring system by managed care organizations matched 134 case patients with HF hospitalization with 134 control patients without HF hospitalization [41]. Case patients experienced gradual weight gain beginning approximately 30 days before hospitalization. Within 7 days of hospitalization, weight patterns between case and control patients began to diverge more substantially with greater weight gain strongly associated with a greater odds ratio for hospitalization for ADHF (>2–5 lbs. HR 2.77; >5–10 lbs. HR 4.46; >10 lbs. HR 5.65). However, only 46% of case patients hospitalized for ADHF gained more than two pounds suggesting that in approximately half of patients, weight gain was not the precipitating cause of hospitalization.

Implantable hemodynamic monitor data in patients with chronic heart failure from the Chronicle Offers Management to Patients with Advanced Signs and Symptoms of Heart Failure (COMPASS-HF) trial provide insight into the time course and pathophysiology of the transition from stable heart failure to ADHF. Earlier studies demonstrated that daily activity, exercise and change in body position caused rapid, large and transient increases in estimated pulmonary artery diastolic pressure (ePADP) in the range of 10–40 mmHg. Increases in ePADP could occur over seconds to minutes with change in body position and exercise. Although these activities could be associated with transient dyspnea, they did not lead to hospitalization for ADHF [42–45]. In a sub-study from COMPASS-HF, ambulatory patients with NYHA FC III—IV heart failure due to either systolic or diastolic dysfunction transmitted hemodynamic data at least weekly. The investigators found that estimated pulmonary artery diastolic pressure (ePADP), right ventricular systolic pressure (RVSP) and right ventricular diastolic pressure (RVDP) were elevated in ambulatory patients with systolic and diastolic heart failure. In patients with systolic and diastolic heart failure, increases in median and minimum ePADP, RVSP and RVDP were seen several weeks (and especially within a week) prior to a hypervolemic heart failure-related event (unexpected hospitalization, emergency room visit, or urgent clinic visit requiring intravenous therapy). These changes were not seen in patients free of a heart failure related event (HFRA). Interestingly, no significant change in weight was seen in patients with an HFRA [46].

A subsequent analysis from the COMPASS-HF study looked at the relationship between three pressure variables measured by an implantable hemodynamic monitor and the development of a HFRE in ambulatory patients with NYHA FC III-IV heart failure. Pressure variables assessed included peak ePADP at the time of a HFRE, change in ePADP from baseline to peak ePADP, and the area under the ePAD pressure-time curve from baseline to peak pressure. Peak ePAD and change in ePAD were not closely associated with the development of an HFRA. However, the area under the ePAD pressure-time curve was strongly associated with the development of a HFRE. It appears that small changes in ePAD sustained over time most strongly correlated with an HFRE [47]. This data suggests that the accumulation of lung water rather than total body salt and water results in hospitalization for ADHF.

These studies do not negate the importance of following serial weights in patients at risk for ADHF. Although it is common to have patients present with ADHF without an antecedent gain in weight, patients with heart failure who do gain weight are at a significantly increased risk of hospitalization.

Hypertension, Increased Systemic Vascular Resistance and Arterial Stiffness

Elevated blood pressure is found in 50% of patients with ADHF on initial presentation. In the ADHERE registry the mean first systolic blood pressure was 144 mmHg and 50% of patients had an initial systolic blood pressure greater than 140 mmHg [10]. In OPTIMIZE-HF, the mean systolic pressure at admission was 143 mmHg and 25% of patients had an initial systolic pressure >161 mmHg [18]. Admission hypertension was associated with female gender, black race, HFpEF and a non-ischemic etiology of heart failure [18]. Some of the patients in each of these registries received medical therapy by emergency medical services before arriving to the ED suggesting that initial blood pressure prior to treatment was actually higher than reported in the registries. In a study of all patients seen for ADHF at a single city hospital over a 3 month period, first blood pressure was recorded before initiation of therapy at the first patient encounter either in the ambulance or ED. Mean blood pressure was 164/88. Seventy five percent of patients had a systolic BP >140 mmHg. Fifty percent of patients had a mean blood pressure >113 mmHg and the mean systolic blood pressure in the highest quartile of mean blood pressures was 212 mmHg [48].

A study of patients who presented with acute pulmonary edema followed hemodynamic parameters using a pulmonary artery catheter for 24 h after presentation. Patients who developed recurrent pulmonary edema after initial stabilization were noted to have a marked, rapid increase in systemic vascular resistance and decrease in cardiac index that preceded an increase in pulmonary capillary wedge pressure. These hemodynamic changes were not seen in patients who did not have recurrent pulmonary edema. The only hemodynamic variable at baseline that predicted recurrent pulmonary edema was low cardiac power index (CPI = cardiovascular flow × mean forward pressure = cardiac index × mean arterial pressure) [49].

These data suggest that high blood pressure and elevated systemic vascular resistance play an important role in the development of ADHF. Many patients with hypertension at the time of hospitalization have a prompt reduction in blood pressure and improvement in symptoms shortly after receiving intravenous diuretics [50, 51]. Some of these patients may have reactive hypertension driven by a response to increased filling pressures and activation of the RAAS and the sympathetic nervous system in the setting of contractile reserve. Some patients may develop acute heart failure in response to elevated blood pressure and systemic vascular resistance in the setting of significant impairment of systolic function that results in an acute decrease in stroke volume, increase in mitral regurgitation, a rapid increase in left atrial pressure and pulmonary congestion in the absence of systemic congestion. It is also possible that an acute decrease in venous capacitance mediated by sympathetic nervous system activation could acutely increase venous return to the heart causing an acute increase in filling pressures.

Balmain compared arterial compliance, microvascular function and venous capacitance in patients with HFpEF, HFrEF, and normal controls [52]. Arterial compliance was significantly lower in patients with HFpEF than in patients with HFrEF and normal controls. Patients with HFpEF and HFrEF had impaired endothelial dependent and independent microvascular vasodilation. Patients with HFrEF had higher venous capacitance than either patients with HFpEF or controls. Higher venous capacitance may result in a greater capacity for the circulation to accommodate greater blood volume without an increase in right atrial and left ventricular end-diastolic pressures. The "normal" venous capacitance of patients with HFpEF may be pathologic and contribute to the development of pulmonary congestion in these patients.

It is unclear what mediates the dynamic change in systemic vascular resistance (and possible acute decrease in venous capacitance) in some patients with ADHF. Age and disease-related increases in arterial stiffness, activation of the RAAS and the sympathetic nervous system, and acute inflammatory activation may all contribute to the transient increase in systemic vascular resistance. This increase in SVR may cause "afterload mismatch" with a decline in stroke volume, and increase in functional mitral regurgitation and an acute rise in left atrial pressure that leads to volume redistribution into the lungs and pulmonary congestion [30, 52–54].

An analysis from the OPTIMIZE-HF registry looked at the impact of admission systolic blood pressure on in-hospital mortality in the entire cohort (48,612 patients) and on post-discharge outcomes in the pre-specified subgroup who were followed for 60–90 days after discharge (5791 patients) [18]. Patients were divided into quartiles by SBP at time of hospital admission (<120, 120–139, 140–161, >161 mmHg). Higher systolic blood pressure at admission was associated with lower in-hospital mortality rates (7.2%, 3.6%, 2.5%, and 1.7%, respectively by quartile of increasing blood pressure). Post-discharge mortality rates in the follow-up cohort were similarly lower in patients with higher admission systolic BP (14%, 8.4%, 6.0%, and 5.4% by quartile of increasing blood pressure). A number of other studies have also demonstrated the prognostic importance of systolic blood pressure in ADHF across a broad range of blood pressures [55–57] In these studies, the adjusted relative risk for mortality have ranged from 0.76 to 0.9 for each 10 mmHg increase in systolic blood pressure.

The consistent relationship between systolic blood pressure and survival suggests an important difference in the pathophysiology of ADHF in patients with high vs. normal or low systolic blood pressure. High blood pressure is more common in advanced age, women, blacks, patients with a non-ischemic cause of heart failure and patients with HFpEF. Patients with elevated SBP on presentation have more pulmonary congestion and respiratory compromise than patients with normal SBP but have more rapid improvement with treatment. Elevated SBP tends to improve rapidly in patients with high admission SBP. Congestive symptoms, which are more common in patients with elevated SBP at admission, become less common prior to discharge when compared to patients with normal or low admission SBP. Elevated SBP is an important reflection of contractile reserve which, like maximum oxygen consumption during cardiopulmonary exercise testing, is a powerful predictor of survival. These observations have led to the suggestion that initial treatment of ADHF be based on presenting SBP with patients divided into three groups: hypertensive (SBP >140 mmHg); normotensive (SBP 100–140 mmHg); and hypotensive (SBP <100 mmHg) based on the initial BP in the ambulance or ED [18, 30, 58, 59].

Pulmonary Manifestations of Acute Versus Chronic Heart Failure

Eighty-nine percent of patients with ADHF have dyspnea on presentation [8]. Two thirds of patients admitted to the hospital with ADHF have pulmonary rales [8, 18]. Two thirds of patients have lower extremity edema (LE) [8, 18]. However, most patients admitted to the hospital do not have reduced oxygen saturation and only a small percentage of patients with ADHF present with acute pulmonary edema (16% in EHFS II). Patients with chronic heart failure may have symptoms of dyspnea without evidence of pulmonary congestion on exam or chest radiograph despite having a high pulmonary capillary wedge pressure (PCWP). Patients with new onset heart failure develop pulmonary edema at pulmonary capillary wedge pressures of approximately 25 mmHg while some patients with chronic heart failure are ambulatory without pulmonary rales despite having wedge pressures of 35–40 mmHg [35, 36, 60].

A number of mechanisms have been proposed to explain the disparity in pulmonary manifestations in patients with acute or recent onset heart failure and patients with chronic heart failure. It has been suggested that lymphatic enlargement seen on post-mortem examination of patients with chronic heart failure may protect from the development of alveolar edema although data supporting this concept has been inconsistent [37, 38].

Pathologic specimens from patients with chronic heart failure, especially studies of patients with mitral stenosis, help explain the difference in presentation in patients with new onset versus longstanding heart failure. At a microscopic level, many specimens demonstrate alveolar fibrosis. Electron micrographs show thickening of the capillary endothelial and alveolar epithelial cell basement membranes. These changes are thought to reduce the permeability of the alveolar-capillary membrane to water and prevent the formation of pulmonary edema. In addition, pulmonary arteries and arterioles develop intimal fibrosis and medial hypertrophy with extension to the small arterioles. Pulmonary veins are thick-walled and lymphatic vessels are dilated and occasionally muscularized [35, 36, 61].

In experimental models of chronic heart failure, there is thickening of the alveolar and capillary basal laminae with pericyte and type IV collagen infiltration of the alveolar-capillary barrier. Alveolar-capillary remodeling leads to a chronic reduction in alveolar capillary membrane conductance, capillary filtration and lung diffusion capacity [35, 36, 40, 62–64]. Wall thickness-lumen ratio is increased in small pulmonary arterioles and venules with an increase in arterial and venous resistance. The vascular remodeling leads to increased vascular resistance [35, 36, 62–64]. These remodeling changes may protect against alveolar edema on the one hand but may impede gas exchange on the other.

There is also likely a difference in alveolar fluid clearance in acute versus chronic heart failure which protects against the development of alveolar edema in chronic heart failure. Alveolar fluid clearance is decreased in the setting of acutely elevated left atrial pressure. However, with chronic elevation of PCWP, alveolar fluid clearance is increased likely secondary to upregulation of active sodium transport [36, 39, 40].

Lower Extremity Edema

Lower extremity edema is a manifestation of severe fluid retention with an increase in total body salt and water and transfer of fluid into the tissues. Tissue edema forms when capillary hydrostatic pressure is greater than plasma colloid pressure by an amount sufficient to cause transudation from the capillary space into the interstitial space at a rate that exceeds the rate at which lymphatics can drain away the interstitial fluid. The rate of edema formation depends on capillary pressure (which is affected by position and right atrial pressure) and capillary permeability [32].

Myocardial Injury

Coronary artery disease (CAD) is present in 50–70% of patients who present with ADHF [10, 11, 14, 15]. In OPTIMIZE-HF, patients with CAD had a higher inpatient mortality rate (3.7% vs. 2.9%) and a higher 60–90 day post-discharge mortality rate (9.2% vs 6.9%) [65]. In EHFS II, ACS was the precipitating factor in 42% of patients who presented with new onset heart failure and 23% of patients who had preexisting heart failure [16]. Approximately 10–20% of patients with ACS have associated heart failure on presentation and another 10% develop heart failure during hospitalization [66].

Cardiac troponin (either T or I) has a high clinical sensitivity and near absolute specificity for myocardial injury [67, 68]. The presence of measurable cardiac troponin (cTn) is abnormal and indicative of myocardial injury. Typically, the patient with ACS precipitating heart failure will have precordial pain, characteristic ST segment elevations on ECG and significant cTn elevations (cTn I > 1.0 ng/ml or mcg/L). However, in ADHF, troponin elevation may be seen in patients with or without ACS and with or without significant obstructive coronary artery disease. There has been a consistent association between elevate cTn and in-hospital mortality.

The reported prevalence of detectable troponin in ADHF has been variable and has depended on the population studied, cTn assay used and cTn threshold considered positive. An analysis from the ADHERE Registry found that an elevated troponin I $\geq$ 1.0 mcg/L or a troponin T $\geq$ 0.1 mcg/liter was found in 6.2% of 67,924 patients who had a troponin an admission and a creatinine <2.0 mg/dL. 53% of troponin positive patients and 52% of troponin negative patients had ischemic heart disease reported as the cause of ADHF. Ischemic heart failure was not a useful discriminator of troponin status. Patients who had a positive troponin had lower systolic blood pressure on admission, lower ejection fraction and higher in-hospital mortality (8.0% vs 2.7%) compared to patients with a negative troponin. The risk adjusted odds ratio for death among patients with a positive troponin was 2.55 ($P < 0.001$). When mortality was assessed by quartiles of cardiac troponin, there was a progressive increase in in-hospital mortality from quartile one to quartile four (from the lowest to highest troponin quartile) [69].

The Enhanced Feedback for Effective Cardiac Treatment (EFFECT) study was a population-based quality improvement initiative that evaluated patients hospitalized with heart failure at 103 acute care hospitals in Ontario, Canada. The EFFECT investigators looked at the relationship between troponin I > 0.5 mcg/L and all-cause mortality in 2025 patients hospitalized for heart failure. Elevated troponin occurred in 34.5% of patients and was an independent predictor of mortality with an adjusted hazard ratio of 1.49 ($p < 0.001$). Adjustment for the presence of reduced ejection fraction had no significant impact on the estimate of risk. As in the analysis from ADHERE, there was a relationship between troponin I level and mortality that persisted after adjusting for confounding variables such that the hazard ratio for mortality increased with each quartile of troponin elevation. In addition, the association between troponin and mortality was similar for patients with and without other clinical features of acute myocardial ischemia [70].

This data demonstrates that myocardial injury, independent of ACS, occurs in a significant number of patients with ADHF with or without coronary artery disease and that myocardial injury plays an important role in the development of acute heart failure. A number of mechanisms underlying cTn release have been proposed. The Carvedilol Hibernation Reversible Ischemia

(CHRISTMAS) trial reported that 60% of patients with heart failure and CAD had hibernating myocardium [71]. Hibernating myocardium may be at risk for injury due to focal myocardial ischemia (especially subendocardial ischemia) in the setting of elevated left ventricular end-diastolic pressure, hypotension with reduced myocardial perfusion, tachycardia, or medications that increase contractility. Patients without CAD may be at risk for injury due to the same hemodynamic conditions. Proposed mechanisms of myocardial injury other than myocardial ischemia in patients with and without CAD include: cardiomyocyte damage from inflammatory cytokines or oxidative stress, altered calcium handling, apoptosis, and release of intact troponin or troponin fragments from viable cardiomyocytes [69, 70, 72].

Conclusions

Acute decompensated heart failure is defined as the new onset or recurrence of heart failure signs and symptoms that require urgent or emergent treatment and that result in hospitalization. This syndrome is common and expensive. Recent large multicenter observational registries have improved our understanding of the demographics, clinical characteristics, comorbidities, management patterns and outcomes of patients admitted with ADHF. ADHF disproportionately affects the elderly. Most patients have a history of hypertension and half of patients have an elevated systolic blood pressure on presentation. Approximately half of the patients with ADHF have normal or near normal left ventricular ejection fraction. Coronary artery disease (CAD) is present in 50–70% of patients who present with ADHF and ACS is the most common precipitating factor in patients who presented with de novo heart failure.

ADHF is a syndrome due to a broad range of cardiovascular disorders. The underlying causes are heterogeneous but most patients seek medical attention because of dyspnea due to elevated left atrial and pulmonary capillary wedge pressure. The pathophysiology of dyspnea in ADHF is complex and multifactorial and impacted by the time course of volume overload, the presence of rapid elevations in systemic vascular resistance and left atrial pressure, and the chronicity of elevated PCWP.

References

1. Go AS, Mozaffarian D, Roger VL, Benjamin EJ, Berry JD, Blaha MJ, et al; American Heart Association Statistics Committee and Stroke Statistics Subcommittee. Heart disease and stroke statistics—2014 update: a report from the American Heart Association. Circulation. 2014;129(3):e28–e292. https://doi.org/10.1161/01.cir.0000441139.02102.80. Epub 2013 Dec 18.
2. Dickstein K, Cohen-Solal A, Filippatos G, McMurray JJ, Ponikowski P, Poole-Wilson PA, et al; ESC Committee for Practice Guidelines (CPG). ESC guidelines for the diagnosis and treatment of acute and chronic heart failure 2008: the task force for the diagnosis and treatment of acute and chronic heart failure 2008 of the European Society of Cardiology. Developed in collaboration with the Heart Failure Association of the ESC (HFA) and endorsed by the European Society of Intensive Care Medicine (ESICM). Eur Heart J. 2008;29(19):2388–442. https://doi.org/10.1093/eurheartj/ehn309. Epub 2008 Sep 17.
3. National Heart Lung and Blood Institute. People Science Health. What is heart failure? Available from: http://www.nhlbi.nih.gov/health/health-topics/topics/hf/. Accessed Feb 2012.
4. Hall MJ, DeFrances CJ, Williams SN, et al. National hospital discharge survey: 2007 summary. National health statistics reports; no 29. National Center for Health Statistics: Hyattsville; 2010. Available from: http://www.cdc.gov/nchs/data/nhsr/nhsr029.pdf
5. Gheorghiade M, Pang PS. Acute heart failure syndromes. J Am Coll Cardiol. 2009;53(7):557–73. https://doi.org/10.1016/j.jacc.2008.10.041.
6. Gheorghiade M, Zannad F, Sopko G, Klein L, Piña IL, Konstam MA, et al.; International Working Group on acute heart failure syndromes. Acute heart failure syndromes: current state and framework for future research. Circulation. 2005;112(25):3958–68.
7. Fang J, Mensah GA, Croft JB, Keenan NL. Heart failure-related hospitalization in the U.S., 1979 to 2004. J Am Coll Cardiol. 2008;52(6):428–34. https://doi.org/10.1016/j.jacc.2008.03.061.
8. Chen J, Normand SL, Wang Y, Krumholz HM. National and regional trends in heart failure hos-

pitalization and mortality rates for Medicare beneficiaries, 1998–2008. JAMA. 2011;306(15):1669–78. https://doi.org/10.1001/jama.2011.1474.
9. Fonarow GC, Abraham WT, Albert NM, Gattis WA, Gheorghiade M, Greenberg B, et al. Organized program to initiate lifesaving treatment in hospitalized patients with heart failure (OPTIMIZE-HF): rationale and design. Am Heart J. 2004;148(1):43–51.
10. Adams KF, Fonarow GC, Emerman CL, LeJemtel TH, Costanzo MR, Abraham WT, et al; ADHERE Scientific Advisory Committee and Investigators. Characteristics and outcomes of patients hospitalized for heart failure in the United States: rationale, design, and preliminary observations from the first 100,000 cases in the Acute Decompensated Heart Failure National Registry (ADHERE). Am Heart J. 2005;149(2):209–16.
11. Fonarow GC, Heywood JT, Heidenreich PA, Lopatin M, Yancy CW, ADHERE Scientific Advisory Committee and Investigators. Temporal trends in clinical characteristics, treatments, and outcomes for heart failure hospitalizations, 2002 to 2004: findings from Acute Decompensated Heart Failure National Registry (ADHERE). Am Heart J. 2007;153(6):1021–8.
12. Fonarow GC, Corday E, ADHERE Scientific Advisory Committee. Overview of acutely decompensated congestive heart failure (ADHF): a report from the ADHERE registry. Heart Fail Rev. 2004;9(3):179–85.
13. Cleland JG, Swedberg K, Cohen-Solal A, Cosin-Aguilar J, Dietz R, Follath F, et al; The Euro Heart Failure Survey of the EUROHEART survey programme. A survey on the quality of care among patients with heart failure in Europe. The Study Group on Diagnosis of the Working Group on Heart Failure of the European Society of Cardiology. The Medicines Evaluation Group Centre for Health Economics University of York. Eur J Heart Fail. 2000;2(2):123–32.
14. Cleland JG, Swedberg K, Follath F, Komajda M, Cohen-Solal A, Aguilar JC, et al; Study Group on Diagnosis of the Working Group on Heart Failure of the European Society of Cardiology. The EuroHeart Failure survey programme—a survey on the quality of care among patients with heart failure in Europe. Part 1: patient characteristics and diagnosis. Eur Heart J. 2003;24(5):442–63.
15. Komajda M, Follath F, Swedberg K, Cleland J, Aguilar JC, Cohen-Solal A, et al; Study Group on Diagnosis of the Working Group on Heart Failure of the European Society of Cardiology. The EuroHeart Failure Survey programme—a survey on the quality of care among patients with heart failure in Europe. Part 2: treatment. Eur Heart J. 2003;24(5):464–74.
16. Nieminen MS, Brutsaert D, Dickstein K, Drexler H, Follath F, Harjola VP, et al; EuroHeart Survey Investigators; Heart Failure Association, European Society of Cardiology. EuroHeart Failure Survey II (EHFS II): a survey on hospitalized acute heart failure patients: description of population Eur Heart J. 2006;27(22):2725–36. Epub 2006 Sep 25.
17. Fonarow GC, Abraham WT, Albert NM, Stough WG, Gheorghiade M, Greenberg BH, et al; OPTIMIZE-HF Investigators and Hospitals. Age- and gender-related differences in quality of care and outcomes of patients hospitalized with heart failure (from OPTIMIZE-HF). Am J Cardiol. 2009;104(1):107–15. https://doi.org/10.1016/j.amjcard.2009.02.057.
18. Gheorghiade M, Abraham WT, Albert NM, Greenberg BH, O'Connor CM, She L, et al; OPTIMIZE-HF Investigators and Coordinators. Systolic blood pressure at admission, clinical characteristics, and outcomes in patients hospitalized with acute heart failure. JAMA. 2006;296(18):2217–26.
19. Yancy CW, Lopatin M, Stevenson LW, De Marco T, Fonarow GC, ADHERE Scientific Advisory Committee and Investigators. Clinical presentation, management, and in-hospital outcomes of patients admitted with acute decompensated heart failure with preserved systolic function: a report from the Acute Decompensated Heart Failure National Registry (ADHERE) database. J Am Coll Cardiol. 2006;47(1):76–84.
20. Fonarow GC, Stough WG, Abraham WT, Albert NM, Gheorghiade M, Greenberg BH, et al; OPTIMIZE-HF Investigators and Hospitals. Characteristics, treatments, and outcomes of patients with preserved systolic function hospitalized for heart failure: a report from the OPTIMIZE-HF Registry. J Am Coll Cardiol 2007;50(8):768–777.
21. Lenzen MJ, op Reimer WJMS, Boersma E, Vantrimpont PJMJ, Follath F, Swedberg K, Cleland J, Komajda M, et al. Differences between patients with a preserved and a depressed left ventricular function: a report from the EuroHeart Failure Survey. Eur Heart J. 2004;25(14):1214–20.
22. Yancy CW, Abraham WT, Albert NM, Clare R, Stough WG, Gheorghiade M, et al. Quality of care of and outcomes for African Americans hospitalized with heart failure: findings from the OPTIMIZE-HF (Organized Program to Initiate Lifesaving Treatment in Hospitalized Patients With Heart Failure) registry. J Am Coll Cardiol. 2008;51(17):1675–84. https://doi.org/10.1016/j.jacc.2008.01.028.
23. Jencks SF, Williams MV, Coleman EA. Rehospitalizations among patients in the Medicare fee-for-service program. N Engl J Med. 2009;360(14):1418–28. https://doi.org/10.1056/NEJMsa0803563.
24. Heidenreich PA, Sahay A, Kapoor JR, Pham MX, Massie B. Divergent trends in survival and readmission following a hospitalization for heart failure in the Veterans Affairs health care system 2002 to 2006.

J Am Coll Cardiol. 2010;56(5):362–8. https://doi.org/10.1016/j.jacc.2010.02.053.
25. Bueno H, Ross JS, Wang Y, Chen J, Vidán MT, Normand SL, et al. Trends in length of stay and short-term outcomes among Medicare patients hospitalized for heart failure, 1993–2006. JAMA. 2010;303(21):2141–7. https://doi.org/10.1001/jama.2010.748.
26. Tuppin P, Cuerq A, de Peretti C, Fagot-Campagna A, Danchin N, Juillière Y, et al. Two-year outcome of patients after a first hospitalization for heart failure: a national observational study. Arch Cardiovasc Dis. 2014;107(3):158–68. https://doi.org/10.1016/j.acvd.2014.01.012. Epub 2014 Mar 21
27. Jessup M, Abraham WT, Casey DE, Feldman AM, Francis GS, Ganiats TG, et al. focused update: ACCF/AHA guidelines for the diagnosis and management of heart failure in adults: a report of the American College of Cardiology Foundation/American Heart Association Task Force on Practice Guidelines: developed in collaboration with the International Society for Heart and Lung Transplantation. Circulation. 2009;119(14):1977–2016. https://doi.org/10.1161/CIRCULATIONAHA.109.192064. Epub 2009 Mar 26
28. Kaul P, Ezekowitz JA, Armstrong PW, Leung BK, Savu A, Welsh RC, et al. Incidence of heart failure and mortality after acute coronary syndromes. Am Heart J. 2013;165(3):379–85.e2. https://doi.org/10.1016/j.ahj.2012.12.005. Epub 2013 Jan 22
29. Steg PG, Dabbous OH, Feldman LJ, Cohen-Solal A, Aumont MC, López-Sendón J, et al; Global Registry of Acute Coronary Events Investigators. Determinants and prognostic impact of heart failure complicating acute coronary syndromes: observations from the Global Registry of Acute Coronary Events (GRACE). Circulation. 2004;109(4):494–9. Epub 2004 Jan 26.
30. Weintraub NL, Collins SP, Pang PS, Levy PD, Anderson AS, Arslanian-Engoren C, et al; American Heart Association Council on Clinical Cardiology and Council on Cardiopulmonary, Critical Care, Perioperative and Resuscitation. Acute heart failure syndromes: emergency department presentation, treatment, and disposition: current approaches and future aims: a scientific statement from the American Heart Association. Circulation. 2010;122(19):1975–96. https://doi.org/10.1161/CIR.0b013e3181f9a223. Epub 2010 Oct 11.
31. Campbell RT, Jhund PS, Castagno D, Hawkins NM, Petrie MC, McMurray J. What have we learned about patients with heart failure and preserved ejection fraction from DIG-PEF, CHARM-preserved, and I-PRESERVE? J Am Coll Cardiol. 2012;60(23):2349–56. https://doi.org/10.1016/j.jacc.2012.04.064. Epub 2012 Nov 7
32. Clark AL, Cleland JG. Causes and treatment of oedema in patients with heart failure. Nat Rev Cardiol. 2013;10(3):156–70. https://doi.org/10.1038/nrcardio.2012.191. Epub 2013 Jan 15
33. ter Maaten JM, Valente MA, Damman K, Hillege HL, Navis G, Voors AA. Diuretic response in acute heart failure-pathophysiology, evaluation, and therapy. Nat Rev Cardiol. 2015;12(3):184–92. https://doi.org/10.1038/nrcardio.2014.215. Epub 2015 Jan 6
34. Ronco C, Cicoira M, McCullough PA. Cardiorenal syndrome type 1: pathophysiological crosstalk leading to combined heart and kidney dysfunction in the setting of acutely decompensated heart failure. J Am Coll Cardiol. 2012;60(12):1031–42. https://doi.org/10.1016/j.jacc.2012.01.077. Epub 2012 Jul 25
35. Gehlbach BK, Geppert E. The pulmonary manifestations of left heart failure. Chest. 2004;125(2):669–82.
36. Guazzi M. Alveolar gas diffusion abnormalities in heart failure. J Card Fail. 2008;14(8):695–702. https://doi.org/10.1016/j.cardfail.2008.06.004. Epub 2008 Jul 18
37. Uhley HN, Leeds SE, Sampson JJ, Friedman M. Role of pulmonary lymphatics in chronic pulmonary edema. Circ Res. 1962;11:966–70.
38. Mackersie RC, Christensen J, Lewis FR. The role of pulmonary lymphatics in the clearance of hydrostatic pulmonary edema. J Surg Res. 1987;43(6):495–504.
39. Hochberg I, Abassi Z, Azzam ZS. Patterns of alveolar fluid clearance in heart failure. Int J Cardiol. 2008;130(2):125–30. https://doi.org/10.1016/j.ijcard.2008.03.015. Epub 2008 Jun 24
40. Guazzi M, Phillips SA, Arena R, Lavie CJ. Endothelial dysfunction and lung capillary injury in cardiovascular diseases. Prog Cardiovasc Dis. 2015;57(5):454–62. https://doi.org/10.1016/j.pcad.2014.11.003. Epub 2014 Nov 12
41. Chaudhry S, Wang Y, Concato J, Gill TM, Krumholz HM. Patterns of weight change preceding hospitalization for heart failure. Circulation. 2007;116(14):1549–54. Epub 2007 Sep 10
42. Adamson PB, Magalski A, Braunschweig F, Böhm M, Reynolds D, Steinhaus D, et al. Ongoing right ventricular hemodynamics in heart failure: clinical value of measurements derived from an implantable monitoring system. J Am Coll Cardiol. 2003;41(4):565–71.
43. Ohlsson A, Steinhaus D, Kjellström B, Ryden L, Bennett T. Central hemodynamic responses during serial exercise tests in heart failure patients using implantable hemodynamic monitors. Eur J Heart Fail. 2003;5(3):253–9.
44. Adamson PB, Kjellström B, Braunschweig F, Magalski A, Linde C, Kolodiezj A, et al. Ambulatory hemodynamic monitoring from an implanted device: components of continuous 24-hour pressures that correlate to supine resting conditions and acute right heart catheterization. Congest Heart Fail. 2006;12(1):14–9.
45. Aaron MF, Aranda JM, Renlund DG, Fonarow GC, Feldman DS, Cho YK, et al. The effect of postural

changes on intracardiac filling pressures [abstract]. J Card Fail. 2008;14:S28.
46. Zile MR, Bennett TD, St John Sutton M, Cho YK, Adamson PB, Aaron MF, et al. Transition from chronic compensated to acute decompensated heart failure: pathophysiological insights obtained from continuous monitoring of intracardiac pressures. Circulation. 2008;118(14):1433–41. https://doi.org/10.1161/CIRCULATIONAHA.108.783910. Epub 2008 Sep 15
47. Zile MR, Adamson PB, Cho YK, Bennett TD, Bourge RC, Aaron MF, et al. Hemodynamic factors associated with acute decompensated heart failure: part 1—insights into pathophysiology. J Card Fail. 2011;17(4):282–91. https://doi.org/10.1016/j.cardfail.2011.01.010. Epub 2011 Feb 26
48. Milo-Cotter O, Adams KF, O'Connor CM, Uriel N, Kaluski E, Felker GM, et al. Acute heart failure associated with high admission blood pressure—a distinct vascular disorder? Eur J Heart Fail. 2007;9(2):178–83. Epub 2006 Jul 31
49. Cotter G, Moshkovitz Y, Milovanov O, Salah A, Blatt A, Krakover R, et al. Acute heart failure: a novel approach to its pathogenesis and treatment. Eur J Heart Fail. 2002;4(3):227–34.
50. Kaluski E, Kobrin I, Zimlichman R, Marmor A, Krakov O, Milo O, et al. RITZ-5: randomized intravenous TeZosentan (an endothelin-A/B antagonist) for the treatment of pulmonary edema: a prospective, multicenter, double-blind, placebo-controlled study. J Am Coll Cardiol. 2003;41(2):204–10.
51. Mebazaa A, Pang PS, Tavares M, Collins SP, Storrow AB, Laribi S, et al. The impact of early standard therapy on dyspnoea in patients with acute heart failure: the URGENT-dyspnoea study. Eur Heart J. 2010;31(7):832–41. https://doi.org/10.1093/eurheartj/ehp458. Epub 2009 Nov 11
52. Balmain S, Padmanabhan N, Ferrell WR, Morton JJ, McMurray JJ. Differences in arterial compliance, microvascular function and venous capacitance between patients with heart failure and either preserved or reduced left ventricular systolic function. Eur J Heart Fail. 2007;9(9):865–71. Epub 2007 Jul 19
53. Cotter G, Metra M, Milo-Cotter O, Dittrich HC, Gheorghiade M. Fluid overload in acute heart failure—re-distribution and other mechanisms beyond fluid accumulation. Eur J Heart Fail. 2008;10(2):165–9. https://doi.org/10.1016/j.ejheart.2008.01.007.
54. Cotter G, Felker GM, Adams KF, Milo-Cotter O, O'Connor CM. The pathophysiology of acute heart failure—is it all about fluid accumulation? Am Heart J. 2008;155(1):9–18.
55. Felker GM, Leimberger JD, Califf RM, Cuffe MS, Massie BM, Adams KF Jr, et al. Risk stratification after hospitalization for decompensated heart failure. J Card Fail. 2004;10(6):460–6.
56. Fonarow GC, Adams JKF, Abraham WT, Yancy CW, Boscardin WJ, ADHERE Scientific Advisory Committee, Study Group, Investigators. Risk stratification for in-hospital mortality in acutely decompensated heart failure: classification and regression tree analysis. JAMA. 2005;293(5):572–80.
57. Lee DS, Austin PC, Rouleau JL, Liu PP, Naimark D, Tu JV. Predicting mortality among patients hospitalized for heart failure: derivation and validation of a clinical model. JAMA. 2003;290(19):2581–7.
58. Collins S, Storrow AB, Kirk JD, Pang PS, Diercks DB, Gheorghiade M. Beyond pulmonary edema: diagnostic, risk stratification, and treatment challenges of acute heart failure management in the emergency department. Ann Emerg Med. 2008;51(1):45–57. Epub 2007 Sep 14
59. Collins S, Storrow AB, Albert NM, Butler J, Ezekowitz J, Felker GM, et al; SAEM/HFSA Acute Heart Failure Working Group. Early management of patients with acute heart failure: state of the art and future directions. A consensus document from the society for academic emergency medicine/heart failure society of America acute heart failure working group. J Card Fail. 2015;21(1):27–43. https://doi.org/10.1016/j.cardfail.2014.07.003. Epub 2014 Jul 18.
60. Stevenson LW, Perloff JK. The limited reliability of physical signs for estimating hemodynamics in chronic heart failure. JAMA. 1989;261(6):884–8.
61. Kay JM, Edwards FR. Ultrastructure of the alveolar-capillary wall in mitral stenosis. J Pathol. 1973;111(4):239–45.
62. Kingsbury MP, Huang W, Donnelly JL, Jackson E, Needham E, Turner MA, Sheridan DJ. Structural remodelling of lungs in chronic heart failure. Basic Res Cardiol. 2003;98(5):295–303. Epub 2003 May 16
63. Huang W, Kingsbury MP, Turner MA, Donnelly JL, Flores NA, Sheridan DJ. Capillary filtration is reduced in lungs adapted to chronic heart failure: morphological and haemodynamic correlates. Cardiovasc Res. 2001;49(1):207–17.
64. Davies SW, Bailey J, Keegan J, Balcon R, Rudd RM, Lipkin DP. Reduced pulmonary microvascular permeability in severe chronic left heart failure. Am Heart J. 1992;124(1):137–42.
65. Rossi JS, Flaherty JD, Fonarow GC, Nunez E, Gattis Stough W, Abraham WT, et al. Influence of coronary artery disease and coronary revascularization status on outcomes in patients with acute heart failure syndromes: a report from OPTIMIZE-HF (Organized Program to Initiate Lifesaving Treatment in Hospitalized Patients with Heart Failure). Eur J Heart Fail. 2008;10(12):1215–23. https://doi.org/10.1016/j.ejheart.2008.09.009. Epub 2008 Nov 8
66. Flaherty JD, Bax JJ, De Luca L, Rossi JS, Davidson CJ, Filippatos G, et al.; Acute Heart Failure Syndromes International Working Group. Acute heart failure syndromes in patients with coronary artery disease early assessment and treatment. J Am Coll Cardiol. 2009;53(3):254–63.

67. Thygesen K, Alpert JS, White HD, Joint ESC/ACCF/AHA/WHF Task Force for the Redefinition of Myocardial Infarction, Jaffe AS, Apple FS, Galvani M, Katus HA, Newby LK, Ravkilde J, et al. Universal definition of myocardial infarction. Circulation. 2007;116(22):2634–53. Epub 2007 Oct 19
68. Kociol RD, Pang PS, Gheorghiade M, Fonarow GC, O'Connor CM, Felker GM. Troponin elevation in heart failure prevalence, mechanisms, and clinical implications. J Am Coll Cardiol. 2010;56(14):1071–8. https://doi.org/10.1016/j.jacc.2010.06.016.
69. Peacock 4th WF, De Marco T, Fonarow GC, Diercks D, Wynne J, Apple FS, Wu AH, ADHERE Investigators. Cardiac troponin and outcome in acute heart failure. N Engl J Med. 2008;358(20):2117–26. https://doi.org/10.1056/NEJMoa0706824.
70. You JJ, Austin PC, Alter DA, Ko DT, Tu JV. Relation between cardiac troponin I and mortality in acute decompensated heart failure. Am Heart J. 2007;153(4):462–70.
71. Cleland JG, Pennell DJ, Ray SG, Coats AJ, Macfarlane PW, Murray GD, et al; Carvedilol Hibernating Reversible Ischaemia Trial: Marker of Success Investigators. Myocardial viability as a determinant of the ejection fraction response to carvedilol in patients with heart failure (CHRISTMAS trial): randomised controlled trial. Lancet. 2003;362(9377):14–21.
72. Beohar N, Erdogan AK, Lee DC, Sabbah HN, Kern MJ, Teerlink J, et al. Acute heart failure syndromes and coronary perfusion. J Am Coll Cardiol. 2008;52(1):13–6. https://doi.org/10.1016/j.jacc.2008.03.037.

Acute Decompensated Heart Failure: Presentation, Physical Exam, and Laboratory Evaluation

11

Daniel Fishbein

Presentation of Patients with ADHF

ADHF may be a manifestation of any abnormality of cardiovascular function. Most patients have a prior history of heart failure. Patients with chronic heart failure may have a history of gradually worsening symptoms of pulmonary and systemic venous congestion over several days to weeks or may have more rapid development of symptoms commonly associated with a clear precipitant (examples: new onset atrial fibrillation with rapid ventricular response in a patient with HFpEF; ACS in a patient with an ischemic cardiomyopathy). Approximately 25% of patients with ADHF have new onset or *de novo* heart failure—many of these patients have associated ACS or poorly controlled hypertension [1].

A minority of patients present with acute pulmonary edema. Patients with pulmonary edema have severe respiratory distress, tachypnea, tachycardia, hypoxemia, pulmonary rales, and radiographic evidence of pulmonary congestion. Some patients may need mechanical ventilation. The onset is frequently acute and associated with severe hypertension or atrial tachyarrhythmia (especially in patients with preserved systolic function) In EHFS II 16% of patients presented with acute pulmonary edema [2]. In OPTIMIZE-HF, 2.5% of patients presented in acute pulmonary edema [3]. In the ADHERE Registry, 4.5% of patients required mechanical ventilation during hospitalization [4]. In ADHERE, the percentage of patients who required mechanical ventilation decreased from 5.3% to 3.4% over 3 years (January 2002 to December 2004) [5].

A minority of patients present with cardiogenic shock. Cardiogenic shock is generally associated with heart failure complicating ACS. The ADHERE and OPTIMIZE registries did not specifically describe patients as having cardiogenic shock. In OPTIMIZE, 10% of patients had a systolic BP <105 mmHg [6]. In ADHERE, 3% of patients had an initial systolic BP <90 mmHg [5]. In EHFS II, 4% of patients admitted with heart failure presented with cardiogenic shock [7].

Symptoms

Patients with heart failure commonly present with dyspnea at rest or with exertion. Other common symptoms include lower extremity edema, fatigue, orthopnea and paroxysmal dyspnea. In ADHERE, 89% of patients had dyspnea, 34% of patients had dyspnea at rest, 65% had peripheral edema and 31% of patients had fatigue [4]. In OPTIMIZE-HF, 61% of patients had dyspnea on exertion, 44% of patients had dyspnea at rest, and 65% of patients had edema [6].

D. Fishbein (✉)
Department of Medicine, Division of Cardiology, University of Washington Medical Center, Seattle, WA, USA
e-mail: dfish@uw.edu

H. J. Eisen (ed.), *Heart Failure I*, https://doi.org/10.1007/978-3-032-12626-9_11

Patients may be unable to sleep flat because of shortness of breath (orthopnea) and some patients may have an acute increase in dyspnea with any degree of recumbence. Orthopnea is a sensitive and specific symptom of elevated filling pressures. In a study of patients with chronic heart failure, orthopnea was reported by 39/43 patients who had a PCWP ≥22 mmHg [8]. In the Evaluation Study of Congestive Heart Failure and Pulmonary Artery Catheterization (ESCAPE) trial, orthopnea ≥2 pillows was the only finding on history that was associated with a PCWP ≥30 mmHg [9]. The symptom of orthopnea can also be seen in patients with central obesity, ascites, esophageal reflux, obstructive airway disease or emphysema. Paroxysmal nocturnal dyspnea (PND) may be a more specific symptom of decompensated heart failure and pulmonary congestion. Typically, the patient with PND is awakened acutely several hours after retiring by symptoms of severe shortness of breath and air hunger. Patients often feel the need to sit up, get out of bed, or seek fresh air from an open window. Symptoms generally resolve within 10–20 min. Nocturnal or exertional cough or wheezing may also be a manifestation of pulmonary congestion.

Patients with systemic venous congestion may have symptoms of lower extremity edema, abdominal fullness or distention, early satiety, nausea, poor appetite and right upper quadrant abdominal pain. Edema is a common finding in patients with ADHF. Edema is, however, not a specific finding for heart failure as patients may have edema from other causes (see below under "Physical Examination") [10, 11].

Patients with low cardiac output may have symptoms of severe fatigue, poor appetite, exertional light headedness and manifestations of cerebral hypoperfusion including impaired mentation, agitation, and irritability [12]. Some patients complain of very bright or very "white" vision in association with low blood pressure and/or low cardiac output. Exertional presyncope or syncope may also be a manifestation of low cardiac output.

Physical Examination

A careful physical examination is an essential component of the evaluation of the patient presenting with shortness of breath. The physical examination is critical in establishing the diagnosis of heart failure and in assessing the severity of disease, the presence and severity of systemic and pulmonary venous congestion, the adequacy of cardiac output and end-organ perfusion, the severity of respiratory compromise and the need for emergent intervention. In addition, the exam provides insights into the underlying cause of heart failure and the presence of reversible conditions that may have contributed to heart failure decompensation.

An assessment should be made of the patient's general appearance, vital signs including O_2 saturation by finger oximetry and neurologic status. In addition, an examination of the heart, neck veins, lungs, abdomen, lower extremities and carotid and peripheral pulses should be performed.

General Examination and Vital Signs

General examination and vital signs provide insight into the presence and severity of heart failure. Patients may have evidence of respiratory distress with tachypnea, hypoxemia on pulse oximetry, inability to speak in full sentences, inability to lie flat, agitation, and use of accessory muscles of respiration. Observation of coughing or wheezing, especially with walking or while recumbent suggests the presence of pulmonary congestion. Respiratory rate is important and should be counted rather than estimated. Tachypnea may reflect severe pulmonary congestion, pulmonary edema and/or respiratory failure. The presence of Cheyne-Stokes respirations suggests that the patient has chronic severe heart failure.

Tachycardia may reflect low cardiac output, sympathetic nervous system activation, or a supraventricular arrhythmia that may be a heart failure precipitant. An irregular pulse may be due to premature ventricular beats or preexisting or new onset atrial fibrillation. An elevated temperature suggests infection as a possible contributor to heart failure decompensation. Temperature <36 °C has been shown to be associated with a 51% higher risk of the composite of HF rehospitalization or CV death when compared with the index group of patients with temperature >36.5 °C in the Efficacy of Vasopressin Antagonism in Heart Failure Outcome Study with Tolvaptan (EVEREST) trial [13].

In acute heart failure, systolic and mean blood pressures are important in guiding the choice of initial therapies including vasodilators, inotropic agents, vasopressors, intra-aortic balloon pump therapy or mechanical circulatory support. Low blood pressure, especially if associated with low pulse pressure, tachycardia and cool distal extremities, is a sign of low cardiac output and inadequate systemic perfusion. Low blood pressure is unusual in patients with ADHF but when present, identifies a patient at high risk of in-hospital mortality who may need more intensive care including admission to the CCU, treatment with inotropic agents (or vasopressors), and/or support with an intra-aortic balloon pump [6, 14]. As heart failure progresses, systolic blood pressure decreases, diastolic blood pressure is unchanged and pulse pressure (systolic blood pressure-diastolic blood pressure) decreases. A pulse pressure/systolic pressure ratio (referred to as the "proportional pulse pressure") of less than 0.25 suggests that the patient has a cardiac index of less than 2.2 L/min/m^2 [15].

Approximately half of patients with ADHF have an initial systolic blood pressure of >140 mmHg. Patients who present with hypertension may have pulmonary congestion related to volume redistribution due to a mismatch between rapidly increasing blood pressure and impaired contractile reserve rather than total body fluid accumulation. These patients may have more severe pulmonary congestion and less volume overload than normotensive patients with ADHF. These patients generally benefit from parenteral diuretics but may also benefit from early initiation of vasodilator therapy [16–22].

Agitation or altered mental status should raise concern about brain hypoperfusion due to severely reduced cardiac output, even in the setting of normal blood pressure. Patients with low cardiac output may also have cool distal extremities, diaphoresis, pallor, tachypnea, dyspnea at rest, low systolic blood pressure, low pulse pressure, and low proportional pulse pressure. Feeling the skin of the hands and feet can give important information about systemic perfusion and the presence of systemic vasoconstriction. The temperature of the hands/feet should be compared to that of the upper arm/leg. Relative coolness of the distal extremities suggests low cardiac output [15, 23]. Some authors have suggested that feeling the temperature of the forearms and calves rather than hands and feet (which may be cool from anxiety) may be more specific for assessment of systemic perfusion [15].

Assessment for Pulmonary and Systemic Venous Congestion

An important goal of the initial physical exam is to identify and quantitate pulmonary and systemic venous congestion. Historically, four signs have been used to determine whether cardiac filling pressures are elevated including the presence of: jugular venous distention, pulmonary rales, a ventricular gallop (S3) and lower extremity edema.

Lung examination provides insight into the cause of dyspnea, volume status and the presence of pulmonary congestion. Percussion of the posterior chest may elicit dullness at one or both bases indicating the presence of a pleural effusion. Patients may also have associated decreased breath sounds. Pleural effusion is generally a manifestation of elevated right and left sided filling pressures. Bilateral pleural effusions are more common than unilateral effusions. When a unilateral effusion is present in a patient with ADHF, it is generally on the right. An isolated left pleural effusion is an unusual manifestation of decompensated heart failure.

Pulmonary crackles (or rales) are caused by transudation of fluid from the pulmonary capillaries into the alveolar space. Crackles due to heart failure generally are audible from the base upward and do not clear with cough or deep inspiration. Patients with chronic heart failure may not have rales despite significantly elevated pulmonary capillary wedge pressure and clinical decompensation [8]. The absence of rales in patients with chronic heart failure does not exclude decompensated heart failure as a cause of worsening dyspnea. Rales may be due to other pulmonary pathology. Rales associated with atelectasis are generally coarse and clear with cough or deep inspiration. Rales associated with pneumonia may be heard at locations other than the bases, are frequently unilateral and commonly associated with fever, leukocytosis, and other findings of pulmonary consolidation such as bronchial breath sounds and egophony. Patients with ADHF may present with "cardiac asthma" with wheezing and decreased airflow. Cardiac asthma is probably caused by a combination of reflex bronchoconstriction in response to elevated pulmonary and bronchial vascular pressure, obstruction from intraluminal edema fluid, and bronchial mucosal swelling [24].

Lower extremity edema is a common finding in patients with ADHF. In patients with chronic heart failure, edema may be absent despite symptoms of dyspnea and elevated pulmonary capillary wedge pressure [8]. Edema is not a specific finding for heart failure as patients may have edema from other causes including venous insufficiency, cirrhosis, hypoalbuminemia, kidney disease including nephrotic syndrome, pregnancy, and treatment with a number of medications including calcium channel blockers (particularly dihydropyridines, e.g. amlodipine, nifedipine), thiazolidinediones, docetaxel, gabapentin, pregabalin, nonsteroidal anti-inflammatory drugs (NSAIDs), glucocorticoids, fludrocortisone, and vasodilators (hydralazine, minoxidil, diazoxide; less frequent—alpha1 blockers, and methyldopa). However, edema is a specific finding of heart failure when associated with elevated jugular venous pressure [10, 11].

The jugular venous pressure (JVP) is the single most important finding in the assessment of intravascular volume status. JVP provides a direct measurement of right atrial (RA) pressure, an estimate of right ventricular filling pressure and some insight into pulmonary capillary wedge and left atrial pressures. JVP is measured as the vertical distance from the mid right atrium to the top of the observable column of blood (or meniscus) in the internal jugular vein and is expressed in centimeters of water.

A number of methods have been suggested to estimate JVP. Assessment of JVP may be made with the upper torso of the patient elevated at 30–45°. When assessing JVP, it is important that the height of the meniscus of the internal jugular vein be clearly identified. In patients with ADHF, a meniscus may not be seen at 30–45° because of high JVP. It is recommended that JVP be assessed at both 30–45° and 90° (sitting upright) to avoid underestimating filling pressures [15, 25]. The position of the right atrium can be estimated to be at the intersection of the fourth or fifth intercostal space and the mid-axillary line. The JVP can be estimated by measuring the vertical distance from the position of the right atrium to the top of the meniscus. Alternatively, the position of the right atrium can be estimated to be 5 cm below the angle of Louis. Using this method, JVP can be estimated to be the vertical distance from the angle of Louis to the meniscus plus 5 cm of water.

Another alternative is to measure JVP in the upright sitting position. In most patients, the distance from the right atrium to the clavicle is 10 cm in the upright position. If a meniscus is seen above the clavicle, the patient has an elevated JVP. The JVP is 10 cm plus the measured distance from the clavicle to the observed meniscus. This method gives JVP <10 cm of water, 10–12 cm, 12–14 cm, etc. This method is less cumbersome, is more accurate, and has less intra- and inter-observer variability and avoids underestimating JVP. If a meniscus is not observed in the upright position, assessment of JVP should then be made at progressively decreasing elevations of the torso above supine. If a meniscus is not seen while lying flat, the patient may be volume depleted [15, 25].

Some studies have found poor inter-observer reliability in the assessment of JVP by ED physicians [26]. A study of patients with heart failure that compared estimates of JVP by exam, estimates of RA pressure by echo and RA pressure measured by a pulmonary artery catheter in patients with heart failure found that clinical assessment of JVP accurately estimated normal RA pressure but tended to underestimate RA pressure in patients with elevated RA pressure [27]. Others have suggested that physical examination is helpful in determining whether central venous pressure is high or low but not in assessing a specific pressure [28, 29].

In the ESCAPE trial, estimates of JVP by physical exam recorded on initial history and physical exam were compared with RA pressure on invasive hemodynamic monitoring in 194 patients with chronic severe symptomatic heart failure randomized to the PA catheter group [9]. Estimated JVP (in cm of water) was converted to RA pressure (in mmHg) by multiplying JVP (in cm of water) by 0.736, the ratio of the density of water relative to the density of mercury. (1 cm of water equals 0.736 mmHg.) Measured right atrial pressure was less than 8 mmHg in 82% of patients (9/11) who had an estimated JVP of less than 8 mmHg. Measured RA pressure was ≥8 mmHg in 82% (149/181) of patients who had an estimated JVP ≥8 mmHg. Measured right atrial pressure was >12 mmHg in 70% (80 of 114) of patients who had an estimated JVP of >12 mmHg.

Elevated JVP is helpful in predicting elevated pulmonary capillary wedge pressure. In the ESCAPE trial, estimated RA pressure ≥12 mmHg was strongly associated with PCWP ≥30 mmHg with an odds ratio of 4.6 [9]. In a study of 1000 patients with advanced heart failure undergoing transplant evaluation, 79% of patients had concordance of right atrial and pulmonary capillary wedge pressures defined as an RAP ≥10 mmHg with a PCWP ≥22 mmHg [30]. An RA pressure of ≥10 mmHg had a positive predictive value of 88% to identify a PCWP ≥22 mmHg. In another study of 4079 potential transplant candidates, elevated pressures were defined as RAP ≥10 mmHg and PCWP ≥22 mmHg. Pressures were described as "concordant" if the RA and PCWP were both either high or low. The frequency of concordant pressures over three sequential 4 year periods was 74%, 72%, and 73% [31]. In another study of 537 patients hospitalized for ADHF who underwent right heart catheterization, 36% of patients had concordant low filling pressures (RA <10 mmHg; PCWP <22 mmHg) and 36% of patients had concordant high filling pressures (RA ≥10 mmHg; PCWP ≥22 mmHg [32]. Fifteen percent of patients had RA <10 with PCWP ≥22 mmHg ("High-Left Mismatch") and 13% of patients had RA ≥10 mmHg and PCWP <22 mmHg ("High-Right Mismatch").

On multivariate analysis, patients with a history of symptomatic heart failure who were enrolled in the Studies of Left Ventricular Function (SOLVD) treatment trial and who had elevated JVP had an increased risk of hospitalization for heart failure, death or hospitalization for heart failure, and death from pump failure [33].

In patients with chronic severe heart failure, findings of volume overload (rales, elevated JVP and lower extremity edema) identify patients with an elevated PCWP. However, rales, elevated JVP and lower extremity edema may be absent despite an elevated PCWP. In a study of 50 patients with chronic heart failure, physical findings of heart failure (rales, elevated JVP and lower extremity edema) were compared with hemodynamic measurements. All 10 patients with lower extremity edema had an RA pressure ≥10 mmHg. All patients with an RA pressure ≥10 mmHg had an elevated PCWP ≥22 mmHg. JVP was the most sensitive finding on exam for elevated PCWP. No patient with edema, rales or elevated JVP had a wedge pressure <22 mmHg. However, 18/43 patients (42%) with PCWP ≥22 mmHg and 8/18 (44%) of patients with PCWP ≥35 mmHg had no findings of volume overload on physical exam [8].

In ADHF, the apical impulse may be displaced leftward indicating cardiac enlargement. A late diastolic gallop (S4) may be heard, especially in patients with heart failure with preserved systolic function in sinus rhythm. An early diastolic gallop (S3) may be heard in patients with heart failure and systolic dysfunction. There is conflicting evidence whether an S3 is specific for elevated LVEDP [8, 34] but its presence reliably predicts the presence of left ventricular dysfunction [8,

34]. A holosystolic murmur of functional mitral regurgitation is common in patients with ADHF and systolic dysfunction. Patients with biventricular dysfunction, pulmonary hypertension or isolated right heart failure may have a murmur of tricuspid regurgitation. This can be distinguished from a murmur of mitral regurgitation by the location of the murmur at the left sternal border and an increase in the intensity of the murmur with inspiration.

Wang et al. reviewed 22 studies of patients who presented to the emergency department with dyspnea to assess the usefulness of history, symptoms, physical findings, and routine diagnostic studies (chest radiograph, electrocardiogram and serum B-type natriuretic peptide) to differentiate heart failure from other causes of dyspnea. Many clinical characteristics increased the probability that dyspnea was caused by heart failure. The finding in each category that best predicted that dyspnea was not due to heart failure was the *presence* of: a past history of heart failure; the symptom of paroxysmal nocturnal dyspnea; sign of a third heart sound; chest radiograph showing pulmonary venous congestion; and electrocardiogram showing atrial fibrillation. The finding in each category that best predicted that dyspnea was not due to heart failure was the *absence* of: a past history of heart failure; the symptom of dyspnea on exertion; rales on physical exam; chest radiograph showing cardiomegaly; and any abnormality on electrocardiogram [35].

Many heart failure practitioners have found a 2 × 2 dichotomous matrix based on a clinical assessment of volume status (congestion/no congestion) ("wet" or "dry") and systemic perfusion (adequate perfusion/clinically important hypoperfusion) ("warm" or "cold") to be useful in characterizing the clinical status of patients with ADHF and in developing a therapeutic plan [36]. See Fig. 2.1 in Chap. 2 [37]. Signs, symptoms and laboratory data that suggest a patient is congested or "wet" include: dyspnea at rest or with exertion, orthopnea, PND, lower extremity swelling, abdominal distention, unexplained weight gain, rales, jugular venous distention, hepatojugular reflux, hepatomegaly, ascites, peripheral edema and elevated B-type natriuretic peptide (BNP) or n-terminal pro-BNP. Signs and symptoms that suggest a patient has compromised perfusion or is "cold" include: a narrow pulse pressure, a proportional pulse pressure of <0.25, pulsus alternans, symptomatic hypotension (without orthostasis), cool distal extremities, anxiety and impaired mentation.

A prospective analysis of 452 patients admitted to an academic heart failure service found that clinical assessment of a patient's hemodynamic profile could be used to predict outcomes. Patients with initial "warm-wet" and "cold-wet" profiles had an increased risk of death or urgent transplant on multivariate analysis (HR 2.48; $P = 0.003$). These profiles were also associated with an increased risk of death or urgent transplant when patients with NHYA FC III (HR 2.23, $p = 0.026$) and NYHA FC IV (HR 2.73, $p = 0.009$) symptoms were analyzed separately [23]. In the ESCAPE trial, clinician determined "cold" vs. "warm" profile was associated with a lower median measured cardiac index in the "cold" patients (1.75 vs. 2.0 L/min/m^2; $p = 0.004$). On Cox regression analysis, "cold" or "wet" profiles at the time of discharge conveyed a 50% increased risk of death or rehospitalization [9].

Patients with right heart failure may have a right-sided S3, increased intensity of the pulmonic component of the second heart sound (in patients with pulmonary hypertension), a murmur of tricuspid regurgitation, hepatomegaly and ascites. A pulsatile liver may be palpable in patients with severe tricuspid regurgitation.

Initial Laboratory Evaluation

The initial evaluation of the patient presenting with ADHF should include laboratory studies which help confirm heart failure as the cause of the presenting symptoms; identify underlying conditions that may be a cause of heart failure or may precipitate heart failure decompensation; help assess the severity of underlying end-organ dysfunction; and identify conditions which may be immediately life threatening and require urgent treatment.

Serum Electrolytes

Minor abnormalities of serum electrolytes are common in patients with ADHF and may be due to neurohormonal activation, low cardiac output, or heart failure medications. The reported incidence of hyponatremia defined as a serum sodium ≤135 mEq/L varies widely between 7.7% and 45% [38, 39]. In EHFS I, 20% of patients were hyponatremic [37]. Hypokalemia is common in patients treated with loop diuretics. Hyperkalemia occurs in approximately 8% of patients with ADHF in the setting of chronic heart failure and is associated with treatment with angiotensin converting enzyme inhibitors (ACEIs), angiotensin receptor blockers (ARBs), mineralocorticoid antagonists (MRAs), potassium supplementation, potassium sparing diuretics, and chronic or acute renal insufficiency [39, 40]. Diabetes is common in patients with ADHF (44% in ADHERE; 41.5% in OPTIMIZE) and poor glycemic control may accompany or contribute to ADHF [41].

Blood Urea Nitrogen (BUN) and Creatinine

Renal dysfunction is common in patients with ADHF. In the ADHERE Registry, chronic renal insufficiency was reported in 30% of patients. Nine percent of patients had a creatinine on admission of >3.0 mg/dL and 21% had a creatinine >2.0 mg/dL. Five percent were on chronic dialysis [1]. In OPTIMIZE-HF, the mean creatinine was 1.8 mg/dL [6]. In EHFS I, renal dysfunction was reported to have complicated management in 18% of patients. Serum creatinine was ≥150 μmol/l (1.7 mg/dL) in 16% of patients and ≥ 200 μmol/l (2.3 mg/dL) in 7% [2]. In a nationwide, prospective, observational study of 206 cardiology centers with intensive cardiac care units in Italy, 47% of patients admitted with acute heart failure had renal dysfunction defined as creatinine ≥1.5 mg % (mg/dL) [39].

Patients with HF commonly have risk factors associated with both heart and kidney disease including diabetes mellitus, hypertension and vascular disease. Elevated BUN and creatinine may be manifestations of renal hypoperfusion in the setting of low cardiac output or in the setting of marked neurohormonal activation even in the face of normal cardiac output and normal or elevated filling pressures. Elevated BUN and creatinine may also be a manifestation of hypovolemia with low filling pressures in the setting of diuretic therapy. The BUN/creatinine ratio may be elevated in the setting of low cardiac output, neurohormonal activation or volume depletion. In each of these conditions, the proximal tubular absorption of sodium is increased. This is accompanied by reabsorption of BUN but not creatinine. Treatment with ACEIs or ARBs may also contribute to renal dysfunction particularly in the setting of renal artery stenosis, severe chronic heart failure or volume depletion [42, 43]. It has been our observation that lower urinary tract obstruction is a common reversible cause of abnormal renal function in older men with ADHF.

Hematologic Measures

Anemia is common in patients with ADHF. The World Health Organization defines anemia as hemoglobin (Hgb) <13.0 g/dL in men and <12.0 g/dL in women. In clinical trials and large HF registries, the prevalence of anemia has ranged from 15% to 61% overall and from 14% to 70% among hospitalized patients [44]. In a meta-analysis of 34 cohort studies or retrospective analyses of randomized controlled trials in HF which included 153,180 patients, 37.2% of patients were anemic. Anemia was associated with an increased risk of mortality in patients with HFrEF and HFpEF with an adjusted hazard ratio of 1.46 [45].

In the OPTIMIZE—HF registry, half of the patients had a hemoglobin <12.1 g/dL and 25% had a hemoglobin of 5–10.7 g/dL. Patients with low hemoglobin tended to be older, female, and Caucasian and more commonly had preserved systolic function and elevated creatinine. Low hemoglobin was associated with higher in-hospital mortality, longer hospital length of stay and more readmissions at 90 days [46]. In EHFS

I, a hemoglobin <11 g/dL was reported in 18% of men and 23% of women [2]. In patients with ADHF in Italy, a hemoglobin <12 g/dL was present in 46% of patients [39]. In a large population-based cohort of Canadian patients discharged after hospitalization for new onset HF, 17% had anemia, 58% of whom had anemia of chronic disease. Anemic patients were more likely to be older, female, and have a history of chronic renal insufficiency or hypertension. Anemic patients had a significantly greater risk-adjusted mortality (HR = 1.34) compared with non-anemic patients [47]. In the EVEREST Trial, 34% of patients with systolic dysfunction hospitalized for ADHF were anemic at baseline. 73% of patients who were anemic at baseline were anemic at discharge or day 7 and 6% of patients without anemia developed anemia by discharge or day 7. Anemia at discharge but not on admission was associated with an increased risk of long-term all-cause mortality and short-term (≤100 days post-discharge) cardiovascular mortality or CHF hospitalization [48].

Anemia in heart failure is multifactorial [44]. In patients with acute decompensation, plasma expansion due to salt and water overload may cause dilutional anemia [49, 50]. Anemia may also be caused by renal dysfunction with inappropriate erythropoietin production, pro-inflammatory cytokine activation with anemia of chronic disease, iron deficiency and defective iron utilization [44, 51]. In a community based study of patients with HF due to systolic dysfunction, the relationship between anemia and renal insufficiency was explored. Anemia was present in 32% of patients. Low serum iron or low ferritin was found in 43% of patients with anemia. Renal dysfunction (defined as a glomerular filtration rate <60 ml/min by the Modification of Diet in Renal Disease (MDRD) equation) was present in 54% of patients. Forty-one percent of patients with renal dysfunction and 22% of patients without renal dysfunction were anemic. Anemia and renal dysfunction independently predicted mortality and the effects were additive [52]. In patients hospitalized for ADHF who had a thorough evaluation for underlying causes of anemia (defined as hemoglobin <12 g/dL in men and <11.5 g/dL in women), iron deficiency was the most common cause of anemia with depleted iron stores found in 73% of anemic patients on bone marrow aspiration. Serum ferritin was not a reliable marker of iron deficiency in this study [53].

Low "relative lymphocyte count" or "lymphocyte ratio" (total number of lymphocytes/total number of leukocytes ×100) is an independent predictor of mortality in outpatients with heart failure [54]. In the EVEREST trial, patients with low relative lymphocyte count tended to be older, more likely to be male, had higher rates of comorbid disease and were more likely to have a history of prior myocardial infarction and coronary revascularization. Patients with low relative lymphocyte ratio had significantly lower presenting systolic and diastolic blood pressure, higher mean heart rates, lower serum sodium levels, higher blood urea nitrogen, and higher natriuretic peptide levels. These patients were less likely to receive evidence-based HF medications. After adjusting for multiple risk factors, relative lymphocyte count <15.4% was an independent predictor of all-cause mortality and cardiovascular mortality or HF hospitalization in the first 100 days following discharge [55].

In the Preliminary study of RELAXin in Acute Heart Failure (Pre-RELAX-AHF), patients admitted with acute heart failure, SBP ≥125 mmHg, and BNP ≥350 pg/ml were randomized to the vasodilator relaxin or placebo. Patients with a lymphocyte ratio <13% had similar baseline characteristics as patients with a lymphocyte ratio >13% but had less improvement in dyspnea, greater worsening of HF, longer initial length of stay, fewer days alive and out of the hospital and greater risk for all-cause mortality at 60 and 180 days [56].

Liver Function Tests (LFTs)

Up to 60% of patients hospitalized with ADHF have mild liver function test abnormalities. Elevation of all liver function tests, and especially γ-glutamyl transferase (GGT) and total bilirubin (Tbili), are associated with high central venous pressure (CVP). Only elevated transaminases and Tbili are associated with both high CVP and low cardiac output [57].

In the EVEREST trial, the most common LFT abnormality was an elevation in GGT which occurred in 60% of patients. Other LFT abnormalities were common and included elevation of alanine aminotransferase (ALT) in 21% of patients, aspartate aminotransferase (AST) in 21%, alkaline phosphatase in 23%, and total bilirubin (Tbili) in 26% and decreased albumin in 17%. LFT abnormalities were minor in most patients. Tbili was the only LFT abnormality to decrease from admission to discharge. All LFTs except albumin improved following discharge. Lower baseline albumin and elevated Tbili were both associated with an increased risk for all-cause mortality. In-hospital decreases in albumin or increases in Tbili were associated with higher rates of both all-cause mortality and HF rehospitalization [58].

Two specific conditions affecting the liver, congestive hepatopathy and ischemic hepatitis (or "shock liver") have been described in patients with heart failure. Congestive hepatopathy refers to a spectrum of chronic liver injury that is caused by chronic passive hepatic congestion in the setting of elevated right atrial pressure. Congestive hepatopathy occurs most commonly in conditions associated with chronically elevated right atrial pressure including: severe right-sided or biventricular heart failure, severe tricuspid regurgitation, cor pulmonale, severe pulmonary hypertension, restrictive cardiomyopathy, pericardial constriction, and congenital heart disease with Fontan reconstruction. Untreated congestion can result in hepatic fibrosis and, eventually cardiac cirrhosis. Laboratory testing generally shows mild non-specific increases in transaminases generally not more than 2–3 times the upper limit of normal, mildly increased Tbili generally <3 mg/dL (predominantly unconjugated), and normal or slightly elevated alkaline phosphatase (which helps differentiate congestion from biliary obstruction). Hepatic synthetic function is usually normal or only slightly impaired. Serum albumin is usually normal or slightly reduced. The international normalized ratio (INR) is rarely increased above 1.5 [59, 60].

Ischemic hepatitis (or "shock liver") refers to a condition of diffuse hepatocellular injury caused by impaired perfusion to the liver. This most commonly occurs in the setting of cardiogenic shock. It can also occur in patients without hypotension but with severe heart failure, marked reduction in cardiac output and elevated right sided filling pressures. The diagnosis is defined by the appropriate clinical setting of cardiac, circulatory or pulmonary failure, marked increases in serum aminotransferase levels generally greater than 20 times the upper limit of normal, and exclusion of other causes of acute liver injury. AST, ALT and lactic dehydrogenase (LDH) levels are markedly elevated. The ALT/LDH ratio is generally less than 1.5 which helps distinguish ischemic injury from other forms of acute hepatic injury. Tbili is also increased but generally not above 4 times the upper limit of normal. Alkaline phosphatase may be normal or mildly elevated. INR, which is a marker of synthetic liver function, may be elevated in the setting of severe liver injury. ALT, AST and LDH generally peak 1–3 days after the precipitating event and return to normal in 7–10 days after improvement in systemic perfusion. Patients who present with ADHF and marked elevation of AST, ALT, and LDH generally require hemodynamic monitoring, support with inotropes, and consideration of IABP or other mechanical circulatory support [59, 60].

Natriuretic Peptides

B-type natriuretic peptide (BNP) is a member of a family of three natriuretic hormones that share a common 17-amino-acid ring structure. BNP is primarily synthesized in the ventricles although can be synthesized in the atria. BNP is synthesized and released in response to increased wall stress resulting from an increase in intra-cardiac filling pressures. In response to increased wall stress, pre-proBNP is synthesized in cardiac myocytes and cleaved to $proBNP_{1-108}$ which is released from the myocyte. $ProBNP_{1-108}$ is subsequently cleaved to BNP_{1-32} which is biologically active and N-terminal proBNP (NT-proBNP) which is biologically inactive. The biologic actions of BNP are mediated by membrane bound natriuretic peptide receptors. The biologic effects of BNP include vasodilation, natriuresis, diuresis and antagonism of activation of the renin-angiotensin-aldosterone system (RAAS). Both BNP an NT-proBNP are elevated in ADHF and the magnitude of the elevation parallels the elevation of left ventricular filling pressure [61, 62].

Both BNP and NT-proBNP levels have been shown to be useful in identifying heart failure as the underlying cause of symptoms in patients who present to the emergency department (ED) with shortness of breath. The Breathing Not Properly (BNP) study was a large multicenter observational evaluation of 1586 patients who presented to the ED with acute dyspnea who had a prospective BNP level obtained. ED physicians, who were blinded to the results of the BNP measurement, assessed the probability that heart failure was the cause of the patient's symptoms. Two cardiologists (also blinded to the results of the BNP measurements) reviewed all medical records and independently classified the diagnosis as: dyspnea due to congestive heart failure; acute dyspnea due to non-cardiac causes in a patient with a history of left ventricular dysfunction; or dyspnea not due to congestive heart failure. Using a BNP cutoff of 100 pg/mL, BNP had a sensitivity, specificity, negative predictive and positive predictive value of 90%, 76%, 79%, and 89%, respectively. BNP had a higher diagnostic accuracy than the ED physician with an area under the receiver-operator curve of 0.91. In multiple logistic regression analysis, an elevated BNP was the strongest predictor of heart failure with an odds ratio of 29.5. BNP was predictive of heart failure in patients with reduced or preserved ventricular function [63].

The ProBNP Investigation of Dyspnea in the ED (PRIDE) was a similar study using NT-proBNP in 600 patients who presented to a single institution with dyspnea. NT-proBNP levels at cut points of >450 pg/ml for patients <50 years of age and >900 pg/ml for patients ≥50 years of age were highly sensitive and specific for the diagnosis of acute heart failure. An NT-proBNP <300 pg/ml was best for ruling out heart failure and had a negative predictive value of 99%. NT-proBNP was the strongest independent predictor of a final diagnosis of heart failure with an odds ratio of 44 and was superior to clinical judgment alone. NT-proBNP combined with clinical judgment was superior to either alone in diagnosing heart failure. The investigators suggested a single cut point of <300 pg/ml to rule out heart failure and two cut points based on age to rule in a diagnosis of heart failure (>450 pg/ml in patients <50 years of age and >900 pg/ml in patients ≥50 years of age) [64]. Other authors have suggested using either an age-independent cut point of >900 pg/ml or a more accurate age-stratified approach of 450/900/1800 for patients ages <50, 50–75, and >75 years [65–67].

Patients with chronic heart failure may have elevated BNP or NT-proBNP levels despite normal volume status. Increases above an established patient-specific "euvolemic" BNP or NT-proBNP level may help identify worsening volume overload in individual patients. However, the biologic variability of both markers complicates interpreting serial BNPs. BNP may need to change by 70% and NT-proBNP by 50% to be helpful diagnostically [66, 68, 69].

In general, BNP and NT-proBNP have similar diagnostic utility. Both are particularly good at ruling out heart failure at levels <100 pg/ml for BNP and <300 pg/ml for NT-proBNP. NT-proBNP levels are increased to a greater degree in advanced age and renal insufficiency. Both can be elevated in the absence of heart failure in a number of conditions including: acute coronary syndromes, chronic heart failure without volume overload, advanced age, renal dysfunction, pulmonary disease, acute hemodynamically significant pulmonary embolism, high output states including sepsis, cirrhosis and hyperthyroidism, and atrial fibrillation. BNP and NT-proBNP are commonly not elevated in obese patients with volume overload. Other conditions in which levels are lower than expected include heart failure from mitral stenosis, acute mitral regurgitation, cardiac tamponade and pericardial constriction [61, 66].

Troponins

Measurement of circulating cardiac troponin (cTn) plays an important role in the diagnosis of ACS and should be obtained in all patients with ADHF on presentation to the emergency department [70]. Cardiac troponin (either T or I) has near absolute specificity for myocardial injury and high clinical sensitivity [71, 72]. The presence of measurable cTn is abnormal and indicative of myocardial injury. Typically, a patient with an acute coronary syndrome (ACS) precipitating heart failure will have precordial pain, characteristic ST segment elevations on ECG and significant cTn elevations (cTn I >1.0 ng/ml). However, in acute heart failure, troponin elevation may be seen in patients with and without ACS and with and without significant obstructive coronary artery disease suggesting that mechanisms other than focal myocardial ischemia/injury may be responsible for troponin release in some patients. The reported prevalence of elevated (defined as "detectable") troponin has varied widely in patients with ADHF depending on the population studied and on the sensitivity of the assay used [72].

Electrocardiography (ECG)

One of the primary goals of the initial evaluation of patients with ADHF is to promptly identify an acute coronary syndrome using history, electrocardiography and serum biomarkers. In EHFS II, 11.1% of patients had evidence of an ST segment elevation myocardial infarction, 10.0% had a non-STEMI and 9.1% had unstable angina [2]. The presence of ST segment elevation and elevated troponin is diagnostic for an acute coronary syndrome [73]. ACS may be more difficult to diagnose in the setting of non-specific ST-T wave abnormalities [74].

The electrocardiogram is abnormal in many patients with ADHF. An abnormal ECG defined as the presence of atrial fibrillation or flutter, left or right bundle branch block, evidence of past myocardial infarction or ST-segment deviation had a sensitivity of 58% and specificity of 78% to identify HF in a group of 880 patients who presented to the ED with acute dyspnea at one of 7 academic medical centers [75].

Sinus tachycardia is common. Atrial fibrillation (AF) is present in approximately 30–40% of patients admitted with ADHF [6, 7, 39, 76–80].

QRS prolongation (QRS >120 ms) is also common. Of 2962 patients enrolled in the EVEREST Trial without a pacemaker or implantable cardioverter-defibrillator (ICD), 1321 (45%) had a QRS duration ≥120 ms. LBBB was present in 909 patients (30.6%). QRS prolongation was independently associated with an increased risk of all-cause mortality and cardiovascular death or HF hospitalization (HR = 1.24 and 1.28, respectively) [81]. The incidence of LBBB has been reported to be lower (16–17%) in other reports [82, 83].

Electrocardiography may offer clues to the cause of heart failure. Patients may have pathologic Q waves indicative of an ischemic cardiomyopathy. Evidence of left ventricular hypertrophy may be present in patients with hypertensive heart disease, aortic stenosis or hypertrophic cardiomyopathy. Patients with cardiac amyloidosis may have low voltage with or without pathologic Q waves ("pseudo-infarction" pattern).

Chest Radiography

A chest radiograph should be obtained in all patients presenting with acute shortness of breath or suspicion of ADHF. A number of radiographic findings may be present in patients with ADHF including cardiomegaly, cephalization of the pulmonary vasculature, interstitial lung edema, alveolar edema, and pleural effusion(s). Heart size on chest radiography is assessed by calculating the cardiothoracic ratio (CTR) which is determined by dividing the largest horizontal width of the heart by the widest internal diameter of the thorax on a posterior-anterior chest film. A normal CTR is less than 0.5. CTR is abnormal in 57–71% of patients with chronic heart failure due to systolic dysfunction [84]. CTR may be less predictive of cardiomegaly in patients with chronic obstructive lung disease as the lung volumes are increase and the diaphragms are flattened.

Evaluation of the pulmonary vasculature and parenchyma is important in patients presenting with acute shortness of breath. It is best to evaluate pulmonary vascularity in the upright position. If the lung is divided into three zones vertically from the mediastinum to the periphery (chest wall), the major pulmonary arteries are located centrally around the hila, the midsize pulmonary arteries are easily visualized in the mid-zone and the small arteries and arterioles are located in the outer zone and are generally not visualized on chest radiograph. Normally, the visible small and mid-size arteries in the mid-zone have sharp definable margins. The lungs may also be divided into three regions horizontally from the diaphragms to the apices. In the upright position, the arteries in the lower region of the lung are generally larger than those in the upper region. This finding is related to the effect of gravity on the distribution of pulmonary blood flow and is not seen on supine CXR. In the setting of elevated left atrial pressure, especially in patients with chronic heart failure, there is redistribution of lung perfusion toward the apical regions. The lower zone vessels appear equal or smaller in diameter compared to the upper zone vessels. This finding is called "cephalization" or "inversion", is best correlated with measures of pulmonary vascular resistance and is likely due to vasoconstriction of lower zone vessels [85, 86].

As PCWP increases, the mid-zone vessels become less distinct due to extravasation of fluid into the pulmonary interstitium. Interstitial fluid may also be seen as small well-defined reticulonodular (reticular, nodular or both) infiltrates seen in both the central and peripheral zones. Fine horizontal pleural-based linear densities may be seen in the periphery of the lung and represent interstitial fluid that accumulates in the septae between anatomic lung lobules (referred to as "Kerley B" or septal lines). This pattern of interstitial edema may progress to alveolar edema characterized by alveolar filling by transudated fluid. Alveolar edema is a bilateral process but may only involve parts of each lung. Alveolar edema causes poorly defined but homogeneous lung opacities that become progressively denser as edema worsens. Air bronchograms may be present as fluid filled alveoli outline air filled bronchi [87].

Pleural effusions may also be present. Effusions are generally bilateral. When unilateral, the effusion is more commonly present on the right.

The characteristic findings of heart failure on chest radiograph may not be present in all patients with ADHF. In patients with emphysema or pulmonary fibrosis, the pulmonary vascular pattern is abnormal at baseline and may not change in a predictable way in the setting of volume overload. Patients with chronic heart failure and chronically elevated pulmonary capillary wedge pressure may not have an abnormal pulmonary vascular pattern and may not develop interstitial or alveolar edema despite significantly elevated pulmonary capillary wedge pressure [88].

In the ADHERE Registry, 18.7% of 85,376 patients (approximately one of every five patients) with a hospital discharge diagnosis of heart failure had no radiographic findings of heart failure (interstitial edema, pulmonary edema, or vascular congestion) on initial chest radiograph. Patients without signs of congestion on initial ED radiograph were more likely to have an ED non-heart failure diagnosis than patients with signs of congestion (13.0 vs 23.3%) [89].

An analysis of 880 patients presenting with acute dyspnea to the emergency departments of seven teaching hospitals found that elevated BNP and radiographic findings of cardiomegaly, cephalization and interstitial edema added significant predictive information in the diagnosis of heart failure. Radiographic findings that were assessed included: cardiomegaly, cephalization, interstitial edema, alveolar edema, pleural effusion, hyperinflated lungs, and evidence of pneumonia. Of the patients evaluated for shortness of breath, 68% were diagnosed with acute heart failure. The radiographic finding of cardiomegaly had a sensitivity of 79% and specificity of 80%. Cephalization, interstitial edema and alveolar edema were all highly specific (96–99%) but insensitive (6–41%). Cardiomegaly, cephalization, interstitial edema and alveolar edema all added significant, predictive information to historical and clinical predictors of heart failure [75].

Conclusions

Most patients with heart failure present with dyspnea at rest or with exertion and lower extremity edema. Some patients present with symptoms and ECG findings consistent with an acute coronary syndrome. A small percentage of patients present with acute pulmonary edema or cardiogenic shock.

The physical examination is critical in establishing the diagnosis of heart failure and in assessing the severity of disease, the presence and severity of systemic and pulmonary venous congestion, the adequacy of cardiac output and end-organ perfusion, the severity of respiratory compromise and the need for emergent intervention. In addition, the exam provides insights into the underlying cause of heart failure and the presence of reversible conditions that may have contributed to heart failure decompensation. Assessment of mental status, respiratory rate, oxygen saturation, blood pressure, jugular venous pressure, presence of pulmonary rales and presence of lower extremity edema are especially important components of the exam.

An ECG and measurement of circulating cardiac troponin are important in the diagnosis of ACS. BNP and NT-proBNP are useful in identifying heart failure as the underlying cause of symptoms in patients who present to the emergency department with shortness of breath.

References

1. Adams KF, Fonarow GC, Emerman CL, LeJemtel TH, Costanzo MR, Abraham WT, ADHERE Scientific Advisory Committee and Investigators, et al. Characteristics and outcomes of patients hospitalized for heart failure in the United States: rationale, design, and preliminary observations from the first 100,000 cases in the Acute Decompensated Heart Failure National Registry (ADHERE). Am Heart J. 2005;149(2):209–16.
2. Cleland JG, Swedberg K, Follath F, Komajda M, Cohen-Solal A, Aguilar JC, Study Group on Diagnosis of the Working Group on Heart Failure of the European Society of Cardiology, et al. The EuroHeart Failure survey programme– a survey on the quality of care among patients with heart failure in Europe. Part 1: patient characteristics and diagnosis. Eur Heart J. 2003;24(5):442–63.
3. Fonarow GC, Stough WG, Abraham WT, Albert NM, Gheorghiade M, Greenberg BH, OPTIMIZE-HF Investigators and Hospitals, et al. Characteristics, treatments, and outcomes of patients with preserved systolic function hospitalized for heart failure: a report from the OPTIMIZE-HF registry. J Am Coll Cardiol. 2007;50(8):768–77.
4. Fonarow GC, Corday E, ADHERE Scientific Advisory Committee. Overview of acutely decompensated congestive heart failure (ADHF): a report from the ADHERE registry. Heart Fail Rev. 2004;9(3):179–85. CrossRef PubMed
5. Fonarow GC, Heywood JT, Heidenreich PA, Lopatin M, Yancy CW, ADHERE Scientific Advisory Committee and Investigators. Temporal trends in clinical characteristics, treatments, and outcomes for heart failure hospitalizations, 2002 to 2004: findings from acute decompensated heart failure National Registry (ADHERE). Am Heart J. 2007;153(6):1021–8. CrossRef PubMed.
6. Gheorghiade M, Abraham WT, Albert NM, Greenberg BH, O'Connor CM, She L, OPTIMIZE-HF Investigators and Coordinators, et al. Systolic blood pressure at admission, clinical characteristics, and outcomes in patients hospitalized with acute heart failure. JAMA. 2006;296(18):2217–26.
7. Nieminen MS, Brutsaert D, Dickstein K, Drexler H, Follath F, Harjola VP, EuroHeart Survey Investigators; Heart Failure Association, European Society of Cardiology, et al. EuroHeart Failure Survey II (EHFS II): a survey on hospitalized acute heart failure patients: description of population. Eur Heart J. 2006;27(22):2725–36. Epub 2006 Sep 25.
8. Stevenson LW, Perloff JK. The limited reliability of physical signs for estimating hemodynamics in chronic heart failure. JAMA. 1989;261(6):884–8. PubMed PMID 2913385. CrossRef PubMed.
9. Drazner MH, Hellkamp AS, Leier CV, Shah MR, Miller LW, Russell SD, et al. Value of clinician assessment of hemodynamics in advanced heart failure: the ESCAPE trial. Circ Heart Fail. 2008;1(3):170–7. https://doi.org/10.1161/CIRCHEARTFAILURE.108.769778. CrossRef PubMed PubMedCentral.
10. Ely JW, Osheroff JA, Chambliss ML, Ebell MH. Approach to leg edema of unclear etiology. J

Am Board Fam Med. 2006;19(2):148–60. CrossRef PubMed.
11. Heart Failure Society of America, Lindenfeld J, Albert NM, Boehmer JP, Collins SP, Ezekowitz JA, Givertz MM, et al. HFSA 2010 comprehensive heart failure practice guideline. Section 12: evaluation and management of patients with acute decompensated heart failure. J Card Fail. 2010;16(6):e131–56. https://doi.org/10.1016/j.cardfail.2010.04.004. CrossRef.
12. Leier CV, Silver MA, Massie BM, Young JB, Fowler MB, Ventura HO, Hershberger RE. Nuggets, pearls, and vignettes of master heart failure clinicians. Part 1 – the medical history. Congest Heart Fail. 2001;7(5):245–9. CrossRef PubMed.
13. Payvar S, Spertus JA, Miller AB, Casscells SW, Pang PS, Zannad F, Efficacy of Vasopressin Antagonism in Heart Failure Outcome Study with Tolvaptan (EVEREST) Investigators, et al. Association of low body temperature and poor outcomes in patients admitted with worsening heart failure: a substudy of the efficacy of vasopressin antagonism in heart failure outcome study with Tolvaptan (EVEREST) trial. Eur J Heart Fail. 2013;15(12):1382–9. https://doi.org/10.1093/eurjhf/hft113. Epub 2013 Jul 15.
14. Gheorghiade M, Vaduganathan M, Ambrosy A, Böhm M, Campia U, Cleland JG, et al. Current management and future directions for the treatment of patients hospitalized for heart failure with low blood pressure. Heart Fail Rev. 2013;18(2):107–22. https://doi.org/10.1007/s10741-012-9315-1. CrossRef PubMed.
15. Leier CV, Young JB, Levine TB, Pina I, Armsrtrong W, Fowler MB, et al. Nuggest, pearls, and vignettes of master heart failure clinicians. Part 2—the physical examination. Congest Heart Fail. 2001;7(6):297–308. PubMed PMID 11828174. CrossRef PubMed.
16. Weintraub NL, Collins SP, Pang PS, Levy PD, Anderson AS, Arslanian-Engoren C, American Heart Association Council on Clinical Cardiology and Council on Cardiopulmonary, Critical Care, Perioperative and Resuscitation, et al. Acute heart failure syndromes: emergency department presentation, treatment, and disposition: current approaches and future aims: a scientific statement from the American Heart Association. Circulation. 2010;122(19):1975–96. https://doi.org/10.1161/CIR.0b013e3181f9a223. Epub 2010 Oct 11.
17. Cotter G, Metra M, Milo-Cotter O, Dittrich HC, Gheorghiade M. Fluid overload in acute heart failure–re-distribution and other mechanisms beyond fluid accumulation. Eur J Heart Fail. 2008;10(2):165–9. https://doi.org/10.1016/j.ejheart.2008.01.007. CrossRef PubMed.
18. Cotter G, Felker GM, Adams KF, Milo-Cotter O, O'Connor CM. The pathophysiology of acute heart failure–is it all about fluid accumulation? Am Heart J. 2008;155(1):9–18. CrossRef PubMed.
19. Collins S, Storrow AB, Albert NM, Butler J, Ezekowitz J, Felker GM, SAEM/HFSA Acute Heart Failure Working Group, et al. Early management of patients with acute heart failure: state of the art and future directions. A consensus document from the society for academic emergency medicine/heart failure society of America acute heart failure working group. J Card Fail. 2015;21(1):27–43. https://doi.org/10.1016/j.cardfail.2014.07.003. Epub 2014 Jul 18.
20. Peacock WF, Chandra A, Char D, Collins S, Der Sahakian G, Ding L, et al. Clevidipine in acute heart failure: results of the a study of blood pressure control in acute heart failure-a pilot study (PRONTO). Am Heart J. 2014;167(4):529–36. https://doi.org/10.1016/j.ahj.2013.12.023. Epub 2014 Jan 15. CrossRef PubMed.
21. Cotter G, Metzkor E, Kaluski E, Faigenberg Z, Miller R, Simovitz A, et al. Randomised trial of high-dose isosorbide dinitrate plus low-dose furosemide versus high-dose furosemide plus low-dose isosorbide dinitrate in severe pulmonary oedema. Lancet. 1998;351(9100):389–93. CrossRef PubMed.
22. Levy P, Compton S, Welch R, Delgado G, Jennett A, Penugonda N, et al. Treatment of severe decompensated heart failure with high-dose intravenous nitroglycerin: a feasibility and outcome analysis. Ann Emerg Med. 2007;50(2):144–52. Epub 2007 May 23. CrossRef PubMed.
23. Nohria A, Tsang SW, Fang JC, Lewis EF, Jarcho JA, Mudge GH, et al. Clinical assessment identifies hemodynamic profiles that predict outcomes in patients admitted with heart failure. J Am Coll Cardiol. 2003;41(10):1797–804. PubMed PMID 12767667. CrossRef PubMed.
24. Gehlbach BK, Geppert E. The pulmonary manifestations of left heart failure. Chest. 2004;125(2):669–82. CrossRef PubMed.
25. Leier CV, Chatterjee K. The physical examination in heart failure–part I. Congest Heart Fail. 2007;13(1):41–7. CrossRef PubMed.
26. Chaudhry A, Singer AJ, Chohan J, Russo V, Lee C. Interrater reliability of hemodynamic profiling of patients with heart failure in the ED. Am J Emerg Med. 2008;26(2):196–201. https://doi.org/10.1016/j.ajem.2007.04.029. CrossRef PubMed.
27. Stein JH, Neumann A, Marcus RH. Comparison of estimates of right atrial pressure by physical examination and echocardiography in patients with congestive heart failure and reasons for discrepancies. Am J Cardiol. 1997;80(12):1615–8. CrossRef PubMed.
28. McGee SR. Physical examination of venous pressure: a critical review. Am Heart J. 1998;136(1):10–8. CrossRef PubMed.
29. Cook DJ, Simel DL. The rational clinical examination. Does this patient have abnormal central venous pressure? JAMA. 1996;275(8):630–4. CrossRef PubMed.
30. Drazner MH, Hamilton MA, Fonarow G, Creaser J, Flavell C, Stevenson LW, et al. Relationship between right and left-sided filling pressures in 1000 patients with advanced heart failure. J Heart Lung Transplant.

1999;18(11):1126–32. PubMed PMID 10598737. CrossRef PubMed.
31. Drazner MH, Brown RN, Kaiser PA, Cabuay B, Lewis NP, Semigran MJ, et al. Relationship of right-and left-sided filling pressures in patients with advanced heart failure: a 14-year multi-institutional analysis. J Heart Lung Transplant. 2012;31(1):67–72. PubMed PMID 22071240. CrossRef PubMed.
32. Campbell P, Drazner MH, Kato M, Lakdawala N, Palardy M, Nohria A, et al. Mismatch of right- and left-sided filling pressures in chronic heart failure. J Card Fail. 2011;17(7):561–8. PubMed PMID 21703528. CrossRef PubMed.
33. Drazner MH, Rame JE, Stevenson LW, Dries DL. Prognostic importance of elevated jugular venous pressure and a third heart sound in patients with heart failure. N Engl J Med. 2001;345(8):574–81. PubMed PMID 11529211. CrossRef PubMed.
34. Marcus GM, Gerber IL, McKeown BH, Vessey JC, Jordan MV, Huddleston M, et al. Association between phonocardiographic third and fourth heart sounds and objective measures of left ventricular function. JAMA. 2005;293(18):2238–44. CrossRef PubMed.
35. Wang CS, FitzGerald JM, Schulzer M, Mak E, Ayas NT. Does this dyspneic patient in the emergency department have congestive heart failure? JAMA. 2005;294(15):1944–56. CrossRef PubMed.
36. Grady KL, Dracup K, Kennedy G, Moser DK, Piano M, Stevenson LW, et al. Team management of patients with heart failure: a statement for healthcare professionals from the cardiovascular nursing Council of the American Heart Association. Circulation. 2000;102(19):2443–56. PubMed PMID 11067802. CrossRef PubMed.
37. Dickstein K, Cohen-Solal A, Filippatos G, McMurray JJ, Ponikowski P, Poole-Wilson PA, et al. ESC Committee for practice guidelines (CPG). ESC guidelines for the diagnosis and treatment of acute and chronic heart failure 2008: the task force for the diagnosis and treatment of acute and chronic heart failure 2008 of the European Society of Cardiology. Developed in collaboration with the heart failure association of the ESC (HFA) and endorsed by the European Society of Intensive Care Medicine (ESICM). Eur Heart J. 2008;29(19):2388–442. https://doi.org/10.1093/eurheartj/ehn309. Epub 2008 Sep 17.
38. Hauptman PJ, Burnett J, Gheorghiade M, Grinfeld L, Konstam MA, Kostic D, Everest Investigators, et al. Clinical course of patients with hyponatremia and decompensated systolic heart failure and the effect of vasopressin receptor antagonism with tolvaptan. J Card Fail. 2013;19(6):390–7. https://doi.org/10.1016/j.cardfail.2013.04.001. Epub 2013 May 14.PMID:23743487 [PubMed – indexed for MEDLINE]. CrossRef PubMed.
39. Tavazzi L, Maggioni AP, Lucci D, Cacciatore G, Ansalone G, Oliva F, Porcu M. Italian survey on acute heart failure investigators. Nationwide survey on acute heart failure in cardiology ward services in Italy. Eur Heart J. 2006;27(10):1207–15. Epub 2006 Apr 7. PMID:16603579 [PubMed – indexed for MEDLINE 1].
40. Juurlink DN, Mamdani MM, Lee DS, Kopp A, Austin PC, Laupacis A, Redelmeier DA. Rates of hyperkalemia after publication of the randomized aldactone evaluation study. N Engl J Med. 2004;351(6):543–51. CrossRef PubMed.
41. Greenberg BH, Abraham WT, Albert NM, Chiswell K, Clare R, Stough WG, et al. Influence of diabetes on characteristics and outcomes in patients hospitalized with heart failure: a report from the organized program to initiate lifesaving treatment in hospitalized patients with heart failure (OPTIMIZE-HF). Am Heart J. 2007;154(2):277.e1–8. CrossRef.
42. Ronco C, Haapio M, House AA, Anavekar N, Bellomo R. Cardiorenal syndrome. J Am Coll Cardiol. 2008;52(19):1527–39. https://doi.org/10.1016/j.jacc.2008.07.051. CrossRef PubMed.
43. McCullough PA, Kellum JA, Haase M, Müller C, Damman K, Murray PT, et al. Pathophysiology of the cardiorenal syndromes: executive summary from the eleventh consensus conference of the acute dialysis quality initiative (ADQI). Contrib Nephrol. 2013;182:82–98. https://doi.org/10.1159/000349966. Epub 2013 May 13. CrossRef PubMed.
44. Anand IS. Anemia and chronic heart failure implications and treatment options. J Am Coll Cardiol. 2008;52(7):501–11. https://doi.org/10.1016/j.jacc.2008.04.044. CrossRef PubMed.
45. Groenveld HF, Januzzi JL, Damman K, van Wijngaarden J, Hillege HL, van Veldhuisen DJ, van der Meer P. Anemia and mortality in heart failure patients a systematic review and meta-analysis. J Am Coll Cardiol. 2008;52(10):818–27. https://doi.org/10.1016/j.jacc.2008.04.061. CrossRef PubMed.
46. Young JB, Abraham WT, Albert NM, Gattis Stough W, Gheorghiade M, Greenberg BH, OPTIMIZE-HF Investigators and Coordinators, et al. Relation of low hemoglobin and anemia to morbidity and mortality in patients hospitalized with heart failure (insight from the OPTIMIZE-HF registry). Am J Cardiol. 2008;101(2):223–30. https://doi.org/10.1016/j.amjcard.2007.07.067.
47. Ezekowitz JA, McAlister FA, Armstrong PW. Anemia is common in heart failure and is associated with poor outcomes: insights from a cohort of 12 065 patients with new-onset heart failure. Circulation. 2003;107(2):223–5. CrossRef PubMed.
48. Mentz RJ, Greene SJ, Ambrosy AP, Vaduganathan M, Subacius HP, Swedberg K, et al. Clinical profile and prognostic value of anemia at the time of admission and discharge among patients hospitalized for heart failure with reduced ejection fraction: findings from the EVEREST trial. Circ Heart Fail. 2014;7(3):401–8. https://doi.org/10.1161/CIRCHEARTFAILURE.113.000840. Epub 2014 Apr 15. CrossRef PubMed PubMedCentral.

49. Abramov D, Cohen RS, Katz SD, Mancini D, Maurer MS. Comparison of blood volume characteristics in anemic patients with low versus preserved left ventricular ejection fractions. Am J Cardiol. 2008;102(8):1069–72. https://doi.org/10.1016/j.amjcard.2008.05.058. Epub 2008 Jul 31. CrossRef PubMed PubMedCentral.
50. Androne AS, Katz SD, Lund L, LaManca J, Hudaihed A, Hryniewicz K, Mancini DM. Hemodilution is common in patients with advanced heart failure. Circulation. 2003;107(2):226–9. PMID:12538419 [PubMed – indexed for MEDLINE]. CrossRef PubMed.
51. Okonko DO, Mandal AK, Missouris CG, Poole-Wilson PA. Disordered iron homeostasis in chronic heart failure: prevalence, predictors, and relation to anemia, exercise capacity, and survival. J Am Coll Cardiol. 2011;58(12):1241–51. https://doi.org/10.1016/j.jacc.2011.04.040. CrossRef PubMed.
52. de Silva R, Rigby AS, Witte KK, Nikitin NP, Tin L, Goode K, et al. Anemia, renal dysfunction, and their interaction in patients with chronic heart failure. Am J Cardiol. 2006;98(3):391–8. Epub 2006 Jun 12. CrossRef PubMed.
53. Nanas JN, Matsouka C, Karageorgopoulos D, Leonti A, Tsolakis E, Drakos SG, et al. Etiology of anemia in patients with advanced heart failure. J Am Coll Cardiol. 2006;48(12):2485–9. Epub 2006 Nov 28. PMID: 17174186. CrossRef PubMed.
54. Huehnergarth KV, Mozaffarian D, Sullivan MD, Crane BA, Wilkinson CW, Lawler RL, et al. Usefulness of relative lymphocyte count as an independent predictor of death/urgent transplant in heart failure. Am J Cardiol. 2005;95(12):1492–5. CrossRef PubMed.
55. Vaduganathan M, Ambrosy AP, Greene SJ, Mentz RJ, Subacius HP, et al. EVEREST trial investigators. Predictive value of low relative lymphocyte count in patients hospitalized for heart failure with reduced ejection fraction: insights from the EVEREST trial. Circ Heart Fail. 2012;5(6):750–8. https://doi.org/10.1161/CIRCHEARTFAILURE.112.970525. Epub 2012 Oct 9.
56. Milo-Cotter O, Teerlink JR, Metra M, Felker GM, Ponikowski P, Voors AA, et al. Low lymphocyte ratio as a novel prognostic factor in acute heart failure: results from the pre-RELAX-AHF study. Cardiology. 2010;117(3):190–6. https://doi.org/10.1159/000321416. Epub 2010 Nov 17. CrossRef PubMed.
57. van Deursen VM, Damman K, Hillege HL, van Beek AP, van Veldhuisen DJ, Voors AA. Abnormal liver function in relation to hemodynamic profile in heart failure patients. J Card Fail. 2010;16(1):84–90. https://doi.org/10.1016/j.cardfail.2009.08.002. Epub 2009 Sep 26. CrossRef PubMed.
58. Ambrosy AP, Vaduganathan M, Huffman MD, Khan S, Kwasny MJ, Fought AJ, EVEREST trial investigators, et al. Clinical course and predictive value of liver function tests in patients hospitalized for worsening heart failure with reduced ejection fraction: an analysis of the EVEREST trial. Eur J Heart Fail. 2012;14(3):302–11.
59. Weisberg IS, Jacobson IM. Cardiovascular diseases and the liver. Clin Liver Dis. 2011;15(1):1–20. https://doi.org/10.1016/j.cld.2010.09.010. Review. PMID: 21111990. CrossRef PubMed.
60. Kavoliuniene A, Vaitiekiene A, Cesnaite G. Congestive hepatopathy and hypoxic hepatitis in heart failure: a cardiologist's point of view. Int J Cardiol. 2013;166(3):554–8. https://doi.org/10.1016/j.ijcard.2012.05.003. Epub 2012 May 30. Review. PMID: 22656043. CrossRef PubMed.
61. Daniels LB, Maisel AS. Natriuretic peptides. J Am Coll Cardiol. 2007;50(25):2357–68. CrossRef PubMed.
62. Silver MA, Maisel A, Yancy CW, McCullough PA, Burnett JC Jr, GS F, et al. BNP consensus panel BNP consensus panel 2004: a clinical approach for the diagnostic, prognostic, screening, treatment monitoring, and therapeutic roles of natriuretic peptides in cardiovascular diseases. Congest Heart Fail. 2004;10(5 Suppl 3):1–30. CrossRef.
63. Maisel AS, Krishnaswamy P, Nowak RM, McCord J, Hollander JE, Duc P, Breathing Not Properly Multinational Study Investigators, et al. Rapid measurement of B-type natriuretic peptide in the emergency diagnosis of heart failure. N Engl J Med. 2002;347(3):161–7.
64. Januzzi JL Jr, Camargo CA, Anwaruddin S, Baggish AL, Chen AA, Krauser DG, et al. The N-terminal pro-BNP investigation of dyspnea in the emergency department (PRIDE) study. Am J Cardiol. 2005;95(8):948–54. CrossRef PubMed.
65. Januzzi JL Jr, Chen-Tournoux AA, Moe G. Amino-terminal pro-B-type natriuretic peptide testing for the diagnosis or exclusion of heart failure in patients with acute symptoms. Am J Cardiol. 2008;101(3A):29–38. https://doi.org/10.1016/j.amjcard.2007.11.017. CrossRef PubMed.
66. Maisel A, Mueller C, Adams K Jr, Anker SD, Aspromonte N, Cleland JG, et al. State of the art: using natriuretic peptide levels in clinical practice. Eur J Heart Fail. 2008;10(9):824–39. https://doi.org/10.1016/j.ejheart.2008.07.014. Epub 2008 Aug 29. CrossRef PubMed.
67. Gopal DJ, Iqbal MN, Maisel A. Updating the role of natriuretic peptide levels in cardiovascular disease. Postgrad Med. 2011;123(6):102–13. https://doi.org/10.3810/pgm.2011.11.2500. CrossRef PubMed.
68. O'Hanlon R, O'Shea P, Ledwidge M, O'Loughlin C, Lange S, Conlon C, et al. The biologic variability of B-type natriuretic peptide and N-terminal pro-B-type natriuretic peptide in stable heart failure patients. J Card Fail. 2007;13(1):50–5. CrossRef PubMed.

69. Wu AH. Serial testing of B-type natriuretic peptide and NTpro-BNP for monitoring therapy of heart failure: the role of biologic variation in the interpretation of results. Am Heart J. 2006;152(5):828–34. CrossRef PubMed.
70. Yancy CW, Jessup M, Bozkurt B, Butler J, Casey DE Jr, Drazner MH, American College of Cardiology Foundation/American Heart Association Task Force on Practice Guidelines, et al. 2013 ACCF/AHA guideline for the management of heart failure: a report of the American College of Cardiology Foundation/American Heart Association task force on practice guidelines. Circulation. 2013;128(16):e240–327. https://doi.org/10.1161/CIR.0b013e31829e8776. Epub 2013 Jun 5.
71. Thygesen K, Alpert JS, White HD, Joint ESC/ACCF/AHA/WHF Task Force for the Redefinition of Myocardial Infarction, Jaffe AS, Apple FS, Galvani M, Katus HA, Newby LK, Ravkilde J, et al. Universal definition of myocardial infarction. Circulation. 2007;116(22):2634–53. Epub 2007 Oct 19.
72. Kociol RD, Pang PS, Gheorghiade M, Fonarow GC, O'Connor CM, Felker GM. Troponin elevation in heart failure prevalence, mechanisms, and clinical implications. J Am Coll Cardiol. 2010;56(14):1071–8. https://doi.org/10.1016/j.jacc.2010.06.016. CrossRef PubMed.
73. O'Gara PT, Kushner FG, Ascheim DD, Casey DE Jr, Chung MK, American College of Cardiology Foundation/American Heart Association Task Force on Practice Guidelines, et al. 2013 ACCF/AHA guideline for the management of ST-elevation myocardial infarction: a report of the American College of Cardiology Foundation/American Heart Association task force on practice guidelines. Circulation. 2013;127(4):e362–425. https://doi.org/10.1161/CIR.0b013e3182742cf6. Epub 2012 Dec 17. No abstract available. Erratum in: Circulation. 2013 Dec 24;128(25):e481.
74. Anderson JL, Adams CD, Antman EM, Bridges CR, Califf RM, Casey DE Jr, American College of Cardiology Foundation/American Heart Association Task Force on Practice Guidelines, et al. 2012 ACCF/AHA focused update incorporated into the ACCF/AHA 2007 guidelines for the management of patients with unstable angina/non-ST-elevation myocardial infarction: a report of the American College of Cardiology Foundation/American Heart Association task force on practice guidelines. Circulation. 2013;127(23):e663–828. https://doi.org/10.1161/CIR.0b013e31828478ac. Epub 2013 Apr 29. No abstract available. Erratum in: Circulation. 2013 Jun 18;127(24):e863–4.
75. Knudsen CW, Omland T, Clopton P, Westheim A, Abraham WT, Storrow AB, et al. Diagnostic value of B-type natriuretic peptide and chest radiographic findings in patients with acute dyspnea. Am J Med. 2004;116(6):363–8. CrossRef PubMed.
76. Cleland JG, Swedberg K, Cohen-Solal A, Cosin-Aguilar J, Dietz R, Follath F, et al. The euro heart failure survey of the EUROHEART survey programme. A survey on the quality of care among patients with heart failure in Europe. The study group on diagnosis of the working group on heart failure of the European Society of Cardiology. The medicines evaluation Group Centre for Health Economics University of York. Eur J Heart Fail. 2000;2(2):123–32. CrossRef PubMed.
77. Publication Committee for the VMAC Investigators (Vasodilatation in the Management of Acute CHF). Intravenous nesiritide vs nitroglycerin for treatment of decompensated congestive heart failure: a randomized controlled trial. JAMA. 2002;287(12):1531–40.
78. Cuffe MS, Califf RM, Adams KF Jr, Benza R, Bourge R, Colucci WS, Outcomes of a Prospective Trial of Intravenous Milrinone for Exacerbations of Chronic Heart Failure (OPTIME-CHF) Investigators, et al. Short-term intravenous milrinone for acute exacerbation of chronic heart failure: a randomized controlled trial. JAMA. 2002;287(12):1541–7. CrossRef PubMed.
79. McManus DD, Saczynski JS, Lessard D, Kinno M, Pidikiti R, Esa N, et al. Recent trends in the incidence, treatment, and prognosis of patients with heart failure and atrial fibrillation (the Worcester heart failure study). Am J Cardiol. 2013;111(10):1460–5. https://doi.org/10.1016/j.amjcard.2013.01.298. CrossRef PubMed PubMedCentral.
80. Mountantonakis SE, Grau-Sepulveda MV, Bhatt DL, Hernandez AF, Peterson ED, Fonarow GC. Presence of atrial fibrillation is independently associated with adverse outcomes in patients hospitalized with heart failure: an analysis of get with the guidelines-heart failure. Circ Heart Fail. 2012;5(2):191–201. https://doi.org/10.1161/CIRCHEARTFAILURE.111.965681. Epub 2012 Feb 23. CrossRef PubMed.
81. Wang NC, Maggioni AP, Konstam MA, Zannad F, Krasa HB, Burnett JC Jr, Efficacy of Vasopressin Antagonism in Heart Failure Outcome Study With Tolvaptan (EVEREST) Investigators, et al. Clinical implications of QRS duration in patients hospitalized with worsening heart failure and reduced left ventricular ejection fraction. JAMA. 2008;299(22):2656–66. https://doi.org/10.1001/jama.299.22.2656.
82. Chioncel O, Vinereanu D, Datcu M, Ionescu DD, Capalneanu R, Brukner I, et al. The Romanian acute heart failure syndromes (RO-AHFS) registry. Am Heart J. 2011;162(1):142–53.e1. https://doi.org/10.1016/j.ahj.2011.03.033. Epub 2011 Jun 15.
83. Huvelle E, Fay R, Alla F, Cohen Solal A, Mebazaa A, Zannad F. Left bundle branch block and mortality in patients with acute heart failure syndrome: a substudy of the EFICA cohort. Eur J Heart Fail. 2010;12(2):156–63. https://doi.org/10.1093/eurjhf/hfp180. Epub 2009 Dec 21. CrossRef PubMed.

84. Petrie MC. It cannot be cardiac failure because the heart is not enlarged on the chest X-ray. Eur J Heart Fail. 2003;5(2):117–9. CrossRef PubMed.
85. Pistolesi M, Miniati M, Bonsignore M, Andreotti F, Di Ricco G, Marini C. Factors affecting regional pulmonary blood flow in chronic ischemic heart disease. J Thorac Imaging. 1988;3(3):65–72. CrossRef PubMed.
86. Ketai LH, Godwin JD. A new view of pulmonary edema and acute respiratory distress syndrome. J Thorac Imaging. 1998;13(3):147–71. CrossRef PubMed.
87. Connolly MA. Black, white, and shades of gray: common abnormalities in chest radiographs. AACN Clin Issues. 2001;12(2):259–69; quiz 330-2. CrossRef PubMed.
88. Chakko S, Woska D, Martinez H, de Marchena E, Futterman L, Kessler KM, Myerberg RJ. Clinical, radiographic, and hemodynamic correlations in chronic congestive heart failure: conflicting results may lead to inappropriate care. Am J Med. 1991;90(3):353–9. CrossRef PubMed.
89. Collins SP, Lindsell CJ, Storrow AB, Abraham WT, ADHERE Scientific Advisory Committee, Investigators and Study Group. Prevalence of negative chest radiography results in the emergency department patient with decompensated heart failure. Ann Emerg Med. 2006;47(1):13–8. Epub 2005 Jun 20.

12 Acute Decompensated Heart Failure: Treatment Guidelines

Daniel Fishbein

Treatment of ADHF: Review of ACCF/AHA, ESC and HFSA Guidelines

Comprehensive guidelines for the management of ADHF have been published including: the American College of Cardiology Foundation/American Heart Association (ACCF/AHA) Guidelines for the Management of Heart Failure [1], the Heart Failure Society of America (HFSA) Comprehensive Practice Guidelines [2, 3], and the European Society of Cardiology (ESC) Task Force Guidelines [4].

There are three phases in the evaluation and management of patients who present with ADHF including [2, 5, 6]:

1. Initial assessment, monitoring, treatment and disposition. This phase generally occurs in the emergency department (ED).
2. Ongoing assessment and treatment. This phase generally occurs in a critical care or telemetry unit. Goals of treatment are to relieve congestion, initiate and/or optimize guideline determined medical therapy (GDMT), and further evaluate and address reversible factors that cause or worsen heart failure.
3. Discharge planning and post-discharge follow up.

Initial Assessment and Treatment in the Emergency Department

A number of important issues need to be addressed as part of the initial assessment of a patient who presents to the ED with the primary symptom of dyspnea. These issues need to be addressed concurrently and often, treatment needs to be initiated in parallel with the ongoing diagnostic evaluation:

1. Is the patient's condition immediately life-threatening because of hypoxia, respiratory failure, hypotension, systemic hypoperfusion, bradyarrhythmia and/or tachyarrhythmia? Does the patient need mechanical ventilation, intravenous vasoactive medications, an intra-aortic balloon pump or other mechanical circulatory support, ventricular pacing, or cardioversion?
2. Is the patient having an acute coronary syndrome precipitating heart failure? Does the patient need to go emergently to the cardiac catheterization laboratory for percutaneous coronary intervention (PCI)?
3. Does the patient have heart failure? Is there an alternative cause of symptoms?

D. Fishbein (✉)
Department of Medicine, Division of Cardiology, University of Washington Medical Center, Seattle, WA, USA
e-mail: dfish@uw.edu

H. J. Eisen (ed.), *Heart Failure I*, https://doi.org/10.1007/978-3-032-12626-9_12

4. Are there precipitating factors that have caused or contributed to acute heart failure decompensation?
5. Relieve symptoms rapidly while avoiding harm. Improvement in symptoms generally requires relief of pulmonary congestion and improvement in elevated blood pressure without causing hypotension, arrhythmia, electrolyte abnormality, renal dysfunction, myocardial injury or respiratory compromise.
6. Does the patient need to be admitted to the hospital (CCU or telemetry floor), observed further in the ED, admitted to an observation unit, or discharged to home?

Initial Triage

Patients who present with acute dyspnea need to be assessed for the presence of pulmonary or hemodynamic instability that may require emergent intervention. Patients who present with tachypnea, hypoxia not readily corrected with nasal oxygen, respiratory distress or mental status changes may need emergent intervention with noninvasive ventilation or endotracheal intubation. While arterial blood gas determination is not routine in the assessment of most patients presenting with ADHF, it should be obtained in the patient with impending respiratory failure or severe lung disease. Endotracheal intubation and mechanical ventilation should be considered in patients with respiratory acidosis.

In EHFS II, ACS was the precipitating factor in 42% of patients who presented with new onset heart failure and 23% of patients who had preexisting heart failure. Patients with ACS generally present with precordial chest pain [7]. A 12-lead ECG is a critical part of the early evaluation of patients with suspected ADHF as the presence of ST segment elevation (or new LBBB) in the setting of an elevated troponin is an indication for emergent coronary intervention as outlined in recent consensus documents [1, 8]. Patients may have ST segment depression and /or T wave inversion that, combined with clinical symptoms suggestive of ischemia and elevated troponin, are indicative of ACS [9]. ST-T wave changes alone may not be diagnostic of coronary ischemia or infarction and may be seen in other conditions including acute pericarditis, early repolarization patterns, LBBB, LV hypertrophy, and Brugada syndrome [10]. The ECG is helpful in identifying underlying heart rhythm abnormalities which may need urgent treatment (e.g. atrial fibrillation with rapid ventricular response, ventricular tachycardia, heart block).

Abnormal ECG findings are not helpful in discriminating HF from other causes of dyspnea (sensitivity 0.5, specificity 0.78 and positive likelihood ratio of 2.2). Atrial fibrillation, however, has a specificity of 0.93 and a positive likelihood ratio of 3.8 [11]. However, it is unlikely for patients with systolic dysfunction to have an entirely normal ECG. In a screening study of 534 patients with suspected heart failure, 96 patients had systolic dysfunction on echocardiography. Of these, 90 had major electrocardiographic abnormalities (atrial fibrillation, previous myocardial infarction, left ventricular hypertrophy, bundle branch block, or left axis deviation); none had a normal electrocardiogram. Of 438 patients with normal left ventricular systolic function, 169 had major electrocardiographic abnormalities [12].

Patients with STEMI, acute decompensation of chronic heart failure or acute heart failure due to myocardial inflammation may present with hypotension, evidence of compromised end-organ perfusion and pulmonary congestion. These patients commonly have sinus tachycardia, hypotension, a narrow pulse pressure, and evidence of pulmonary and systemic venous congestion. This subset of critically ill patients may need inotropic and/or vasopressor support, pulmonary artery catheterization to guide therapy and mechanical support with an IABP, Impella, TandemHeart, or extracorporeal life support (ECLS) [8].

Determination of either BNP or NT-proBNP is recommended in patients with dyspnea and signs and symptoms consistent with heart failure. The use of either biomarker is most helpful when there is an intermediate pretest probability of heart failure and the values are either very low or very high. Age, gender, renal function and obesity may affect natriuretic peptide levels. Levels should not be interpreted in isolation but rather, in the context of the broader clinical evaluation.

A BNP level <100 pg/mL has a sensitivity, specificity, negative predictive and positive predictive value of 90%, 76%, 79%, and 89%, respectively [13]. BNP levels tend to increase with age. In patients less than 70 years of age, a BNP level >400 pg/mL has a sensitivity of 60%, specificity of 95%, positive predictive value of 86%, negative predictive value of 81% and diagnostic accuracy of 82%. In patients ≥70 years of age, a BNP level >400 pg/mL has a sensitivity of 65%, specificity of 83%, positive predictive value of 86%, negative predictive value of 60% and diagnostic accuracy of 72% [14]. Approximately 75% of patients who present with acute dyspnea will have either low (<100 pg/mL) or high (>400–500 pg/mL) BNP levels. In general, in patients who present to the ED with dyspnea, if the BNP is <100 pg/ml, heart failure is unlikely to be the cause of dyspnea. If the BNP is >500 pg/ml, HF is likely with a positive predictive value of 90%. With BNP levels between 100–500 pg/ml, alternative causes of increased BNP need to be considered including stable chronic LV dysfunction, RV failure due to cor pulmonale, acute pulmonary embolism or renal insufficiency. Patients may present with HF and normal BNP levels in the following settings: flash pulmonary edema within 1–2 h of onset, HF upstream from the left ventricle, (e.g., acute papillary muscle rupture with acute mitral regurgitation), and obesity. In patients with a body mass index >35 kg/m^2, a BNP cutoff of 60 pg/mL has been recommended to rule out and 200 pg/mL to rule in HF as the cause of acute dyspnea. In general, BNP is elevated in the setting of chronic renal insufficiency. It may be reasonable to recalibrate the BNP cutoff to 200–225 pg/mL in patients with an estimated glomerular filtration rate of <60 mL/min to rule out heart failure. BNP levels are lower in obese people with and without heart failure. There seems to be a linear decrease in BNP level with increasing BMI [15, 16]. In general, in patients with chronic heart failure, changes of >50% from baseline represent worsening heart failure. However, significant variation in levels can occur in the same patient and individual differences in NP do not necessarily represent an acute clinical event. There is a substantial grey zone in interpreting the results [17].

An NT-proBNP <300 pg/ml has a 99% negative predictive value to exclude heart failure in patients who present with dyspnea. This is independent of age and BMI [18]. An NT-proBNP >900 pg/mL has a sensitivity of 90%, specificity of 85% and positive predictive value of 76% to predict heart failure as the cause of dyspnea [19]. Age stratification of NT-proBNP using cut points of 450, 900, and 1800 pg/ml for age groups of <50, 50–75, and >75 years, respectively reduces false-negative findings in younger patients, reduces false-positive findings in older patients, and improves the overall positive predictive value without a change in overall sensitivity or specificity. These cut-points have a 90% sensitivity and 84% specificity for acute HF [20, 21] and are predictive of acute heart failure across a wide range of BMIs [22].

Initial Treatment

The HFSA and ESC guidelines recommend that oxygen should be administered by nasal cannula or face mask in patients with hypoxia but is not recommended in the absence of hypoxia. The HFSA and ESC guidelines recommend the use of non-invasive positive pressure ventilation for patients with severe dyspnea and clinical evidence of pulmonary edema [2, 4]. The ESC guidelines specifically recommend non-invasive ventilation in patients with dyspnea, evidence of pulmonary edema and a respiratory rate of >20 breaths/minute.

The ESC Guidelines recommend that IV morphine sulfate (MS) should be considered, especially in anxious, restless or distressed patients to relieve these symptoms and improve breathlessness. However, the HFSA guidelines recommend that if used at all, MS should be used with caution given recent data demonstrating an association between MS use and adverse outcomes.

Treatment with an intravenous loop diuretic is consistently recommended in the ACCF/AHA,

ESC and HFSA guidelines as first line treatment in the initial management of patients with ADHF and that diuretic therapy should be initiated in the ED without delay [1, 2, 4]. Although there are no randomized placebo-controlled clinical trials to establish the safety and efficacy of diuretics in ADHF, extensive observational experience has shown that diuretics relieve congestion and improve symptoms. The impact of diuretic therapy on mortality has not been adequately studied.

The HFSA Guidelines do not make specific recommendations about initial diuretic dose. The ACCF/AHA Guidelines recommend that in patients already receiving a loop diuretic, the initial diuretic dose should equal or exceed their chronic oral daily dose and be given either as intermittent intravenous boluses or continuous infusion [1]. The ESC Guidelines recommend that an initial dose of furosemide 20–40 mg IV (or 0.5–1.0 mg bumetanide IV or 10–20 mg of torsemide IV) be given on admission. In patients with evidence of volume overload, a higher dose of parenteral diuretic may be considered based on renal function and history of chronic oral diuretic use. Continuous infusion may also be considered after an initial starting bolus dose. ESC recommends that the total furosemide dose should remain <100 mg in the first 6 h and 240 mg during the first 24 h [5].

Table 12.1 Recommendations for hospitalizing patients presenting with ADHF

Recommendation	Clinical circumstance
Hospitalization recommended	Evidence of severely decompensated HF, including:
	Hypotension
	Worsening renal function
	Altered mentation
	Dyspnea at rest
	Typically reflected by resting tachypnea; less commonly reflected by oxygen saturation <90%
	Hemodynamically significant arrhythmia; including new onset of rapid atrial fibrillation
	Acute coronary syndromes
Hospitalization should be considered	Worsened congestion
	Even without dyspnea
	Signs and symptoms of pulmonary or systemic congestion; even in the absence of weight gain
	Major electrolyte disturbance
	Associated comorbid conditions:
	Pneumonia
	Pulmonary embolus
	Diabetic ketoacidosis
	Symptoms suggestive of transient ischemic accident or stroke
	Repeated ICD firings
	Previously undiagnosed HF with signs and symptoms of systemic or pulmonary congestion

Reprinted from Lindenfeld et al. [2]

Indications for Hospitalization

Recommendations for hospitalization from the HFSA Guidelines are summarized in Table 12.1 [2]. A recently published consensus document from the Society for Academic Emergency Medicine/Heart Failure Society of America Acute Heart Failure Working Group has suggested that ED patients with ADHF can be divided into three groups based on risk profile, presence of co-morbidities, initial response to therapy in the ED and barriers to self-care [23]. Patients at high risk for mortality or serious adverse events (those with low blood pressure, hypoxia, renal insufficiency or myocardial ischemia/infarction) should be admitted to the CCU.

Identifying Precipitating Causes of Acute HF Decompensation

An essential task in the evaluation of a patient who presents with acute decompensated heart failure is to identify new or chronic issues/conditions that may cause, precipitate or contribute to heart failure decompensation. This should be done early in the evaluation so that appropriate therapies can be initiated, symptoms can be alleviated more rapidly, reversible myocardial dysfunction can be treated and recurrent heart failure hospitalizations can be prevented. Table 12.2 summarizes conditions that can cause or contribute to the development of acute decompensated heart failure.

Table 12.2 Possible precipitating causes of heart failure decompensation

Coronary artery disease
Myocardial ischemia
ACS
Mechanical complications of AMI (VSD, MR)
Valvular disease
Mitral regurgitation: worsening chronic or acute
Progressive aortic stenosis
Worsening tricuspid insufficiency
Aortic insufficiency
Endocarditis
Aortic dissection
Progressive cardiac dysfunction
Progression of underlying cardiac dysfunction
Physical, emotional or environmental stress
Cardiac toxins—alcohol, cocaine, methamphetamines, chemotherapy
RV pacing
Persistent tachycardia
Frequent PVCs
Myocardial disease
Lymphocytic myocarditis
Giant cell myocarditis
Post-partum cardiomyopathy
Sarcoid
Uncontrolled high blood pressure
Dietary and medication adherence
Excessive salt and water intake
Medication nonadherence
Iatrogenic volume expansion
Arrhythmia
Atrial fibrillation
Atrial flutter
Other supraventricular arrhythmia
Recurrent ventricular tachycardia
Bradycardia-sinus node dysfunction, heart block, AF with slow ventricular response
Recent onset LBBB
Non-cardiac conditions
Systemic infection: sepsis, pneumonia, URI, UTI, viral infection (especially influenza)
Renal insufficiency
Thyroid disorders
Anemia
COPD/asthma
Sleep apnea
Pulmonary embolism
AV shunts
Urinary outlet obstruction
Tamponade
Iron deficiency
CVA
Depression, dementia, and cognitive impairment
Recent addition of medications with negative inotropic effects:
Calcium channel blockers: especially the non-dihydropyridines verapamil and diltiazem

(continued)

Table 12.2 (continued)

Class Ia, Ic and III antiarrhythmic medications:
Quinidine, procainamide, disopyramide, flecainide, sotalol, propafenone, dronedarone
β-adrenergic blocking agents
Non-cardiac medications that promote sodium retention:
Nonsteroidal anti-inflammatory drugs
COX-2 inhibitors
Corticosteroids
Thiazolidinediones
Pregabalin
Chemotherapy
Anthracyclines
Monoclonal antibodies—Trastuzumab and Bevacizumab
Taxanes—paclitaxel and docetaxel
Cyclophosphamide
Small tyrosine kinase inhibitors—Sunitinib, sorafenib, imatinib

Co-morbid conditions are common and play a significant role in hospitalization for ADHF. In the OPTIMIZE-HF registry, one or more precipitating factors were identified in 61.3% of patients admitted with ADHF. The most common precipitating factors included: pneumonia/respiratory process (15.3%), ischemia/acute coronary syndrome (14.7%), arrhythmia (13.5%), and poorly controlled hypertension (10.7%). Nonadherence to medications was identified in 8.9% and nonadherence to diet was identified in 5.2% [24].

Coronary Artery Disease

Coronary artery disease is present in approximately 50–70% of patients with ADHF [7, 25–30]. Patients may present with ACS complicated by heart failure or ADHF with underlying CAD.

ACS Complicated by Heart Failure

Approximately 10–20% of patients with ACS have associated heart failure on presentation and another 10% of ACS patients develop heart failure during hospitalization. Patients with ACS due to a STEMI typically have chest pain, diagnostic ECG changes and high levels of biomarkers consistent with substantial myocardial injury [29]. Patients with heart failure complicating an STEMI (either on presentation or developing later after hospitalization) have significantly increased in-hospital and post-discharge mortality compared to patients without heart failure [29–32]. Patients with ACS who develop heart failure after admission are at greater risk than patients with ACS who have heart failure on presentation [30, 32]. The severity of heart failure measured by the Killip classification is a powerful predictor of mortality in patients with heart failure complicating ACS. Patients with Killip class II or III are 4 times more likely to die during hospitalization compared with Killip class I patients while patients with Killip class IV (cardiogenic shock) are 10 times more likely [30, 32]. Patients with heart failure and unstable angina have also been found have a significant fourfold increase in mortality compared to similar patients without HF [31].

The Global Registry of Acute Coronary Events (GRACE) enrolled 16,166 patients with ACS. Patients who presented with HF complicating ACS had lower rates of catheterization and PCI and were less likely to receive β-blockers and statins [31]. In the National Registry of Myocardial Infarction (NRMI), patients with HF complicating ACS were less likely to receive aspirin, heparin, intravenous nitroglycerine and β-blockers compared to patients with ACS without heart failure. In addition, patients with heart failure were less likely to undergo PCI or CABG compared with patients without heart failure on presentation (40% vs 20%) [32].

An analysis of the Can Rapid Risk Stratification of Unstable Angina Patients Suppress Outcomes with Early Implementation of the American College of Cardiology/American Heart Association (ACC/AHA) Guidelines (CRUSADE) initiative (2.8% of patients had HF) demonstrated that patients with a non-STEMI with heart failure with preserved EF had a significantly higher mortality rate than patients without HF and preserved systolic function and a similar mortality to patients with no HF and systolic dysfunction. Patients with both HF and systolic dysfunction had the highest mortality (1.5% vs 5.7% vs 5.8% vs 10.7%). Cardiac catheterization and PCI rates were lower for patients without heart failure with systolic dysfunction and with HF with or without systolic dysfunction. Patients with HF received aspirin, clopidogrel, glycoprotein IIb/IIIa inhibitors, heparin, B-blockers and statins less frequently than patients with no HF and preserved systolic function [33].

There is broad consensus that patients with HF complicating ACS should undergo urgent coronary angiography and coronary intervention in the catheterization laboratory [1, 2, 9, 34, 35].

ADHF with Underlying CAD

It has been estimated that 50–70% of patients with ADHF have concomitant coronary artery disease. Registry data suggest that CAD is associated with higher in-hospital and post-discharge mortality rates. In the OPTIMIZE-HF Registry, in-hospital mortality rates were 3.75% vs 2.9% and post-discharge 60–90 day mortality rates were 9.2 vs 6.9% in patients with CAD vs no CAD [36].

In multicenter registries of patients admitted with ADHF, rates of diagnostic coronary angiography are relatively low overall: OPTIMIZE –HF 8.7% [36]; ADHERE 10% [25]; EHFS 16% [27]; and EHFS II 36.5% (EHFS II reported angiography within a year of hospitalization) [7]. In OPTIMIZE-HF, 18.6% of patients presenting with de novo heart failure underwent coronary angiography [36]. Rates of coronary revascularization were relatively low: ADHERE 8.1% PCI, 1.8% CABG [25]; EHFS PCI 4%, CABG 3% [27]; EHFS II PCI 8.4%, CABG 1.8% [7]; OPTIMIZE-HF 1.3% PCI, 1.0% CABG [37].

In OPTIMIZE-HF, patients with CAD who did not undergo revascularization had a higher post-discharge mortality compared to patients without CAD (10.6% vs 6.9%). Patients who did undergo revascularization during HF hospitalization had a similar post-discharge mortality compared to patients without CAD [36].

The data from the OPTIMIZE-HF registry was analyzed to determine if the performance of coronary angiography during the index HF hospitalization had an impact on care and post-discharge outcome [37]. 8.7% of all patients underwent coronary angiography. 27.5% of patients who underwent angiography also had in-hospital revascularization. Patients with CAD who underwent angiography were more likely to be treated with aspirin, statins, B-blockers, and angiotensin converting enzyme inhibitors at the time of discharge. In patients with CAD, the use of in-hospital coronary angiography was associated with a significantly lower mortality and rate of rehospitalization in the first 60–90 days after adjustment for multiple comorbidities (mortality HR 0.31; $p = 0.004$; death or rehospitalization HR 0.65; $p = 0.003$) when compared to patients with CAD who did not undergo coronary angiography. This data suggests that early coronary angiography and revascularization may be beneficial in patients admitted to the hospital with CAD and ADHF.

These results were registry based and may not account for unmeasured variables or selection biases. In the randomize Surgical Treatment for Ischemic Heart Failure (STICH) trial, there was no difference in death from any cause in patients with LVEF ≤35% and coronary artery disease amenable to CABG randomized to medical therapy or medical therapy plus CABG on intention to treat analysis. However, when early crossovers were considered, "on-therapy" CABG was associated with a lower mortality at 5 years (25% vs 42%; HR 0.50; $p = 0.008$). Myocardial viability or inducible myocardial ischemia did not identify patients with a differential survival benefit from CABG compared to medical therapy alone [38–40].

Practice guidelines provide recommendations on the use of coronary angiography in the evaluation of patients with chronic heart failure. However, they do not give specific recommendations about the timing of invasive evaluation of coronary anatomy and specifically do not provide recommendations about indications for coronary angiography in patients hospitalized for ADHF. Given the absence of definitive data concerning coronary angiography and revascularization in ADHF, decisions should be individualized based on patient preference, symptoms, clinical presentation, comorbidities, candidacy for revascularization and willingness to undergo revascularization [1, 2]. In general, coronary angiography is recommended for patients with heart failure and symptoms suggestive of angina to assess for the possibility of revascularization. Non-invasive imaging *or* coronary angiography is recommended for patients with new onset heart failure, no angina and unknown CAD status and patients with new or worsening heart failure without obvious cause, no angina and known CAD [2].

Uncontrolled Hypertension

Hypertension is an important precipitant of decompensated heart failure, especially among blacks, women and patients with HFpEF. In the OPTIMIZE-HF registry, poorly controlled hypertension was a precipitating factor in 10.7% of patients [24]. In the ADHERE Registry, almost 50% of patients admitted with decompensated heart failure has an initial blood pressure of >140/90 mmHg [25]. Medical non-adherence with antihypertensive medications may result in an abrupt increase in blood pressure and precipitate worsening heart failure or acute pulmonary edema [1, 41].

Arrhythmia

Arrhythmia was a precipitating factor of heart failure decompensation in 13.5% of patients enrolled in the OPTIMIZE-HF registry [24]. Atrial fibrillation (AF) is present in approximately 30–40% of patients hospitalized with ADHF [7, 27, 35, 42–45]. New onset or newly diagnosed AF has been reported to occur in approximately 20% percent of patients admitted with ADHF [35, 44, 45]. AF is associated with the loss of coordinated atrial contraction. In patients with heart failure and especially in patients with HFpEF, this may be associated with significantly decreased left ventricular filling, increased PCWP and decreased cardiac output. In AF with rapid ventricular response, ventricular filling is further compromised and myocardial ischemia and/or pulmonary edema may be precipitated [46, 47].

Atrial flutter, other supraventricular tachyarrhythmias and ventricular tachycardia may also precipitate acute heart failure. Frequent premature ventricular contractions (PVCs) may be associated with a distinct cardiomyopathy (PVC-related cardiomyopathy) or worsening heart failure and LV dysfunction in the setting of a preexisting cardiomyopathy. In general, a PVC burden of approximately 20–24% of all QRS complexes on a 24 h Holter monitor identifies a patient with LV systolic dysfunction who may improve with PVC ablation [48–51].

Medication and Dietary Non-adherence

Excessive sodium and fluid intake may contribute to heart failure decompensation. In the OPTIMIZE-HF Registry, non-adherence to diet was identified as a precipitating factor in 5.2% of patients hospitalized for ADHF. Non-adherence to medication was a precipitating factor in 8.9% of patients [24]. Non-adherence with diet or HF medication has been reported to be an even more common precipitating factor in some single-center studies [52, 53]. Factors that have been associated with medical non-adherence include more advanced NYHA functional class, minority ethnicity, lower financial status, and lack of perceived social support. Patient perception of barriers to medication adherence may also be fundamental to poor adherence. Frequently reported barriers include: forgetting to take medication, cost, too many pills taken per day, too frequent medication schedule and the belief that skipping one dose of medication will not have an adverse impact on the patient's condition [54, 55].

Patients with heart failure commonly have excessive and bothersome thirst mediated by activation of central arterial volume receptors and increased levels of angiotensin II both of which stimulate thirst centers in the brain. This leads to excessive sodium and water intake [56–59]. This is a particularly difficult issue in patients with severe heart failure who are not able to be treated with an ACE inhibitor or ARB at reasonable or target dose. In addition, older patients commonly have chemosensory deficits that decrease salt detection and sensitivity and increase salt affinity and intake. Salt affinity may be modifiable toward normal after >2 months of sodium restriction [60]. Patients may also be unaware of the salt content of foods they are consuming or may feel that they do not need to limit sodium intake. A careful review of the patient's history of dietary intake of sodium and free water (including "hidden" sources of free water such as fruit) is an important part of the assessment of patients admitted with ADHF.

Pneumonia or Other Pulmonary Processes

Pneumonia and other acute respiratory processes were the most common precipitating factor (15.3%) identified in patients hospitalized for ADHF in the OPTIMIZE-HF registry [24]. Pulmonary infections may alter pulmonary function, cause hypoxia, and increase metabolic demands and are poorly tolerated by patients with heart failure. Pulmonary congestion in a patient with chronic obstructive pulmonary disease can compromise already marginal pulmonary function. Patients with heart failure are hypercoagulable and pulmonary embolus may be a cause of HF decompensation [61–64]. Sleep disordered breathing is very common in patients with heart failure. It may worsen heart failure by causing hypoxia, increasing sympathetic nervous system activation and causing or worsening systemic hypertension. Sleep disordered breathing has also been associated with left ventricular remodeling, endothelial dysfunction with progression of coronary artery disease, left ventricular hypertrophy and atrial fibrillation [65–67].

Infection

Systemic bacterial or viral infection (pneumonia, urinary tract infection, influenza) are common precipitants of worsening heart failure. Infections increase metabolic demands. In addition, sepsis can cause reversible myocardial dysfunction likely mediated by release of pro-inflammatory cytokines [68, 69].

Thyroid Disease

Hypothyroidism and hyperthyroidism can cause or worsen heart failure. All patients seen for ADHF should have thyroid function studies obtained on admission. Approximately 20% of patients admitted with ADHF are treated for thyroid disease and should have their therapy reevaluated during hospitalization [70, 71]. Amiodarone-induced hyperthyroidism (AIT) can cause severe worsening of heart failure with or without new or worsening arrhythmias and can be difficult to treat. The clinical presentation of AIT is variable and is often similar to other forms of thyrotoxicosis. However, AIT often occurs in elderly patients and may be "apathetic" with atypical symptoms such as reduced appetite and depression and absence of hyperactivity, tremor, nervousness and heat intolerance [72].

Medications

A number of non-cardiac medications can precipitate worsening heart failure. Non-steroidal anti-inflammatory drugs and COX-2 inhibitors inhibit the physiologic production of vasodilatory and natriuretic prostanoids in the kidney and promote sodium and water retention, worsen renal function, inhibit the effect of ACE inhibitors, contribute to diuretic resistance and are associated with a significantly increased risk of hospitalization for heart failure [73].

The thiazolidinediones (TZD), (pioglitazone and rosiglitazone) used to treat diabetes, have been associated with the development of lower extremity edema and new or worsening heart failure [74]. These side effects are primarily due to fluid retention caused by TZD stimulation of the peroxisome proliferator-activated receptor-gamma (PPARγ). PPARγ-mediated activation of the collecting duct epithelium's sodium channel (ENaC) and stimulation of sodium transporters in the proximal tubule contribute to salt and water retention [75, 76]. In addition, TZDs reduce systemic vascular resistance and may cause fluid extravasation by exposing the capillaries of the lower extremities to higher perfusion pressures. TZDs also increase the concentration of vascular endothelial growth factor which is a potent inducer of vascular permeability which may predispose patients to edema [77].

Insulin can also cause sodium retention mediated by stimulation of a broad range of sodium transporters in the proximal tubule, loop of Henle and distal tubule [74]. Pregabalin, which is frequently used to treat diabetic peripheral neuropathic pain, has also been reported to precipitate heart failure decompensation [78].

Cardiotoxicity is a common complication of many conventional and targeted biological anticancer medications [79–83]. Cocaine, excessive alcohol intake, and methamphetamine are associated with worsening heart failure [84–89].

A number of cardiac medications have negative inotropic properties and can worsen heart failure. Recent initiation or uptitration of β-blockers has been associated with worsening heart failure, especially in patients with severe ventricular dysfunction and those recently treated with inotropic agents. Calcium channel blockers (CCBs), especially the non-dihydropyridine CCBs, have been associated with worsening heart failure. A large number of antiarrhythmic agents may also precipitate worsening heart failure including quinidine, procainamide, disopyramide, flecainide, sotalol, propanone, and dronedarone.

Right Ventricular (RV) Pacing

Right ventricular pacing can lead to abnormal electrical and mechanical activation patterns (referred to as ventricular "dyssynchrony") which lead to adverse effects on left ventricular performance and hemodynamics, subsequent adverse effects on cardiac structure and function, and clinical heart failure.

Patients with a single lead pacemaker or ICD may develop gradually progressive sinus bradycardia in response to beta blocker or amiodarone therapy and present with worsening heart failure in the setting of recent onset ventricular pacing. A similar scenario may be seen in patients who develop atrial fibrillation with a slow ventricular response in the setting of beta blockade or amiodarone therapy. These patients may improve by pacemaker reprogramming that minimizes RV pacing or an upgrade to a device that provides biventricular pacing [90, 91].

Renal Dysfunction

Renal dysfunction is common in patients with ADHF. In the ADHERE registry, chronic renal insufficiency was reported in 30% of patients and 21% had a creatinine >2.0 mg/dL [25]. In OPTIMIZE-HF, the mean creatinine was 1.8 mg/dL [92]. Elevated BUN and creatinine may be manifestations of renal hypoperfusion in the setting of low cardiac output, high filling pressures and/or neurohormonal activation. In HF, renal cortical blood flow is especially decreased and tubulointerstitial damage may develop due to decreased local renal perfusion and increased venous congestion. Albuminuria can occur in heart failure and is a manifestation of both a loss of glomerular integrity and tubular damage. A high albumin load may also contribute to tubular damage [93]. In addition, patients with heart failure commonly have risk factors for both cardiac and renal disease including diabetes and hypertension that may contribute to renal insufficiency independent of hemodynamic derangements from heart failure. A gradual or acute reduction in renal function will decrease renal clearance of sodium and water, worsen diuretic resistance, contribute to inadequate blood pressure control, contribute to hyperkalemia, and worsen anemia all of which will contribute to worsening HF.

Benign prostatic hypertrophy is common in men over the age of 50 years and may contribute to urinary obstruction, impaired renal function and worsening heart failure in men with ADHF. The prevalence of histologically diagnosed prostatic hyperplasia increases from 40 to 50 percent in men age 51 to 60 years, to over 80 percent in men older than age 80 years [94]. A population based study from Olmstead County, Minnesota found that moderate to severe lower urinary tract obstructive symptoms were present in 13% of men 40–49 years and 28% of those older than 70 years [95]. An evaluation for urinary obstruction can easily performed using bladder scanning. We have found that routine bladder scanning of men hospitalized with ADHF who have an elevated creatinine or diuretic resistance is helpful in identifying lower urinary tract obstruction. Relief of urinary obstruction with placement of a urinary catheter commonly results in improvements in renal function, diuretic resistance, pulmonary and systemic venous congestion and heart failure symptoms.

Ongoing Assessment and Treatment

The goals of treatment for patients admitted with ADHF from the HFSA guidelines are summarized in Table 12.3 [2].

Most patients have a significant improvement within 1–6 h after diuretic administration [96]. However, when diuresis is inadequate to relieve symptoms, the ACCF/AHA, HFSA, and ESC guidelines recommend giving a higher dose of diuretic or adding a second thiazide or thiazide-like diuretic (hydrochlorothiazide, chlorothiazide or metolazone). The HFSA and ESC guidelines also recommend considering use of a continuous infusion of a loop diuretic. The ACCF/AHA guidelines note that low-dose dopamine added to loop diuretic therapy may be considered to improve diuresis and preserve renal function.

Table 12.3 HFSA treatment goals for patients admitted for ADHF

HFSA treatment goals for patients admitted for ADHF [2]
Improve symptoms, especially congestion and low-output symptoms
Restore normal oxygenation
Optimize volume status
Identify etiology
Identify and address precipitating factors
Optimize chronic oral therapy
Minimize side effects
Identify patients who might benefit from revascularization
Identify patients who might benefit from device therapy
Identify risk of thromboembolism and need for anticoagulant therapy
Educate patients concerning medications and self-management of HF
Consider and, where possible, initiate a disease management program

Reprinted from Lindenfeld et al. [2]
HFSA Heart Failure Society of America

The ACCF/AHA, HFSA, and ESC guidelines suggest that veno-venous ultrafiltration may be considered in volume overloaded patients to treat congestive symptoms and relieve volume overload. The ACCF/AHA guidelines suggest that UF may be appropriate "for patients with refractory congestion not responding to medical therapy". The HFSA guidelines state that UF "may be considered in lieu of diuretics".

The ACCF/ACC, HFSA, and ESC guidelines emphasize the importance of careful monitoring of vital signs, signs and symptoms of congestion, urine output, electrolytes and renal function after initiation of diuretic therapy. Excessive diuresis may result in hypotension and a reduction in cardiac output. During loop diuretic-induced natriuresis, intravascular volume is generally maintained by vascular "refilling' or re-equilibration as interstitial fluid moves from the interstitial space to the intravascular space. The rate of refilling varies among patients. During brisk diuresis, it is possible for the rate of diuresis to exceed the rate of refilling. This may result in low intravascular volume, inadequate cardiac filling, and hypotension despite persistent volume overload. Patients with HPpEF are at greater risk of diuretic-induced hypotension—these patients tend to be less volume overloaded and have a steep diastolic filling curve so that moderate reductions in intravascular volume may result in significant reductions in cardiac filling and cardiac output. Patients with infiltrative or restrictive cardiomyopathy may have diuretic induced hypotension in the setting of continued volume overload as elevated ventricular filling pressures are needed to maintain normal cardiac output [2, 97]. Diuresis that results in a decrease in ventricular filling pressures makes patients more sensitive to the hypotensive effects of other vasodilators used in the routine treatment of heart failure.

The ACCF/AHA and HFSA guidelines recommend that in the absence of symptomatic hypotension, intravenous nitroglycerine or nitroprusside may be considered as an addition to diuretic therapy for relief of dyspnea in patients with ADHF. Blood pressure should be monitored frequently and the vasodilator should be stopped or dose decreased if symptomatic hypotension occurs. The ESC Guidelines recommend NTG or nitroprusside in patients with pulmonary congestion/edema provided SBP >110 mmHg to reduce pulmonary capillary wedge pressure. Caution is advised when using nitroprusside in patients with acute myocardial infarction.

The ACCF/AHA and HFSA guidelines suggest that the use of the intravenous inotropes dobutamine, milrinone, and dopamine (ACCF/AHA only) be limited to patients with LV dilation, LV systolic dysfunction and evidence of low cardiac output or end-organ dysfunction. Commonly, these patients will have low blood pressure and evidence of hypoperfusion manifest by cold clammy skin, cool distal extremities, decreased urine output and altered mentation. These agents may also be appropriate in patients who have evidence of elevated filling pressures and an inadequate response to diuretics and parenteral vasodilators or who have worsening renal function in response to diuretic therapy [2, 98]. The guidelines emphasize that there is no evidence to support the routine use of inotropic therapy in patients with acute decompensated heart failure. Patients treated with an inotrope should have frequent blood pressure monitoring and continuous cardiac rhythm monitoring as treatment with these agents has been associated with hypotension and an increased risk of atrial and ventricular arrhythmias. In the ESC guidelines, inotropic agents are not recommended unless the patient is hypotensive (systolic blood pressure of <85 mmHg) and has evidence of hypoperfusion.

The ACCF/AHA guidelines recommend that guideline determined medical therapy (GDMT) including ACEI or ARB, β-blocker and MRA be continued in patients with HFrEF hospitalized with ADHF in the absence of hemodynamic instability, worsening renal function or hypokalemia. In addition, the ACCF/AHA guidelines recommend that medications on admission be reassessed during the ADHF hospitalization and that GDMT be initiated in patients who have HFrEF who are not receiving appropriate GDMT. The HFSA guidelines recommend that "near optimal" pharmacologic therapy, including ACEI and β-blocker, be achieved during the heart failure hospitalization. The ESC guidelines recommend that ACEI or ARB, β-blocker, and MRA be initiated and up-titrated as appropriate in patients with HFrEF and that digoxin may provide symptom benefit and reduce the risk of HF hospitalization in patients with severe systolic HF.

The HFSA guidelines recommend fluid restriction of <2 L/day in patients with ADHF with moderate hyponatremia (serum sodium <130 mEq/L). Stricter fluid restriction may be considered in patients with more severe hyponatremia (serum sodium <125 mEq/L). The ACCF/AHA guidelines recommend fluid restriction and optimization of medications that modulate the RAAS and decrease thirst in patients hospitalized for ADHF who have hyponatremia. These guidelines also recommend consideration of a vasopressin antagonist in patients hospitalized with ADHF who have persistent severe hyponatremia and volume overload (hypervolemic hyponatremia) who are at risk for or are having cognitive symptoms despite water restriction and optimization of GDMT.

The ACCF/AHA and ECS guidelines do not recommend the routine use of invasive hemodynamic monitoring with pulmonary artery catheterization in patients hospitalized for ADHF. PA catheterization should be considered in a patient: who is refractory to pharmacologic therapy; who has persistent clinically significant hypotension; who has significantly worsening renal function in response to therapy; or whose volume status and cardiac filling pressures are uncertain.

The ACCF/AHA, ECS and HFSA guidelines all recommend that patients hospitalized with ADHF who are not already anticoagulated receive venous thromboembolism (VTE) prophylaxis with an anticoagulant medication provided there are no contraindications to anticoagulation and in whom the risk-benefit ratio is favorable (ACCF/AHA). The HFSA guidelines recommend VTE prophylaxis with a mechanical device (intermittent pneumatic compression devices or graded compression stockings) in patients hospitalized with ADHF who have a contraindication to anticoagulation.

References

1. Yancy CW, Jessup M, Bozkurt B, Butler J, Casey Jr DE, Drazner MH, et al.; American College of Cardiology Foundation/American Heart Association Task Force on Practice Guidelines. 2013 ACCF/AHA guideline for the management of heart failure: a report of the American College of Cardiology Foundation/ American Heart Association Task Force on practice guidelines. Circulation. 2013;128(16):e240–327. https://doi.org/10.1161/CIR.0b013e31829e8776. Epub 2013 Jun 5.
2. Lindenfeld J, Albert NM, Boehmer JP, Collins SP, Ezekowitz JA, Givertz MM, et al.; Heart Failure Society of America, HFSA. Comprehensive heart failure practice guideline. Section 12: evaluation and management of patients with acute decompensated heart failure. J Card Fail. 2010;16(6):e131–56. doi:https://doi.org/10.1016/j.cardfail.2010.04.004.
3. Givertz MM, Teerlink JR, Albert NM, Westlake Canary CA, Collins SP, Colvin-Adams M, et al. Acute decompensated heart failure: update on new and emerging evidence and directions for future research. J Card Fail. 2013;19(6):371–89. https://doi.org/10.1016/j.cardfail.2013.04.002.
4. McMurray JJ, Adamopoulos S, Anker SD, Auricchio A, Böhm M, Dickstein K, et al; Task Force for the Diagnosis and Treatment of Acute and Chronic Heart Failure 2012 of the European Society of Cardiology, Bax JJ, Baumgartner H, Ceconi C, Dean V, Deaton C, et al; ESC Committee for Practice Guidelines. ESC guidelines for the diagnosis and treatment of acute and chronic heart failure 2012: The Task Force for the Diagnosis and Treatment of Acute and Chronic Heart Failure 2012 of the European Society of Cardiology. Developed in collaboration with the Heart Failure Association (HFA) of the ESC. Eur J Heart Fail. 2012;14(8):803–69. https://doi.org/10.1093/eurjhf/hfs105. No abstract available. Erratum in: Eur J Heart Fail. 2013;15(3):361.
5. Dickstein K, Cohen-Solal A, Filippatos G, McMurray JJV, Ponikowski P, Poole-Wilson PA, et al. ESC Committee for Practice Guidelines (CPG); ESC Guidelines for the diagnosis and treatment of acute and chronic heart failure 2008: the Task Force for the Diagnosis and Treatment of Acute and Chronic Heart Failure 2008 of the European Society of Cardiology. Developed in collaboration with the Heart Failure Association of the ESC (HFA) and endorsed by the European Society of Intensive Care Medicine (ESICM). Eur Heart J. 2008;29(19):2388–442. https://doi.org/10.1093/eurheartj/ehn309. Epub 2008 Sep 17.
6. Weintraub NL, Collins SP, Pang PS, Levy PD, Anderson AS, Arslanian-Engoren C, et al; American Heart Association Council on Clinical Cardiology and Council on Cardiopulmonary, Critical Care, Perioperative and Resuscitation. Acute heart failure syndromes: emergency department presentation, treatment, and disposition: current approaches and future aims: a scientific statement from the American Heart Association. Circulation. 2010;122(19):1975–96. https://doi.org/10.1161/CIR.0b013e3181f9a223. Epub 2010 Oct 11.
7. Nieminen MS, Brutsaert D, Dickstein K, Drexler H, Follath F, Harjola VP, et al.; EuroHeart Survey Investigators; heart failure association, European Society of Cardiology. EuroHeart Failure Survey II (EHFS II): a survey on hospitalized acute heart failure patients: description of population. Eur Heart J. 2006;27(22):2725–36. Epub 2006 Sep 25.
8. O'Gara PT, Kushner FG, Ascheim DD, Casey DE Jr, Chung MK, et al.; American College of Cardiology Foundation/American Heart Association Task Force on Practice Guidelines. 2013 ACCF/AHA guideline for the management of ST-elevation myocardial infarction: a report of the American College of Cardiology Foundation/American Heart Association Task Force on Practice Guidelines. Circulation. 2013;127(4):e362–425. https://doi.org/10.1161/CIR.0b013e3182742cf6. Epub 2012 Dec 17. No abstract available. Erratum in: Circulation. 2013 Dec 24;128(25):e481.
9. Anderson JL, Adams CD, Antman EM, Bridges CR, Califf RM, Casey DE Jr, et al.; American College of Cardiology Foundation/American Heart Association Task Force on Practice Guidelines. 2012 ACCF/AHA focused update incorporated into the ACCF/AHA 2007 guidelines for the management of patients with unstable angina/non-ST-elevation myocardial infarction: a report of the American College of Cardiology Foundation/American Heart Association Task Force on Practice Guidelines. Circulation. 2013;127(23):e663–828. doi: https://doi.org/10.1161/CIR.0b013e31828478ac. Epub 2013 Apr 29. No abstract available. Erratum in: Circulation. 2013;127(24):e863–4.
10. Thygesen K, Alpert JS, White HD; Joint ESC/ ACCF/AHA/WHF Task Force for the Redefinition of Myocardial Infarction, Jaffe AS, Apple FS, Galvani M, Katus HA, Newby LK, Ravkilde J, et al. Universal definition of myocardial infarction. Circulation. 2007;116(22):2634–53. Epub 2007 Oct 19.
11. Wang CS, FitzGerald JM, Schulzer M, Mak E, Ayas NT. Does this dyspneic patient in the emergency department have congestive heart failure? JAMA. 2005;294(15):1944–56.
12. Davie AP, Francis CM, Love MP, Caruana L, Starkey IR, Shaw TR, et al. Value of the electrocardiogram in

identifying heart failure due to left ventricular systolic dysfunction. BMJ. 1996;312(7025):222.
13. Maisel AS, Krishnaswamy P, Nowak RM, McCord J, Hollander JE, Duc P, et al; Breathing Not Properly Multinational Study Investigators. Rapid measurement of B-type natriuretic peptide in the emergency diagnosis of heart failure. N Engl J Med. 2002;347(3):161–7.
14. Maisel AS, Clopton P, Krishnaswamy P, Nowak RM, McCord J, Hollander JE, et al; BNP Multinational Study Investigators. Impact of age, race, and sex on the ability of B-type natriuretic peptide to aid in the emergency diagnosis of heart failure: results from the breathing not properly (BNP) multinational study. Am Heart J. 2004;147(6):1078–84.
15. Wang TJ, Larson MG, Levy D, Benjamin EJ, Leip EP, Wilson PW, Vasan RS. Impact of obesity on plasma natriuretic peptide levels. Circulation. 2004;109(5):594–600.
16. Peacock WF, Mueller C, Disomma S, Maisel A. Emergency department perspectives on B-type natriuretic peptide utility. Congest Heart Fail. 2008;14(4 Suppl 1):17–20. Review
17. Maisel A, Mueller C, Adams JK, Anker SD, Aspromonte N, Cleland JG, et al. State of the art: using natriuretic peptide levels in clinical practice. Eur J Heart Fail. 2008;10(9):824–39. https://doi.org/10.1016/j.ejheart.2008.07.014. Epub 2008 Aug 29
18. Bayes-Genis A, Lloyd-Jones DM, van Kimmenade RR, Lainchbury JG, Richards AM, Ordoñez-Llanos J, et al. Effect of body mass index on diagnostic and prognostic usefulness of amino-terminal pro-brain natriuretic peptide in patients with acute dyspnea. Arch Intern Med. 2007;167(4):400–7.
19. Januzzi JL Jr, Camargo CA, Anwaruddin S, Baggish AL, Chen AA, Krauser DG, et al. The N-terminal Pro-BNP investigation of dyspnea in the emergency department (PRIDE) study. Am J Cardiol. 2005;95(8):948–54.
20. Januzzi JJL, Chen-Tournoux AA, Moe G. Amino-terminal pro-B-type natriuretic peptide testing for the diagnosis or exclusion of heart failure in patients with acute symptoms. Am J Cardiol. 2008;101(3A):29–38. https://doi.org/10.1016/j.amjcard.2007.11.017.
21. Collins SP, Lindsell CJ, Storrow AB, Abraham WT; ADHERE Scientific Advisory Committee, Investigators and Study Group. Prevalence of negative chest radiography results in the emergency department patient with decompensated heart failure. Ann Emerg Med. 2006;47(1):13–8. Epub 2005 Jun 20.
22. Januzzi JL, van Kimmenade R, Lainchbury J, Bayes-Genis A, Ordonez-Llanos J, Santalo-Bel M, et al. NT-proBNP testing for diagnosis and short-term prognosis in acute destabilized heart failure: an international pooled analysis of 1256 patients: the International Collaborative of NT-proBNP Study. Eur Heart J. 2006;27(3):330–7. Epub 2005 Nov 17
23. Collins S, Storrow AB, Albert NM, Butler J, Ezekowitz J, Felker GM, et al; SAEM/HFSA Acute Heart Failure Working Group. Early management of patients with acute heart failure: state of the art and future directions. A consensus document from the society for academic emergency medicine/heart failure society of America acute heart failure working group. J Card Fail. 2015;21(1):27–43. https://doi.org/10.1016/j.cardfail.2014.07.003. Epub 2014 Jul 18.
24. Fonarow GC, Abraham WT, Albert NM, Stough WG, Gheorghiade M, Greenberg BH, et al; OPTIMIZE-HF Investigators and Hospitals. Factors identified as precipitating hospital admissions for heart failure and clinical outcomes: findings from OPTIMIZE-HF. Arch Intern Med. 2008;168(8):847–54. https://doi.org/10.1001/archinte.168.8.847.
25. Adams KF, Fonarow GC, Emerman CL, LeJemtel TH, Costanzo MR, Abraham WT, et al.; ADHERE Scientific Advisory Committee and Investigators. Characteristics and outcomes of patients hospitalized for heart failure in the United States: rationale, design, and preliminary observations from the first 100,000 cases in the Acute Decompensated Heart Failure National Registry (ADHERE). Am Heart J. 2005;149(2):209–16.
26. Fonarow GC, Heywood JT, Heidenreich PA, Lopatin M, Yancy CW; ADHERE Scientific Advisory Committee and Investigators. Temporal trends in clinical characteristics, treatments, and outcomes for heart failure hospitalizations, 2002 to 2004: findings from Acute Decompensated Heart Failure National Registry (ADHERE). Am Heart J. 2007;153(6):1021–8.
27. Cleland JG, Swedberg K, Follath F, Komajda M, Cohen-Solal A, Aguilar JC, et al.; Study Group on Diagnosis of the Working Group on Heart Failure of the European Society of Cardiology. The EuroHeart Failure survey programme-- a survey on the quality of care among patients with heart failure in Europe. Part 1: patient characteristics and diagnosis. Eur Heart J. 2003;24(5):442–63.
28. Fonarow GC, Abraham WT, Albert NM, Stough WG, Gheorghiade M, Greenberg BH, et al; OPTIMIZE-HF Investigators and Hospitals. Age- and gender-related differences in quality of care and outcomes of patients hospitalized with heart failure (from OPTIMIZE-HF). Am J Cardiol 2009;104(1):107–15. https://doi.org/10.1016/j.amjcard.2009.02.057.
29. Gheorghiade M, Sopko G, De Luca L, Velazquez EJ, Parker JD, Binkley PF, et al. Navigating the crossroads of coronary artery disease and heart failure. Circulation. 2006;114(11):1202–13.
30. Flaherty JD, Bax JJ, De Luca L, Rossi JS, Davidson CJ, Filippatos G, et al; Acute Heart Failure Syndromes International Working Group. Acute heart failure syndromes in patients with coronary artery disease early assessment and treatment. J Am Coll Cardiol. 2009;53(3):254–63. https://doi.org/10.1016/j.jacc.2008.08.072.
31. Steg PG, Dabbous OH, Feldman LJ, Cohen-Solal A, Aumont MC, López-Sendón J, Global Registry of Acute Coronary Events Investigators, et al.

Determinants and prognostic impact of heart failure complicating acute coronary syndromes: observations from the Global Registry of Acute Coronary Events (GRACE). Circulation. 2004;109(4):494–9. Epub 2004 Jan 26
32. Wu AH, Parsons L, Every NR, Bates ER, Second National Registry of Myocardial Infarction. Hospital outcomes in patients presenting with congestive heart failure complicating acute myocardial infarction: a report from the Second National Registry of Myocardial Infarction (NRMI-2). J Am Coll Cardiol. 2002;40(8):1389–94.
33. Spencer FA, Meyer TE, Gore JM, Goldberg RJ. Heterogeneity in the management and outcomes of patients with acute myocardial infarction complicated by heart failure: the National Registry of Myocardial Infarction. Circulation. 2002;105(22):2605–10.
34. Cuffe MS, Califf RM, Adams KF Jr, Benza R, Bourge R, Colucci WS, et al; Outcomes of a Prospective Trial of Intravenous Milrinone for Exacerbations of Chronic Heart Failure (OPTIME-CHF) Investigators. Short-term intravenous milrinone for acute exacerbation of chronic heart failure: a randomized controlled trial. JAMA. 2002;287(12):1541–7.
35. McManus DD, Saczynski JS, Lessard D, Kinno M, Pidikiti R, Esa N, et al. Recent trends in the incidence, treatment, and prognosis of patients with heart failure and atrial fibrillation (the Worcester Heart Failure Study). Am J Cardiol. 2013;111(10):1460–5. https://doi.org/10.1016/j.amjcard.2013.01.298.
36. Rossi JS, Flaherty JD, Fonarow GC, Nunez E, Gattis Stough W, Abraham WT, et al. Influence of coronary artery disease and coronary revascularization status on outcomes in patients with acute heart failure syndromes: a report from OPTIMIZE-HF (Organized Program to Initiate Lifesaving Treatment in Hospitalized Patients with Heart Failure). Eur J Heart Fail. 2008;10(12):1215–23. https://doi.org/10.1016/j.ejheart.2008.09.009. Epub 2008 Nov 8. Now #62
37. Flaherty JD, Rossi JS, Fonarow GC, Nunez E, Stough WG, Abraham WT, et al. Influence of coronary angiography on the utilization of therapies in patients with acute heart failure syndromes: findings from Organized Program to Initiate Lifesaving Treatment in Hospitalized Patients with Heart Failure (OPTIMIZE-HF). Am Heart J. 2009;157(6):1018–25. https://doi.org/10.1016/j.ahj.2009.03.011. Epub 2009 Apr 23
38. Velazquez EJ, Lee KL, Deja MA, Jain A, Sopko G, Marchenko A, STICH Investigators, et al. Coronary-artery bypass surgery in patients with left ventricular dysfunction. N Engl J Med. 2011;364(17):1607–16. https://doi.org/10.1056/NEJMoa1100356. Epub 2011 Apr 4
39. Bonow RO, Maurer G, Lee KL, Holly TA, Binkley PF, Desvigne-Nickens P, STICH Trial Investigators, et al. Myocardial viability and survival in ischemic left ventricular dysfunction. N Engl J Med. 2011;364(17):1617–25. https://doi.org/10.1056/NEJMoa1100358. Epub 2011 Apr 4
40. Panza JA, Holly TA, Asch FM, She L, Pellikka PA, Velazquez EJ. Inducible myocardial ischemia and outcomes in patients with coronary artery disease and left ventricular dysfunction. J Am Coll Cardiol. 2013;61(18):1860–70. https://doi.org/10.1016/j.jacc.2013.02.014. Epub 2013 Mar 7
41. Gandhi SK, Powers JC, Nomeir AM, Fowle K, Kitzman DW, Rankin KM, Little WC. The pathogenesis of acute pulmonary edema associated with hypertension. N Engl J Med. 2001;344(1):17–22.
42. Fonarow GC, Stough WG, Abraham WT, Albert NM, Gheorghiade M, Greenberg BH, OPTIMIZE-HF Investigators and Hospitals, et al. Characteristics, treatments, and outcomes of patients with preserved systolic function hospitalized for heart failure: a report from the OPTIMIZE-HF Registry. J Am Coll Cardiol. 2007;50(8):768–77.
43. Tavazzi L, Maggioni AP, Lucci D, Cacciatore G, Ansalone G, Oliva F, Porcu M, Italian survey on Acute Heart Failure Investigators. Nationwide survey on acute heart failure in cardiology ward services in Italy. Eur Heart J. 2006;27(10):1207–15. Epub 2006 Apr 7. PubMed – indexed for MEDLINE 1
44. Mountantonakis SE, Grau-Sepulveda MV, Bhatt DL, Hernandez AF, Peterson ED, Fonarow GC. Presence of atrial fibrillation is independently associated with adverse outcomes in patients hospitalized with heart failure: an analysis of get with the guidelines-heart failure. Circ Heart Fail. 2012;5(2):191–201. https://doi.org/10.1161/CIRCHEARTFAILURE.111.965681. Epub 2012 Feb 23
45. Ambrosy AP, Fonarow GC, Butler J, Chioncel O, Greene SJ, Vaduganathan M, et al. The global health and economic burden of hospitalizations for heart failure: lessons learned from hospitalized heart failure registries. J Am Coll Cardiol. 2014;63(12):1123–33. https://doi.org/10.1016/j.jacc.2013.11.053. Epub 2014 Feb 5
46. Rosca M, Lancellotti P, Popescu BA, Piérard LA. Left atrial function: pathophysiology, echocardiographic assessment, and clinical applications. Heart. 2011;97(23):1982–9. https://doi.org/10.1136/heartjnl-2011-300069.
47. Melenovsky V, Hwang SJ, Redfield MM, Zakeri R, Lin G, Borlaug BA. Left atrial remodeling and function in advanced heart failure with preserved or reduced ejection fraction. Circ Heart Fail. 2015;8(2):295–303. https://doi.org/10.1161/CIRCHEARTFAILURE.114.001667. Epub 2015 Jan 15
48. Eugenio PL. Frequent premature ventricular contractions: an electrical link to cardiomyopathy. Cardiol Rev. 2015;32:168.
49. El Kadri M, Yokokawa M, Labounty T, Mueller G, Crawford T, Good E, et al. Effect of ablation of frequent premature ventricular complexes on left ventricular function in patients with nonischemic cardiomyopathy. Heart Rhythm. 2015;12(4):706–13. https://doi.org/10.1016/j.hrthm.2014.12.017. Epub 2014 Dec 16

50. Kumar S, Stevenson WG, John RM. Catheter ablation for premature ventricular contractions and ventricular tachycardia in patients with heart failure. Curr Cardiol Rep. 2014;16(9):522. https://doi.org/10.1007/s11886-014-0522-3.
51. Baman TS, Lange DC, Ilg KJ, Gupta SK, Liu TY, Alguire C, et al. Relationship between burden of premature ventricular complexes and left ventricular function. Heart Rhythm. 2010;7(7):865–9. https://doi.org/10.1016/j.hrthm.2010.03.036. Epub 2010 Mar 27
52. Michalsen A, König G, Thimme W. Preventable causative factors leading to hospital admission with decompensated heart failure. Heart. 1998;80(5):437–41.
53. Diaz A, Ciocchini C, Esperatti M, Becerra A, Mainardi S, Farah A. Precipitating factors leading to decompensation of chronic heart failure in the elderly patient in South-American community hospital. J Geriatr Cardiol. 2011;8(1):12–4. https://doi.org/10.3724/SP.J.1263.2011.00012.
54. Wu JR, Moser DK, Chung ML, Lennie TA. Predictors of medication adherence using a multidimensional adherence model in patients with heart failure. J Card Fail. 2008;14(7):603–14. https://doi.org/10.1016/j.cardfail.2008.02.011. Epub 2008 May 27
55. Mathes T, Jaschinski T, Pieper D. Adherence influencing factors—a systematic review of systematic reviews. Arch Public Health. 2014;72(1):37. https://doi.org/10.1186/2049-3258-72-37. eCollection 2014
56. Waldréus N, Hahn RG, Jaarsma T. Thirst in heart failure: a systematic literature review. Eur J Heart Fail. 2013;15(2):141–9. https://doi.org/10.1093/eurjhf/hfs174. Epub 2012 Nov 23
57. Coble JP, Grobe JL, Johnson AK, Sigmund CD. Mechanisms of brain renin angiotensin system-induced drinking and blood pressure: importance of the subfornical organ. Am J Phys Regul Integr Comp Phys. 2015;308(4):R238–49. https://doi.org/10.1152/ajpregu.00486.2014. Epub 2014 Dec 17
58. Menani JV, De Luca Jr LA, Johnson AK. Role of the lateral parabrachial nucleus in the control of sodium appetite. Am J Phys Regul Integr Comp Phys. 2014;306(4):R201–10. https://doi.org/10.1152/ajpregu.00251.2012. Epub 2014 Jan 8
59. Bourque CW. Central mechanisms of osmosensation and systemic osmoregulation. Nat Rev Neurosci. 2008;9(7):519–31. https://doi.org/10.1038/nrn2400. Epub 2008 May 29
60. Wessler JD, Hummel SL, Maurer MS. Dietary interventions for heart failure in older adults: re-emergence of the hedonic shift. Prog Cardiovasc Dis. 2014;57(2):160–7. https://doi.org/10.1016/j.pcad.2014.03.007. Epub 2014 Mar 12
61. Cugno M, Mari D, Meroni PL, Gronda E, Vicari F, Frigerio M, et al. Haemostatic and inflammatory biomarkers in advanced chronic heart failure: role of oral anticoagulants and successful heart transplantation. Br J Haematol. 2004;126(1):85–92.
62. Lip GY, Gibbs CR. Does heart failure confer a hypercoagulable state? Virchow's triad revisited. J Am Coll Cardiol. 1999;33(5):1424–6.
63. de Peuter OR, Kok WE, Torp-Pedersen C, Büller HR, Kamphuisen PW. Systolic heart failure: a prothrombotic state. Semin Thromb Hemost. 2009;35(5):497–504. https://doi.org/10.1055/s--0029-1234145. Epub 2009 Sep 8
64. Stein PD, Sostman HD, Hull RD, Goodman LR, Leeper KV Jr, Gottschalk A, et al. Diagnosis of pulmonary embolism in the coronary care unit. Am J Cardiol. 2009;103(6):881–6. https://doi.org/10.1016/j.amjcard.2008.11.040. Epub 2009 Jan 24
65. Costanzo MR, Khayat R, Ponikowski P, Augostini R, Stellbrink C, Mianulli M, Abraham WT. Mechanisms and clinical consequences of untreated central sleep apnea in heart failure. J Am Coll Cardiol. 2015;65(1):72–84. https://doi.org/10.1016/j.jacc.2014.10.025.
66. Valdivia-Arenas MA, Powers M, Khayat RN. Sleep-disordered breathing in patients with decompensated heart failure. Heart Fail Rev. 2009;14(3):183–93. https://doi.org/10.1007/s10741-008-9103-0. Epub 2008 Aug 29
67. Khayat R, Jarjoura D, Porter K, Sow A, Wannemacher J, Dohar R, et al. Sleep disordered breathing and post-discharge mortality in patients with acute heart failure. Eur Heart J. 2015;36:1463–9.
68. Zanotti-Cavazzoni SL, Hollenberg SM. Cardiac dysfunction in severe sepsis and septic shock. Curr Opin Crit Care. 2009;15(5):392–7. https://doi.org/10.1097/MCC.0b013e3283307a4e.
69. Flynn A, Chokkalingam Mani B, Mather PJ. Sepsis-induced cardiomyopathy: a review of pathophysiologic mechanisms. Heart Fail Rev. 2010;15(6):605–11. https://doi.org/10.1007/s10741-010-9176-4.
70. Klein I, Danzi S. Thyroid disease and the heart. Circulation. 2007;116(15):1725–35.
71. Cooper DS, Biondi B. Subclinical thyroid disease. Lancet. 2012;379(9821):1142–54. https://doi.org/10.1016/S0140-6736(11)60276-6. Epub 2012 Jan 23
72. Bogazzi F, Tomisti L, Bartalena L, Aghini-Lombardi F, Martino E. Amiodarone and the thyroid: a 2012 update. J Endocrinol Investig. 2012;35(3):340–8. https://doi.org/10.3275/8298. Epub 2012 Mar 19
73. Bhala N, Emberson J, Merhi A, Abramson S, Arber N, et al; Coxib and traditional NSAID Trialists' (CNT) Collaboration. Vascular and upper gastrointestinal effects of non-steroidal anti-inflammatory drugs: meta-analyses of individual participant data from randomised trials. Lancet. 2013;382(9894) https://doi.org/10.1016/S0140-6736(13)60900-9. Epub 2013 May 30.
74. Gilbert RE, Krum H. Heart failure in diabetes: effects of anti-hyperglycaemic drug therapy. Lancet. 2015;385(9982):2107–17. https://doi.org/10.1016/S0140-6736(14)61402-1.
75. Guan Y, Hao C, Cha DR, Rao R, Lu W, Kohan DE, et al. Thiazolidinediones expand body fluid volume through PPARgamma stimulation of ENaC-mediated

renal salt absorption. Nat Med. 2005;11(8):861–6. Epub 2005 Jul 10
76. Seki G, Endo Y, Suzuki M, Yamada H, Horita S, Fujita T. Role of renal proximal tubule transport in thiazolidinedione-induced volume expansion. World J Nephrol. 2012;1(5):146–50. https://doi.org/10.5527/wjn.v1.i5.146.
77. Emoto M, Fukuda N, Nakamori Y, Taguchi A, Okuya S, Oka Y, Tanizawa Y. Plasma concentrations of vascular endothelial growth factor are associated with peripheral oedema in patients treated with thiazolidinedione. Diabetologia. 2006;49(9):2217–8. Epub 2006 Jul 1
78. Murphy N, Mockler M, Ryder M, Ledwidge M, McDonald K. Decompensation of chronic heart failure associated with pregabalin in patients with neuropathic pain. J Card Fail. 2007;13(3):227–9.
79. Curigliano G, Mayer EL, Burstein HJ, Winer EP, Goldhirsch A. Cardiac toxicity from systemic cancer therapy: a comprehensive review. Prog Cardiovasc Dis. 2010;53(2):94–104. https://doi.org/10.1016/j.pcad.2010.05.006.
80. Berardi R, Caramanti M, Savini A, Chiorrini S, Pierantoni C, Onofri A, et al. State of the art for cardiotoxicity due to chemotherapy and to targeted therapies: a literature review. Crit Rev Oncol Hematol. 2013;88(1):75–86. https://doi.org/10.1016/j.critrevonc.2013.02.007. Epub 2013 Mar 21
81. Albini A, Pennesi G, Donatelli F, Cammarota R, De Flora S, Noonan DM. Cardiotoxicity of anticancer drugs: the need for cardio-oncology and cardio-oncological prevention. J Natl Cancer Inst. 2010;102(1):14–25. https://doi.org/10.1093/jnci/djp440. Epub 2009 Dec 10
82. Bhave M, Akhter N, Rosen ST. Cardiovascular toxicity of biologic agents for cancer therapy. Oncology (Williston Park). 2014;28(6):482–90.
83. Accordino MK, Neugut AI, Hershman DL. Cardiac effects of anticancer therapy in the elderly. J Clin Oncol. 2014;32(24):2654–61. https://doi.org/10.1200/JCO.2013.55.0459. Epub 2014 Jul 28
84. Iacovoni A, De Maria R, Gavazzi A. Alcoholic cardiomyopathy. J Cardiovasc Med (Hagerstown). 2010;11(12):884–92. https://doi.org/10.2459/JCM.0b013e32833833a3.
85. Awtry EH, Philippides GJ. Alcoholic and cocaine-associated cardiomyopathies. Prog Cardiovasc Dis. 2010;52(4):289–99. https://doi.org/10.1016/j.pcad.2009.11.004.
86. Maraj S, Figueredo VM, Lynn MD. Cocaine and the heart. Clin Cardiol. 2010;33(5):264–9. https://doi.org/10.1002/clc.20746.
87. Phillips K, Luk A, Soor GS, Abraham JR, Leong S, Butany J. Cocaine cardiotoxicity: a review of the pathophysiology, pathology, and treatment options. Am J Cardiovasc Drugs. 2009;9(3):177–96. https://doi.org/10.2165/00129784-200909030-00005.
88. Figueredo VM. Chemical cardiomyopathies: the negative effects of medications and nonprescribed drugs on the heart. Am J Med. 2011;124(6):480–8. https://doi.org/10.1016/j.amjmed.2010.11.031.
89. Won S, Hong RA, Shohet RV, Seto TB, Parikh NI. Methamphetamine-associated cardiomyopathy. Clin Cardiol. 2013;36(12):737–42. https://doi.org/10.1002/clc.22195. Epub 2013 Aug 27
90. Tops LF, Schalij MJ, Bax JJ. The effects of right ventricular apical pacing on ventricular function and dyssynchrony implications for therapy. J Am Coll Cardiol. 2009;54(9):764–76. https://doi.org/10.1016/j.jacc.2009.06.006.
91. Akerström F, Pachón M, Puchol A, Jiménez-López J, Segovia D, Rodríguez-Padial L, Arias MA. Chronic right ventricular apical pacing: adverse effects and current therapeutic strategies to minimize them. Int J Cardiol. 2014;173(3):351–60. https://doi.org/10.1016/j.ijcard.2014.03.079. Epub 2014 Mar 20
92. Gheorghiade M, Abraham WT, Albert NM, Greenberg BH, O'Connor CM, She L, et al; OPTIMIZE-HF Investigators and Coordinators. Systolic blood pressure at admission, clinical characteristics, and outcomes in patients hospitalized with acute heart failure. JAMA. 2006;296(18):2217–26.
93. Damman K, Voors AA, Navis G, van Veldhuisen DJ, Hillege HL. The cardiorenal syndrome in heart failure. Prog Cardiovasc Dis. 2011;54(2):144–53. https://doi.org/10.1016/j.pcad.2011.01.003.
94. Berry SJ, Coffey DS, Walsh PC, Ewing LL. The development of human benign prostatic hyperplasia with age. J Urol. 1984;132(3):474–9.
95. Chute CG, Panser LA, Girman CJ, Oesterling JE, Guess HA, Jacobsen SJ, Lieber MM. The prevalence of prostatism: a population-based survey of urinary symptoms. J Urol. 1993;150(1):85–9.
96. Mebazaa A, Pang PS, Tavares M, Collins SP, Storrow AB, Laribi S, et al. The impact of early standard therapy on dyspnoea in patients with acute heart failure: the URGENT-dyspnoea study. Eur Heart J. 2010;31(7):832–41. https://doi.org/10.1093/eurheartj/ehp458. Epub 2009 Nov 11
97. Stevenson LW, Tillisch JH. Maintenance of cardiac output with normal filling pressures in patients with dilated heart failure. Circulation. 1986;74(6):1303–8.
98. Hunt SA, Abraham WT, Chin MH, Feldman AM, Francis GS, Ganiats TG, et al. 2009 focused update incorporated into the ACC/AHA 2005 Guidelines for the Diagnosis and Management of Heart Failure in Adults: a report of the American College of Cardiology Foundation/American Heart Association Task Force on Practice Guidelines: developed in collaboration with the International Society for Heart and Lung Transplantation. Circulation. 2009;119(14):e391–479. https://doi.org/10.1161/CIRCULATIONAHA.109.192065. Epub 2009 Mar 26

13 Acute Decompensated Heart Failure: Treatment—Specific Therapies

Daniel Fishbein

There have been few prospective randomized clinical trials conducted to guide treatment of patients with ADHF. Many of the guideline recommendations are based on broad clinical experience, registry data, meta-analyses, and a limited number of prospective, randomized clinical trials.

Oxygen

Routine administration of oxygen is recommended in patients with hypoxia (ESC, ACC/AHA, and HFSA guidelines). While there are no randomized trials of oxygen in ADHF, improvement in systemic and myocardial oxygenation would be expected to improve symptoms and clinical status of the patient with ADHF. Supplemental oxygen is recommended for patients with acute myocardial infarction complicated by heart failure. In some patients, oxygen may lower elevated pulmonary vascular resistance and improve right heart failure. However, routine administration of oxygen in the presence of normal oxygen saturations on room air is not recommended. In patients with a history of chronic obstructive pulmonary disease, high concentrations of oxygen can result in respiratory depression and worsening hypercapnia. High concentrations of inhaled oxygen have been shown to decrease cardiac output and increase systemic vascular resistance in patients with stable mild-moderate heart failure and LV systolic dysfunction [1].

Morphine

Morphine has been used in patients with ADHF for decades. Proposed mechanisms of benefit include reduction in dyspnea and anxiety, a resulting decrease in sympathetic tone with a reduction in afterload, and venodilation with a reduction in preload [2]. Venodilation seems to be mediated by histamine release and not by opiate receptors [3]. There is some controversy about whether morphine reduces left sided filling pressures in ADHF [4]. Morphine causes nausea and reduces respiratory drive. Despite long-standing practice, there is little prospective data to support the use of morphine in ADHF. Several studies have suggested an increase in adverse events in patients with ADHF treated with morphine [5, 6]. An analysis from the ADHERE registry found that treatment with intravenous morphine was a predictor of in-hospital adverse events [7]. Patients who received morphine were more likely to require mechanical ventilation (15.4% vs 2.8%), had a longer median hospitalization (5.6 days vs 4.2 days), more ICU admissions (38.7% vs 14.4%), and had a greater

D. Fishbein (✉)
Department of Medicine, Division of Cardiology, University of Washington Medical Center, Seattle, WA, USA
e-mail: dfish@uw.edu

H. J. Eisen (ed.), *Heart Failure I*, https://doi.org/10.1007/978-3-032-12626-9_13

in-hospital mortality (13.0% vs 2.4%) (all $p < 0.001$). After risk adjustment and exclusion of ventilated patients, morphine remained an independent predictor of mortality with a HR of 4.84 ($p < 0.001$). Despite risk adjustment, some of this data may be confounded by the likelihood that patients who received morphine were sicker. The HFSA Guidelines recommend caution "that if used at all, [morphine] should be used with caution, especially in patients with abnormal mental status or impaired respiratory drive" [8].

Noninvasive Ventilation (NIV)

Patients with severe decompensated heart failure may present with acute respiratory distress and severe hypoxia related to extravasation of fluid into the alveoli, dilution of surfactant, decrease in oxygen uptake, alveolar collapse, intrapulmonary shunting and VQ mismatch. Positive pressure ventilation decreases work of breathing, improves oxygenation, improves lung compliance by recruiting previously collapsed alveoli, reduces respiratory distress, reduces afterload and improves cardiac output [9]. Patients with ADHF and acute cardiogenic pulmonary edema may be supported with noninvasive methods of ventilation (NIV) also known as noninvasive positive pressure ventilation (NPPV).

There are two common methods of delivering NIV. Continuous positive airway pressure (CPAP) maintains the same positive pressure throughout the respiratory cycle. Noninvasive intermittent positive pressure ventilation (NIPPV), also referred to as bi-level noninvasive pressure support ventilation (NIPSV), increases airway pressure more during inspiration than expiration.

Several meta-analyses of predominantly small single-center randomized trials that compared NIV with standard therapy in patients with acute cardiogenic pulmonary edema found that NIV significantly reduced mortality and the need for intubation/mechanical ventilation. The level of evidence was greater for CPAP than NIPPV [10, 11]. In an analysis of three studies comparing CPAP with NIPPV in acute cardiogenic pulmonary edema, estimates of the incidence of new myocardial infarction were increased in the NIPPV group (relative risk 1.99; $p = 0.03$) [11]. This finding was driven by the results from a small study of 27 patients with acute pulmonary edema randomized to CPAP or NIPPV [12].

The Three Interventions in Cardiogenic Pulmonary Oedema (3CPO) trial randomized 1069 patients with acute cardiogenic pulmonary edema to standard oxygen therapy, CPAP, or NIPPV. There was no difference in 7-day mortality between patients receiving standard oxygen therapy and those receiving NIV. There was no difference in the combined end point of death or intubation at 7 days between the patients randomized to CPAP or NIPPV. NIV was associated with greater mean improvements at 1 h after initiation of therapy in patient-reported dyspnea, heart rate, acidosis, and hypercapnea. Patients receiving standard oxygen therapy and those receiving NIV had similar rates of endo tracheal intubation, admission to the critical care unit, and myocardial infarction. Patients receiving CPAP and those receiving NIPPV also had similar rates of these outcomes. There were no differences in the rates of myocardial infarction between the three groups. There was no difference in the rate of myocardial infarction when standard oxygen therapy was compared with NIV and when CPAP was compared with NIPPV [13]. One of the criticisms of the 3CPO Trial was the lower than expected rate of intubation (2.8%) and the lower than expected 7-day mortality (9.8%) in the control group. There was a 15.3% crossover rate between standard therapy and NIV. The lower event rates decreased the power of the study to show a difference between standard oxygen therapy and NIV. It is possible that the population studied was not sick enough to show a benefit from NIV and that those patients with more severe compromise in the control group crossed over to NIV support [14].

Two subsequent meta-analyses that included patients in the 3CPO Trial found that NIV reduced morality and endotracheal intubation when compared with standard therapy in patients with acute cardiogenic pulmonary edema [14, 15]. The Cochran analysis suggested that CPAP should be considered the first option in the selection of NIV in light of more robust evidence of safety and effectiveness when compared with NIPPV.

A recent meta-analysis of randomized studies compared out-of-hospital NIV with "standard" therapy for treatment of adults with severe respiratory distress. NIV used by emergency medical services for treatment of patients in respiratory distress reduced in-hospital mortality (RR = 0.58) and the need for endotracheal intubation (RR = 0.37) when compared with standard therapy. Four of seven studies in the analysis included only patients with suspected acute cardiogenic pulmonary edema. An additional two studies included patients with cardiogenic pulmonary edema and other causes of respiratory distress [16].

The HFSA Practice Guidelines recommend that the "use of non-invasive positive pressure ventilation may be considered for severely dyspneic patients with clinical evidence of pulmonary edema" (Strength of Evidence A). The ESC guidelines suggest that NIV may be used as adjunctive therapy to relieve symptoms in patients with pulmonary edema and severe respiratory distress or patients who fail to improve with pharmacologic therapy.

Contraindications to NIV include: immediate need for intubation; inability to cooperate because of anxiety, decreased level of consciousness or severe cognitive impairment; inability to tolerate the mask; and vomiting. Adverse effects include: worsening of severe right heart failure; hypercapnia; anxiety; claustrophobia; pneumothorax; and aspiration. Caution should be exercised in patients with cardiogenic shock, COPD, or severe right heart failure [17]. Endotracheal intubation and mechanical ventilation should be reserved for patients with: respiratory failure leading to hypercapnia and respiratory acidosis; hypoxia that cannot be corrected with oxygen by nasal cannula, mask or NIV; physical exhaustion; diminished consciousness; and/or inability to maintain or protect their airway [18].

Diuretic Therapy

Diuretics differ in their site and mechanism of action and in their impact on sodium and water excretion. Diuretics are classified by their site of action in the nephron (loop diuretics), chemical structure (thiazides), mode of action (MRAs, carbonic anhydrase inhibitors), and/or specific physiologic effects (potassium sparing diuretics). Figure 13.1 outlines the site of action in the nephron of each class of diuretic [19].

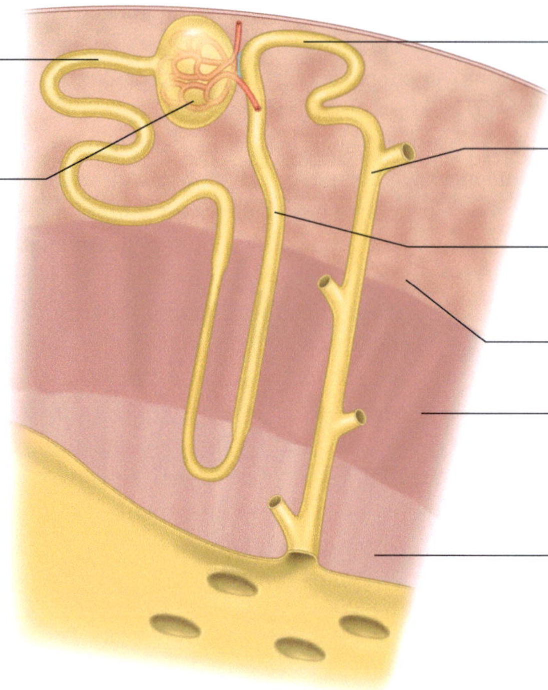

Fig. 13.1 Schematic diagram of the nephron demonstrating the site of action of diuretics [19]

Loop Diuretics (LD)

Pharmacokinetics/Pharmacology

LDs are first line therapy in the treatment of patients with ADHF. Of all diuretic classes, LDs have the most immediate onset of action when given intravenously and the greatest impact on sodium and water excretion. Furosemide, bumetanide, and torsemide are sulfonamide loop diuretics that reversibly bind to and reversibly inhibit the Na^+: K^+:$2Cl^-$ co-transporter on the apical membrane of epithelial cells in the thick ascending limb of the loop of Henle. LDs inhibit sodium transport at this site in the nephron. Loop diuretics can increase sodium excretion by as much as 20–25% of filtered sodium and augment excretion of both sodium and water. Inhibition of the co-transporter also inhibits reabsorption of calcium and magnesium. The increased sodium delivered to the distal convoluted tubule significantly increases the excretion of urinary potassium via the sodium potassium co-transporter. This effect is amplified by elevated levels of aldosterone typically seen in patients with ADHF. Loop diuretics indirectly decrease the reabsorption of water in the collecting ducts by decreasing the concentration of sodium in the medullary interstitium resulting in a decrease in the driving force for water reabsorption in the collecting duct. Urine produced in response to LDs is mildly hypotonic when compared with plasma [19–26].

Ethacrynic acid is a non-sulfonamide loop diuretic that inhibits reabsorption of sodium and chloride in the ascending loop of Henle and distal renal tubule by interfering with the chloride-binding co-transport system, causing increased excretion of water, sodium, chloride, magnesium, and calcium. Ethacrynic is a less effective diuretic than the other three loop diuretics, is probably more ototoxic at high doses, and is cumbersome to administer intravenously because of its relative insolubility. Its use is limited to patients who have an allergy to sulfonamide LDs [27].

An adequate intraluminal concentration of diuretic is needed for LDs to be effective. Because LDs are extensively bound to plasma proteins, delivery to the loop of Henley by glomerular filtration is limited. LDs are secreted into the intraluminal space of the nephron by the organic acid transport system in the proximal tubule. Intraluminal concentration is dependent on dose, bioavailability, adequate renal blood flow and adequate proximal tubule secretory function. Secretion into the proximal tubule may be impaired in heart failure by a decrease in renal plasma flow. In addition, in renal insufficiency, the accumulation of organic anions (e.g., blood urea nitrogen) competes with LDs for the receptor sites of the organic anion transporter. Higher doses are required to overcome this competitive inhibition and to obtain therapeutic urinary concentrations in patients with heart failure and renal impairment [20, 25].

Loop diuretics have an "S" shaped dose-response curve characterized by a threshold concentration below which no diuresis occurs (the minimal effective concentration), a steep increase in dose response, and a concentration ceiling above which no additional diuretic effect is seen. Diuretic effect is dependent on achieving an adequate or "threshold" intraluminal concentration of diuretic in the thick ascending limb of the loop of Henle. In heart failure, the dose response curve is shifted downward and to the right so that a higher concentration of LD is needed to induce a diuresis and the peak response is decreased (see Fig. 13.2) [23].

The dose response curve has a number of clinical implications. First, there is a threshold concentration of LD that needs to be achieved at the active site to elicit any diuretic response. Diuretic doses that achieve intraluminal concentrations below threshold are ineffective so that it is important to demonstrate a response to a specific dose of LD rather than give an inadequate dose more frequently. Because of individual differences in diuretic sensitivity and pharmacokinetics, the dose that achieves threshold concentrations differs among patients. Second, the diuretic ceiling limits the maximal effect of increasing diuretic dose. A ceiling dose of diuretic can be identified in individual patients (the lowest dose of LD that elicits a maximal response). If additional diuresis is needed, the dosing frequency should be increased rather than increasing the LD dose above the ceiling dose [19, 25].

When a bolus of LD is administered, there is generally a diuretic response within 30 minutes that peaks in 1 hour provided that the intraluminal concentration of diuretic is above the threshold concentration in the loop of Henle. When the intraluminal concentration of LD declines below the threshold concentration, urinary excretion of

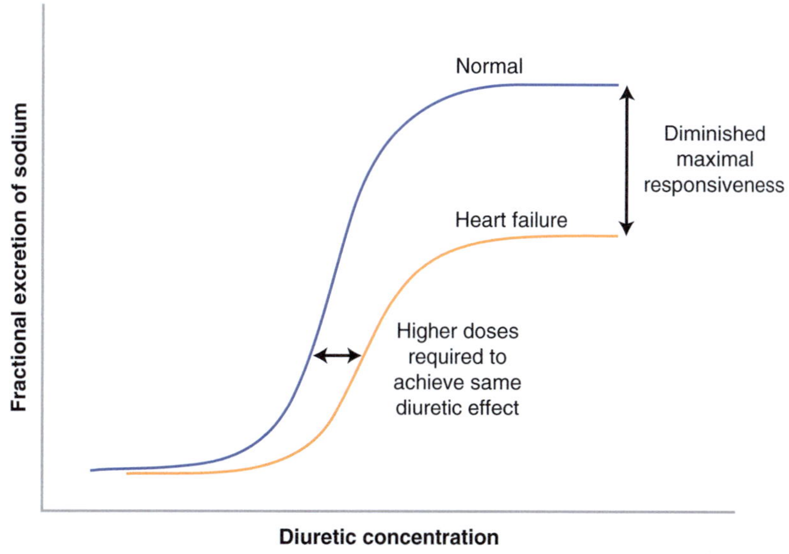

Fig. 13.2 Schematic of doseresponse curve of loop diuretics in heart failure patients compared with normal controls [23]

sodium stops and compensatory sodium retention occurs (post-diuretic salt retention or "rebound") until another diuretic dose is administered and threshold concentration is again achieved. It takes four half-lives for LDs to reach steady state so that administration at a frequency of longer than 4 half-lives will allow for a period of "post-diuretic sodium retention" [23]. Diuretic rebound is directly related to sodium and water excretion and can be prevented by replacement of excreted sodium with normal saline. If dietary intake is not limited, diuretic-induced net sodium excretion may be nullified by post-diuretic salt retention. This phenomenon suggests that in patients hospitalized with ADHF, sodium intake should be restricted and LDs should be given at least 2–3 times/day or administered as a continuous infusion [19, 21, 26, 28].

Two forms of diuretic tolerance have been described. Acute tolerance develops within the first several days of LD therapy and refers to a progressive time-dependent decline in sodium excretion in response to the same dose of LD. This form of early tolerance has been referred to as the "breaking phenomenon". A number of studies have demonstrated decreases in mean blood pressure and eGFR and increases in renin, angiotensin II, aldosterone and plasma norepinephrine levels after a single dose of IV furosemide. The pathophysiology of early tolerance is likely multi-factorial with contributions from: a decrease in renal blood flow mediated by hypotension, increased angiotensin II and sympathetic activation; increases in renin, angiotensin II and aldosterone levels; an increase in sodium reabsorption in the proximal tubule mediated by angiotensin II; and an increase in distal sodium absorption mediated by aldosterone [25, 26, 29]. The release of adenosine by the macula densa/juxtaglomerular apparatus in response to a LD-induced increase in sodium chloride concentration in the distal loop of Henley may contribute to early tolerance by reducing renal blood flow and GFR [30–32]. In addition, vasopressin-induced upregulation of the Na^+: K^+:$2Cl^-$ co-transporter may also contribute to tolerance [33].

A second type of LD tolerance occurs with chronic administration of LD. With LD administration, the nephron distal to the loop of Henle is flooded with solute. This causes diuretic-induced hypertrophy of the distal convoluted tubule and functional changes in the distal nephron that result in increased sodium reabsorption in the distal nephron. This attenuates loop diuretic-induced sodium and water excretion [20, 23].

Furosemide, bumetanide, and torsemide all act by reversibly inhibiting the Na^+:K^+: $2Cl^-$ co-transporter in the ascending limb of the loop of Henle. They differ primarily in oral bioavailability, dose, metabolism, relative potency and duration of action. Furosemide is the most commonly used diuretic in patients with ADHF. In the ADHERE Registry, 84% of patients received IV furosemide, 7% received IV bumetanide and 2% received IV torsemide [34]. All of the loop diuretics (including ethacrynic acid) are extensively bound to plasma proteins, have limited glomerular filtration and are secreted into the intraluminal space of the nephron by the organic acid transport system in the proximal tubule. Furosemide has the most variable bioavailability ranging from 40–70% of the oral dose. The bioavailability of bumetanide and torsemide are 80–100% of the oral dose. Furosemide is metabolized and excreted by the kidney. Bumetanide and torsemide are primarily metabolized by the liver. The onset of diuretic effect when given intravenously is 5 min for furosemide, 2–3 min for bumetanide and 10 min for torsemide. The onset of diuretic effect when given orally is 30–60 min for all three LDs. Furosemide has a half-life of 1.5–2 h, bumetanide 0.8 (range 0.3–1.5) h and torsemide 3.5 h. The duration of action of furosemide is 6–8 h; bumetanide 4–6 h and torsemide 12 h (range 6–16). Furosemide and bumetanide are available for oral and intravenous administration while torsemide is currently available only for oral administration in the United States. The relative potency of LDs given intravenously is furosemide 40 mg: bumetanide 1 mg: torsemide 20 mg. IV to PO conversion is 1:2 for furosemide and 1:1 for bumetanide and torsemide [35–38]. Table 13.1 summarizes the pharmacokinetics of the sulfonamide loop diuretics [24, 39].

Ethacrynic acid has a bioavailability of 100% of the oral dose, is significantly protein bound

Table 13.1 Pharmacokinetics of the loop diuretics [24]

Property	Furosemide	Bumetanide	Torsemide
Relative IV potency, mg	40	1	20
Bioavailability, %	10–100 (average, 50)	80–100	80–100
Oral to intravenous conversion	2:1	1:1	1:1
Initial outpatient total daily oral dose, mg	20–40	0.5–1	5–10
Maintenance outpatient total daily oral dose, mg	40–240	1–5	10–200
Onset, min			
Oral	30–60	30–60	30–60
Intravenous	5	2–3	10
Peak serum concentration after oral administration, h	1	1–2	1
Affected by food	Yes	Yes	No
Metabolism	50% renal conjugation	50% hepatic	80% hepatic
Half-life, h			
Normal	1.5–2	1	3–4
Renal dysfunction	2.8	1.6	4–5
Hepatic dysfunction	2.5	2.3	8
Heart failure	2.7	1.3	6
Average duration of effect, h	6–8	4–6	6–8
Approximate cost of oral 30-day supply (community pharmacy), $	4	4	19–23

Reprinted from Felker and Mentz [23], with permission from Elsevier

and is secreted into the proximal tubule via the organic acid transporter. It has a half-life of approximately 1 h, duration of action of 4–6 h, and potency relative to IV furosemide of 0.7 [24].

Hemodynamic Effects

Loop diuretics should be given intravenously in ADHF as the bioavailability of furosemide is highly variable and the absorption of all loop diuretics may be impeded by bowel edema or intestinal hypoperfusion [40]. Loop diuretics have a number of benefits in volume-overloaded patients with ADHF. Intravenous administration of an effective dose of loop diuretic generally results in a diuretic effect that peaks within an hour of administration [19, 23, 24, 38]. Diuretic induced excretion of sodium and water affects a reduction in right- and left-sided filling pressures with a decrease in pulmonary and systemic venous congestion and a decrease in left ventricular dilation. In patients with LV systolic dysfunction and volume overload, the left ventricle is operating on the flat part of the LV performance curve where stroke volume is relatively independent of LV filling pressures. Diuretic induced reductions in LV filling pressure generally do not cause hypotension or a reduction in stroke volume or cardiac index [41]. Diuretic-related reduction in left and right sided ventricular filling pressures is associated with an improvement in stroke volume and cardiac output related to: a decrease in functional mitral and tricuspid regurgitation; a decrease in right ventricular volume with relief of ventricular-interdependent LV compression; improved endocardial blood flow; and a reduction in LV wall tension resulting in a decrease in myocardial oxygen consumption. The reduction in wall tension may be particularly important in patients with coronary artery disease. The associated reduction in secondary mitral regurgitation and left ventricular wall tension results in an improvement in cardiac output and overall myocardial performance [42–45].

Loop diuretics also have hemodynamic effects independent of their diuretic effects. Several studies have suggested that administration of an intravenous loop diuretic results in an early reduction in pulmonary capillary wedge pressure that may be independent of diuretic effect [46–48]. This effect is likely due to dose-dependent direct venodilation mediated by the release of vasodilatory prostaglandins [49, 50]. These findings may explain why LDs can produce clinically significant reductions in left- and right-sided filling pressures and improvement in symptoms in as little as 15 min after administration [47].

In contrast, in some patients, IV loop diuretics may cause an early increase in systemic vascular resistance and systolic blood pressure. This effect is not mediated by a direct vascular effect but rather, by neurohormonal activation of the sympathetic nervous system and RAAS [42, 43, 50]. In a study of the hemodynamic and neurohormonal responses to IV furosemide in 15 patients with severe chronic heart failure, mean arterial pressure, heart rate, systemic vascular resistance, and left ventricular filling pressure increased and stroke volume index decreased 20 min after the administration of intravenous furosemide. These changes were associated with increases in plasma norepinephrine, plasma renin activity and plasma arginine vasopressin. At 2 h, patients had diuresed and had a reduction in filling pressures to below baseline. Neurohormone levels returned toward baseline [51]. In another study, neurohormonal activation was followed in 34 patients admitted with acute decompensation of chronic HFrEF. Patients were treated with hemodynamically guided therapy with diuretics and sodium nitroprusside titrated to reduce filling pressures and lower systemic vascular resistance. Patients were then transitioned to oral therapy. Neurohormone levels were obtained at baseline, during parenteral treatment (mean 1.4 days) and after transition to oral therapy (mean 3.4 days). Filling pressures (PCWP 31 to 18 mmHg; RA 15 to 8 mmHg) and cardiac index (1.7 to 2.6 L/min/m^2) improved during treatment with parenteral medications. Plasma norepinephrine levels did not change during parenteral therapy but decreased after transition to oral medication. Plasma aldosterone and plasma renin activity increased during parenteral therapy. Aldosterone levels returned to baseline and plasma renin activity remained elevated after transition to oral medication. Plasma endothelin levels decreased during parenteral therapy and remained lower after transition to oral medication [52]. These observations support the early use of a vasodilator added to a diuretic to attenuate the effects of LD-induced neurohormonal activation.

LD Dose and Mode of Administration

There has been little prospective evidence to guide diuretic use in ADHF. It has been hypothesized that the continuous infusion of a loop diuretic should avoid the periods of ineffective diuretic concentration in the loop of Henle seen with intermittent bolus therapy and should result in greater diuresis. It has also been suggested that continuous infusion should be associated with fewer electrolyte abnormalities, preservation of renal function and a shorter length of stay. A Cochran review published in 2005 compared intermittent bolus administration with continuous intravenous infusion of loop diuretics in eight studies of a total of 254 patients. The studies were small (8–107 patients) and heterogeneous. There were significant differences among the studies with respect to diuretic dose, method of administration, follow-up period and clinical outcomes reported [53]. The authors concluded that the data were insufficient to assess the merits of the two methods of LD administration.

The Diuretic Optimization Strategies in Acute Heart Failure (DOSE) trial was a multicenter, randomized, controlled, double-blind trial that assessed the effect of diuretic dose and mode of administration in patients admitted with ADHF [54]. 308 patients hospitalized for ADHF with a history of chronic heart failure treated with an oral loop diuretic at a daily dose of furosemide of 80–240 mg/day or equivalent for at least one month prior to hospitalization were enrolled in the study. Using a 2 × 2 factorial design, patients were randomized in a 1:1:1:1 ratio to receive furosemide administered intravenously by means of either a bolus every 12 h or continuous infusion and with either a low dose (equivalent to the patient's previous oral dose) or a high dose (2.5 times the previous oral dose). Dose adjustments could be made at 48 h. There were two co-primary end-points: patients' global assessment of symptoms, quantified as the area under the curve on a visual-analogue scale over the course of 72 h (the efficacy end-point); and the change in the serum creatinine level from baseline to 72 h (the safety end-point). There was no significant difference in the patients' global assessment of symptoms or mean change in creatinine between the bolus and continuous infusion groups. Patients in the bolus therapy group were more likely to require an increase in furosemide dose at 48 h. There was a non-significant trend toward greater improvement in symptoms assessed by the visual analogue scale in the high dose group compared to the low dose group ($P = 0.06$). The high dose strategy was associated with greater relief of dyspnea ($P = 0.04$), greater fluid ($p = 0.001$) and weight ($p = 0.01$) loss and fewer adverse events ($p = 0.033$). Patients in the high dose group were less likely to require an increase in furosemide dose and more likely to be changed to oral therapy at the 48-h reevaluation. There were more cases of ventricular tachycardia and myocardial infarction with bolus than with continuous infusion and with the low-dose strategy than with the high-dose strategy. A higher proportion of patients in the high dose group met the pre-specified secondary safety end-point of an increase in serum creatinine of more than 0.3 mg per deciliter at any time during the 72 h after randomization. Although prior studies have suggested that an increase in creatinine during hospitalization for ADHF is associated with worse long-term outcome [55, 56], there was no evidence of worse clinical outcome in the high dose group at 60 days. This is consistent with other reports that found that a transient increase in creatinine during hospitalization may not be associated with poorer outcomes after discharge [57, 58].

Two recent meta-analyses that included the results from the DOSE Trial compared the efficacy of continuous infusion versus IV bolus of loop diuretics in patients hospitalized with ADHF. One meta-analysis included ten randomized controlled trials with a total of 518 patients in the analysis. Continuous infusion of diuretics was associated with a significantly greater weight loss compared with bolus injection but no significant differences in urine output, the incidence of electrolyte abnormality, change in creatinine level, hospital length of stay, the incidence of ototoxicity, cardiac mortality, or all-cause mortality [59]. The second meta-analysis included 7 crossover and 8 parallel-arm randomized trials in adults with a total of 844 patients in the analysis. 8/15 studies included patients with ADHF, 3 included ICU patients, 2 included cardiac surgery patients and 2 included patients with chronic kidney disease. A non-significant net increase in daily urine output was seen with continuous infusion diuretic therapy. When the 8 studies that included an initial loading dose were analyzed, continuous loop diuretic infusion was associated with a significant net increase in daily urine output of 294 ml/day and a significant net negative weight loss of 0.78 kg when compared with intermittent infusion [60].

The optimal dose of LD is uncertain and needs to be individualized based on age, prior diuretic use, severity of heart failure, the presence of impaired systemic perfusion, creatinine and estimated glomerular filtration rate calculated using either the Cockroft-Gault (CG) or the Modified Diet in Renal Disease (MDRD) equations. Diuretics should be given at a dose and frequency sufficient to relieve symptoms and signs of congestion and normalize volume status without causing excessively rapid reduction in intravascular volume or clinically significant electrolyte abnormalities [8].

The ACCF/ACC guidelines recommend that in patients already receiving a loop diuretic, the initial diuretic dose should equal or exceed their chronic oral daily dose and be given either as intermittent intravenous boluses or continuous infusion [28]. The ESC guidelines recommend that an initial dose of furosemide 20–40 mg IV (or 0.5–1.0 mg bumetanide or 10–20 mg of torsemide) be given on admission; in patients with evidence of volume overload, the dose of parenteral diuretic may be higher based on renal function and a history of chronic oral diuretic use [18]. Continuous infusion may also be considered after an initial starting bolus dose. The ESC recommends that the total furosemide dose should remain <100 mg in the first 6 h and

Table 13.2 Standardizing care for acute decompensated heart failure in a large megatrial: The approach for the Acute Studies of Clinical Effectiveness of Nesiritide in Subjects with Decompensated Heart Failure (ASCEND-HF) [61]

Creatinine clearance[a]	Patient	Initial IV dose[b]	Maintenance dose
>60 ml/(min 1.73m^2)	New-onset HF or no maintenance diuretic therapy	Furosemide 20–40 mg 2–3 times daily	Lowest diuretic dose that allows for clinical stability is the ideal dose
	Established HF or chronic oral diuretic therapy	Furosemide bolus equivalent to oral dose	
<60 mL/(min 1.73m^2)	New-onset HF or no maintenance diuretic therapy	Furosemide 20–80 mg 2–3 times daily	
	Established HF or chronic oral diuretic therapy	Furosemide bolus equivalent to oral dose	

Reprinted from Ezekowitz et al. [61], with permission from Elsevier

[a]Creatinine clearance is calculated from the Cockroft-Gault or Modified Diet in Renal Disease formula

[b]Intravenous continuous furosemide at doses of 5 to 20 mg/h is also an option See text for details

<240 mg during the first 24 h. Diuretic dosing guidelines from the ASCEND-HF trial based on creatinine clearance and the chronicity of heart failure are summarized in Table 13.2 [61]. The recommended doses of LDs given by continuous infusion are summarized in Table 13.3 [23, 62].

Table 13.3 Continuous infusion with as needed uptitration [23]

IV loading dose (mg)		Infusion rate (mg/h)		
Creatinine clearance	All GFRs	<25	25–75	>75
Furosemide	40	20, then 40	10, then 20	10
Bumetanide	1	1, then 2	0.5, then 1	0.5
Torsemide	20	10, then 20	5, then 10	5

Reprinted with permission from Brater [22], with permission from Elsevier

Note: Before increasing to a higher infusion rate, a repeat loading dose should be administered

Response to Therapy

There is conflicting data concerning the rapidity of response to parenteral diuretics in patients with ADHF. There is a general understanding that most patients have a rapid and significant improvement in dyspnea after administration of a parenteral diuretic although not all studies confirm this [8, 63]. In the Value of Endothelin Receptor Inhibition With Tezosentan in Acute Heart Failure (VERITAS) trial, patients admitted to the hospital with acute heart failure, dyspnea, tachypnea and evidence of volume overload or LV systolic dysfunction were treated with standard heart failure therapy which consisted mostly of parenteral diuretics and randomized to an infusion of tezosentan, an intravenous short-acting endothelin receptor antagonist, or placebo. The primary end-point was the change in dyspnea over the first 24 h measured at 3, 6 and 24 h using a visual analog scale. There were rapid and significant improvements in dyspnea in the placebo and tezosentan groups at 3, 6, and 24 h. Interestingly, these changes were associated with small changes in hemodynamic parameters. In the placebo group, baseline PCWP was 25.6 mmHg and decreased by 1.5, 1.9, and 2.9 mmHg at 3, 6, and 24 h, respectively. Baseline RAP was 15.9 mmHg and changed by 0.8, −0.2 and 0.7 mmHg at 3, 6, and 24 h respectively. Baseline cardiac index was 2.01 L/min/m^2 and increased by 0.18, 0.18 and 0.15 L/min/m^2 at 3, 6, and 24 h, respectively. Baseline systemic vascular resistance was 1813 dyne-sec/cm^5 and changed by −157, −54 and 136 dyne-sec/cm^5 at 3, 6, and 24 h [64].

In the Efficacy of Vasopressin Antagonism in Heart Failure Outcome Study with Tolvaptan (EVEREST) trial, patients with chronic heart failure and systolic dysfunction who were hospitalized for worsening HF received standard therapy for acute heart failure and were randomized to receive tolvaptan, an oral non-peptide selective V_2-receptor antagonist or placebo. Approximately

2/3 of the placebo patients reported mild, moderate or marked improvement in dyspnea but only one third of patients reported moderate or marked improvement in dyspnea at day 1 of the study. Physician assessment of signs and symptoms of heart failure on day 1 noted improvement in dyspnea in 47.1% of patients, orthopnea in 59.2%; JVD in 43.8%; rales in 43.7% and edema in 52.6% [65].

The rate of dyspnea relief was reviewed in a post hoc analysis of data from the Placebo-controlled Randomized study of the selective A1 adenosine receptor antagonist rolofylline for patients hospitalized with acute heart failure and volume Overload to assess Treatment Effect on Congestion and renal funcTion (PROTECT) clinical trial pilot study. In PROTECT, patients with acute heart failure and mild to moderate renal impairment defined as an eGFR of 20–80 mL/min using the Cockcroft-Gault equation with dyspnea at rest or with minimal activity, signs and symptoms of volume overload and an elevated BNP or NT-pro-BNP were randomized within 24 h of presentation to treatment with placebo or one of three doses of rolofylline, a selective A1 adenosine receptor antagonist. Dyspnea relief was defined as a moderate to marked improvement in dyspnea using a seven-point Likert scale and occurred in the placebo group in 49%, 64%, 78%, and 75% of patients at 24 h, 48 h, day 7 and day 14, respectively. Improvement at 24 and 48 h was associated with greater improvement in patient-reported general wellbeing, and greater decreases from baseline in edema, rales, jugular venous distention and orthopnea. Patients with relief of dyspnea did not have a greater decrease in weight compared to patients without relief of dyspnea [66].

The frequency of early dyspnea relief was assessed in the Preliminary study of RELAX in Acute Heart Failure (Pre-RELAX-AHF) study. Patients in Pre-RELAX-HF had acute heart failure, evidence of volume overload, a systolic blood pressure of >125 mmHg, and impaired renal function with an eGFR of 30–75 ml/min/1.73 m^2 calculated using the simplified Modification of Diet in Renal Disease (sMDRD) equation. Patients were randomized to placebo or one of four doses of relaxin, a naturally occurring peptide vasodilator. Early dyspnea relief was defined as moderate or marked improvement in dyspnea assessed by the Likert scale at 6, 12, and 24 h after the start of study medication. Moderate or marked improvement in dyspnea at 6, 12 and 24 h was observed in only 23% of patients in the placebo group. 70% of all patients had moderate or marked improvement in dyspnea at 14 days. Improvement in dyspnea was correlated with improvements in general well-being measured by a visual analogue scale, orthopnea, dyspnea on exertion, edema, and rales but not with improvements in JVP or weight. Early dyspnea relief was predicted by a higher initial systolic blood pressure and respiratory rate [67].

The Ularitide Global Evaluation in Acute Decompensated Heart Failure (URGENT) Dyspnoea study was an international, multicenter, observational cohort study of 524 acute heart failure patients managed conventionally and enrolled within 1 h of first hospital medical evaluation [68]. The primary outcome was patient assessed dyspnea at 6 h measured by a 5-point Likert scale. Dyspnea improvement was reported in 76% of patients after 6 h of standard therapy.

LD Side Effects

Excessive Diuresis

Excessive diuresis may result in hypotension and a reduction in cardiac output. During LD-induced natriuresis, intravascular volume is generally maintained by vascular "refilling" or equilibration as interstitial fluid moves into the intravascular space. The rate of refilling varies among patients. During brisk diuresis, it is possible for the rate of volume loss to exceed the rate of refilling. This may result in low intravascular volume, inadequate cardiac filling, and hypotension despite persistent volume overload.

Patients with HPpEF are at greater risk of diuretic-induced hypotension. These patients tend to be less volume overloaded and have a steep diastolic filling curve so that moderate reductions in intravascular volume may result in significant reductions in cardiac filling and cardiac output. Patients with infiltrative or restrictive cardiomyopathy may have diuretic-induced hypotension in the setting of continued volume overload as elevated ventricular filling pressures are needed to maintain normal cardiac output [41]. Diuresis that results in a decrease in ventricular filling pressures may makes patients more sensitive to the hypotensive effects of other vasodilators used in the routine treatment of heart failure.

Electrolyte Abnormalities

LDs cause urinary losses of potassium due to augmented distal tubular secretion of potassium in response to increased distal tubular sodium reabsorption (creating a lumen negative gradient that favors potassium secretion) and secondary hyperaldosteronism. Electrolytes need to be monitored frequently, especially early during the period when diuresis is most significant. Hypokalemia should be treated promptly with either oral or intravenous potassium supplementation. Electrolytes should be monitored at least daily during hospitalization and more frequently if potassium supplementation is needed. Patients also need to be monitored for the development of hyperkalemia which may develop later during hospitalization as a result of less daily diuresis, fixed dosing of potassium supplementation, the initiation or uptitration of angiotensin converting enzyme inhibitors (ACEI), angiotensin receptor blockers (ARBs), and/or mineralocorticoid receptor blockers (MRAs), and the development of renal insufficiency.

LDs also cause hypomagnesemia. 70% of filtered magnesium is reabsorbed in the thick ascending limb of the loop of Henle. Inhibition of the Na^+: K^+:$2Cl^-$ cotransporter decreases the lumen positive charge in this segment and reduces the driving force for paracellular magnesium reabsorption. Hypomagnesemia can be associated with arrhythmia and can exacerbate diuretic-induced hypokalemia. Monitoring magnesium levels is indicated in patients admitted with ADHF.

Hypersensitivity Reactions

Furosemide, bumetanide and torsemide are sulfonamides and can cause hypersensitivity reactions which are usually manifest as rash or, rarely, acute interstitial nephritis. All three medications have chemical similarities to sulfonamide antibiotics, sulfonylureas, carbonic anhydrase inhibitors, and thiazide diuretics. There is little evidence that sensitivity to a sulfonamide antibiotic predicts sensitivity to a loop diuretic beyond the finding that patients who have a reaction to one medication are at increased risk of reactions to medications in general [69–72]. Despite this data, the United Stated Food and Drug Administration approved product information for bumetanide and torsemide caution: "Patients allergic to sulfonamides may show hypersensitivity to Bumex" [73] and "Torsemide Tablets are contraindicated in patients with known hypersensitivity to torsemide or to sulfonylureas" [74].

Ethacrynic acid is a loop diuretic without a sulfhydryl group. It can be used safely in patients with hypersensitivity to furosemide, bumetanide or torsemide. The major limitation to using ethacrynic acid is that it is significantly less effective than the other LDs in facilitating sodium excretion.

Ototoxicity

Furosemide can cause dose-related ototoxicity with tinnitus and/or clinical or subclinical hearing loss [75–78]. Permanent hearing loss can occur but is unusual. Ototoxicity of LDs is related to the blood level of the drug. Rapid infusion or use of large parenteral doses, especially in the setting of renal insufficiency, increases the risk of toxicity. Reducing the infusion rate or changing to oral administration reduces the risk of ototoxicity. It is recommended that infusion rates of furosemide should not exceed 4 mg/min in adults [79]. The risk of ototoxicity is also increased in the setting of hypoproteinemia, or concomitant use of other ototoxic drugs such as aminoglycosides or ethacrynic acid. Hearing impairment may be associated with high dose intravenous bumetanide although bumetanide is probably less ototoxic than furosemide. Ototoxicity is less common with torsemide than with furosemide or bumetanide. Ethacrynic acid can also cause ototoxicity. The mechanism differs from that of furosemide. Hearing loss from ethacrynic acid is more commonly irreversible [75].

Muscle Pain: Bumetanide

Diffuse muscle pain is a limiting side effect of high dose intravenous bumetanide. Pain can be severe and is reversible with reduction in dose or discontinuation of the medication. Muscle pain is not associated with elevations in skeletal muscle enzymes. Dosing of torsemide is not limited by muscle pain.

Other Diuretic Classes

Carbonic Anhydrase Inhibitors

The zinc metalloenzyme carbonic anhydrase plays a key role in $NaHCO_3^-$ resorption and acid secretion in the proximal tubule and, to a lesser extent, in the collecting duct. Acetazolamide is the prototype of a group of carbonic acid inhibitors and the only one used in clinical practice. Acetazolamide inhibits the absorption of $NaHCO_3^-$ in the proximal tubule. In the absence of another diuretic that inhibits sodium reabsorption in the distal nephron, treatment with acetazolamide does not cause a significant diuresis. It does however, cause significant excretion of HCO3 $^-$, an increase in urinary pH, significant excretion of potassium and metabolic acidosis [80]. Acetazolamide has been shown to cause a marked natriuresis when added to either hydrochlorothiazide or furosemide in patients resistant to either diuretic and who have a low fractional excretion of sodium [81]. However, its use is limited by the development of metabolic acidosis. In clinical practice, acetazolamide is only used in ADHF in the setting of marked diuretic-induced normokalemic, hypochloremic metabolic acidosis [82].

Thiazide and Thiazide-Like Diuretics

Benzothiadiazides were the first drugs to inhibit the Na^+-Cl^- cotransporter in the distal convoluted tubule. This class of medication came to be known as thiazide diuretics (hydrochlorothiazide, chlorothiazide). Subsequently, drugs that were pharmacologically similar to thiazides and inhibited the Na^+-Cl^-cotransporter were termed thiazide—like diuretics (metolazone, chlorthalidone) [27]. Thiazide diuretics inhibit the Na^+-Cl^- cotransporter in the distal convoluted tubule and promote Na^+ and Cl^- excretion. Thiazides are only moderately effective diuretics—they block the reabsorption of 5–10% of filtered sodium compared with LDs which block 25% of filtered sodium. Thiazides are ineffective as monotherapy in the treatment of more than mild heart failure and are not used as single agents in the treatment of ADHF. However, thiazide diuretics are very useful when added to LDs in treating patients with ADHF who remain volume overloaded despite appropriate treatment with adequately dosed LD (see below). Side effects from thiazide diuretics include hypokalemia, hyponatremia (unrelated to arginine vasopressin release), metabolic alkalosis, hypomagnesemia, hypercalcemia and hyperuricemia [23, 25, 83].

Potassium Sparing Diuretics

Triamterene and amiloride have the same mechanism of action and are the only drugs in this class. Spironolactone and eplerenone also decrease the excretion of potassium but are more appropriately classified as mineralocorticoid receptor antagonists (see below). Triamterene and amiloride block epithelial Na^+ channels (amiloride-sensitive Na + channels or ENaC) in the luminal membrane of principal cells in the late distal tubule and collecting duct. The effect of ENaC blockade on lumen negative voltage decreases potassium (and H^+, Ca^{2+} and Mg^{2+}) excretion and increases serum potassium concentration. Na^+ excretion is minimally increased (2%

of filtered load of sodium). The major side effect of this class of medication is the risk of hyperkalemia. As a result, these medications are contraindicated in in patients with hyperkalemia or patients with conditions that put them at risk of hyperkalemia including renal insufficiency, treatment with ACEI or ARB, treatment with potassium supplements, or treatment with MRAs. In light of their modest natriuretic effects and risk of hyperkalemia, triamterene and amiloride have little use in the treatment of patients with ADHF [25, 27].

Mineralocorticoid Receptor Antagonists (MRAs)

Aldosterone is a steroid hormone with mineralocorticoid effects that is primarily produced in the renal cortex. Aldosterone plays a major role in the control of sodium and potassium homeostasis by increasing sodium and water resorption and increasing K^+ and H^+ excretion. Aldosterone binds to cytosolic mineralocorticoid receptors (MRs) with high aldosterone affinity in epithelial cells in the late distal convoluted tubule and collecting duct. MRs are members of the superfamily of receptors for steroid hormones, thyroid hormones, vitamin D and retinoids. When aldosterone binds to MR, the MR-aldosterone complex translocates to the nucleus and binds to specific DNA sequences that regulate the expression of multiple gene products. Transepithelial NaCl transport is enhanced. The resulting increase in lumen-negative transepithelial voltage increases the driving force for K^+ and H^+ secretion into the tubular lumen. The genomic effects of aldosterone take several hours to begin to take effect. Aldosterone also has non-genomic effects that are fast acting (occur within minutes) and are probably mediated by binding to plasma membrane MRs. These effects have not been well characterized but probably include an increase in blood pressure that is independent of sodium retention [27, 84, 85].

The MRAs spironolactone and eplerenone competitively inhibit the binding of aldosterone to the MR. The effects on urinary excretion of sodium are similar to those of the renal epithelial Na^+ channel inhibitors. However, unlike the effects of Na^+ channel inhibitors, the clinical effects of MRAs are dependent on endogenous aldosterone levels. Aldosterone levels are increased in heart failure despite treatment with ACEI or ARB and are increased further after administration of loop diuretics [86]. The higher the aldosterone level, the greater the impact of MRAs on urinary excretion. In the Randomized Aldactone Evaluation Study (RALES), spironolactone 25 mg daily did not increase urinary sodium excretion [87]. However, there is literature suggesting that higher doses (50–100 mg daily) of spironolactone significantly increase urinary excretion of sodium when added to standard therapy in patients with ADHF [88, 89].

MR antagonists are the only diuretics that do not require access to the tubular lumen to induce a diuresis. Spironolactone is absorbed partially (~65%), is metabolized extensively by the liver, undergoes enterohepatic recirculation, is highly protein bound, and has a short half-life of ~1.6 h. The half-life is prolonged to 9 h in patients with cirrhosis. Eplerenone has good oral availability, is eliminated primarily by metabolism by CYP3A4 to inactive metabolites, and has a half-life of ~5 h.

MRAs are generally not used as diuretics in ADHF. They may be used to attenuate potassium losses from LD therapy. They should be initiated or continued during ADHF hospitalization as guideline directed medical therapy for their long-term benefit in patients with HFrEF (see below) [90].

The major side effect of MRAs is life-threatening hyperkalemia. Because spironolactone has affinity for other steroid receptors (progesterone and androgen receptors), it may cause gynecomastia, impotence, decreased libido, hirsutism, and menstrual irregularities. Eplerenone has very low affinity for androgen and progesterone receptors and generally does not cause these side effects.

Monitoring Response to Diuretic Therapy

A primary goal in the treatment of patients with ADHF is to relieve symptoms associated with pulmonary and systemic venous congestion without causing excessively rapid diuresis resulting in hypotension, renal insufficiency or electrolyte abnormalities. Patients with ADHF need to be carefully monitored for: persistent or worsening signs and symptoms of heart failure; respiratory compromise; adequacy of diuresis; oxygenation; adequate end-organ perfusion; hypotension; worsening renal function; and electrolyte abnormalities. The ACCF/AHA Guidelines recommend that patients should be followed with careful measurement of fluid intake and output, vital signs, daily weight, careful clinical assessment of signs and symptoms of congestion and systemic perfusion, and daily electrolytes and creatinine [28].

Routine use of a Foley catheter is not recommended for monitoring urine output. There should be a high index of suspicion for bladder outlet obstruction particularly in older men. Determining a post-void urine residual volume should be considered in middle age and older men and all patients with renal insufficiency or diuretic resistance. Placement of a catheter is recommended when close monitoring of urine output is needed or if bladder outlet obstruction may be contributing to renal insufficiency and diuretic resistance. Recommendations for patient monitoring are summarized in Table 13.4 [8, 28].

Table 13.4 Patient monitoring during treatment for ADHF [8]

Monitoring recommendations for patients hospitalized with ADHF		
Frequency	Value	Specifies
At least daily	Weight	Determine after voiding in the morning Account for possible increased food intake due to improved appetite
At least daily	Fluid intake and output	
More than daily	Vital signs	Orthostatic blood pressure if indicated Oxygen saturation daily until stable
At least daily	Signs	Edema Ascites Pulmonary rales Hepatomegaly Increased JVP Hepatojuglar reflux Liver tenderness
At least daily	Symptoms	Orthopnea PND or cough Nocturnal cough Dyspnea Fatigue, lightheadedness
At least daily	Electrolytes	Potassium Sodium
At least daily	Renal function	BUN Serum Creatinine[a]

Reprinted from Heart Failure Society of America et al. [8], pp. e1–e194, © 2010, with permission from Elsevier
[a]See background section for addictional recommendations on laboratory evaluations

One of the primary goals of care in a patient hospitalized with ADHF is sustained decongestion. The ACCF/AHA Guidelines recommend that patients receive intravenous diuretics until congestion resolves at which time, oral diuretics should be initiated with a goal of maintaining volume status. Generally, patients are transitioned to oral diuretics by using the total daily dose of IV diuretic to calculate the initial total daily dose of oral diuretic. The conversion of IV to oral diuretic dose is 1:1 for bumetanide and torsemide and 1:2 for furosemide. The calculated total daily dose of oral diuretic should be divided in half and given twice daily. Patients should be observed for at least 24 h after transition to oral diuretics to ensure that volume status, serum potassium and renal function remain stable. Patients with a history of diuretic resistance or persistent congestion may not tolerate the transition to oral diuretics because of recurrent or worsening volume overload. Conversely, patients may become more responsive to diuretics as volume overload improves and guideline directed medical therapy is initiated or uptitrated. These patients may develop low blood pressure, orthostatic symptoms, hypokalemia, hyperkalemia and/or worsening renal function. Because of these possibilities, oral diuretics need to be carefully titrated after the transition from IV diuretics using signs and symptoms of congestion and volume depletion, careful monitoring of daily weight and fluid intake and output, and changes in electrolytes and renal function.

Determining whether a patient continues to be volume overloaded can be challenging. In the OPTIMIZE-HF Registry, 50% of patients lost less than ≤2 kg and 25% of patients lost no weight during heart failure hospitalization. At *discharge*, one quarter had lower extremity edema, 15% had rales, and half had persistent symptoms. This data suggests that a significant proportion of patients hospitalized for ADHF remain congested at discharge [91]. In a post-hoc analysis of the placebo group in the EVEREST trial, a modified composite congestion score (CCS) was calculated by summing individual scores for orthopnea, JVD and pedal edema that were graded daily on a 0–3 scale of clinician-investigator determined severity (total possible score 0–9) [92]. The median CCS score decreased from a mean of 4 at baseline to 1 at discharge. At discharge, nearly three quarters of study participants had a CCS of 0–1 and less than 10% of patients had a CCS > 3. Each CCS point >0 was associated with a hazard ratio of 1.34 and 1.16 for mortality at 30 days and for the study period, respectively (median follow up was 9.9 months). Patients with a CCS of 0 at discharge experienced a heart failure rehospitalization rate of 26.2% and all-cause mortality rate of 19.1% during the follow-up period. Patients with CCS scores of 1 or 3–9 at discharge had HF rehospitalization rates of 34.9% and 34.7%, respectively and an all-cause mortality rates of 24.8% and 42.8%, respectively.

Some patients, especially those with HFpEF, have no or little history of weight gain prior to hospitalization and may have an improvement in symptoms with improvement in blood pressure and little diuresis. However, it is notable that in the OPTIMIZE-HF registry, patients with HFpEF had a similar distribution of weight loss, symptom improvement, and frequency of edema and rales at discharge compared with patients with HFrEF [91].

The data concerning the relationship between weight loss, net fluid loss, dyspnea relief and clinical outcomes in patients hospitalized for ADHF is conflicting. In the EVEREST trial, there was a correlation between weight loss and patient assessed dyspnea relief [93]. The Ultrafiltration versus Intravenous Diuretics for Patients Hospitalized for Acute Decompensated Congestive Heart Failure (UNLOAD) trial compared ultrafiltration (UF) with IV diuretic therapy in patients with ADHF. In the patients randomized to UF, there was a greater reduction in body weight, greater fluid loss and a reduction in rehospitalization and unscheduled clinic visits, but no difference in dyspnea score when compared with the IV diuretic arm [94]. In the ESCAPE trial, there was no association between weight loss and clinical events (days alive out of the hospital in the first 6 months; death; death or rehospitalization; and death, rehospitalization, or cardiac transplantation) although patients with the greatest weight loss had a significantly decreased orthopnea score [95]. In the PROTECT Trial, there was a strong association with weight loss, early dyspnea relief and reduced early post-discharge mortality [96]. In the Pre-RELAX-AHF study, there was an association between sustained relief of dyspnea at 5 days and reduced 30-day mortality [67]. Data from the Diuretic Optimization Strategy Evaluation in Acute Heart Failure (DOSE-AHF) trial found that weight loss, fluid loss and NT-proBNP reduction at 72 h did not correlate with dyspnea relief but did correlate with improved outcomes at 60 days. Improvement in dyspnea was associated with a small improvement in clinical outcomes [97].

These data challenge the idea that weight loss is a sufficient surrogate marker for adequate decongestion and suggest that careful evaluation of symptoms, physical findings, laboratory measures, weight change and net fluid balance need to be considered when assessing volume status and diuretic dosing [28, 97]. The diagnostic value of clinical markers of congestion from a scientific statement from the Acute Heart Failure Committee of the Heart Failure Association of the European Society of Cardiology is summarized in Table 13.5 [98].

Table 13.5 Diagnostic value of clinical markers of congestion [98]

Sign or symptom	Sensitivity	Specificity	PPV	NPV
Dyspnoea on exertion	66	52	45	27
Orthopnoea	66	47	61	37
Oedema	46	73	79	46
Resting JVD	70	79	85	62
S3	73	42	66	44
Chest X-ray				
Cardiomegaly	97	10	61	–
Redistribution	60	68	75	52
Interstitial oedema	60	73	78	53
Pleural effusion	43	79	76	47

JVD jugular venous distension, *S3* third heart sound, *PPV* positive predictive value, *NPV* negative predictive value. All numbers are expressed as percentages.

Hemoconcentration (HC)

Several studies have suggested that hemoconcentration (an increase in low hemoglobin or a relative increase in the cellular elements in blood) is a surrogate marker for intravascular volume status and may be a useful indicator of adequate decongestion in patients hospitalized for ADHF [99, 100]. A post-hoc analysis from the ESCAPE trial assessed the impact of hemoconcentration on outcome [58]. Three hundred thirty-six of 433 randomized patients who had paired baseline and pre-discharge hematocrit, albumin or total protein values were included in the analysis. Baseline to discharge differences in the laboratory values that fell within the top tertile of the group were defined as indicators of hemoconcentration. Patients with ≥2 paired laboratory values in the top tertile were considered to have evidence of hemoconcentration. The group of patients with evidence of HC received higher doses of diuretics, lost more weight and fluid and had greater reductions in filling pressures. HC was strongly associated with worsening renal function whereas changes in RA and PCWP were not associated with worsening renal function. HC was strongly associated with a lower 180-day mortality rate that persisted after adjustment for baseline differences in risk (HR 0.16; P = 0.001).

A post hoc analysis of 1969 patients enrolled in the PROTECT study assessed the relationship between the change in hematocrit during heart failure hospitalization and outcome [101]. Anemia at baseline was defined, according to the World Health Organization (WHO) criteria, as a baseline hemoglobin level of <13 g/dl for men and < 12 g/dl for women and was present in 50.3% of patients. Hemoconcentration was defined as an increase in hemoglobin levels between baseline and day 7 and was seen in 69.1% of patients. HC was associated with better renal function at baseline, more weight loss and greater deterioration in renal function. The total dose of diuretics was *lower* in the patients with HC. Greater weight loss and better baseline renal function were associated with a more rapid increase in hemoglobin concentration. The absolute change in hemoglobin was an independent predictor of outcome. There was a 34% reduction in all-cause mortality at 180 days for each gram/dl increase in hemoglobin between baseline and day 7.

A retrospective analysis of 1684 patients assigned to the placebo arm in the EVEREST trial found that 26% of patients had evidence of hemoconcentration defined as a ≥ 3% absolute increase in hematocrit between baseline and discharge or day 7 [102]. Patients with greater increases in hematocrit tended to have better baseline renal function. HC was associated with a greater risk of in-hospital worsening of renal function, which generally returned to baseline at 4 weeks after discharge. Patients with HC were less likely to have clinical congestion at discharge, and experienced greater in-hospital decreases in body weight and natriuretic peptide levels. After adjustment for baseline clinical risk factors, every 5% absolute increase in in-hospital hematocrit change was associated with a 19% reduction in all-cause mortality following discharge over an average follow up 9.9 months. HCT change was also associated with a significantly decreased risk of cardiovascular mortality or HF hospitalization at ≤100 days following randomization (HR 0.73). In the Korean Heart Failure (KorHF) Registry, HC (defined as an increase in hemoglobin levels between admission and discharge) occurred in 43% of patients and was found to be an independent negative predictor of the combined primary end-point of all-cause mortality and HF hospitalization after adjusting for other HF risk factors (HR = 0.671; $P < 0.001$) [103].

There may be a difference in the prognostic value of hemoconcentration based on when it occurs during the HF hospitalization. In a single center study of 845 patients hospitalized for ADHF, hemoconcentration (defined as an increase in both hemoglobin and hematocrit) occurred in 422 patients. HC was defined as "early" or "late" based on whether the maximal increase in hemoglobin and hematocrit occurred in the first or second half of the hospitalization. Early and late patients had similar baseline characteristics, cumulative in-hospital diuretic administration, and degree of worsening renal function. Late patients had higher average daily loop diuretic doses, greater weight loss, later transition to oral diuretics, and shorter length of stay. Late HC was associated with a significant survival advantage over a median follow-up of 3.4 years compared with early HC (HR: 0.73, $p = 0.026$) and no HC (HR: 0.74; $p = 0.0090$). Early HC was not associated with a survival advantage [104].

This data suggests that more complete decongestion is associated with a better post-discharge prognosis and that HC may be a reasonable surrogate for assessing the adequacy of decongestion during an admission for decompensated heart failure. However, the data supporting the use of HC to guide therapy have significant limitations. A prospective randomized study comparing HC with usual clinical care as a therapeutic strategy to guide treatment has not been performed. It is possible that patients with HC are healthier and more diuretic responsive. Most of the data comes from studies of patients with HFrEF. Because HC has been variably defined, it is unclear what degree of change in hemoglobin, hematocrit or both is clinically significant [99]. Also, in some patients, the absence of hemoconcentration may not reflect residual volume overload but instead, occult blood loss, poor nutritional status, medications, or the effects of serial phlebotomy. Therefore, the data do not support the routine intensification of diuretic therapy in patients who do not demonstrate an increase in hemoglobin or hematocrit [105].

Natriuretic-Peptide (NP) Guided Therapy

NP levels are important markers of risk that add prognostic information in ambulatory patients with chronic HF and in hospitalized patients with ADHF [8, 106, 107]. In addition, the pre-discharge NP and change in NP from admission to discharge provide additional independent information that helps identify patients at risk for hospitalization or death after discharge [108–110].

However, it is not clear if serial NP measurements are useful in guiding therapy in patients hospitalized with acute heart failure. The Rapid Emergency Department Heart Failure Outpatients Trial (REDHOT II) was a multicenter, prospective randomized controlled study of 447 patients hospitalized with acute heart failure randomized to serial BNP testing at 3, 6, 9, and 12 h, then daily versus standard care. No difference was found between the two groups with respect to length of stay, in-hospital mortality, 30-day mortality, or readmission rate [111]. The HFSA and ACCF/AHA guidelines do not recommend the use serial NP testing to guide therapy in patients hospitalized with acute heart failure [8, 28].

Pulmonary Artery Catheterization (PAC)

Invasive hemodynamic monitoring (IHM) with a pulmonary artery catheter (PAC) has been used in small non-randomized studies to guide diuretic and vasodilator therapy to achieve pre-specified near normal filling pressures in patients with severe refractory heart failure. This approach resulted in sustained improvements in hemodynamics, severity of mitral regurgitation, exercise tolerance and symptoms [45, 112, 113].

The Evaluation Study of Congestive Heart Failure and Pulmonary Artery Catheterization (ESCAPE) trial evaluated whether the routine use of a PAC was safe and improved clinical outcomes in patients with ADHF [114]. Four hundred forty-three patients with severe symptomatic heart failure at 26 sites were randomized to receive therapy guided by clinical assessment and PAC or clinical assessment alone. The target patient was sufficiently ill with advanced heart failure to make the use of the PAC reasonable, but also sufficiently stable to make crossover to PAC for urgent management unlikely. Patients who were felt to require a PAC for management of heart failure were not included in the study but were included in a PAC registry. The goal of treatment in both groups was resolution of clinical signs and symptoms of congestion, particularly jugular venous pressure elevation, edema, and orthopnea. Additional goals in the PAC group included achieving a pulmonary capillary wedge pressure of 15 mm Hg and a right atrial pressure of 8 mm Hg. Medications were not specified, but inotrope use was explicitly discouraged. The patient population was a particularly ill group as reflected by an average LVEF 19%, urea nitrogen 35 mg/dL, creatinine1.5 mg/dL, RAP 14 mmHg, PCWP 25 mmHg, and cardiac index 1.9 l/min/m^2.

Treatment in both groups led to substantial reductions in symptoms, JVP and edema. The use of a PAC did not significantly affect the primary end-point of number of days alive and out of the hospital during the first six months. There was no difference between groups with respect to number of days hospitalized, mortality at 180 days, or in-hospital plus 30-day mortality. Exercise and quality of life end- points improved in both groups with a trend toward greater improvement in the PAC group. The Minnesota Living with Heart Failure questionnaire improved in both groups with greater improvement in the PAC group at 1 but not 6 months. The time trade-off tool showed great improvement for the PAC group compared with the clinical assessment group at all time points suggesting a greater improvement in quality of life. There was a consistent trend of greater improvement in clinical status in patients in whom therapy had been adjusted using PAC. There were no deaths related to PAC use. Adverse events specifically attributable to PACs occurred in 9/215 (4.2%) patients and included: PAC-related infection (4 patients), bleeding (2 patients), catheter knotting (2 patients), pulmonary infarction/hemorrhage (2 patients) and ventricular tachycardia (1 patient).

The neutral findings from ESCAPE are consistent with recent meta-analysis data concerning the use of PACs in more diverse populations of patients in the critical care setting [115, 116]. These findings cannot be extrapolated to all patients in the critical care setting as patients enrolled in ESCAPE and other randomized studies were not felt to require invasive hemodynamic monitoring—that is, physicians had clinical equipoise about the need for a PAC.

Complications associated with the use of PACs include hematoma, pneumothorax, infection, pulmonary infarction, pulmonary hemorrhage, hemothorax, arterial puncture, catheter knotting, heart block in the setting of LBBB, and ventricular tachycardia. In the UK multicenter randomized Pulmonary Artery Catheters in Management of Patients in Intensive Care (PAC-Man) trial, the incidence of complications directly attributable to PAC insertion was significantly higher (10%) than in the ESCAPE trail (4.2%). However, the patients enrolled in the PAC-Man trial were significantly sicker than those in ESCAPE: 65% had multi-system organ failure; only 11% had decompensated heart failure; and the in-hospital mortality rate was 66% in the control group [117].

The HFSA, ACCF/AHA, and ESC guidelines do not recommend the routine use of invasive hemodynamic monitoring in ADHF but do outline indications for PAC in carefully selected patients [8, 28, 118]. IHM should be considered in patients whose volume status and filling pressures are uncertain. In addition, placement of a PA catheter should be strongly considered in patients who are hypotensive, in cardiogenic shock, are unresponsive to initial medical therapy, or who develop clinically significant hypotension and/or significant worsening of renal function during initial treatment for ADHF. IHM will help identify patients who have hypotension because of low filling pressures, can guide the use of higher dose diuretic therapy and/or parenteral vasodilator therapy in patients with marginal blood pressure and persistent pulmonary congestion, and can indicate the need for inotropic therapy in patients with end-organ dysfunction, hypotension or worsening renal failure. IHM is indicated in patients with persistent severe symptoms despite adjustment of recommended therapies. In addition, invasive measurement of hemodynamics is indicated in patients being considered for heart transplantation to determine PA pressures, pulmonary vascular resistance, and transpulmonary gradient and in patients being considered for a long-term left ventricular assist device to better assess right ventricular performance [8, 119].

Diuretic Resistance

An impaired response to loop diuretics is seen in some patients with ADHF and is referred to as diuretic resistance (DR). Estimating an accurate incidence of diuretic resistance among patients with ADHF is hindered by the absence of a uniformly accepted definition. Probably the most commonly cited definition is "failure to decongest despite adequate and escalating doses of diuretics" [120]. Other definitions include measures of sodium excretion or volume loss related to the amount of furosemide administered [20]. A practical definition may be: persistent volume overload despite administration of 160 to 320 mg of furosemide or LD equivalent given intravenously over a 24-h period [83]. DR is more common in patients with diabetes, atherosclerotic disease, lower eGFR, high BUN and/or low systolic BP and is associated with greater risk of death and heart failure rehospitalization [121, 122].

DR results from the interplay between the pathophysiology of sodium retention in heart failure and the renal and neurohormonal responses to diuretic therapy. As described above, the diuretic response curve in heart failure is shifted downward and to the right so that the intraluminal threshold for diuresis is increased and the maximal effect or "ceiling" is reduced. DR represents a further shift downward and to the right of the response curve. The pathophysiology of DR is multifactorial. Potential causes include: changes in cardiac and renal hemodynamics (see below); decreased delivery of LDs to the proximal tubule as a result of decreased renal blood flow or decreased secretion of LDs into the proximal tubule due competition with organic acids (e.g. BUN) for binding sites on the organic acid transport system; the "breaking phenomenon" (see above); activation of the RAAS and sympathetic nervous system resulting in decreased renal blood flow; and an increase in the absorption of sodium at tubular sites not blocked by LDs including the proximal tubule (mediated by increases in angiotensin II) and the distal tubule and proximal collecting duct (mediated by increases in aldosterone) despite optimal doses of neurohormonal antagonists [86, 123]. Chronically, hypertrophy and hyperfunction of the tubular cells in the nephron distal to the loop of Henle occurs which results in enhanced sodium retention [25, 26].

Venous Congestion

There is increasing evidence that elevated central venous pressure and elevated intra-abdominal pressure (IAP) contribute to diuretic resistance and worsening renal function in patients with ADHF. This has been appreciated since 1950 [124]. A retrospective review of 2557 patients who underwent right heart catheterization at a single academic medical center found that elevated CVP was the only hemodynamic parameter that was associated with low eGFR on multivariate analysis [125]. In another study, 51 patients with heart failure underwent pulmonary artery catheterization. GFR and renal blood flow were assessed by (125)I-Iothalamate and (131) I-Hippuran clearances, respectively. High right atrial pressure had little impact on GFR in patients with normal or high renal blood flow but was associated with a significant reduction in GFR in patients with low renal blood flow [126]. In a study of 145 consecutive patients admitted with ADHF treated with intensive medical therapy guided by hemodynamic monitoring using a pulmonary artery catheter, elevated CVP on admission (and after intensive medical therapy) was the only hemodynamic measure that was associated with worsening renal function defined as increase in serum creatinine of ≥0.3 mg/dL. There was an incremental risk of worsening renal function with increasing CVP; 75% of patients with baseline CVP > 24 mmHg developed worsening renal function during hospitalization [127].

Mullens measured intraabdominal pressure (IAP) serially using a transvesicle technique [128, 129] in 40 patients admitted for treatment of ADHF. 60% of patients had increased intraabdominal pressure (>7 mmHg) and 10% had intraabdominal hypertension (≥12 mmHg). Increased IAP was associated with worse renal function at baseline. Intensive medical therapy resulted in improved hemodynamics and lower IAP. There was a strong correlation noted between reduction in IAP and improvement in renal function in patients with elevated IAP at baseline [130]. In a small group of patients hospitalized for ADHF who had increased IAP and ascites who developed progressive elevation in serum creatinine in response to intravenous loop diuretics, mechanical fluid removal by paracentesis decreased IAP and improved renal function [131].

These data suggest that high right atrial pressure and elevated intraabdominal pressure contribute to renal dysfunction and diuretic resistance in patients with ADHF. Elevated IAP may compress the renal veins, the ureters or the renal parenchyma and probably impacts intraglomerular hemodynamics. Glomerular filtration pressure can be calculated by subtracting proximal tubular pressure (which can be estimated by IAP) from mean blood pressure. The renal filtration gradient, which strongly correlates with GFR, is calculated by subtracting proximal tubular pressure from glomerular filtration pressure (mean blood pressure—2 IAP). As IAP increases, especially in patients with relatively low mean arterial pressure, GFR significantly decreases [130].

Cardiorenal Syndrome (CRS)

Combined disorders of cardiac and renal function are classified as cardiorenal syndromes. CRS Type 1 is defined by the development of acute kidney injury occurring in the setting of an acute cardiac illness, most commonly ADHF. It occurs in approximately 25–30% of patients hospitalized for ADHF. The most commonly used criteria to identify patients with CRS Type 1 are an increase in serum creatinine >0.3 mg/dL or a reduction in eGFR of 20–25%. Risk factors for developing CRS include prior heart failure, male gender, diabetes, admission creatinine ≥1.5 mg/dL, and hypertension [132, 133]. The clinical syndrome is characterized by a rise in serum creatinine (generally within the first 3 days of hospitalization), oliguria and diuretic resistance with or without worsening HF symptoms. While alterations in renal hemodynamics including renal hypoperfusion, low systemic blood pressure and elevated venous congestion play a role in diuretic resistance and renal insufficiency in ADHF, changes in renal hemodynamics alone do not account for this syndrome. In an analysis from the ESCAPE trial, no correlation was found between any baseline hemodynamic parameter or change in hemodynamic parameter and the development of worsening renal function during heart failure hospitalization [134]. In an analysis of hemodynamic data from patients enrolled in the Vasodilation in Management of Acute Congestive Heart Failure (VMAC) trial who had undergone right heart catheterization, no correlation was found between worsening renal function and baseline right atrial pressure (RAP) or change in RAP. Smaller net fluid loss in the first 24 h was strongly associated with an increased risk of developing worsening renal function [135]. Emerging evidence suggests that the pathophysiology of CRS Type I is multifactorial, involves complex heart and renal crosstalk and is mediated by hemodynamic changes, neurohormonal activation, inflammation, immune cell signaling, hypothalamic-pituitary stress reaction, systemic endotoxin exposure from the abdominal viscera, and oxidative stress resulting in bidirectional organ injury. This pathophysiology is incompletely understood and definitive approaches to treatment have not been established [32, 122, 136–138].

Diuretic Resistance-Treatment Strategies

A number of treatment strategies have been found to be useful in patients with diuretic resistance. Diuretics should be given intravenously to avoid issues of decreased or delayed absorption because of intestinal edema. Escalating doses of IV diuretics should be administered to insure that the patient is diuretic resistant and not undertreated. Diuretics should be dosed at least 2–3 times a day or given as a continuous infusion to insure that the time of sub-threshold diuretic concentration in the loop of Henle is kept at a minimum. Data from several studies suggest that continuous infusion of loop diuretics improves diuresis and renal function when compared to bolus therapy [139, 140]. These results were not confirmed in the DOSE trial.

Combined Diuretic Therapy (CDT)

The addition of an oral or intravenous thiazide diuretic has been shown to be helpful in patients with diuretic resistance. Thiazide diuretics are weak natriuretic agents that block only 5–10% of filtered sodium when used as monotherapy. They are ineffective as single agents in the treatment of patients with moderate to severe heart failure. However, in the setting of LD therapy, sodium delivery to the distal tubule increases significantly. Hypertrophy and hyperfunction of the distal nephron contribute to diuretic resistance. Blocking sodium uptake using TD has been shown to increase diuresis significantly. The combination of diuretics that act at different sites in the nephron has been termed "sequential nephron blockade". Generally, it is appropriate to consider adding a TD when adequate diuresis has not been achieved despite an intravenous dose of furosemide of 180–360 mg daily (or other LD equivalent). There is little evidence to suggest that one TD is superior to another when used in combination with an intravenous LD. It has been suggested that metolazone is superior to other TDs in patients with renal insufficiency but other TDs have been shown to be effective in this patient population. Traditionally, TDs have been given 30 min before LD administration. However, this dosing regimen has not been studied—most studies of CDT looked at the effect of giving an LD and TD at the same time [20, 83, 141, 142].

The most serious complication of CDT is hypokalemia which can be profound. Hyponatremia is common. Hypomagnesemia can occur and may make hypokalemia worse. Occasionally, CDT results in a marked diuresis which may result in hypotension. Electrolytes, renal function, urine output and vital signs need to be followed closely.

Ultrafiltration (UF)

Ultrafiltration (UF) is the process of extracorporeal removal of plasma water from whole blood using a semipermeable membrane that allows for the removal of fluid in response to a transmembrane pressure gradient generated either by arterial pressure (in the case of arterial-venous ultrafiltration) or by an extracorporeal pump (in the case of veno-venous ultrafiltration). Blood is removed from and then returned to the circulation after passing through a UF filter. The fluid removed is isotonic with plasma. In the past, the use of UF was limited by machines that required high flow rates, large extracorporeal blood volumes and the use of large bore intravenous catheters. With contemporary UF devices (Aquadex System 100), veno-venous ultrafiltration can be performed using a double lumen venous catheter placed centrally or peripherally that can accommodate 10–40 ml/min of blood flow. Therapeutic anticoagulation using continuous infusion heparin is recommended to avoid clotting the UF filter. UF can be performed at the bedside without the need for specialized personnel. The total extracorporeal blood volume is 33 cc. Pump blood flow can be adjusted to between 10–40 ml/min. Fluid removal can range from 10–500 ml/h [23, 143, 144].

UF removes fluid from the intravascular space. The reduction in blood volume results in a decrease in intraluminal hydrostatic pressure that promotes movement of fluid from the interstitial to the intravascular space. This preserves intravascular volume and maintains adequate intracardiac filling pressures, cardiac output and systemic blood pressure. Ultrafiltration can safely remove fluid in patients with volume overload provided that the rate of fluid removal does not exceed the rate at which extravascular fluid is reabsorbed into the intravascular space (the plasma refill rate or PRR). The PRR is proportional to the trans-capillary pressure gradient (the net difference between intraluminal and interstitial oncotic and hydrostatic pressure gradients) and the permeability of the capillary membrane. The plasma refill rate is approximately 15 ml/min but is variable among patients and changes in the same patient in response to heart failure treatment [23, 143, 144].

UF has been shown in patients with refractory heart failure to lower right atrial and pulmonary capillary wedge pressure and increase cardiac output and stroke volume without changing mean arterial pressure, heart rate or plasma volume [145]. One study compared UF with continuous infusion of furosemide with a goal of achieving a 50% reduction in RA pressure in 16 patients with ADHF. The UF and furosemide patients had a similar reduction in RA and PCW pressures immediately after treatment. Both groups had elevation in plasma renin activity, norepinephrine and aldosterone levels immediately after treatment. At day 4, the UF group demonstrated a sustained reduction in filling pressures while the furosemide group had a return of filling pressures to baseline. In addition, by day 2, plasma renal activity, plasma norepinephrine levels, and aldosterone levels decreased to below baseline in the UF group but remained elevated in the furosemide group. These differences in filling pressures and neurohormone levels were sustained for three months [146]. These observations led to the hypothesis that ultrafiltration may be superior to IV diuretic therapy in avoiding diuretic-induced neurohormonal activation.

The Relief for Acutely Fluid-Overloaded Patients with Decompensated Congestive Heart Failure (RAPID-CHF) trial was a small multicenter study that compared a single 8-h session of UF with usual care to usual care alone in 40 patients hospitalized for ADHF who had evidence of significant volume overload on physical exam. The primary end-point was weight loss 24 h after the time of enrollment. Ultrafiltration was successfully performed in 18 of the 20 patients assigned to UF group. Fluid removal after 24 h was 4650 ml in the UF group and 2838 ml in the usual care groups ($p = 0.001$). Weight loss after 24 h, the primary end-point, was 2.5 kg in the UF group and 1.86 kg in the usual care group ($p = 0.240$). UF was well tolerated. Dyspnea and CHF symptoms were significantly improved in the UF group compared to usual care at 48 h. There were greater improvements in global CHF and dyspnea assessments in the UF group compared with the usual care group at 48 h. There was no difference in the median length of stay between the study groups [147].

The Ultrafiltration versus Intravenous Diuretics for Patients Hospitalized for Acute Decompensated Congestive Heart Failure (UNLOAD) trial tested the hypothesis that veno-venous ultrafiltration is superior to intravenous diuretics in patients hospitalized with ADHF [94]. 200 patients hospitalized with ADHF who had evidence of volume overload were randomized within 24 h of admission to parenteral diuretics or ultrafiltration without concomitant diuretic therapy. The duration and rate (up to 500 ml/h) of fluid removal were decided by the treating physician. The minimum daily intravenous diuretic dose had to be at least twice the before-hospitalization daily oral dose. The primary efficacy end-points were weight loss and patients' dyspnea assessment 48 h after randomization. The primary safety endpoints were: changes in serum blood urea nitrogen, creatinine, and electrolytes assessed at entry and at intervals up to 90 days after enrollment; and episodes of hypotension within 48 h of randomization.

Weight loss at 48 h was greater in the ultrafiltration group (5.0 kg vs 3.1 kg; p = 0.001). Dyspnea score improved to a similar degree in the two treatment arms. Changes in serum creatinine were similar in the two groups. Serum potassium <3.5 mEq/L was more common in the diuretic group than in the ultrafiltration group (12% vs 1%, P = 0.018). There was no difference in the length of index hospitalization. Fewer patients in the ultrafiltration group required vasoactive drugs at 48 h. At 90 days, the ultrafiltration group had fewer patients rehospitalized for HF (18% vs 32%; p = 0.037). New York Heart Association functional class, Minnesota Living with Heart Failure scores, 6 -minute walk distance, Global Assessment scores and B-type natriuretic peptide levels were similarly improved in both groups at discharge and at 30 and 90 days.

The Cardiorenal Rescue Study in Acute Decompensated Heart Failure (CARRESS-HF) compared veno-venous ultrafiltration to diuretic-based stepped pharmacologic therapy in patients hospitalized for ADHF who had worsening renal function and persistent congestion [148]. Patients could be considered for inclusion in the trial if they were hospitalized for ADHF, had worsened renal function defined as an increase in serum creatinine of at least 0.3 mg/dL within 12 weeks before or 10 days after the index admission for heart failure and had evidence of persistent congestion (defined by at least two of the following: at least 2+ peripheral edema, jugular venous pressure greater than 10 cm of water, or pulmonary edema or pleural effusions on chest radiography). There was no exclusion criterion based on ejection fraction. Patients with a serum creatinine level > 3.5 mg/dL at the time of admission and those receiving intravenous vasodilators or inotropic agents were excluded from the study. Patients were randomized in a 1:1 ratio to ultrafiltration using the Aquadex System 100 with fluid removal at a rate of 200 ml per hour without concomitant diuretic therapy or stepped pharmacologic therapy targeted to achieve a daily urine output of 3–5 l and that could include bolus furosemide, continuous infusion furosemide, a thiazide diuretic, metolazone, dopamine or dobutamine at 2 mcg/kg/min, and nitroglycerine or nesiritide. The primary end point was the bivariate change from baseline in the serum creatinine level and body weight, assessed 96 h after random assignment. Patients were followed for 60 days.

UF was found inferior to pharmacologic therapy due to an increase in creatinine in the ultrafiltration group (+0.23 vs −0.04; p = 0.003). There was no difference between treatment groups with respect to change in weight. A higher percentage of patients in the ultrafiltration group than in the pharmacologic-therapy group had a serious adverse event (72% vs. 57%, P = 0.03) predominantly related to bleeding complications, renal failure and infection. There was no difference in the estimated 60-day mortality rate or the composite rate of death or hospitalization for heart failure. At 96 h and at day 7 or hospital discharge, there were no significant between group differences in scores on the dyspnea and global well-being visual-analogue scales. Clinical decongestion at 96 h (defined as JVP < 8 cm of water, no more than trace peripheral edema, and the absence of orthopnea) occurred in 9% of patients with pharmacologic therapy and 10% of patients with ultrafiltration.

Ultrafiltration has not been established as first line therapy to treat volume overload in ADHF in light of cost, the need for veno-venous access, provider experience, the need for specially trained nursing support, and the lack of benefit in randomized trials comparing UF to standard therapy. The ACCF/AHA and HFSA guidelines suggest that UF may be considered for patients with obvious volume overload in lieu of diuretics or for patients with refractory congestion not responding to medical therapy [8, 28]. Providers should be aware that initiating UF in patients with significant or progressive renal insufficiency, diuretic resistance, and refractory volume overload may cause worsening renal function and the need for chronic renal replacement therapy.

Parenteral Vasodilators

Vasodilators have a role in the management of patients with ADHF, especially in patients with hypertension on presentation, in patients without hypotension and with systolic dysfunction who have severe symptomatic volume overload and in patients who do not respond promptly to diuretic therapy alone in the absence of hypotension. Three parenteral vasodilators are appropriate in the treatment of ADHF: nitroglycerine, sodium nitroprusside and nesiritide. Vasodilators decrease preload and afterload to varying degrees, increase stroke volume, and decrease functional mitral regurgitation. Guidelines from the ACCF/AHA and HFSA endorse the use of nitroglycerine, nitroprusside, or nesiritide as additions to diuretic therapy for relief of congestive symptoms in the absence of hypotension [8, 28]. The use of IV nitroglycerine in the absence of hypotension is also endorsed by guidelines from the ESC and the American College of Emergency Physicians [118, 149]. The 2012 ESC guidelines suggest that: "an IV infusion of a nitrate should be considered in patients with pulmonary congestion/edema and a systolic blood pressure of >110 mmHg, who do not have severe mitral or aortic stenosis, to reduce pulmonary capillary wedge pressure and systemic vascular resistance. Nitrates may also relieve dyspnea and congestion. Symptoms and blood pressure should be monitored frequently during administration of IV nitrates" [118]. The HFSA Guidelines suggest that intravenous vasodilators (nitroprusside, nitroglycerin, or nesiritide) may be considered in patients with ADHF who have persistent severe HF despite aggressive treatment with diuretics and standard oral therapies. It should be noted that only 18% of patients enrolled in the ADHERE registry received IV vasodilators and < 1% of patients receive nitroprusside [150].

Nitroglycerin, nitroprusside and nesiritide all act by activating soluble guanylate cyclase in smooth muscle cells. The resulting increase in intracellular cyclic guanosine monophosphate (cGMP) results in vasodilation. The physiologic effect may be predominantly venodilation (NTG) or so called "balanced" arterial and venous dilation (SNP, nesiritide, and higher dose NTG). Most studies of vasodilator therapy in ADHF have looked at short-term hemodynamic endpoints. These studies suggest that vasodilator therapy is associated with an improvement in hemodynamic parameters with a reduction in right atrial and pulmonary capillary wedge pressures, a reduction in the severity of mitral regurgitation and an increase in cardiac output. Reasonable goals for the use of vasodilator therapy include: more rapid relief of dyspnea; control of blood pressure in the patient presenting with ADHF and hypertension; improvement of symptoms in patients with an inadequate response to diuretic therapy; treatment of myocardial ischemia (with NTG); and improvement in hemodynamics while transitioning to oral heart failure medication [45, 61, 151–156].

Hypotension is the most important limitation of using vasodilators in heart failure. Vasodilators should be avoided in patients with a systolic blood pressure of <90–110 mmHg or mean blood pressures of less than 65 mmHg. Blood pressure should be monitored frequently and the vasodilator should be discontinued if hypotension develops. Vasodilator therapy may be reinitiated at a lower dose once hypotension resolves. Because volume depleted patients are at significant risk of developing hypotension with vasodilator therapy, it is important to establish that the patient is volume overloaded prior to starting any of these medications. Vasodilators should be used with caution in patients with HFpEF as these patients are more preload sensitive. Vasodilators should also be used with caution, if at all, in patients with significant aortic or mitral stenosis [8, 118, 157].

Organic Nitrates/Nitroglycerine

Nitroglycerine and other organic nitrates are pro-drugs that are converted to nitric oxide and other NO-containing compounds. NO stimulates the enzyme guanylate cyclase which in turn increases the production of cyclic guanosine monophosphate (cGMP) in the vascular wall. Increases in cGMP reduce cytosolic calcium levels by decreasing the release of calcium from the cytoplasmic reticulum and by reducing calcium influx from the extracellular space. In addition, NO-mediated increases in intracellular cGMP activate protein kinase G (PKG) which also plays an important role in mediating nitrate-mediated vasorelaxation. These changes lead to smooth muscle relaxation and venous and arterial vasodilation [153–158]. Endothelial release of prostacyclin may also contribute to the vascular effects [159]. The exact mechanism of the process of biotransformation from nitroglycerine to NO is incompletely understood. Some studies suggest that NTG is hydrolyzed by hepatic glutathione–organic nitrate reductase. Other data suggest that mitochondrial aldehyde dehydrogenase (ALDH-2) mediates NTG biotransformation [160].

Organic nitrates can be administered sublingually, orally, by inhalation, transdermally, or intravenously. At low dose (30–40 μg/min), intravenous NTG predominantly causes venodilation. At higher doses, NTG also causes arterial and coronary vasodilation [158]. The onset of the hemodynamic effects of NTG is immediate. The offset is also rapid. NTG has an elimination half-life of 3 minutes. Nitrates are cleared by extraction in the vasculature, hydrolysis in the blood, and metabolism by glutathione-nitrate reductase in the liver. Glass bottles and non-polyvinyl chloride plastic tubing must be used to avoid absorption onto plastic surfaces. The drug is generally initiated at an infusion rate of 10 mcg/min and increased in increments of 5–10 μg/min every 3–5 minutes titrated to relief of symptoms of angina or dyspnea, reduction in PCWP, change in systolic blood pressure, or drug related side effects [17]. The maximum dose is between 200–500 mcg/min [153, 161].

The hemodynamic effects of a therapeutic dose of NTG in patients with heart failure due to systolic dysfunction include reductions in right- and left-sided filling pressures, pulmonary and systemic vascular resistance, and systolic blood pressure. Cardiac output generally improves due to a reduction in systemic vascular resistance and the severity of mitral regurgitation [152, 153, 161]. In some patients, there may also be an improvement in myocardial ischemia related to NTG-mediated dilation of epicardial coronary arteries and reductions in preload and afterload.

There is evidence that the vasodilator response and hemodynamic effects of organic nitrates are attenuated in patients with heart failure. This is referred to as “nitrate resistance”. Up to 50% of patients with heart failure do not have a significant reduction in PCWP with conventional doses of nitrate (e.g. isosorbide dinitrate 40 mg orally) [162–165]. Nitrate resistance can be overcome with increasing doses of nitrate but approximately 20% of patients do not have a hemodynamic response to NTG regardless of dose [165, 166]. Nitrate resistance appears to be more common in patients with high right atrial pressure and/or significant edema. Proposed mechanisms for nitrate resistance include: an increase in sodium and water in the vascular wall; mechanical compression of arterioles by excessive interstitial fluid [164]; sulfhydryl group deficiency [167]; and neurohormonal activation leading to vasoconstriction with attenuation of the vasodilatory effects of nitrates [161]. Patients who do not have hemodynamic or clinical benefit at doses of IV NTG of greater than 200 mcg/min should be considered non-responders and are not expected to have clinical benefit from further dose escalation.

In addition, there is substantial evidence that treatment of ADHF with nitroglycerine is limited by the development of early tolerance that results in a marked attenuation of the initial hemodynamic response and occurs in as little as 12–24 h after NTG initiation [161, 168, 169]. Early tolerance occurs in about half of patients and cannot be predicted by baseline hemodynamic measurements, the magnitude of the initial change in hemodynamics in response to

NTG or baseline or treatment plasma levels of epinephrine, norepinephrine or renin [170]. A number of mechanisms have been proposed to explain nitrate tolerance including: early volume expansion after NTG initiation; neurohormonal activation in response to NTG administration (RAAS, sympathetic nervous system, arginine vasopressin, endothelin); sulfhydryl group depletion; nitrate-mediated increases in vascular superoxide/peroxynitrite production; impairment of nitrate biotransformation; and abnormalities of nitric oxide signal transduction including desensitization of soluble guanylate cyclase and increased phosphodiesterase activity [161, 168–170]. Data suggests that volume expansion, neurohormonal activation and sulfhydryl depletion are less likely to play an important role in the development of nitrate tolerance [161, 165, 171–174].

A number of strategies have been proposed to avoid nitrate tolerance. Sulfhydryl group repletion has been proposed for the prevention of tolerance [168]. This has not been supported by studies of concomitant treatment with the sulfhydryl group donor N-acetylcysteine or the sulfhydryl-containing ACE inhibitor captopril [171, 173, 175]. Hydralazine has been shown to prevent the development of NTG tolerance in both experimental models and patients with congestive heart failure [176–178]. It has been suggested that hydralazine prevents tolerance by preventing NTG-induced increases in vascular superoxide/peroxynitrite production or by scavenging vascular superoxide/peroxynitrite. The African American Heart Failure Trial (A-HeFT) demonstrated an improvement in survival and a decrease in hospitalization in patients with chronic HFrEF with hydralazine and isosorbide dinitrate added to standard heart failure therapy compared with chronic heart failure therapy alone [179]. The use of hydralazine and ISDN has not been investigated in patients with ADHF. The strategy of a > 12-h nitrate free interval used to prevent tolerance in patients with chronic stable angina or chronic heart failure is not practical in the treatment of ADHF.

Randomized Clinical Trials of Nitrates in ADHF

A prospective randomized trial studied the benefit of furosemide and isosorbide dinitrate in 104 patients who presented to mobile emergency units with pulmonary edema and oxygen saturations of less than 90% [180]. All patients were treated with oxygen, morphine sulfate 3 mg bolus and furosemide 40 mg IV and then randomized to high dose isosorbide dinitrate (3 mg bolus administered intravenously every 5 min) or high dose furosemide (80 mg IV every 15 min and isosorbide dinitrate infusion at 1 mg/h (16 mcg/min) increased by 1 mg/h every 10 min. Treatment was continued in both groups until oxygen saturation increased to at least 96% or mean arterial blood pressure decreased by at least 30% or to lower than 90 mm Hg. The main end-points were death, need for mechanical ventilation, and myocardial infarction. The group that received high dose nitrates had significantly fewer myocardial infarctions (17% vs 37%; p = 0.047) and less need for mechanical ventilation (13% vs 40%; p = 0.0041). In addition, there were significantly greater improvements in heart rate, respiratory rate and oxygenation in the high dose nitrate group. Limitations of the study were that it was not blinded, it was conducted in an ambulatory out of hospital setting, and that a significant number of patients who were screened for enrollment did not meet the inclusion criteria and were excluded from randomization.

The Vasodilation in the Management of Acute Congestive Heart Failure (VMAC) Trial was a complex, randomized, multicenter, double blind, double-dummy, controlled trial of 489 patients with ADHF [181]. The study included patients with preserved and depressed systolic function and patients with and without coronary artery disease. 246 patients underwent right heart catheterization at the discretion of the investigator (the catheterized stratum). Patients were randomized to receive intravenous NTG, intravenous nesiritide or placebo added to standard therapy for the first 3 h followed by nesiritide or NTG added to standard therapy for 24 h (the patients in the initial placebo group were again randomized to nesiritide or NTG at 3 h.) Nesiritide was administered as a 2 mcg/kg bolus followed by a fixed-dose infusion of 0.01 mcg/kg/min infusion. The dose could be increased every 3 h up to 0.03 mcg/kg/min. The NTG dose was not dictated by protocol but was determined by the investigator and could be changed throughout the study period at the discretion of the investigator. The primary end-points of the trial were change in PCWP at 3 h in the catheterized stratum and patient self-evaluation of dyspnea at 3 h in the catheterized and non-catheterized strata. Secondary end-points included comparisons of hemodynamic and clinical effects between nesiritide and NTG groups at 24 h. At 3 h, the mean dose of NTG was 42 mcg/min in the catheterized patients and 29 mcg/min in the non-catheterized patients. At 24 h, the mean dose of NTG in the catheterized patients increased to 55 mcg/min, but did not change in the non-catheterized patients. Only 23/273 patients in the nesiritide arm had an increase in nesiritide dose. At 3 h, there was a greater reduction in PCWP in the nesiritide group compared to both the placebo ($P < 0.001$) and NTG groups ($P = 0.03$). PCWP decreased by 5.8 mmHg in the nesiritide group; 3.8 mmHg in the NTG group; and 2 mmHg in the placebo group. The difference in PCWP between NTG and placebo was not significant. At 3 h, there was greater improvement in dyspnea when nesiritide was compared to placebo but not to NTG. There was no difference in dyspnea or global clinical assessment between NTG and placebo. At 24 h, there was a greater reduction in PCWP in the nesiritide group compared with the NTG group (−8.2 vs −6.3 mmHg; $p < 0.05$) but no difference in dyspnea and only a modest difference in improvement in global clinical status favoring nesiritide.

The most important limitation in the use of NTG is dose-related hypotension. Hypotension can develop in volume depleted patients or in patients in whom cardiac output is critically dependent on preload (e.g., aortic stenosis, restrictive cardiomyopathy, RV infarction). Sublingual nitroglycerin may rarely produce bradycardia and hypotension, probably due to activation of the Bezold-Jarisch reflex. Side effects of NTG include headache and abdominal pain. Serious side effects are unusual. NTG use is contraindicated in patients who have recently taken one of the phosphodiesterase type 5 (PDE5) inhibitors (sildenafil, vardenafil, tadalafil, avanafil) used to treat erectile dysfunction or pulmonary hypertension because of the risk sustained hypotension. Approximately 20% of patients with heart failure are resistant to the hemodynamic effects of any dose of NTG [8, 182, 183].

The preferred dose and route of administration of nitrates have not been established. A common approach is to give nitrates at progressive dose increments with a goal of reducing mean blood pressure by 10 mmHg while maintaining systolic blood pressure > 90 mmHg. Invasive hemodynamic monitoring is not needed. IV administration is preferred by most HF specialists. Starting nitroglycerin at 10–20 mcg/min and increasing dose up to physiologic effect up to a maximum of 200 mcg/min or isosorbide dinitrate 1–10 mg/h are common dosing regimens [61]. NTG should not be abruptly withdrawn in patients with ADHF as this may precipitate reflex vasoconstriction with acute decompensation.

Sodium Nitroprusside

Nitroprusside (SNP) is a powerful "balanced" nitrovasodilator affecting both arterial and venous vasodilation. It is a water-soluble sodium salt comprised of Fe^{2+} complexed with nitric oxide (NO) and five cyanide anions. It functions as a pro-drug in that it reacts with sulfhydryl groups on erythrocytes, albumin and other proteins to form nitrosothiol and ultimately NO in the vasculature. The mechanism of release of NO is not entirely clear. NO activates the guanylyl cyclase–cyclic GMP–PKG pathway which, in turn, results in vascular smooth muscle relaxation and venous and arterial vasodilation. Dilation of arterial résistance vessels reduces LV afterload. The venodilator effect increases venous capacitance and decreases preload. Infusion results in a reduction in RA pressure, PCWP, systemic vascular resistance and pulmonary vascular resistance, an increase in stroke volume and cardiac output, reduction in secondary mitral regurgitation and little change in heart rate. In general, in patients with severe heart failure, nitroprusside increases cardiac output and renal blood flow, and improves GFR and diuretic effectiveness. However, excessive reduction in systemic blood pressure may prevent an increase or result in a decrease in renal blood flow. Nitroprusside generally reduces systolic and diastolic ventricular wall stress and lowers myocardial oxygen consumption [153, 184–186].

Nitroprusside is an unstable molecule that decomposes when exposed to light. The medication must be protected from light to prevent degradation and subsequent rapid cyanide release on administration. The drug is administered as a continuous infusion. The onset of effect is within 30 s of the start of an infusion with peak hemodynamic effect seen within 2 min. The hemodynamic effects resolve within 2 min of stopping the infusion [153, 184–186].

The major side effect of SNP is hypotension which can be rapidly reversed by lowering the dose or discontinuing the medication. Nitroprusside-related hypotension may be harmful in patients with myocardial infarction or ischemia. Nitroprusside may cause coronary steal in patients with coronary artery disease by dilating non-obstructed coronary arteries directing blood away from maximally dilated coronary beds downstream from a flow limiting stenosis. Unlike organic nitrates, tachyphyalaxis to SNP does not occur. Some patients may have rebound elevation of systemic vascular resistance and blood pressure with clinical deterioration after abrupt discontinuation [187]. Therefore, gradual weaning after initiation of oral vasodilator therapy is recommended. Nitroprusside can worsen arterial hypoxemia in patients with chronic obstructive pulmonary disease or pneumonia due to worsening ventilation-perfusion mismatching resulting from nitroprusside-induced reversal of hypoxic pulmonary vasoconstriction with pulmonary arteriolar dilation in in non-ventilated areas. Methemoglobinemia is an unusual complication of treatment with SNP and is due to oxidation of hemoglobin by nitric oxide.

Toxicity from SNP may result from conversion of nitroprusside to cyanide and thiocyanate. Nitroprusside metabolism results in the release of cyanide anions in vivo. Cyanide is generally rapidly metabolized by hepatic rhodanase to thiocyanate which is eliminated in the urine. The elimination half-life for thiocyanate is 3 days in patients with normal renal function but can be much longer in patients with renal insufficiency. Cyanide can also bind to tissue cytochrome oxidase. Accumulation of cyanide leads to severe lactic acidosis and symptoms of restlessness, agitation, and sinus tachycardia. Patients are at risk of cyanide toxicity when SNP is infused at rates >5 mcg/kg/min or administered in the setting of significant hepatic dysfunction. Cyanide toxicity is better correlated with serum rather than whole blood cyanide concentrations. Elevated lactate concentration is an excellent surrogate marker for cyanide toxicity. Cyanide toxicity can be treated by administration of thiosulfate or hydroxycobalamin. These medications are equally effective and have no significant adverse effects [188].

The risk of thiocyanate toxicity increases in patients receiving SNP at rates >3 mcg/kg/min for ≥72 h and in patients with renal insufficiency. Signs and symptoms of thiocyanate toxicity include anorexia, nausea, fatigue, disorientation, and toxic psychosis. Thiocyanate can be removed readily by hemodialysis while cyanide cannot [185]. Thiocyanate and cyanide toxicity are rare in patients receiving ≤3 mcg/kg/min for ≤72 h.

There are a limited number of clinical trials that demonstrate efficacy of SNP in ADHF. A small single center trial of SNP in patients with refractory heart failure demonstrated a consistent reduction in PCWP from a mean of 32.2 to 17.2 mmHg, increase in cardiac output from 2.98 to 5.2 l/min, reduction in mean blood pressure of 15 mmHg, and doubling of forward LVEF and stroke volume with similar responses in patients with and without an ischemic etiology of heart failure [189]. A single center open label randomized controlled trial compared SNP to furosemide in 50 patients with a PCWP >20 mmHg within 24 h of an acute myocardial infarction [190]. Within 1 h, there were greater decreases in PCWP (−9 vs. −4 mmHg) and systemic vascular resistance (−21% vs +10%), and greater increases in cardiac index (+16% vs. −7%) in the SNP group compared with the furosemide group, respectively.

A multi-center randomized placebo-controlled study compared a 48-h infusion of SNP to placebo in 812 men with presumed acute myocardial infarction and a left ventricular filling pressure ≥ 12 mmHg [191]. The mortality rates at 21 days and 13 weeks were not different between groups. The impact of SNP was related to the time of treatment with respect to onset of MI –related pain. Mortality at 13 weeks was higher in the SNP group compared with the placebo group in patients in whom infusions were started within 9 h of the onset of pain but lower in the SNP group compared with placebo in patients in whom infusions were started after 9 h of the onset of pain.

A single-center retrospective review of patients admitted for ADHF who underwent right heart catheterization and were found to have a cardiac index ≤2.0 l/min/m^2 and elevated filling pressures compared outcomes in patients who were or were not treated with SNP [192]. Patients treated with SNP had greater improvement in hemodynamic measurements during hospitalization, higher rates of oral vasodilator prescription at discharge, and lower rates of all-cause mortality at a median follow up of 25.7 months. SNP use was not associated with a higher rate of inotrope use or worsening renal function during hospitalization.

In a series of single center studies, SNP and IV diuretics were used to achieve specific hemodynamic parameters in patients with advanced heart failure many of whom were felt refractory to heart failure medications and were referred for heart transplantation. Using this approach, patients with severe decompensated heart failure having low cardiac outputs and high filling pressures on right heart catheterization were treated with IV diuretics and sodium nitroprusside adjusted to achieve specific hemodynamic goals defined as: PCWP ≤15–18 mmHg, right atrial pressure ≤ 8 mmHg, decrease in mean pulmonary artery pressure by at least 20%, improvement in cardiac index to ≥2.2 l/min/m^2 or systemic vascular resistance to 1000–1200 dynes/sec cm^{-5}, while maintaining a mean arterial pressure > 65 mmHg or systolic blood pressure ≥ 80 mmHg [44]. Parenteral therapy was replaced with oral vasodilator and diuretic therapy tailored to maintain hemodynamic goals. Using this approach, goals for cardiac output, pulmonary capillary wedge pressure, and systemic vascular resistance could be achieved by intravenous followed by oral therapy in the majority of patients [193].

Intensive reduction in systemic vascular resistance and ventricular filling pressures was accompanied by a reduction in LV end-diastolic and end-systolic volumes, no change in LFEF, a decrease in total stroke volume but a 40% increase in forward stroke volume, and significant decreases in mitral and tricuspid regurgitation [45]. Improvements in hemodynamic parameters including near normal filling pressures were maintained at 8 months. Chronic hemodynamic improvement was accompanied by sustained symptomatic improvement [112]. Improvements in mitral and tricuspid regurgitation and estimated pulmonary artery pressures were sustained at 6 months on oral vasodilators and a flexible diuretic regimen. Further reductions in right atrial and left atrial volumes were also seen [113].

The HFSA, ACCF/AHA and ESC guidelines all endorse the use of nitroprusside to treat ADHF in the absence of symptomatic hypotension [8, 28, 118]. Nitroprusside is particularly useful in severely congested patients in whom rapid reduction of afterload is felt necessary—especially in the setting of hypertension or severe mitral regurgitation. Because of its powerful blood pressure lowering effect, SNP should be used in an intensive care unit setting where frequent blood pressures can be obtained. It can be rapidly titrated to achieve a specific systolic or mean blood pressure starting at doses as low as 0.1 mcg/kg/min and titrating up to as much as 5.0 mcg/kg/min.

Nesiritide

Nesiritide is a recombinant preparation of human B-type natriuretic peptide manufactured for intravenous administration. It has the same 32-amino acid sequence as endogenous BNP produced by the heart. Nesiritide is a balanced vasodilator with arterial and venous vasodilatory properties. Nesiritide binds to the natriuretic peptide receptor-A (NPR-A) which is widely expressed in kidney, lung, adipose, and vascular smooth muscle cells. (NPR-B receptors bind C-type natriuretic peptide and NPR-C receptors do not have a guanylate cyclase domain and function as clearance receptors.) The NPR-A receptor is linked to the cGMP-dependent signaling cascade and mediates many of the cardiovascular and renal effects of the natriuretic peptides. BNP binding to the NPR-A receptor activates the guanylyl cyclase–cyclic GMP–PKG pathway. The mean terminal half-life of nesiritide in patients with heart failure is approximately 18 min. Steady-state infusions of 0.01–0.03 mcg/kg/min increase baseline circulating BNP levels by three to six fold. BNP is metabolized by two mechanisms: binding to the NPR-C receptor with receptor-mediated internalization/degradation and proteolytic cleavage by neutral endopeptidases. Renal clearance plays a minimal role in nesiritide metabolism and medication dosing does not need to be modified for any degree of renal insufficiency [153, 194–197].

Nesiritide infusion is associated with dose-related decreases in systemic vascular resistance, pulmonary vascular resistance, and right atrial and pulmonary capillary wedge pressures and increases in stroke volume and cardiac output without a change in heart rate [198–200]. Nesiritide has been reported to decrease aldosterone [198, 200] and endothelin-1 levels [201] with conflicting reports concerning the impact on plasma norepinephrine levels [198, 201]. Nesiritide exerts vasodilator effects on coronary conductance and resistance vessels, increases coronary blood flow despite a reduction in coronary perfusion pressure and decreases myocardial oxygen consumption [202]. Nesiritide infusion is not associated with an increase in ventricular arrhythmias [203].

The results of clinical trials that have assessed the effect of nesiritide on urine output have been conflicting. In a placebo-controlled trial in which diuretics were held for 4 h prior to and during study drug infusion, patients receiving nesiritide at infusion rates of 0.015 mcg/kg/min or 0.03 mcg/kg/min had significantly greater urine output over a 6-h period compared to patients receiving placebo [200]. In the same report, nesiritide infusions at 0.015 mcg/kg/min or 0.03 mcg/kg/min were compared with placebo but patients could receive diuretics and/or other vasodilators. Intravenous diuretics were given to significantly fewer patients in the nesiritide groups compared with the placebo group [200]. In the Nesiritide Administered Peri-Anesthesia in Patients Undergoing Cardiac Surgery (NAPA) trial, patients with an LVEF<40% undergoing CABG with anticipated use of cardio-pulmonary bypass were randomized to receive fixed dose nesiritide at 0.01 mcg/kg/min or placebo for 24–96 h after induction of anesthesia [204]. Nesiritide was associated with greater urine output (2926 vs 2350 ml) during the initial 24 h after surgery and a shorter hospital stay. In a double-blind, placebo-controlled, crossover study of patients with decompensated heart failure who had an increase in creatinine of ≥0.2 mg/dL and ≥ 10% above baseline within 6 months of enrollment, patients were randomized to a nesiritide bolus of 2 mcg/kg IV bolus followed by an infusion at 0.01 mcg/kg/min or placebo for 24 h on consecutive days [205]. There were no differences in GFR by iothalamate clearance, effective renal plasma flow by para-amino hippurate clearance, urine output, or sodium excretion for any time interval or for the entire 24-h period between the nesiritide and placebo study days.

The Renal Optimization Strategies Evaluation (ROSE) trial was a multicenter, double blind placebo-controlled trial of 360 patients hospitalized with acute heart failure and renal dysfunction (defined as an eGFR of 15–60 mL/min/1.73 m^2 by the MDRD equation) randomized to dopamine 2 mcg/kg/min, nesiritide 0.005 mcg/kg/min without a bolus, or placebo for 72 h.

All patients received open label intravenous loop diuretic treatment with a recommended daily dose of 2.5 times their total daily outpatient diuretic dose. No difference was found between study groups with respect to the two primary end-points: 72-h cumulative urine volume and change in cystatin C level. In addition, there were no between group differences in secondary end-points of measures of decongestion, renal function or clinical outcomes [206].

The Vasodilator in the Management of Acute Heart Failure (VMAC) trial was a complex, multi-center, randomized double-blinded controlled study of nesiritide, nitroglycerine, and placebo added to standard therapy in 489 patients hospitalized for worsening heart failure [181]. The study compared the hemodynamic and clinical effects of nesiritide infusion at 0.01 mcg/kg/min after a bolus of 2 mcg/kg, IV nitroglycerine infusion at a rate determined by the investigator or placebo (see above for details). At 3 and 24 h, nesiritide lowered PCWP more than NTG, but there were no significant differences in patient reported dyspnea and only modest improvement in global clinical status in the nesiritide group.

A limitation of VMAC is that the mean dose of NTG was 42 mcg/min in the catheterized patients and 29 mcg/min in the non-catheterized patients, significantly below the optimal dose of 120–200 mg/min for the treatment of ADHF [161]. One of the sites in VMAC reported their single center results using aggressive up-titration of NTG that achieved a mean dose of 155 mcg/min at 3 h [207]. Nesiritide was associated with an early reduction in PCWP that was sustained over the 24-h study period. There was no evidence of nesiritide tolerance. High dose NTG was associated with a comparable reduction in PCWP that was delayed when compared with nesiritide. The NTG-associated decrease in PCWP was gradually attenuated despite continued up-titration reflecting the early development of NTG tolerance.

A subsequent retrospective pooled analysis of five small randomized trials of nesiritide of varying doses suggested that nesiritide increased the risk of worsening renal failure (defined by an increase in creatinine of greater than 0.5 mg/dL recorded at any time during the inpatient portion of the trial) [208]. Another retrospective pooled analysis of three small randomized trials of nesiritide of varying doses that reported 30-day mortality and did not require inotrope infusion as a control suggested that there was a trend toward increased mortality in the nesiritide treated patients that did not reach statistical significance [209, 210]. Two subsequent meta-analyses of randomized clinical trials of nesiritide did not show an increase in 30-day or 180-day all-cause mortality [211, 212] and did not show a clear relationship between mortality and nesiritide dose [212].

The Acute Study of Clinical Effectiveness of Nesiritide in Decompensated Heart Failure (ASCEND-HF) trial was a multicenter randomized placebo-controlled trial designed to assess the safety and efficacy of nesiritide added to standard therapy compared to placebo added to standard therapy in 7141 patients hospitalized for ADHF [213]. Patients were randomized in a 1:1 ratio to receive placebo or nesiritide. Nesiritide was administered as a continuous IV infusion at a dose of 0.01 mcg/kg/min for 24–164 h. At the discretion of the investigator, patients could receive an optional intravenous bolus of 2 mcg/kg prior to the initiation of the continuous infusion. Co-primary end-points were the change in self-reported dyspnea measured by a 7-point Likert scale at 6 and 24 h and the composite end-point of rehospitalization for heart failure or death within 30 days. Patients assigned to nesiritide more frequently reported improved dyspnea at 6 and 24 h but this difference was small and did not meet the prespecified level for significance. There was no difference in rehospitalization for heart failure or death from any cause at 30 days analyzed separately or as a composite end-point. There was also no difference in the rates of worsening renal function defined as a more than a 25% decrease in the eGFR calculated using the simplified MDRD equation at any time from study drug initiation through day 30 of the trial. The results from ASCEND-HF suggest that nesiritide can be used safely in patients with ADHF but cannot be recommended for routine use in a broad range of patients hospitalized for decompensated heart failure.

The HFSA, ACCF/AHA and ESC guidelines all endorse the use of nesiritide for the rapid improvement of congestive symptoms in patients with ADHF in the absence of symptomatic hypotension [8, 28, 118]. The recommended starting dose of nesiritide is 0.01 mcg/kg/min with or without an initial bolus of 2 mcg/kg. The dose can be increased by 0.005 mcg/kg/min every 3 h up to a maximum of 0.03 mcg/kg/min as tolerated by systemic blood pressure.

The primary side effects of nesiritide are headache and hypotension. In VMAC, headache occurred in 8% of patients. Symptomatic hypotension was reported in 4% of patients receiving nesiritide, was of mild to moderate severity in most patients, and resolved spontaneously after a decrease or discontinuation of medication or following an intravenous fluid bolus of ≤250 mL [181]. Symptomatic hypotension is dose-dependent and was reported in 11% of patients with ADHF during infusion of 0.015 mcg/kg/min and in 17% of patients during an infusion of 0.03 mcg/kg/min [200].

Inotropic Agents

The use of inotropic agents in patients hospitalized for ADHF is relatively common despite a lack of data from clinical trials that establishes safety and efficacy and despite observational data from large clinical registries that raise questions about safety. The most commonly used inotropic agents are dobutamine, dopamine, milrinone, and levosimendan. Dobutamine, dopamine and milrinone increase intracellular cyclic adenosine monophosphate (cAMP) and intracellular calcium concentration. Levosimendan is a calcium sensitizing agent with inotropic and vasodilatory effects. Levosimendan has not been approved for use in the U.S. or Canada. Intravenous inotropic agents may be used to relieve symptoms, improve hemodynamics and improve end-organ function in patients with acute decompensated heart failure with severe systolic dysfunction who have diminished peripheral perfusion and/or hypotension.

Dobutamine

Dobutamine was originally thought to be a selective β1 adrenergic receptor agonist. However, it has become clear that its pharmacologic effects are more complex. Dobutamine is a racemic mixture that stimulates β1, β2 and α1 adrenergic receptors. Its pharmacologic actions are a composite of the dose-related effects of each enantiomer on adrenergic receptors. Its effects are not mediated through endogenous release of norepinephrine and it does not stimulate dopaminergic receptors. Both enantiomers have agonist effects on the β1 adrenergic receptor. (+)-dobutamine is 10 fold more potent than (−)—dobutamine with respect to β1 stimulation. Both isomers have mild agonist effects on the β2 receptor. (−)-dobutamine is an α1 agonist while (+)-dobutamine is a mixed α1 agonist/antagonist.

The primary pharmacologic effect of dobutamine is an increase in myocardial contractility mediated by β1 receptor stimulation. β1 stimulation increases adenylyl cyclase activity resulting in an increase in intracellular cAMP. An increase in intracellular cAMP facilitates calcium release from the sarcoplasmic reticulum and an increase in force generation by contractile proteins. The β1 effects result in positive inotropic effects with resulting increases in stroke volume and cardiac output and some reflex-mediated reduction in systemic vascular resistance. Dobutamine has relatively more inotropic than chronotropic effects when compared with isoproterenol. At equivalent inotropic doses, dobutamine enhances sinus node automaticity less than isoproterenol although has similar effects in increasing AV nodal and intraventricular conduction. The blunted chronotropic response relative to inotropic response is not well understood but may be related to a contribution of cardiac α1 receptor stimulation to inotrope effect. In the peripheral circulation, β2 stimulation can cause vasodilation at low doses. The α1 agonist effect of (−)—dobutamine on the arterial circulation is generally offset by the antagonist effect of (+)-dobutamine and the vasodilator effect of β2 stimulation. However, at higher doses, α-1 adrenergic receptor stimulation may cause venous and arterial vasoconstriction [214–217].

In most patients with heart failure, systolic dysfunction and low cardiac output, treatment with dobutamine results in an increase in stroke volume and cardiac output, a reduction in systemic vascular resistance and a modest reduction in filling pressures. The overall effect on blood pressure is variable depending on the impact on cardiac output, systemic vascular resistance and reflex sympathetic tone. In general, dobutamine causes little change in blood pressure and can be used safely in patients with hypotension. Pulmonary vascular resistance is generally not decreased. An increase in blood pressure may be seen at higher doses [214, 215, 218].

The effects of dobutamine on clinical outcomes have not been studied in prospective randomized controlled clinical trials. Substantial clinical experience suggests that dobutamine improves cardiac output, improves symptoms of low cardiac output and pulmonary congestion, and improves end-organ function in patients with low cardiac output syndrome in the setting of severe left ventricular systolic dysfunction.

Dobutamine has a half-life of 2 min. The onset of effect is rapid. Steady state concentrations are reached within 10 min of starting the infusion. Doses of 2–10 mcg/kg/minute are generally required to have an impact on cardiac output. The ESC guidelines recommend that dobutamine be started at infusion rates of 2–3 mcg/kg/min. The dose can be increased by 1–2 mcg/kg/min based on clinical and hemodynamic response. The maximum recommended dose is 15–20 mcg/kg per minute. However, if a desired response is not achieved with up to 10 mcg/kg per minute, the addition of another inotrope or placement of an intra-aortic balloon pump should be considered. The response to dobutamine is commonly attenuated in patients receiving β-adrenergic blocking agents. In some studies of dobutamine using infusion durations of >24–72 h, cardiac output has been noted to return toward baseline in some patients raising the possibility of pharmacologic tolerance [214, 216].

Side effects of dobutamine include tachycardia (especially in patients with atrial fibrillation), atrial and ventricular arrhythmias, eosinophilia and hypersensitivity myocarditis [203, 219, 220]. Dobutamine increases myocardial oxygen consumption in patients with and without coronary artery disease [218, 221]. In patients with coronary artery disease, the increase in myocardial oxygen consumption may result in myocardial ischemia and worsening hemodynamics. Concern has been raised that dobutamine (and dopamine and milrinone) may cause additional cardiomyocyte damage and ultimately worsen heart failure by causing myocardial ischemia and, perhaps, direct myocyte toxicity [216, 217, 222–224].

Dopamine

Dopamine is an endogenously produced catecholamine. It is a central neurotransmitter that plays an important role in the regulation of movement. It is also produced in the periphery by epithelial cells of the proximal tubule in the kidney and is thought to have local diuretic and natriuretic effects.

The cardiovascular effects of dopamine are mediated by a number of distinct cell surface receptors that vary in their affinity for dopamine and mediate distinct dose-dependent cardiovascular effects. At low dose (≤2 mcg/kg/min), dopamine acts primarily on the vascular dopamine type 1 (D1) receptors in the renal, mesenteric and coronary vasculature leading to vasodilation and natriuresis. D1 binding activates adenyl cyclase and increases intracellular cAMP leading to vasodilation. In addition, activation of D1 receptors in the proximal tubule and thick ascending limb of the loop of Henle inhibits the Na^+-H^+ exchanger and Na^+:K^+:$2Cl^-$ co-transporter facilitating the excretion of urinary sodium. Low-dose dopamine infusion results in an increase in renal blood flow, glomerular filtration rate and natriuresis.

At intermediate doses (2–5 mcg/kg/min), dopamine acts primarily on β1 receptors and facilitates release of norepinephrine from nerve terminals. At this dose, dopamine has a predominant inotropic and chronotropic effect. Cardiac output and heart rate are increased. Systolic blood pressure and pulse pressure are generally increased and diastolic blood pressure remains the same or increases slightly. There is generally little change in peripheral vascular resistance at these doses. At higher doses (>5 mcg/kg/min) dopamine activates α1 receptors which causes arterial vasoconstriction [214, 216, 217].

The effect of dopamine on renal physiology was evaluated in 13 patients with chronic heart failure [225]. Cardiac output, renal artery cross sectional area, renal blood flow, and renal vascular resistance were calculated at baseline and at intravenous dopamine doses of 1, 2, 3, 5, and 10 mcg/kg/min. Cardiac output increased with increasing dose reaching statistical significance at doses of 5 and 10 μg/kg/min with the peak occurring at 10 mcg/kg/min. Renal artery cross-sectional area demonstrated a progressive increase with dose uptitration reaching statistical significance at doses of 5 and 10 μg/kg/min. Renal vascular resistance decreased reaching statistical significance at 2 mcg/kg/min with no difference seen from 2–10 mcg/kg/min. Renal blood flow progressively increased from 2–10 μg/kg/min. The increase in renal blood flow was proportionately larger than corresponding increases in cardiac output and was due primarily to dilation of large conductance and small resistance renal blood vessels.

Despite the demonstrated effect of dopamine on renal blood flow, it has been difficult to demonstrate a clinical benefit of low dose dopamine in prospective randomized clinical trials that studied patients with ADHF. The Dopamine in Acute Decompensated Heart Failure Trials (DAD-HF and DAD-HF II) evaluated the efficacy of adding dopamine to furosemide infusion in patients with ADHF [226, 227]. DAD-HF compared high dose furosemide (40 mg IV bolus followed by a 20 mg/h continuous infusion for 8 h) versus low dose furosemide (40 mg IV bolus followed by a 5 mg/h infusion for 8 h) plus dopamine 5 mcg/kg/min in sixty patients with ADHF. End-points included total diuresis and changes in dyspnea score during the 8-h protocol, worsening renal failure defined as a rise in serum creatinine >0.3 mg/dL from baseline to 24 h, electrolyte balance and 60-day post-discharge outcomes. The low-dose furosemide/dopamine protocol was equally effective as high dose furosemide with respect to diuresis and relief of dyspnea and was associated with less worsening renal failure and hypokalemia but no difference in 60-day mortality or rehospitalization rate. DAD-HF II was a three arm trial that randomized 161 patients with ADHF to an 8-h infusion(s) of: high dose furosemide (20 mg/h continuous infusion); low dose furosemide (5 mg/h continuous infusion) plus dopamine 5 mcg/kg/min; or low dose furosemide (5 mg/h continuous infusion) alone. All patients received furosemide 40 mg IV prior to randomization. No difference was found in the primary end-points of all-cause mortality and heart failure hospitalization at 60-days and one year. There was also no difference in urinary output over 24 h, dyspnea relief, or length of stay. Worsening renal function defined as a rise in serum creatinine ≥0.3 mg/dL from baseline to 24 h was more common in the high dose furosemide group than the low dose furosemide/dopamine or the low dose furosemide groups. The investigators concluded that the addition of low-dose dopamine was not associated with any clinical benefit.

The Renal Optimization Strategies Evaluation (ROSE) trial was a multicenter, double blind placebo-controlled trial of 360 patients hospitalized with acute heart failure and renal dysfunction (defined as an eGFR of 15–60 mL/min/1.73 m^2 by the MDRD equation) randomized to dopamine 2 mcg/kg/min, nesiritide 0.005 mcg/kg/min without a bolus, or placebo for 72 h (see above). No difference was found between study groups with respect to the two primary end-points: 72-h cumulative urine volume and change in cystatin C level. In addition, there were no between-group differences in secondary end-points of measures of decongestion, renal function or clinical outcomes [206].

The ACCF/AHA guidelines suggest that low dose dopamine ≤2 mcg/kg/min may be considered in addition to loop diuretics to improve diuresis and preserve renal function and renal blood flow [28]. The ESC guidelines suggest that dopamine at doses of 2–5 mcg/kg/min may be used as an inotrope in patients with heart failure, volume overload and hypotension [17]. Dopamine may be used to improve renal blood flow and diuresis in patients with decompensated heart failure who have an inadequate response to appropriately dosed intravenous loop diuretic. Dopamine dose should be based on estimated lean body weight and not on actual weight [216]. Dopamine should be administered through a central venous access site to avoid the risk of drug extravasation and ischemic necrosis of surrounding tissues associated with peripheral intravenous administration. Although dopamine increases cardiac output, it does not reduce left ventricular filling pressures and, in some patients, increases filling pressures. Dopamine causes more tachycardia than dobutamine and may precipitate angina in patients with coronary artery disease. It may cause atrial and ventricular arrhythmias [214].

Milrinone

Milrinone is a bipyridine derivative that selectively inhibits phosphodiesterase III (PDE3). Milrinone decreases intracellular cAMP degradation and increases intracellular cAMP which, in turn, increases intracellular calcium in cardiac and smooth muscle cells. Milrinone increases cardiac contractility and improves myocardial relaxation. Milrinone also causes systemic venous and arterial vasodilation and pulmonary arterial vasodilation. Milrinone increases cardiac output, lowers systemic and pulmonary vascular resistance, and decreases left and right ventricular filling pressures. The reductions in systemic and pulmonary vascular resistance and intracardiac filling pressures are greater than those seen with dobutamine at doses that produce similar increases in cardiac output [218]. Milrinone causes less tachycardia than dobutamine and, unlike dobutamine, causes a minimal increase in myocardial oxygen consumption [218, 228, 229]. The effect on systemic blood pressure depends on the increase in cardiac output and the reduction in systemic vascular resistance that occurs with milrinone administration. Vasodilation-mediated decreases in mean arterial pressure are relatively common and may limit the use of milrinone in some patients with low cardiac output and marginal arterial blood pressure. Unlike dobutamine, the effects of milrinone are not mediated by adrenergic receptors. As a result, milrinone may be used instead of dobutamine in patients with low cardiac output syndrome who are being treated with β-adrenergic blocking agents [216, 217].

The recommended dose of milrinone has been a 50 mcg/kg IV bolus followed by an infusion of 0.25–0.75 mcg/kg/min. However, bolus dosing has been associated with symptomatic hypotension. A study that compared the hemodynamic effects of a continuous infusion of 0.5 mcg/kg/min milrinone with or without an initial bolus demonstrated that the maximal effects on cardiac index and PCWP were seen immediately after the initial IV bolus. However, improvement in pulmonary capillary wedge pressure and cardiac output were similar at 2 and 3 h, with or without a bolus [230]. The ACCF/AHA and HFSA guidelines do not recommend a loading dose [8, 28]. The HFSA guidelines recommend that an initial dose of 0.01 mcg/kg/min and final dose of 0.2–0.3 mcg/kg/min be considered [8]. The ACCF/AHA guidelines recommend a maintenance dose of 0.125–0.75 mcg/kg/min [28].

The elimination half-life of milrinone is 2.5 h but is nearly doubled in patients with severe heart failure. Milrinone is predominantly excreted by the kidney so dosage adjustments need to be made for patients with an eGFR <60 mL/min. Major side effects of milrinone include hypotension, atrial fibrillation and ventricular arrhythmias.

Levosimendan

Levosimendan differs from other inotropic agents in that its mechanism for increasing contractility does not involve an increase in intracellular cAMP. Levosimendan is a myofilament calcium sensitizer that interacts with Ca^{2+}-saturated cardiac troponin C (cTNC). cTNC acts as a calcium sensitive "switch" to turn myocardial force production on during systole and off during diastole. Levosimendan binding to cTNC facilitates prolonged interaction between cTNC and troponin I increasing the contractile force generated during systole. Levosimendan does not affect diastolic function. Levosimendan is a vasodilator of systemic, pulmonary and coronary arteries and systemic veins. Vasodilation is probably mediated by opening of adenosine triphosphate (ATP)-sensitive potassium channels in vascular smooth muscle cells which results in smooth muscle relaxation [231]. Levosimendan and its active metabolite OR-1896 are selective inhibitors of PDE3. PDE inhibition probably does not play a role in the vasodilatory or inotropic effects of levosimendan at doses used in clinical practice. The combined inotropic and vasodilatory effects result in an increased force of contraction, increased stroke volume and cardiac output, decreased preload and afterload and decreased PCWP. Levosimendan does not increase myocardial oxygen consumption [231]. The most common side effects are hypotension and headache. Tachycardia is unusual. The incidence of atrial fibrillation and hypokalemia are increased modestly. The elimination half-life of levosimendan is 1–1.5 h. However, the elimination half-life of OR-1896 is 75–80 h so that cardiovascular effects may persist for 75–80 h after discontinuation of infusion [232, 233].

Several adequately powered multicenter randomized controlled clinical trials have assessed the efficacy of levosimendan compared with either placebo or dobutamine in patients with ADHF.

The Survival of Patients With Acute Heart Failure in Need of Intravenous Inotropic Support (SURVIVE) study was a randomized, double-blind trial comparing the efficacy and safety of intravenous levosimendan or dobutamine in 1327 patients hospitalized with acute decompensated heart failure who required inotropic support [234]. No difference was found between treatment groups in the primary end-point of all-cause mortality at 180 days. In addition, no differences were found in a number of secondary end-points including all-cause mortality at 31 days, number of days alive and out of the hospital during 180 days following randomization, patient global assessment, patient assessment of dyspnea at 24 h, and cardiovascular mortality at 180 days.

The Randomized EValuation of Intravenous Levosimendan Efficacy (REVIVE II) trial enrolled 600 patients hospitalized for treatment of ADHF who had an LVEF <35% and who remained dyspneic at rest despite treatment with intravenous diuretics [235]. Patients were randomly assigned to receive a single infusion of levosimendan or placebo, each in addition to local standard treatments for ADHF. The primary end-point evaluated was the distribution of patients characterized as "Improved", "Unchanged", or "Worse" during the first 5 days after randomization based on a composite of patient self-reported global assessment at 6 h, 24 h and 5 days. There was a modest benefit in the primary end-point in the levosimendan group. There was a decrease in length of stay in the levosimendan group but no difference in mortality at 90 days. Treatment with levosimendan was associated with more hypotension and atrial fibrillation.

A meta-analysis of randomized controlled clinical trials of levosimendan evaluated the effect of levosimendan on mortality and length of stay compared to placebo or dobutamine. Data from 5480 patients in 45 randomized clinical trials were analyzed. In 23/48 trials, levosimendan was evaluated in patients with decompensated heart failure and in 17/48 trials, levosimendan was evaluated in patients who underwent cardiothoracic surgery. The analysis found a significant reduction in mortality associated with the use of levosimendan. In addition, a reduction in mortality was found with levosimendan use when studies comparing levosimendan to placebo and levosimendan to dobutamine were analyzed separately. A reduction in mortality was also seen when studies with at least 30, 90, and 180 days of follow up were analyzed. In addition, treatment with levosimendan was associated with a decrease in length of stay [236].

In 2000, levosimendan was approved for use in Sweden. Since then, the drug has been approved in 60 countries worldwide but it remains not licensed in the United States.

Use of Inotropes

The pattern of inotrope use has been described in several North American and European registries of patients admitted to the hospital with acute heart failure syndromes. In the ADHERE registry, 14% of patients were treated with one or more inotropic agents although <3% of the patients in the registry had a systolic blood pressure of <90 mmHg at hospital admission and almost 50% had preserved systolic function. One or more inotropic agents were used in 8% of patients with preserved systolic function (3% dobutamine, 5% dopamine and 1% milrinone) and in 19% of patients with reduced systolic function (11% dobutamine; 10% dopamine; 5% milrinone). Only 8% of patients who received either dobutamine or dopamine had a systolic blood pressure < 90 mmHg. The mean systolic blood pressure on admission was 121.3 (±27.4) mmHg in patients who received milrinone and 124.0 (±29.3) mmHg in patients who received dobutamine [150].

In the OPTIMIZE-HF Registry, intravenous inotropic medications were used in 4% of patients admitted for ADHF who had preserved systolic function and 12% of patients with left ventricular systolic dysfunction [91]. Of the patients enrolled in OPTIMIZE-HF, 15%, 6.5%, 4.5% and 3.2% of patients were treated with an intravenous inotrope in the systolic blood pressure quartiles of <120 mmHg, 120–139 mmHg, 140–161 mmHg, and >161 mmHg, respectively [237]. In the EuroHeart Failure Survey II, of 3580 patients hospitalized with heart failure, ~25–30% of patients were treated with an inotropic agent (10.2% dobutamine; 11.3% dopamine; 3.9% levosimendan). Of patients admitted with "Decompensated Heart Failure" (as opposed to "Cardiogenic Shock" or "Pulmonary Oedema"), ~20–24% of patients were treated with an inotrope (8.6% dobutamine; 8.5% dopamine; 4.4% levosimendan) [238]. In an Italian survey, of 2807 patients hospitalized for ADHF, 25% of patients were treated with an IV inotrope [239].

Several studies have suggested that the use of intravenous inotropic agents in patients with ADHF is associated with an increase in adverse events including symptomatic hypotension, atrial and ventricular arrhythmias and in-hospital and long-term mortality [150, 240–242]. A retrospective observational analysis of data from the ADHERE registry suggested that in-hospital mortality is increased in patients admitted for ADHF who are treated with intravenous inotropic agents. The risk factor and propensity score-adjusted odds ratio for in-hospital mortality was calculated for 15,230 of 65,180 patients in the registry who received nitroglycerine, nesiritide, dobutamine or milrinone during hospitalization for ADHF. The majority of patients included in this analysis had either normal or elevated blood pressure. Treatment with either nesiritide or nitroglycerine was associated with significantly lower in-hospital mortality than either dobutamine or milrinone. The covariate and propensity score adjusted odds ratio for mortality was 0.69 ($p < 0.005$) when nitroglycerine was compared with milrinone and 0.46 ($p < 0.005$) when nitroglycerine was compared with dobutamine [150].

A similar retrospective analysis was performed using data from the University Health System Consortium (UHC) Clinical Database Pharmacy (a database with information from 32 academic hospitals) [240]. 2130 patients were identified who were hospitalized for ADHF and treated with dobutamine, milrinone or nesiritide. Using logistic regression, the relationship between drug therapy and in-hospital mortality was assessed. In-hospital mortality was 10.2%, 7.9% and 2.9% for patients treated with dobutamine, milrinone and nesiritide, respectively. The risk adjusted odds ratio for in-hospital mortality was 3.5 for dobutamine and 3.9 for milrinone when compared with nesiritide.

A retrospective observational analysis was performed using data from the ESCAPE Trial to assess the impact of inpatient inotrope use on 6 month outcomes [241]. Of the 433 patients enrolled, risk-adjusted hazard ratios for 6-month mortality and mortality and rehospitalization were determined for the overall population and for patients treated with an intravenous vasodilator, inotrope or combination of inotrope and vasodilator. Overall 6-month mortality was 19%. When compared to the overall cohort, risk adjusted HR for 6-month mortality was not significantly different for patients treated with vasodilators (HR 1.39, 95% CI 0.64–3.00) but was significantly increased for patients treated with inotropes (HR 2.14, 95% CI 1.10–4.15) and for patients treated with a combination of inotropes and vasodilators (HR 4.81, 95% CI 2.34–9.90). The risk adjusted combined end-point of 6-month mortality or rehospitalization was not significantly increased for patients treated with vasodilators (HR1.2, CI 0.81–1.78) but was significantly increased for patients treated with inotropes (HR 1.96, CI 1.37–2.82) and patients treated with inotropes and vasodilators (HR 2.90, CI 1.88–4.48). On multivariable analysis, impaired renal function and right atrial pressure were significant predictors for the use of inotropes. Renal function and elevated PCWP were predictors for the use of vasodilators. However, the most powerful predictor of inotrope or vasodilator use was the study site and managing physician.

The Outcomes of a Prospective Trial of Intravenous Milrinone for Exacerbations of Chronic Heart Failure (OPTIME-CHF) was a randomize, placebo-controlled, double blind trial that tested the hypothesis that short-term use of milrinone added to standard therapy in patients with chronic heart failure hospitalized for ADHF (but without "low output syndrome") would improve clinical outcomes [243]. The study randomized 951 patients hospitalized with ADHF who did not require intravenous inotropic support to receive a 48-h infusion of milrinone 0.5 mcg/kg/min or saline placebo. No loading dose was administered. The dose could be adjusted downward to 0.375 mcg/kg/min or upward to 0.75 mcg/kg/min at the discretion of the treating physician. Patients were ineligible if the treating physician judged that intravenous inotropic therapy was essential. The primary end-point was the total number of days hospitalized for cardiovascular causes within 60 days after randomization. There was no difference found in the primary endpoint. There were also no differences in in-hospital mortality, 60-day mortality or the composite of death or readmission. Sustained hypotension (systolic blood pressure less than 80 mmHg for greater than 30 min) requiring intervention and new atrial arrhythmias occurred more frequently in patients who received milrinone. There was also an important trend for an increase in ventricular tachycardia or ventricular fibrillation in the milrinone group that approached but did not reach statistical significance ($p = 0.06$). The authors concluded that milrinone was not indicated as adjunctive therapy in patients hospitalized for ADHF.

A post-hoc analysis of the OPTIME-CHF data was performed to assess whether there was an interaction between the effect of short-term milrinone therapy and the etiology of heart failure (ischemic vs. non-ischemic) [242]. Patients with ischemic cardiomyopathy were found to have been adversely affected by milrinone. Patients with ischemic cardiomyopathy who were treated with milrinone had an increase in the primary end-point of days in the hospital or death within 60 days, death or re-hospitalization at 60 days, and in-hospital mortality (5.0% vs 1.6%) when compared to those treated with placebo. Conversely, patients with non-ischemic cardiomyopathy seemed to benefit from milrinone. Non-ischemic patients treated with milrinone as compared with those treated with placebo had lower rates of in-hospital mortality and death or rehospitalization at 60 days.

A number of mechanisms have been proposed to explain the increase in adverse outcomes seen in patients with ADHF who are treated with inotropic agents. These include: cAMP-induced atrial and ventricular arrhythmias; vasodilation with coronary hypoperfusion resulting in myocardial damage; increased myocardial oxygen consumption resulting in myocardial ischemia and myocardial injury; and direct myocyte toxicity possibly mediated by intracellular calcium overload [222, 224].

The ACCF/AHA, HFSA and ESC guidelines endorse the use of inotropes in patients with ADHF who have severe systolic dysfunction, significantly decreased cardiac output, diminished peripheral perfusion and end-organ dysfunction despite adequate or elevated filling pressures [8, 28, 118]. The goals of inotropic therapy are to relieve symptoms, maintain systemic perfusion and preserve end-organ function. Inotropes also may be indicated in fluid overloaded patients who remain volume overloaded despite intravenous diuretics and, if appropriate, intravenous vasodilators. Inotropes may be used as "bridge therapy" in Stage D patients who are awaiting mechanical circulatory support or heart transplantation.

The guidelines note the risk associated with inotropic therapy and recommend continuous heart rhythm monitoring and frequent blood pressure monitoring. The need for management in an intensive care or cardiac care unit should be assessed. Obtaining objective measurements of hemodynamic parameters using a PA catheter to guide therapy should be strongly considered. Lower doses of inotrope are recommended to minimize adverse effects. The continued need for inotropic support (and the possibility of discontinuation) should be regularly assessed. An attempt to wean inotropes should be made after optimization of guideline directed medical therapy.

If an inotrope is indicated in a patient being treated with a β-blocker, milrinone is the preferred agent as its positive inotropic effect is not mediated by β-adrenergic stimulation. There is little data to guide decisions concerning whether to continue chronic β-blocker therapy in a patient who requires inotropic support. It is reasonable to continue the β-blocker without a change in dose or decrease the dose of β-blocker with a plan to increase the dose if the patient improves and the inotrope can be discontinued. In the case of patients with cardiogenic shock, pulmonary edema, hypotension, or manifestations of severe end-organ hypoperfusion, it is reasonable to hold the β-blocker until the patient stabilizes and end-organ function improves [61].

Conclusions

Comprehensive guidelines for the management of ADHF have been published by the American College of Cardiology Foundation/American Heart Association (ACCF/AHA), the Heart Failure Society of America (HFSA), and the European Society of Cardiology (ESC). In general, there are three phases in the evaluation and management of patients who present with ADHF including: initial assessment; ongoing assessment and treatment; and discharge planning. A critical part of the initial assessment is the evaluation for the presence of pulmonary or hemodynamic instability that may require emergent intervention. Assessment for ACS that may require emergent coronary artery angiography and coronary intervention is also an essential component of the initial assessment.

Initial treatment is focused on relieving respiratory distress and correcting hypoxia. Oxygen administered by nasal cannula or face mask is recommended in patients with hypoxia. The use of non-invasive positive pressure ventilation is recommended in patients with severe dyspnea, clinical evidence of pulmonary edema, or persistent hypoxia.

Pharmacologic therapy is focused on relieving pulmonary congestion. Intravenous loop diuretics are first-line therapy. Routine use of invasive hemodynamic monitoring is not indicated and should be reserved for patients in cardiogenic shock, patients who are unresponsive to initial medical therapy, or patients who develop clinically significant hypotension and/or significant worsening of renal function during initial treatment for ADHF. Assessment of the adequacy of decongestion can be challenging and is based on symptom relief and physical exam.

In the absence of hypotension, intravenous nitroglycerine, nitroprusside or nesiritide may be used in patients who do not respond adequately to parenteral diuretics. The use of intravenous inotropes is not indicated in most patients with

ADHF except those with LV systolic dysfunction with cardiogenic shock, evidence of low cardiac output or end-organ dysfunction, hypotension or heart failure unresponsive to diuretics and parenteral vasodilators.

References

1. Park JH, Balmain S, Berry C, Morton JJ, McMurray JJ. Potentially detrimental cardiovascular effects of oxygen in patients with chronic left ventricular systolic dysfunction. Heart. 2010;96(7):533–8. https://doi.org/10.1136/hrt.2009.175257.
2. Vismara LA, Leaman DM, Zelis R. The effects of morphine on venous tone in patients with acute pulmonary edema. Circulation. 1976;54(2):335–7.
3. Grossmann M, Abiose A, Tangphao O, Blaschke TF, Hoffman BB. Morphine-induced venodilation in humans. Clin Pharmacol Ther. 1996;60(5):554–60.
4. Timmis AD, Rothman MT, Henderson MA, Geal PW, Chamberlain DA. Haemodynamic effects of intravenous morphine in patients with acute myocardial infarction complicated by severe left ventricular failure. Br Med J. 1980;280(6219):980–2.
5. Sacchetti A, Ramoska E, Moakes ME, McDermott P, Moyer V. Effect of ED management on ICU use in acute pulmonary edema. Am J Emerg Med. 1999;17(6):571–4.
6. Hoffman JR, Reynolds S. Comparison of nitroglycerin, morphine and furosemide in treatment of presumed pre-hospital pulmonary edema. Chest. 1987;92(4):586–93.
7. Peacock WF, Hollander JE, Diercks DB, Lopatin M, Fonarow G, Emerman CL. Morphine and outcomes in acute decompensated heart failure: an ADHERE analysis. Emerg Med J. 2008;25(4):205–9. https://doi.org/10.1136/emj.2007.050419.
8. Heart Failure Society of America, Lindenfeld J, Albert NM, Boehmer JP, Collins SP, Ezekowitz JA, Givertz MM, et al. HFSA 2010 comprehensive heart failure practice guideline. Section 12: evaluation and management of patients with acute decompensated heart failure. J Card Fail. 2010;16(6):e131–56. https://doi.org/10.1016/j.cardfail.2010.04.004.
9. Kato T, Suda S, Kasai T. Positive airway pressure therapy for heart failure. World J Cardiol. 2014;6(11):1175–91. https://doi.org/10.4330/wjc.v6.i11.1175.
10. Masip J, Roque M, Sánchez B, Fernández R, Subirana M, Expósito JA. Noninvasive ventilation in acute cardiogenic pulmonary edema: systematic review and meta-analysis. JAMA. 2005;294(24):3124–30.
11. Peter JV, Moran JL, Phillips-Hughes J, Graham P, Bersten AD. Effect of non-invasive positive pressure ventilation (NIPPV) on mortality in patients with acute cardiogenic pulmonary oedema: a meta-analysis. Lancet. 2006;367(9517):1155–63. Review.
12. Mehta S, Jay GD, Woolard RH, Hipona RA, Connolly EM, Cimini DM, et al. Randomized, prospective trial of bilevel versus continuous positive airway pressure in acute pulmonary edema. Crit Care Med. 1997;25(4):620–8.
13. Gray A, Goodacre S, Newby DE, Masson M, Sampson F, Nicholl J, 3CPO Trialists. Noninvasive ventilation in acute cardiogenic pulmonary edema. N Engl J Med. 2008;359(2):142–51. https://doi.org/10.1056/NEJMoa0707992.
14. Mariani J, Macchia A, Belziti C, Deabreu M, Gagliardi J, Doval H, et al. Noninvasive ventilation in acute cardiogenic pulmonary edema: a meta-analysis of randomized controlled trials. J Card Fail. 2011;17(10):850–9. https://doi.org/10.1016/j.cardfail.2011.05.010. Epub 2011 Jul 8.
15. Vital FM, Ladeira MT, Atallah AN. Non-invasive positive pressure ventilation (CPAP or bilevel NPPV) for cardiogenic pulmonary oedema. Cochrane Database Syst Rev. 2013;5:CD005351. https://doi.org/10.1002/14651858.CD005351.pub3.
16. Mal S, McLeod S, Iansavichene A, Dukelow A, Lewell M. Effect of out-of-hospital noninvasive positive-pressure support ventilation in adult patients with severe respiratory distress: a systematic review and meta-analysis. Ann Emerg Med. 2014;63(5):600–607.e1. https://doi.org/10.1016/j.annemergmed.2013.11.013. Epub 2013 Dec 15.
17. Dickstein K, Cohen-Solal A, Filippatos G, McMurray JJ, Ponikowski P, Poole-Wilson PA, ESC Committee for Practice Guidelines (CPG), et al. ESC Guidelines for the diagnosis and treatment of acute and chronic heart failure 2008: the Task Force for the diagnosis and treatment of acute and chronic heart failure 2008 of the European Society of Cardiology. Developed in collaboration with the Heart Failure Association of the ESC (HFA) and endorsed by the European Society of Intensive Care Medicine (ESICM). Eur Heart J. 2008;29(19):2388–442. https://doi.org/10.1093/eurheartj/ehn309. Epub 2008 Sep 17.
18. McMurray JJ, Adamopoulos S, Anker SD, Auricchio A, Böhm M, Dickstein K, et al; Task Force for the Diagnosis and Treatment of Acute and Chronic Heart Failure 2012 of the European Society of Cardiology, Bax JJ, Baumgartner H, Ceconi C, Dean V, Deaton C, et al; ESC Committee for Practice Guidelines. ESC guidelines for the diagnosis and treatment of acute and chronic heart failure 2012: The Task Force for the Diagnosis and Treatment of Acute and Chronic Heart Failure 2012 of the European Society of Cardiology. Developed in collaboration with the Heart Failure Association (HFA) of the ESC. Eur J Heart Fail. 2012;14(8):803–69. https://doi.org/10.1093/eurjhf/hfs105. No abstract available. Erratum in: Eur J Heart Fail. 2013 Mar;15(3):361.

19. De Bruyne LKM. Mechanisms and management of diuretic resistance in congestive heart failure. Postgrad Med J. 2003;79(931):268–71.
20. Cleland JG, Coletta A, Witte K. Practical applications of intravenous diuretic therapy in decompensated heart failure. Am J Med. 2006;119(12 Suppl 1):S26–36.
21. Brater DC. Diuretic therapy. N Engl J Med. 1998;339(6):387–95.
22. Brater DC. Update in diuretic therapy: clinical pharmacology. Semin Nephrol. 2011;31(6):483–94. https://doi.org/10.1016/j.semnephrol.2011.09.003. Review.
23. Felker GM, Mentz RJ. Diuretics and ultrafiltration in acute decompensated heart failure. J Am Coll Cardiol. 2012;59(24):2145–53. https://doi.org/10.1016/j.jacc.2011.10.910.
24. Brater DC. Pharmacology of diuretics. Am J Med Sci. 2000;319(1):38–50.
25. Shankar SS, Brater DC. Loop diuretics: from the Na-K-2Cl transporter to clinical use. Am J Physiol Renal Physiol. 2003;284(1):F11–21.
26. Reilly RF, Jackson EK. Chapter 25. Regulation of renal function and vascular volume. In: Brunton LL, Chabner BA, Knollmann BC, editors. Goodman & Gilman's the pharmacological basis of therapeutics. 12th ed. New York: McGraw-Hill; 2011. http://accessmedicine.mhmedical.com/content.aspx?bookid=374&Sectionid=41266232.
27. ter Maaten JM, Valente MA, Damman K, Hillege HL, Navis G, Voors AA. Diuretic response in acute heart failure-pathophysiology, evaluation, and therapy. Nat Rev Cardiol. 2015;12(3):184–92. https://doi.org/10.1038/nrcardio.2014.215. Epub 2015 Jan 6.
28. Yancy CW, Jessup M, Bozkurt B, Butler J, Casey Jr DE, Drazner MH, American College of Cardiology Foundation/American Heart Association Task Force on Practice Guidelines, et al. 2013 ACCF/AHA guideline for the management of heart failure: a report of the American College of Cardiology Foundation/American Heart Association Task Force on practice guidelines. Circulation. 2013;128(16):e240–327. https://doi.org/10.1161/CIR.0b013e31829e8776. Epub 2013 Jun 5.
29. Leto L, Aspromonte N, Feola M. Efficacy and safety of loop diuretic therapy in acute decompensated heart failure: a clinical review. Heart Fail Rev. 2014;19(2):237–46. https://doi.org/10.1007/s10741-012-9354-7.
30. Huang X, Dorhout Mees EJ, Vos PF, Hamza S, Braam B. Everything we always wanted to know about furosemide but were afraid to ask. Am J Physiol Renal Physiol. 2016;310(10):F958–71. https://doi.org/10.1152/ajprenal.00476.2015. Epub 2016 Feb 24.
31. Gottlieb SS, Brater DC, Thomas I, Havranek E, Bourge R, Goldman S, et al. BG9719 (CVT-124), an A1 adenosine receptor antagonist, protects against the decline in renal function observed with diuretic therapy. Circulation. 2002;105(11):1348–53.
32. Liang KV, Williams AW, Greene EL, Redfield MM. Acute decompensated heart failure and the cardiorenal syndrome. Crit Care Med. 2008;36(1 Suppl):S75–88. https://doi.org/10.1097/01.CCM.0000296270.41256.5C.
33. Ares GR, Caceres PS, Ortiz PA. Molecular regulation of NKCC2 in the thick ascending limb. Am J Physiol Renal Physiol. 2011;301(6):F1143–59. https://doi.org/10.1152/ajprenal.00396.2011. Epub 2011 Sep 7.
34. Fonarow GC, Corday E, ADHERE Scientific Advisory Committee. Overview of acutely decompensated congestive heart failure (ADHF): a report from the ADHERE registry. Heart Fail Rev. 2004;9(3):179–85.
35. Buggey J, Mentz RJ, Pitt B, Eisenstein EL, Anstrom KJ, Velazquez EJ, O'Connor CM. A reappraisal of loop diuretic choice in heart failure patients. Am Heart J. 2015;169(3):323–33. https://doi.org/10.1016/j.ahj.2014.12.009. Epub 2015 Jan 6.
36. Knauf H, Mutschler E. Clinical pharmacokinetics and pharmacodynamics of torasemide. Clin Pharmacokinet. 1998;34(1):1–24.
37. Roush GC, Kaur R, Ernst ME. Diuretics: a review and update. Cardiovasc Pharmacol Ther. 2014;19(1):5–13. https://doi.org/10.1177/1074248413497257. Epub 2013 Nov 15.
38. Wargo KA, Banta WM. A comprehensive review of the loop diuretics: should furosemide be first line? Ann Pharmacother. 2009;43(11):1836–47. https://doi.org/10.1345/aph.1M177. Epub 2009 Oct 20.
39. Felker M. Diuretic management in heart failure. Congest Heart Fail. 2010;16(Suppl 1):S68–72.
40. Vasko MR, Cartwright DB, Knochel JP, Nixon JV, Brater DC. Furosemide absorption altered in decompensated congestive heart failure. Ann Intern Med. 1985;102(3):314–8.
41. Stevenson LW, Tillisch JH. Maintenance of cardiac output with normal filling pressures in patients with dilated heart failure. Circulation. 1986;74(6):1303–8.
42. Raftery EB. Haemodynamic effects of diuretics in heart failure. Br Heart J. 1994;72(2 Suppl):S44–7.
43. Nelson GI, Ahuja RC, Silke B, Okoli RC, Hussain M, Taylor SH. Haemodynamic effects of frusemide and its influence on repetitive rapid volume loading in acute myocardial infarction. Eur Heart J. 1983;4(10):706–11.
44. Stevenson LW. Tailored therapy to hemodynamic goals for advanced heart failure. Eur J Heart Fail. 1999;1(3):251–7.
45. Stevenson LW, Bellil D, Grover-McKay M, Brunken RC, Schwaiger M, Tillisch JH, Schelbert HR. Effects of afterload reduction (diuretics and vasodilators) on left ventricular volume and mitral regurgitation in severe congestive heart failure secondary to isch-

emic or idiopathic dilated cardiomyopathy. Am J Cardiol. 1987;60(8):654–8.

46. Dikshit K, Vyden JK, Forrester JS, Chatterjee K, Prakash R, Swan HJ. Renal and extrarenal hemodynamic effects of furosemide in congestive heart failure after acute myocardial infarction. N Engl J Med. 1973;288(21):108.
47. Verma SP, Silke B, Hussain M, Nelson GI, Reynolds GW, Richmond A, Taylor SH. First-line treatment of left ventricular failure complicating acute myocardial infarction: a randomised evaluation of immediate effects of diuretic, venodilator, arteriodilator, and positive inotropic drugs on left ventricular function. J Cardiovasc Pharmacol. 1987;10(1):38–46.
48. Verma SP, Silke B, Reynolds G, Muller P, Frais MA, Taylor SH. Immediate effects of bumetanide on systemic haemodynamics and left ventricular volume in acute and chronic heart failure. Br J Clin Pharmacol. 1987;24(1):21–31.
49. Pickkers P, Dormans TP, Russel FG, Hughes AD, Thien T, Schaper N, Smits P. Direct vascular effects of furosemide in humans. Circulation. 1997;96(6):1847–52.
50. Smits P. Vascular effects of loop diuretics. Cardiovasc Res. 1996;32(6):988–97.
51. Francis GS, Siegel RM, Goldsmith SR, Olivari MT, Levine TB, Cohn JN. Acute vasoconstrictor response to intravenous furosemide in patients with chronic congestive heart failure. Activation of the neurohumoral axis. Ann Intern Med. 1985;103(1):1–6.
52. Johnson W, Omland T, Hall C, Lucas C, Myking OL, Collins C, et al. Neurohormonal activation rapidly decreases after intravenous therapy with diuretics and vasodilators for class IV heart failure. J Am Coll Cardiol. 2002;39(10):1623–9.
53. Salvador DR, Rey NR, Ramos GC, Punzalan FE. Continuous infusion versus bolus injection of loop diuretics in congestive heart failure. Cochrane Database Syst Rev. 2005;3:CD003178.
54. Felker GM, Lee KL, Bull DA, Redfield MM, Stevenson LW, Goldsmith SR, NHLBI Heart Failure Clinical Research Network, et al. Diuretic strategies in patients with acute decompensated heart failure. N Engl J Med. 2011;364(9):797–805. https://doi.org/10.1056/NEJMoa1005419.
55. Givertz MM, Postmus D, Hillege HL, Mansoor GA, Massie BM, Davison BA, et al. Renal function trajectories and clinical outcomes in acute heart failure. Circ Heart Fail. 2014;7(1):59–67. https://doi.org/10.1161/CIRCHEARTFAILURE.113.000556. Epub 2013 Nov 26.
56. Metra M, Nodari S, Parrinello G, Bordonali T, Bugatti S, Danesi R, et al. Worsening renal function in patients hospitalised for acute heart failure: clinical implications and prognostic significance. Eur J Heart Fail. 2008;10(2):188–95. https://doi.org/10.1016/j.ejheart.2008.01.011.
57. Aronson D, Burger AJ. The relationship between transient and persistent worsening renal function and mortality in patients with acute decompensated heart failure. J Card Fail 2010;16(7):541–7. https://doi.org/10.1016/j.cardfail.2010.02.001. Epub 2010 Mar 19.
58. Testani JM, Chen J, McCauley BD, Kimmel SE, Shannon RP. Potential effects of aggressive decongestion during the treatment of decompensated heart failure on renal function and survival. Circulation. 2010;122(3):265–72. https://doi.org/10.1161/CIRCULATIONAHA.109.933275. Epub 2010 Jul 6.
59. Wu MY, Chang NC, Su CL, Hsu YH, Chen TW, Lin YF, et al. Loop diuretic strategies in patients with acute decompensated heart failure: a meta-analysis of randomized controlled trials. J Crit Care. 2014;29(1):2–9. https://doi.org/10.1016/j.jcrc.2013.10.009. Epub 2013 Oct 29.
60. Alqahtani F, Koulouridis I, Susantitaphong P, Dahal K, Jaber BL. A meta-analysis of continuous vs intermittent infusion of loop diuretics in hospitalized patients. J Crit Care. 2014;29(1):10–7. https://doi.org/10.1016/j.jcrc.2013.03.015. Epub 2013 May 14.
61. Ezekowitz JA, Hernandez AF, Starling RC, Yancy CW, Massie B, Hill JA, et al. Standardizing care for acute decompensated heart failure in a large megatrial: the approach for the Acute Studies of Clinical Effectiveness of Nesiritide in Subjects with Decompensated Heart Failure (ASCEND-HF). Am Heart J. 2009;157(2):219–28. https://doi.org/10.1016/j.ahj.2008.10.002. Epub 2008 Nov 28.
62. Michalsen A, König G, Thimme W. Preventable causative factors leading to hospital admission with decompensated heart failure. Heart. 1998;80(5):437–41.
63. McKelvie RS, Moe GW, Ezekowitz JA, Heckman GA, Costigan J, Ducharme A, et al. The 2012 Canadian Cardiovascular Society heart failure management guidelines update: focus on acute and chronic heart failure. Can J Cardiol. 2013;29(2):168–81. https://doi.org/10.1016/j.cjca.2012.10.007. Epub 2012 Nov 30.
64. McMurray JJ, Teerlink JR, Cotter G, Bourge RC, Cleland JG, Jondeau G, VERITAS Investigators, et al. Effects of tezosentan on symptoms and clinical outcomes in patients with acute heart failure: the VERITAS randomized controlled trials. JAMA. 2007;298(17):2009–19.
65. Gheorghiade M, Konstam MA, Burnett Jr JC, Grinfeld L, Maggioni AP, Swedberg K, Efficacy of Vasopressin Antagonism in Heart Failure Outcome Study with Tolvaptan (EVEREST) Investigators, et al. Short-term clinical effects of tolvaptan, an oral vasopressin antagonist, in patients hospitalized for heart failure: the EVEREST Clinical Status Trials. JAMA. 2007;297(12):1332–43. Epub 2007 Mar 25.
66. Metra M, Cleland JG, Weatherley BD, Dittrich HC, Givertz MM, Massie BM, et al. Dyspnoea in patients with acute heart failure: an analysis of its clinical course, determinants, and relationship to 60-day outcomes in the PROTECT pilot study. Eur J Heart Fail. 2010;12(5):499–507. https://doi.org/10.1093/eurjhf/hfq021. Epub 2010 Mar 12. 10.

67. Metra M, Teerlink JR, Felker GM, Greenberg BH, Filippatos G, Ponikowski P, et al. Dyspnoea and worsening heart failure in patients with acute heart failure: results from the Pre-RELAX-AHF study. Eur J Heart Fail. 2010;12(10):1130–9. https://doi.org/10.1093/eurjhf/hfq132. Epub 2010 Aug 22.
68. Felker GM, Leimberger JD, Califf RM, Cuffe MS, Massie BM, Adams KF Jr, et al. Risk stratification after hospitalization for decompensated heart failure. J Card Fail. 2004;10(6):460–6.
69. Knauf H, Mutschler E. Clinical pharmacokinetics and pharmacodynamics of torasemide. Clin Pharmacokinet. 1998;34(1):1–24. Review. Strom BL, Schinnar R, Apter AJ, Margolis DJ, Lautenbach E, Hennessy S, Bilker WB, Pettitt D. Absence of cross-reactivity between sulfonamide antibiotics and sulfonamide nonantibiotics. N Engl J Med. 2003;349(17):1628–35.
70. Strom B, Schinnar R, Apter AJ, Margolis DJ, Lautenbach E, Hennessy S, et al. Absence of cross-reactivity between sulfonamide antibiotics and sulfonamide nonantibiotics. N Engl J Med. 2003;349(17):1628–35.
71. Lee AG, Anderson R, Kardon RH, Wall M. Presumed "sulfa allergy" in patients with intracranial hypertension treated with acetazolamide or furosemide: cross-reactivity, myth or reality? Am J Ophthalmol. 2004;138(1):114–8.
72. Hemstreet BA, Page RL 2nd. Sulfonamide allergies and outcomes related to use of potentially cross-reactive drugs in hospitalized patients. Pharmacotherapy 2006;26(4):551–557.
73. Bumex package insert. www.accessdata.fda.gov/drugsatfda_docs/label/2010/019225s024161.pdf.
74. Torsemide package insert. www.accessdata.fda.gov/drudsatfda_docs/label/2012/020136s014lbl.pdf.
75. Greenberg A. Diuretic complications. Am J Med Sci. 2000;319(1):10–24.
76. Rybak LP. Ototoxicity of loop diuretics. Otolaryngol Clin N Am. 1993;26(5):829–44.
77. Seligmann H, Podoshin L, Ben-David J, Fradis M, Goldsher M. Drug-induced tinnitus and other hearing disorders. Drug Saf. 1996;14(3):198–212.
78. Gerlag PG, van Meijel JJ. High-dose furosemide in the treatment of refractory congestive heart failure. Arch Intern Med. 1988;148(2):286–91.
79. Micromedex Solutions. Truven health analytics 2016.
80. Kassamali R, Sica DA. Acetazolamide: a forgotten diuretic agent. Cardiol Rev. 2011;19(6):276–8. https://doi.org/10.1097/CRD.0b013e31822b4939.
81. Knauf H, Mutschler E. Sequential nephron blockade breaks resistance to diuretics in edematous states. J Cardiovasc Pharmacol. 1997;29(3):367–72.
82. Khan MI. Treatment of refractory congestive heart failure and normokalemic hypochloremic alkalosis with acetazolamide and spironolactone. Can Med Assoc J. 1980;123(9):883–7.
83. Jentzer JC, DeWald TA, Hernandez AF. Combination of loop diuretics with thiazide-type diuretics in heart failure. J Am Coll Cardiol. 2010;56(19):1527–34. https://doi.org/10.1016/j.jacc.2010.06.034.
84. Masoumi A, Ortiz F, Radhakrishnan J, Schrier RW, Colombo PC. Mineralocorticoid receptor antagonists as diuretics: can congestive heart failure learn from liver failure? Heart Fail Rev. 2015;20(3):283–90. https://doi.org/10.1007/s10741-014-9467-2.
85. Bauersachs J, Jaisser F, Toto R. Mineralocorticoid receptor activation and mineralocorticoid receptor antagonist treatment in cardiac and renal diseases. Hypertension. 2015;65(2):257–63. https://doi.org/10.1161/HYPERTENSIONAHA.114.04488. Epub 2014 Nov 3.
86. McKelvie RS, Yusuf S, Pericak D, Avezum A, Burns RJ, Probstfield J, et al. Comparison of candesartan, enalapril, and their combination in congestive heart failure: randomized evaluation of strategies for left ventricular dysfunction (RESOLVD) pilot study. The RESOLVD Pilot Study Investigators. Circulation. 1999;100:1056–64.
87. Pitt B, Zannad F, Remme WJ, Cody R, Castaigne A, Perez A, Palensky J, Wittes J. The effect of spironolactone on morbidity and mortality in patients with severe heart failure. Randomized Aldactone Evaluation Study Investigators. N Engl J Med. 1999;341(10):709–17.
88. van Vliet AA, Donker AJ, Nauta JJ, Verheugt FW. Spironolactone in congestive heart failure refractory to high-dose loop diuretic and low-dose angiotensin-converting enzyme inhibitor. Am J Cardiol. 1993;71(3):21A–8A.
89. Ferreira JP, Santos M, Almeida S, Marques I, Bettencourt P, Carvalho H. Mineralocorticoid receptor antagonism in acutely decompensated chronic heart failure. Eur J Intern Med. 2014;25(1):67–72. https://doi.org/10.1016/j.ejim.2013.08.711. Epub 2013 Sep 23.
90. Butler J, Ezekowitz JA, Collins SP, Givertz MM, Teerlink JR, Walsh MN, et al. Update on aldosterone antagonists use in heart failure with reduced left ventricular ejection fraction. Heart Failure Society of America Guidelines Committee. J Card Fail. 2012;18(4):265–81. https://doi.org/10.1016/j.cardfail.2012.02.005.
91. Fonarow GC, Stough WG, Abraham WT, Albert NM, Gheorghiade M, Greenberg BH, OPTIMIZE-HF Investigators and Hospitals, et al. Characteristics, treatments, and outcomes of patients with preserved systolic function hospitalized for heart failure: a report from the OPTIMIZE-HF Registry. J Am Coll Cardiol. 2007;50(8):768–77.
92. Ambrosy AP, Pang PS, Khan S, Konstam MA, Fonarow GC, Traver B, et al. EVEREST Trial Investigators. Clinical course and predictive value of congestion during hospitalization in patients admitted for worsening signs and symptoms of heart failure with reduced ejection fraction: findings from the EVEREST trial. Eur Heart J. 2013;34(11):835–43. https://doi.org/10.1093/eurheartj/ehs444. Epub 2013 Jan 4.

93. Pang PS, Konstam MA, Krasa HB, Swedberg K, Zannad F, Blair JE, Efficacy of Vasopressin Antagonism in Heart Failure Outcome Study with Tolvaptan (EVEREST) Investigators, et al. Effects of tolvaptan on dyspnoea relief from the EVEREST trials. Eur Heart J. 2009;30(18):2233–40. https://doi.org/10.1093/eurheartj/ehp253. Epub 2009 Jun 27.
94. Costanzo MR, Guglin ME, Saltzberg MT, Jessup ML, Bart BA, UNLOAD Trial Investigators. Ultrafiltration versus intravenous diuretics for patients hospitalized for acute decompensated heart failure. J Am Coll Cardiol. 2007;49(6):675–83.
95. Mehta RH, Rogers JG, Hasselblad V, Tasissa G, Binanay C, Califf RM, O'Connor CM, Evaluation Study of Congestive Heart Failure and Pulmonary Artery Catheterization Effectiveness (ESCAPE) Trial Investigators. Association of weight change with subsequent outcomes in patients hospitalized with acute decompensated heart failure. Am J Cardiol. 2009;103(1):76–81. https://doi.org/10.1016/j.amjcard.2008.08.041. Epub 2008 Oct 7.
96. Metra M, O'Connor CM, Davison BA, Cleland JG, Ponikowski P, Teerlink JR, et al. Early dyspnoea relief in acute heart failure: prevalence, association with mortality, and effect of rolofylline in the PROTECT Study. Eur Heart J. 2011;32(12):1519–34. https://doi.org/10.1093/eurheartj/ehr042. Epub 2011 Mar 8.
97. Kociol RD, McNulty SE, Hernandez AF, Lee KL, Redfield MM, Tracy RP, Braunwald E, O'Connor CM, Felker GM, NHLBI Heart Failure Network Steering Committee and Investigators. Markers of decongestion, dyspnea relief, and clinical outcomes among patients hospitalized with acute heart failure. Circ Heart Fail. 2013;6(2):240–5.
98. Gheorghiade M, Follath F, Ponikowski P, Barsuk JH, Blair JE, Cleland JG, European Society of Intensive Care Medicine, et al. Assessing and grading congestion in acute heart failure: a scientific statement from the acute heart failure committee of the heart failure association of the European Society of Cardiology and endorsed by the European Society of Intensive Care Medicine. Eur J Heart Fail. 2010;12(5):423–33. https://doi.org/10.1093/eurjhf/hfq045. Epub 2010 Mar 30.
99. Vaduganathan M, Greene SJ, Fonarow GC, Voors AA, Butler J, Gheorghiade M. Hemoconcentration-guided diuresis in heart failure. Am J Med. 2014;127(12):1154–9. https://doi.org/10.1016/j.amjmed.2014.06.009. pii: S0002-9343(14)00482-3. [Epub ahead of print].
100. Boyle A, Sobotka PA. Redefining the therapeutic objective in decompensated heart failure: hemoconcentration as a surrogate for plasma refill rate. J Card Fail. 2006;12(4):247–9.
101. van der Meer P, Postmus D, Ponikowski P, Cleland JG, O'Connor CM, Cotter G, et al. The predictive value of short-term changes in hemoglobin concentration in patients presenting with acute decompensated heart failure. J Am Coll Cardiol. 2013;61(19):1973–81. https://doi.org/10.1016/j.jacc.2012.12.050. Epub 2013 Mar 14.
102. Greene SJ, Gheorghiade M, Vaduganathan M, Ambrosy AP, Mentz RJ, Subacius H, EVEREST Trial investigators, et al. Haemoconcentration, renal function, and post-discharge outcomes among patients hospitalized for heart failure with reduced ejection fraction: insights from the EVEREST trial. Eur J Heart Fail 2013;15(12):1401–1411. https://doi.org/10.1093/eurjhf/hft110. Epub 2013 Jul 11.
103. Oh J, Kang SM, Hong N, Youn JC, Han S, Jeon ES, et al. Hemoconcentration is a good prognostic predictor for clinical outcomes in acute heart failure: data from the Korean Heart Failure (KorHF) Registry. Int J Cardiol. 2013;168(5):4739–43. https://doi.org/10.1016/j.ijcard.2013.07.241. Epub 2013 Aug 2.
104. Testani JM, Brisco MA, Chen J, McCauley BD, Parikh CR, Tang WH. Timing of hemoconcentration during treatment of acute decompensated heart failure and subsequent survival: importance of sustained decongestion. J Am Coll Cardiol. 2013;62(6):516–24. https://doi.org/10.1016/j.jacc.2013.05.027. Epub 2013 Jun 7.
105. Desai AS. Hemoglobin concentration in acute decompensated heart failure: a marker of volume status? J Am Coll Cardiol. 2013;61(19):1982–4. https://doi.org/10.1016/j.jacc.2013.02.021. Epub 2013 Mar 14.
106. Desai AS. Are serial BNP measurements useful in heart failure management? Serial natriuretic peptide measurements are not useful in heart failure management: the art of medicine remains long. Circulation 2013;127(4):509–16. discussion 516. https://doi.org/10.1161/CIRCULATIONAHA.112.120493.
107. Doust JA, Pietrzak E, Dobson A, Glasziou P. How well does B-type natriuretic peptide predict death and cardiac events in patients with heart failure: systematic review. BMJ. 2005;330(7492):625.
108. Cheng V, Kazanagra R, Garcia A, Lenert L, Krishnaswamy P, Gardetto N, et al. A rapid bedside test for B-type peptide predicts treatment outcomes in patients admitted for decompensated heart failure: a pilot study. J Am Coll Cardiol. 2001;37(2):386–91.
109. Logeart D, Thabut G, Jourdain P, Chavelas C, Beyne P, Beauvais F, et al. Predischarge B-type natriuretic peptide assay for identifying patients at high risk of re-admission after decompensated heart failure. J Am Coll Cardiol. 2004;43(4):635–41.
110. Gackowski A, Isnard R, Golmard JL, Pousset F, Carayon A, Montalescot G, et al. Comparison of echocardiography and plasma B-type natriuretic peptide for monitoring the response to treatment in acute heart failure. Eur Heart J. 2004;25(20):1788–96.
111. Singer AJ, Birkhahn RH, Guss D, Chandra A, Miller CD, Tiffany B, et al. Rapid Emergency Department Heart Failure Outpatients Trial (REDHOT II): a randomized controlled trial of the effect of serial B-type natriuretic peptide testing on patient management. Circ Heart Fail. 2009;2(4):287–93. https://doi.

org/10.1161/CIRCHEARTFAILURE.108.826685. Epub 2009 May 19.
112. Steimle AE, Stevenson LW, Chelimsky-Fallick C, Fonarow GC, Hamilton MA, Moriguchi JD, et al. Sustained hemodynamic efficacy of therapy tailored to reduce filling pressures in survivors with advanced heart failure. Circulation. 1997;96(4):1165–72.
113. Hamilton MA, Stevenson LW, Child JS, Moriguchi JD, Walden J, Woo M. Sustained reduction in valvular regurgitation and atrial volumes with tailored vasodilator therapy in advanced congestive heart failure secondary to dilated (ischemic or idiopathic) cardiomyopathy. Am J Cardiol. 1991;67(4):259–63.
114. Binanay C, Califf RM, Hasselblad V, O'Connor CM, Shah MR, Sopko G, ESCAPE Investigators and ESCAPE Study Coordinators, et al. Evaluation study of congestive heart failure and pulmonary artery catheterization effectiveness: the ESCAPE trial. JAMA. 2005;294(13):1625–33.
115. Rajaram SS, Desai NK, Kalra A, Gajera M, Cavanaugh SK, Brampton W, et al. Pulmonary artery catheters for adult patients in intensive care. Cochrane Database Syst Rev. 2013;(2):CD003408. https://doi.org/10.1002/14651858.CD003408.pub3.
116. Shah MR, Hasselblad V, Stevenson LW, Binanay C, O'Connor CM, Sopko G, Califf RM. Impact of the pulmonary artery catheter in critically ill patients: meta-analysis of randomized clinical trials. JAMA. 2005;294(13):1664–70.
117. Harvey S, Harrison DA, Singer M, Ashcroft J, Jones CM, Elbourne D, PAC-Man study collaboration, et al. Assessment of the clinical effectiveness of pulmonary artery catheters in management of patients in intensive care (PAC-Man): a randomised controlled trial. Lancet. 2005;366(9484):472–7.
118. Collins SP, Lindsell CJ, Storrow AB, Abraham WT, ADHERE Scientific Advisory Committee, Investigators and Study Group. Prevalence of negative chest radiography results in the emergency department patient with decompensated heart failure. Ann Emerg Med. 2006;47(1):13–8. Epub 2005 Jun 20.
119. Gheorghiade M, Sopko G, De Luca L, Velazquez EJ, Parker JD, Binkley PF, et al. Navigating the crossroads of coronary artery disease and heart failure. Circulation. 2006;114(11):1202–13.
120. Ellison DH. Diuretic therapy and resistance in congestive heart failure. Cardiology. 2001;96(3–4):132–43.
121. Valente MA, Voors AA, Damman K, Van Veldhuisen DJ, Massie BM, O'Connor CM, et al. Diuretic response in acute heart failure: clinical characteristics and prognostic significance. Eur Heart J. 2014;35(19):1284–93. https://doi.org/10.1093/eurheartj/ehu065. Epub 2014 Feb 28.
122. Testani JM, Brisco MA, Turner JM, Spatz ES, Bellumkonda L, Parikh CR, Tang WH. Loop diuretic efficiency: a metric of diuretic responsiveness with prognostic importance in acute decompensated heart failure. Circ Heart Fail. 2014;7(2):261–70. https://doi.org/10.1161/CIRCHEARTFAILURE.113.000895. Epub 2013 Dec 30.
123. Kazory A, Elkayam U. Cardiorenal interactions in acute decompensated heart failure: contemporary concepts facing emerging controversies. J Card Fail. 2014;20(12):1004–11. https://doi.org/10.1016/j.cardfail.2014.09.005. Epub 2014 Sep 16.
124. Maxwell MH, Breed ES, Schwartz IL. Renal venous pressure in chronic congestive heart failure. J Clin Invest. 1950;29(3):342–8.
125. Damman K, van Deursen VM, Navis G, Voors AA, van Veldhuisen DJ, Hillege HL. Increased central venous pressure is associated with impaired renal function and mortality in a broad spectrum of patients with cardiovascular disease. J Am Coll Cardiol. 2009;53(7):582–8. https://doi.org/10.1016/j.jacc.2008.08.080.
126. Damman K, Navis G, Smilde TD, Voors AA, van der Bij W, van Veldhuisen DJ, Hillege HL. Decreased cardiac output, venous congestion and the association with renal impairment in patients with cardiac dysfunction. Eur J Heart Fail. 2007;9(9):872–8. Epub 2007 Jun 22.
127. Mullens W, Abrahams Z, Francis GS, Sokos G, Taylor DO, Starling RC, et al. Importance of venous congestion for worsening of renal function in advanced decompensated heart failure. J Am Coll Cardiol. 2009;53(7):589–96. https://doi.org/10.1016/j.jacc.2008.05.068.
128. Cheatham ML, Safcsak K. Intraabdominal pressure: a revised method for measurement. J Am Coll Surg. 1998;186(3):368–9.
129. Malbrain ML. Different techniques to measure intra-abdominal pressure (IAP): time for a critical re-appraisal. Intensive Care Med. 2004;30(3):357–71. Epub 2004 Jan 17.
130. Mullens W, Abrahams Z, Skouri HN, Francis GS, Taylor DO, Starling RC, et al. Elevated intra-abdominal pressure in acute decompensated heart failure: a potential contributor to worsening renal function? J Am Coll Cardiol. 2008;51(3):300–6. https://doi.org/10.1016/j.jacc.2007.09.043.
131. Mullens W, Abrahams Z, Francis GS, Taylor DO, Starling RC, Tang WH. Prompt reduction in intra-abdominal pressure following large-volume mechanical fluid removal improves renal insufficiency in refractory decompensated heart failure. J Card Fail. 2008;14(6):508–14. https://doi.org/10.1016/j.cardfail.2008.02.010. Epub 2008 May 27.
132. Forman DE, Butler J, Wang Y, Abraham WT, O'Connor CM, Gottlieb SS, et al. Incidence, predictors at admission, and impact of worsening renal function among patients hospitalized with heart failure. J Am Coll Cardiol. 2004;43(1):61–7.
133. Krumholz HM, Chen YT, Vaccarino V, Wang Y, Radford MJ, Bradford WD, Horwitz RI. Correlates and impact on outcomes of worsening renal function in patients > or =65 years of age with heart failure. Am J Cardiol. 2000;85(9):1110–3.

134. Nohria A, Hasselblad V, Stebbins A, Pauly DF, Fonarow GC, Shah M, et al. Cardiorenal interactions: insights from the ESCAPE trial. J Am Coll Cardiol. 2008;51(13):1268–74. https://doi.org/10.1016/j.jacc.2007.08.072.
135. Aronson D, Abassi Z, Allon E, Burger AJ. Fluid loss, venous congestion, and worsening renal function in acute decompensated heart failure. Eur J Heart Fail. 2013;15(6):637–43. https://doi.org/10.1093/eurjhf/hft036. Epub 2013 Mar 8.
136. Ronco C, Cicoira M, McCullough PA. Cardiorenal syndrome type 1: pathophysiological crosstalk leading to combined heart and kidney dysfunction in the setting of acutely decompensated heart failure. J Am Coll Cardiol. 2012;60(12):1031–42. https://doi.org/10.1016/j.jacc.2012.01.077. Epub 2012 Jul 25.
137. Virzì GM, Clementi A, Brocca A, de Cal M, Vescovo G, Granata A, Ronco C. The hemodynamic and non-hemodynamic crosstalk in cardiorenal syndrome type 1. Cardiorenal Med. 2014;4(2):103–12. https://doi.org/10.1159/000362650. Epub 2014 May 14.
138. Husain-Syed F, McCullough PA, Birk HW, Renker M, Brocca A, Seeger W, Ronco C. Cardio-pulmonary-renal interactions: a multidisciplinary approach. J Am Coll Cardiol. 2015;65(22):2433–48. https://doi.org/10.1016/j.jacc.2015.04.024.
139. van Meyel JJ, Smits P, Dormans T, Gerlag PG, Russel FG, Gribnau FW. Continuous infusion of furosemide in the treatment of patients with congestive heart failure and diuretic resistance. J Intern Med. 1994;235(4):329–34.
140. Dormans TP, van Meyel JJ, Gerlag PG, Tan Y, Russel FG, Smits P. Diuretic efficacy of high dose furosemide in severe heart failure: bolus injection versus continuous infusion. J Am Coll Cardiol. 1996;28(2):376–82.
141. Channer KS, McLean KA, Lawson-Matthew P, Richardson M. Combination diuretic treatment in severe heart failure: a randomised controlled trial. Br Heart J. 1994;71(2):146–50.
142. Rosenberg J, Gustafsson F, Galatius S, Hildebrandt PR. Combination therapy with metolazone and loop diuretics in outpatients with refractory heart failure: an observational study and review of the literature. Cardiovasc Drugs Ther. 2005;19(4):301–6.
143. Costanzo MR. Ultrafiltration in the management of heart failure. Curr Opin Crit Care. 2008;14(5):524–30.
144. Costanzo MR, Jessup M. Treatment of congestion in heart failure with diuretics and extracorporeal therapies: effects on symptoms, renal function, and prognosis. Heart Fail Rev. 2012;17(2):313–24.
145. Marenzi G, Lauri G, Grazi M, Assanelli E, Campodonico J, Agostoni P. Circulatory response to fluid overload removal by extracorporeal ultrafiltration in refractory congestive heart failure. J Am Coll Cardiol. 2001;38(4):963–8.
146. Agostoni P, Marenzi G, Lauri G, Perego G, Schianni M, Sganzerla P, Guazzi MD. Sustained improvement in functional capacity after removal of body fluid with isolated ultrafiltration in chronic cardiac insufficiency: failure of furosemide to provide the same result. Am J Med. 1994;96(3):191–9.
147. Bart BA, Boyle A, Bank AJ, Anand I, Olivari MT, Kraemer M, et al. Ultrafiltration versus usual care for hospitalized patients with heart failure: the Relief for Acutely Fluid-Overloaded Patients With Decompensated Congestive Heart Failure (RAPID-CHF) trial. J Am Coll Cardiol. 2005;46(11):2043–6.
148. Bart BA, Goldsmith SR, Lee KL, Givertz MM, O'Connor CM, s. Ultrafiltration in decompensated heart failure with cardiorenal syndrome. N Engl J Med. 2012;367(24):2296–304.
149. Silvers SM, Howell JM, Kosowsky JM, Rokos IC, Jagoda AS, American College of Emergency Physicians. Clinical policy: critical issues in the evaluation and management of adult patients presenting to the emergency department with acute heart failure syndromes. Ann Emerg Med. 2007;49(5):627–69. Epub 2007 Apr 3.
150. Abraham WT, Adams KF, Fonarow GC, Costanzo MR, Berkowitz RL, LeJemtel TH, ADHERE Scientific Advisory Committee and Investigators; ADHERE Study Group, et al. In-hospital mortality in patients with acute decompensated heart failure requiring intravenous vasoactive medications: an analysis from the Acute Decompensated Heart Failure National Registry (ADHERE). J Am Coll Cardiol. 2005;46(1):57–64.
151. Hamilton MA, Stevenson LW, Child JS, Moriguchi JD, Woo M. Acute reduction of atrial overload during vasodilator and diuretic therapy in advanced congestive heart failure. Am J Cardiol. 1990;65(18):1209–12.
152. Leier CV, Bambach D, Thompson MJ, Cattaneo SM, Goldberg RJ, Unverferth DV. Central and regional hemodynamic effects of intravenous isosorbide dinitrate, nitroglycerin and nitroprusside in patients with congestive heart failure. Am J Cardiol. 1981;48(6):1115–23.
153. Elkayam U, Janmohamed M, Habib M, Hatamizadeh P. Vasodilators in the management of acute heart failure. Crit Care Med. 2008;36(1 Suppl):S95–105. https://doi.org/10.1097/01.CCM.0000297161.41559.93.
154. Hollenberg SM. Vasodilators in acute heart failure. Heart Fail Rev. 2007;12(2):143–7.
155. Heart Failure Executive Committee, Peacock WF, Fonarow GC, Heart Failure Diagnosis Subcommittee, Ander DS, Maisel A, Hollander JE, Januzzi Jr JL, Yancy CW, Heart Failure Risk Stratification Subcommittee, Collins SP, Gheorghiade M, Weintraub NL, Storrow AB, Pang PS, Abraham WT, Hiestand B, Heart Failure Treatment Subcommittee, Kirk JD, Filippatos G, Gheorghiade M, Pang PS, Levy P, Amsterdam EA. Society of Chest Pain Centers Recommendations for the evaluation and management of the observation stay acute heart failure patient: a report from the Society of Chest Pain Centers Acute Heart Failure Committee. Crit Pathw

Cardiol. 2008;7(2):83–6. https://doi.org/10.1097/01.hpc.0000317706.54479.a4.
156. Moazemi K, Chana JS, Willard AM, Kocheril AG. Intravenous vasodilator therapy in congestive heart failure. Drugs Aging. 2003;20(7):485–508.
157. Hunt SA, Abraham WT, Chin MH, Feldman AM, Francis GS, Ganiats TG, et al. 2009 focused update incorporated into the ACC/AHA 2005 guidelines for the diagnosis and management of heart failure in adults: a report of the American College of Cardiology Foundation/American Heart Association Task Force on Practice Guidelines: developed in collaboration with the International Society for Heart and Lung Transplantation. Circulation. 2009;119(14):e391–479. https://doi.org/10.1161/CIRCULATIONAHA.109.192065. Epub 2009 Mar 26.
158. Herling IM. Intravenous nitroglycerin: clinical pharmacology and therapeutic considerations. Am Heart J. 1984;108:141–8.
159. De Caterina R, Dorso CR, Tack-Goldman K, Weksler BB. Nitrates and endothelial prostacyclin production: studies in vitro. Circulation. 1985;71(1):176–82.
160. Chen Z, Zhang J, Stamler JS. Identification of the enzymatic mechanism of nitroglycerin bioactivation. Proc Natl Acad Sci USA. 2002;99(12):8306–11. Epub 2002 Jun 4.
161. Elkayam U, Bitar F, Akhter MW, Khan S, Patrus S, Derakhshani M. Intravenous nitroglycerin in the treatment of decompensated heart failure: potential benefits and limitations. J Cardiovasc Pharmacol Ther. 2004;9(4):227–41.
162. Elkayam U. Nitrates in the treatment of congestive heart failure. Am J Cardiol. 1996;77(13):41C–51C.
163. Armstrong PW, Armstrong JA, Marks GS. Pharmacokinetic-hemodynamic studies of intravenous nitroglycerin in congestive cardiac failure. Circulation. 1980;62(1):160–6.
164. Magrini F, Niarchos AP. Ineffectiveness of sublingual nitroglycerin in acute left ventricular failure in the presence of massive peripheral edema. Am J Cardiol. 1980;45(4):841–7.
165. Kulick D, Roth A, McIntosh N, Rahimtoola SH, Elkayam U. Resistance to isosorbide dinitrate in patients with severe chronic heart failure: incidence and attempt at hemodynamic prediction. J Am Coll Cardiol. 1988;12(4):1023–8.
166. Katz SD, Biasucci L, Sabba C, Strom JA, Jondeau G, Galvao M, et al. Impaired endothelium-mediated vasodilation in the peripheral vasculature of patients with congestive heart failure. J Am Coll Cardiol. 1992;19(5):918–25.
167. Mehra A, Shotan A, Ostrzega E, Hsueh W, Vasquez-Johnson J, Elkayam U. Potentiation of isosorbide dinitrate effects with N-acetylcysteine in patients with chronic heart failure. Circulation. 1994;89(6):2595–600.
168. Packer M, Lee WH, Kessler PD, Gottlieb SS, Medina N, Yushak M. Prevention and reversal of nitrate tolerance in patients with congestive heart failure. N Engl J Med. 1987;317(13):799–804.
169. Daiber A, Mülsch A, Hink U, Mollnau H, Warnholtz A, Oelze M, Münzel T. The oxidative stress concept of nitrate tolerance and the antioxidant properties of hydralazine. Am J Cardiol. 2005;96(7B):25i–36i. Epub 2005 Aug 8.
170. Hink U, Oelze M, Kolb P, Bachschmid M, Zou MH, Daiber A, et al. Role for peroxynitrite in the inhibition of prostacyclin synthase in nitrate tolerance. J Am Coll Cardiol. 2003;42(10):1826–34.
171. Dakak N, Makhoul N, Flugelman MY, Merdler A, Shehadeh H, Schneeweiss A, et al. Failure of captopril to prevent nitrate tolerance in congestive heart failure secondary to coronary artery disease. Am J Cardiol. 1990;66(5):608–13.
172. Elkayam U, Kulick D, McIntosh N, Roth A, Hsueh W, Rahimtoola SH. Incidence of early tolerance to hemodynamic effects of continuous infusion of nitroglycerin in patients with coronary artery disease and heart failure. Circulation. 1987;76(3):577–84.
173. Dupuis J, Lalonde G, Lemieux R, Rouleau JL. Tolerance to intravenous nitroglycerin in patients with congestive heart failure: role of increased intravascular volume, neurohumoral activation and lack of prevention with N-acetylcysteine. J Am Coll Cardiol. 1990;16(4):923–31.
174. Elkayam U, Roth A, Henriquez B, Weber L, Tonnemacher D, Rahimtoola SH. Hemodynamic and hormonal effects of high-dose transdermal nitroglycerin in patients with chronic congestive heart failure. Am J Cardiol. 1985;56(8):555–9.
175. Dupuis J, Lalonde G, Bichet D, Rouleau JL. Captopril does not prevent nitroglycerin tolerance in heart failure. Can J Cardiol. 1990;6(7):281–6.
176. Bauer JA, Fung HL. Concurrent hydralazine administration prevents nitroglycerin-induced hemodynamic tolerance in experimental heart failure. Circulation. 1991;84(1):35–9.
177. Daiber A, Oelze M, Coldewey M, Kaiser K, Huth C, Schildknecht S, et al. Hydralazine is a powerful inhibitor of peroxynitrite formation as a possible explanation for its beneficial effects on prognosis in patients with congestive heart failure. Biochem Biophys Res Commun. 2005;338(4):1865–74. Epub 2005 Nov 11.
178. Elkayam U, Bitar F. Effects of nitrates and hydralazine in heart failure: clinical evidence before the african american heart failure trial. Am J Cardiol. 2005;96(7B):37i–43i. Epub 2005 Aug.
179. Taylor AL, Ziesche S, Yancy C, Carson P, D'Agostino Jr R, Ferdinand K, African-American Heart Failure Trial Investigators, et al. Combination of isosorbide dinitrate and hydralazine in blacks with heart failure. N Engl J Med. 2004;351(20):2049–57. Epub 2004 Nov 8.
180. Cotter G, Metzkor E, Kaluski E, Faigenberg Z, Miller R, Simovitz A, et al. Randomised trial of high-dose isosorbide dinitrate plus low-dose furosemide versus high-dose furosemide plus low-dose

isosorbide dinitrate in severe pulmonary oedema. Lancet. 1998;351(9100):389–93.
181. Publication Committee for the VMAC Investigators (Vasodilatation in the Management of Acute CHF). Intravenous nesiritide vs nitroglycerin for treatment of decompensated congestive heart failure: a randomized controlled trial. JAMA. 2002;287(12):1531–40.
182. Elkayam U, for the VMAC Study Group. Superior hemodynamic effect of nesiritide (B-type natriuretic peptide) compared to high dose nitroglycerin (NTG) in patients with decompensated heart failure. NAIP 5th Annual Meeting; 2002, p 7.
183. Fung HL, Bauer JA. Mechanisms of nitrate tolerance. Cardiovasc Drugs Ther. 1994;8(3):489–99.
184. Michel T, Hoffman BB. Chapter 27. Treatment of myocardial ischemia and hypertension. In: Brunton LL, Chabner BA, Knollmann BC, editors. Goodman & Gilman's the pharmacological basis of therapeutics. 12th ed. New York: McGraw-Hill; 2011. http://accessmedicine.mhmedical.com/content.aspx?bookid=374&Sectionid=41266234. Accessed 04 Aug 2015.
185. Hottinger DG, Beebe DS, Kozhimannil T, Prielipp RC, Belani KG. Sodium nitroprusside in 2014: a clinical concepts review. J Anaesthesiol Clin Pharmacol. 2014;30(4):462–71. https://doi.org/10.4103/0970-9185.142799.
186. Carlson MD, Eckman PM. Review of vasodilators in acute decompensated heart failure: the old and the new. J Card Fail. 2013;19(7):478–93. https://doi.org/10.1016/j.cardfail.2013.05.007.
187. Packer M, Meller J, Medina N, Gorlin R, Herman MV. Rebound hemodynamic events after the abrupt withdrawal of nitroprusside in patients with severe chronic heart failure. N Engl J Med. 1979;301(22):1193–7.
188. Reade MC, Davies SR, Morley PT, Dennett J, Jacobs IC, Australian Resuscitation Council. Review article: management of cyanide poisoning. Emerg Med Australas. 2012;24(3):225–38. https://doi.org/10.1111/j.1742-6723.2012.01538.x. Epub 2012 Feb 21.
189. Guiha NH, Cohn JN, Mikulic E, Franciosa JA, Limas CJ. Treatment of refractory heart failure with infusion of nitroprusside. N Engl J Med. 1974;291(12):587–92.
190. Hockings BE, Cope GD, Clarke GM, Taylor RR. Randomized controlled trial of vasodilator therapy after myocardial infarction. Am J Cardiol. 1981;48(2):345–52.
191. Cohn JN, Franciosa JA, Francis GS, Archibald D, Tristani F, Fletcher R, et al. Effect of short-term infusion of sodium nitroprusside on mortality rate in acute myocardial infarction complicated by left ventricular failure: results of a Veterans Administration cooperative study. N Engl J Med. 1982;306(19):1129–35.
192. Mullens W, Abrahams Z, Francis GS, Skouri HN, Starling RC, Young JB, et al. Sodium nitroprusside for advanced low-output heart failure. J Am Coll Cardiol. 2008;52(3):200–7. https://doi.org/10.1016/j.jacc.2008.02.083.
193. Stevenson LW, Dracup KA, Tillisch JH. Efficacy of medical therapy tailored for severe congestive heart failure in patients transferred for urgent cardiac transplantation. Am J Cardiol. 1989;63(7):461–4.
194. Levin ER, Gardner DG, Samson WK. Natriuretic peptides. N Engl J Med. 1998;339(5):321–8.
195. Elkayam U, Akhter MW, Tummala P, Khan S, Singh H. Nesiritide: a new drug for the treatment of decompensated heart failure. J Cardiovasc Pharmacol Ther. 2002;7(3):181–94.
196. Potter LR, Yoder AR, Flora DR, Antos LK, Dickey DM. Natriuretic peptides: their structures, receptors, physiologic functions and therapeutic applications. In: Handb Exp Pharmacol, vol. 191; 2009. p. 341–66. https://doi.org/10.1007/978-3-540-68964-5_15.
197. Potter LR. Natriuretic peptide metabolism, clearance and degradation. FEBS J. 2011;278(11):1808–17. https://doi.org/10.1111/j.1742-4658.2011.08082.x. Epub 2011 Apr 7.
198. Abraham WT, Lowes BD, Ferguson DA, Odom J, Kim JK, Robertson AD, et al. Systemic hemodynamic, neurohormonal, and renal effects of a steady-state infusion of human brain natriuretic peptide in patients with hemodynamically decompensated heart failure. J Card Fail. 1998;4(1):37–44.
199. Mills RM, LeJemtel TH, Horton DP, Liang C, Lang R, Silver MA, et al. Sustained hemodynamic effects of an infusion of nesiritide (human b-type natriuretic peptide) in heart failure: a randomized, double-blind, placebo-controlled clinical trial. Natrecor Study Group. J Am Coll Cardiol. 1999;34(1):155–62.
200. Colucci WS, Elkayam U, Horton DP, Abraham WT, Bourge RC, Johnson AD, et al. Intravenous nesiritide, a natriuretic peptide, in the treatment of decompensated congestive heart failure. Nesiritide Study Group. N Engl J Med. 2000;343(4):246–53.
201. Aronson D, Horton DP, Burger AJ. Effect of nesiritide, B-type natriuretic peptide, on endothelin-1 in patients with decompensated congestive heart failure. J Am Coll Cardiol. 2001;37(2 Suppl A):1A–648A.
202. Michaels AD, Klein A, Madden JA, Chatterjee K. Effects of intravenous nesiritide on human coronary vasomotor regulation and myocardial oxygen uptake. Circulation. 2003;107(21):2697–701. Epub 2003 May 12.
203. Burger AJ, Horton DP, LeJemtel T, Ghali JK, Torre G, Dennish G, Prospective Randomized Evaluation of Cardiac Ectopy with Dobutamine or Natrecor Therapy, et al. Effect of nesiritide (B-type natriuretic peptide) and dobutamine on ventricular arrhythmias in the treatment of patients with acutely decompensated congestive heart failure: the PRECEDENT study. Am Heart J. 2002;144(6):1102–8.
204. Mentzer Jr RM, Oz MC, Sladen RN, Graeve AH, Hebeler Jr RF, Luber Jr JM, Smedira NG, NAPA Investigators. Effects of perioperative nesiritide in patients with left ventricular dysfunction undergoing

cardiac surgery: the NAPA Trial. J Am Coll Cardiol. 2007;49(6):716–26. Epub 2006 Dec 11.
205. Wang DJ, Dowling TC, Meadows D, Ayala T, Marshall J, Minshall S, et al. Nesiritide does not improve renal function in patients with chronic heart failure and worsening serum creatinine. Circulation. 2004;110(12):1620–5. Epub 2004 Aug 30.
206. Chen HH, Anstrom KJ, Givertz MM, Stevenson LW, Semigran MJ, Goldsmith SR, NHLBI Heart Failure Clinical Research Network, et al. Low-dose dopamine or low-dose nesiritide in acute heart failure with renal dysfunction: the ROSE acute heart failure randomized trial. JAMA. 2013;310(23):2533–43. https://doi.org/10.1001/jama.2013.282190.
207. Elkayam U, Akhter MW, Singh H, Khan S, Usman A. Comparison of effects on left ventricular filling pressure of intravenous nesiritide and high-dose nitroglycerin in patients with decompensated heart failure. Am J Cardiol. 2004;93(2):237–40.
208. Sackner-Bernstein JD, Skopicki HA, Aaronson KD. Risk of worsening renal function with nesiritide in patients with acutely decompensated heart failure. Circulation. 2005;111(12):1487–91. Epub 2005 Mar 21.
209. Sackner-Bernstein JD, Kowalski M, Fox M, Aaronson K. Short-term risk of death after treatment with nesiritide for decompensated heart failure: a pooled analysis of randomized controlled trials. JAMA. 2005;293(15):1900–5.
210. Aaronson KD, Sackner-Bernstein J. Risk of death associated with nesiritide in patients with acutely decompensated heart failure. JAMA. 2006;296(12):1465–6.
211. Arora RR, Venkatesh PK, Molnar J. Short and long-term mortality with nesiritide. Am Heart J. 2006;152(6):1084–90.
212. Abraham WT, Trupp RJ, Jarjoura D. Nesiritide in acute decompensated heart failure: a pooled analysis of randomized controlled trials. Clin Cardiol. 2010;33(8):484–9. https://doi.org/10.1002/clc.20793.
213. O'Connor CM, Starling RC, Hernandez AF, Armstrong PW, Dickstein K, Hasselblad V, et al. Effect of nesiritide in patients with acute decompensated heart failure. N Engl J Med. 2011;365(1):32–43. https://doi.org/10.1056/NEJMoa1100171.
214. Westfall TC, Westfall DP. Chapter 12. Adrenergic agonists and antagonists. In: Brunton LL, Chabner BA, Knollmann BC, editors. Goodman & Gilman's the pharmacological basis of therapeutics. 12th ed. New York: McGraw-Hill; 2011. http://accessmedicine.mhmedical.com/content.aspx?bookid=374&Sectionid=41266218. Accessed 28 Mar 2015.
215. Leier CV, Unverferth DV. Drugs five years later. Dobutamine. Ann Intern Med. 1983;99(4):490–6.
216. Bayram M, De Luca L, Massie MB, Gheorghiade M. Reassessment of dobutamine, dopamine, and milrinone in the management of acute heart failure syndromes. Am J Cardiol. 2005;96(6A):47G–58G.
217. Shin DD, Brandimarte F, De Luca L, Sabbah HN, Fonarow GC, Filippatos G, et al. Review of current and investigational pharmacologic agents for acute heart failure syndromes. Am J Cardiol. 2007;99(2A):4A–23A. Epub 2006 Nov 27
218. Monrad ES, Baim DS, Smith HS, Lanque AS. Milrinone, dobutamine, and nitroprusside: comparative effects on hemodynamics and myocardial energetics in patients with severe congestive heart failure. Circulation. 1986;73(3 Pt 2):III168–74.
219. El-Sayed OM, Abdelfattah RR, Barcelona R, Leier CV. Dobutamine-induced eosinophilia. Am J Cardiol. 2004;93(8):1078–9.
220. Takkenberg JJ, Czer LS, Fishbein MC, Luthringer DJ, Quartel AW, Mirocha J, et al. Eosinophilic myocarditis in patients awaiting heart transplantation. Crit Care Med. 2004;32(3):714–21.
221. Beanlands RS, Bach DS, Raylman R, Armstrong WF, Wilson V, Montieth M, et al. Acute effects of dobutamine on myocardial oxygen consumption and cardiac efficiency measured using carbon-11 acetate kinetics in patients with dilated cardiomyopathy. J Am Coll Cardiol. 1993;22(5):1389–98.
222. Schulz R, Rose J, Martin C, Brodde OE, Heusch G. Development of short-term myocardial hibernation. Its limitation by the severity of ischemia and inotropic stimulation. Circulation. 1993;88(2):684–95.
223. Nikolaidis LA, Hentosz T, Doverspike A, Huerbin R, Stolarski C, Shen YT, Shannon RP. Catecholamine stimulation is associated with impaired myocardial O(2) utilization in heart failure. Cardiovasc Res. 2002;53(2):392–404.
224. Teerlink JR, Metra M, Zacà V, Sabbah HN, Cotter G, Gheorghiade M, Cas LD. Agents with inotropic properties for the management of acute heart failure syndromes. Traditional agents and beyond. Heart Fail Rev. 2009;14(4):243–53. https://doi.org/10.1007/s10741-009-9153-y.
225. Elkayam U, Ng TM, Hatamizadeh P, Janmohamed M, Mehra A. Renal vasodilatory action of dopamine in patients with heart failure: magnitude of effect and site of action. Circulation. 2008;117(2):200–5. Epub 2008 Jan 2.
226. Giamouzis G, Butler J, Starling RC, Karayannis G, Nastas J, Parisis C, et al. Impact of dopamine infusion on renal function in hospitalized heart failure patients: results of the Dopamine in Acute Decompensated Heart Failure (DAD-HF) Trial. J Card Fail. 2010;16(12):922–30. https://doi.org/10.1016/j.cardfail.2010.07.246.
227. Triposkiadis FK, Butler J, Karayannis G, Starling RC, Filippatos G, Wolski K, et al. Efficacy and safety of high dose versus low dose furosemide with or without dopamine infusion: the Dopamine in Acute Decompensated Heart Failure II (DAD-HF II) trial. Int J Cardiol. 2014;172(1):115–21. https://doi.org/10.1016/j.ijcard.2013.12.276. Epub 2014 Jan 10.

228. Baim DS. Effect of phosphodiesterase inhibition on myocardial oxygen consumption and coronary blood flow. Am J Cardiol. 1989;63(2):23A–6A.
229. Banfor PN, Preusser LC, Campbell TJ, Marsh KC, Polakowski JS, Reinhart GA, et al. Comparative effects of levosimendan, OR-1896, OR-1855, dobutamine, and milrinone on vascular resistance, indexes of cardiac function, and O2 consumption in dogs. Am J Physiol Heart Circ Physiol. 2008;294(1):H238–48. Epub 2007 Nov 2.
230. Baruch L, Patacsil P, Hameed A, Pina I, Loh E. Pharmacodynamic effects of milrinone with and without a bolus loading infusion. Am Heart J. 2001;141(2):266–73.
231. Papp Z, Édes I, Fruhwald S, De Hert SG, Salmenperä M, Leppikangas H, et al. Levosimendan: molecular mechanisms and clinical implications: consensus of experts on the mechanisms of action of levosimendan. Int J Cardiol. 2012;159(2):82–7. https://doi.org/10.1016/j.ijcard.2011.07.022. Epub 2011 Jul 23.
232. Kivikko M, Antila S, Eha J, Lehtonen L, Pentikäinen PJ. Pharmacokinetics of levosimendan and its metabolites during and after a 24-hour continuous infusion in patients with severe heart failure. Int J Clin Pharmacol Ther. 2002;40(10):465–71.
233. Kivikko M, Lehtonen L. Levosimendan: a new inodilatory drug for the treatment of decompensated heart failure. Curr Pharm Des. 2005;11(4):435–55.
234. Mebazaa A, Nieminen MS, Packer M, Cohen-Solal A, Kleber FX, Pocock SJ, SURVIVE Investigators, et al. Levosimendan vs dobutamine for patients with acute decompensated heart failure: the SURVIVE randomized Trial. JAMA. 2007;297(17):1883–91.
235. Cleland JG, Freemantle N, Coletta AP, Clark AL. Clinical trials update from the American Heart Association: REPAIR-AMI, ASTAMI, JELIS, MEGA, REVIVE-II, SURVIVE, and PROACTIVE. Eur J Heart Fail. 2006;8(1):105–10.
236. Landoni G, Biondi-Zoccai G, Greco M, Greco T, Bignami E, Morelli A, et al. Effects of levosimendan on mortality and hospitalization. A meta-analysis of randomized controlled studies. Crit Care Med. 2012;40(2):634–46. https://doi.org/10.1097/CCM.0b013e318232962a.
237. Gheorghiade M, Abraham WT, Albert NM, Greenberg BH, O'Connor CM, She L, OPTIMIZE-HF Investigators and Coordinators, et al. Systolic blood pressure at admission, clinical characteristics, and outcomes in patients hospitalized with acute heart failure. JAMA. 2006;296(18):2217–26.
238. Nieminen MS, Brutsaert D, Dickstein K, Drexler H, Follath F, Harjola VP, EuroHeart Survey Investigators, Heart Failure Association, European Society of Cardiology, et al. EuroHeart Failure Survey II (EHFS II): a survey on hospitalized acute heart failure patients: description of population. Eur Heart J. 2006;27(22):2725–36. Epub 2006 Sep 25.
239. Tavazzi L, Maggioni AP, Lucci D, Cacciatore G, Ansalone G, Oliva F, Porcu M, Italian survey on Acute Heart Failure Investigators. Nationwide survey on acute heart failure in cardiology ward services in Italy. Eur Heart J. 2006;27(10):1207–15. Epub 2006 Apr 7.
240. Arnold LM, Crouch MA, Carroll NV, Oinonen MJ. Outcomes associated with vasoactive therapy in patients with acute decompensated heart failure. Pharmacotherapy. 2006;26(8):1078–85.
241. Elkayam U, Tasissa G, Binanay C, Stevenson LW, Gheorghiade M, Warnica JW, et al. Use and impact of inotropes and vasodilator therapy in hospitalized patients with severe heart failure. Am Heart J. 2007;153(1):98–104.
242. Felker GM, Benza RL, Chandler AB, Leimberger JD, Cuffe MS, Califf RM, OPTIME-CHF Investigators, et al. Heart failure etiology and response to milrinone in decompensated heart failure: results from the OPTIME-CHF study. J Am Coll Cardiol. 2003;41(6):997–1003.
243. Cuffe MS, Califf RM, Adams Jr KF, Benza R, Bourge R, Colucci WS, Outcomes of a Prospective Trial of Intravenous Milrinone for Exacerbations of Chronic Heart Failure (OPTIME-CHF) Investigators, et al. Short-term intravenous milrinone for acute exacerbation of chronic heart failure: a randomized controlled trial. JAMA. 2002;287(12):1541–7.

14 Acute Decompensated Heart Failure: Treatment with Guideline Directed Medical Therapy and Discharge Planning

Daniel Fishbein

Initiation or Continuation of Guideline Directed Medical Therapy (GDMT)

A number of medications including ACE inhibitors, ARBs, β-blockers, mineralocorticoid receptor antagonists (MRAs), and the combination of hydralazine/isosorbide dinitrate (in black patients) have been shown, in prospective randomized placebo-controlled clinical trials, to improve symptoms, decrease mortality and decrease hospitalization in ambulatory patients with heart failure with reduced ventricular systolic function [1–11]. Randomized studies of these agents have not been conducted in patients hospitalized for ADHF. The ACCF/AHA guidelines recommend that heart failure medications be carefully reviewed on admission and that appropriate changes be made during hospitalization. Chronic maintenance therapy with GDMT should, in general, be continued during hospitalization for ADHF and GDMT should be initiated in patients with ADHF and HFrEF who are not receiving chronic heart failure medications [12]. The HFSA guidelines emphasize that hospitalization for ADHF is an "excellent opportunity" to optimize a patient's chronic oral medical regimen [13]. The ESC guidelines recommend that GDMT should be continued on admission or should be started as soon as possible in patients with HFrEF [14].

D. Fishbein (✉)
Department of Medicine, Division of Cardiology, University of Washington Medical Center, Seattle, WA, USA
e-mail: dfish@uw.edu

Angiotensin Converting Enzyme Inhibitors (ACEI) or Angiotensin Receptor Blockers (ARB)

An attempt should be made during heart failure hospitalization to increase the ACEI or ARB dose to recommended target doses (lisinopril 20–35 mg daily, captopril 50 mg tid, enalapril 10–20 mg bid; losartan 150 qd, candesartan 32 mg qd, valsartan 160 mg bid) as tolerated by blood pressure, serum potassium concentration and renal function. An increased dose of ACE inhibitor or ARB may not be tolerated in patients who have low intracardiac filling pressures as a result of over diuresis. A reduction in the dose of ACEI and ARB should be considered in patients admitted with significant renal dysfunction or hyperkalemia. MRAs should be discontinued before ACEI or ARB in patients with hyperkalemia. An attempt to reinitiate or up titrate these medications should be subsequently considered depending on whether renal function or hyperkalemia improve during hospitalization.

The recommended starting doses of ACE inhibitor or ARB in hospitalized patients not receiving heart failure medications on admission are: captopril 6.25 mg tid, enalapril 2.5 mg

H. J. Eisen (ed.), *Heart Failure I*, https://doi.org/10.1007/978-3-032-12626-9_14

bid, lisinopril 2.5–5.0 mg qd; losartan 50 mg qd, valsartan 40 mg bid, or candesartan 4–8 mg daily [14]. It is reasonable to consider initiating an ACE inhibitor or ARB at half of the recommended starting dose in patients with borderline blood pressure or renal insufficiency. Caution should be used when treating a patient with significant hyperkalemia ($K^+ > 5.0$ mmol/L), significant renal dysfunction (creatinine >2.5 mg/dL or eGFR < 30 mL/min/1.73 m^2), or symptomatic or significant asymptomatic hypotension (systolic blood pressure <90 mmHg). In general, ACEIs or ARBs are not initiated in these settings. The dose of ACE inhibitor or ARB can be cautiously increased daily in the absence of hypotension, worsening renal function or hyperkalemia [12, 14].

Beta-Blockers

In general, β-blockers should not be held nor the dose reduced unless the patient has severe pulmonary congestion, evidence of marginal or low cardiac output or hypotension or if the ADHF hospitalization is felt to have been precipitated by β-blocker initiation or recent dose increase. Data from the Carvedilol or Metoprolol European Trial (COMET) [15], the ESCAPE trial [16], and the OPTIMIZE-HF program [17] all suggest that patients admitted to the hospital for ADHF who have their outpatient chronic β-blocker stopped or who are discharged on a significantly lower dose have a significantly higher risk-adjusted one and 2 year mortality (COMET); a significantly higher risk adjusted rate of rehospitalization or death at 60–90 days (ESCAPE), and a significantly higher risk and propensity adjusted 60–90 day post-discharge mortality (OPTIMIZE-HF).

The ACCF and ESC recommend that β-blocker therapy should be initiated when parenteral diuretics, intravenous vasodilators and inotropic agents have been successfully discontinued [12, 14]. The patient should be hemodynamically stable and volume status should be optimized prior to β-blocker initiation. The initial dose of β-blocker should be small (carvedilol 3.125 mg bid, metoprolol succinate 12.5–25 mg qd, bisoprolol 1.25 mg qd). Caution should also be used when initiating β-blockers in patients who have required treatment with inotropes earlier in their hospitalization [12]. The Initiation Management Predischarge: Process for Assessment of Carvedilol Therapy in Heart Failure (IMPACT-HF) trial was a prospective randomized open-label study in 363 β-blocker naïve patients stabilized after hospitalization for ADHF who were randomized to pre-discharge initiation of β-blocker therapy or post-discharge initiation at the physician's discretion [18]. Patients who had been treated with inotropic therapy during the HF hospitalization were excluded from entering the trial. The primary end-point, treatment with a β-blocker at 60 days after discharge, was significantly greater in the pre-discharge initiation group (91.2% vs 73.4%). No difference was found between groups with respect to side effects or hospital length of stay. Data from the OPTIMIZE-HF registry found that only 56.9% of patients who were eligible for β-blocker therapy were receiving a β-blocker at admission; the mean total daily dose of carvedilol or metoprolol in patients who were receiving a β-blocker was less than half the recommended dose; there was little change in dose during hospitalization or within the first 60–90 days after discharge; and only 17.5% and 7.9% of patients discharged on a β-blocker were at the recommended target dose of carvedilol or metoprolol succinate, respectively [19].

Mineralocorticoid Receptor Antagonists (MRAs)

The MRAs spironolactone and eplerenone have been shown to improve survival in patients with HFrEF and are recommended GDMT in patients with systolic dysfunction. Despite this, data from the Get with the Guidelines-Heart Failure quality improvement registry suggest that only one third of patients eligible for aldosterone antagonist therapy receive an MRA at discharge following hospitalization for ADHF [20]. The ACCF/AHA and ESC guidelines recommend that treatment with an MRA be either continued or initiated in patients with reduced ejection fraction hospitalized for ADHF [12, 14]. The ACCF/AHA guidelines recommend that an MRA should be initiated only if the serum potassium is less than 5 mEq/L [12]. The starting dose for patients with an eGFR ≥ 50 mL/min/1.73 m^2 is 12.5–25 mg qd for spironolactone and 25 mg qd for eplerenone. For patients with an eGFR 30 to 49 mL/min/1.73 m^2, the initial dose should be eplerenone 25 mg once every other day or spironolactone 12.5 mg once daily or every other day. MRAs should not be used in patients being treated with both an ACEI and an ARB. Potassium supplementation should be decreased on initiation of an MRA. Potassium and renal function need to be followed carefully in the hospitalized patient because of ongoing changes in volume status, diuretic dose, ACE inhibitor or ARB dose, systemic perfusion and renal function.

Hydralazine and Nitrates (H/NTG)

Black patients with HFrEF may benefit from the addition of hydralazine and nitrates. The African-American Heart Failure Trial (A-HeFT) randomized 1050 self-identified black patients with systolic dysfunction and NYHA Class III or IV heart failure symptoms who were receiving standard therapy for heart failure for at least 3 months to receive either a fixed dose of isosorbide dinitrate plus hydralazine or placebo [1]. The study was terminated prematurely because of a significantly lower mortality in the hydralazine/nitrate group compared to the control group (6.2% vs 10.2%; HR 0.57). In addition, there was a 33% relative risk reduction in the rate of first hospitalization for heart failure and an improvement in quality of life score assessed by the Minnesota Living with Heart Failure questionnaire. Both the ACCF/AHA and HFSA guidelines recommend the combination of hydralazine/nitrates as part of GDMT in self-identified black patients with symptomatic HFrEF [12, 13]. Despite these guidelines, an analysis from the Get with The Guidelines-Heart Failure registry found that of 11,185 African American patients admitted with HFrEF who were eligible for hydralazine/nitrate therapy, only 22.4% received H/NTG on discharge [21].

An attempt should be made to insure that the doses of GDMT be optimized during the heart failure hospitalization and after discharge. A study of initiation and persistence of GDMT in 107,092 patients discharged after first hospitalization for heart failure in Denmark from 1995–2004 demonstrated that treatment with ACEI or ARB, β-blocker or MRA was initiated in 43%, 27% and 19% of patients, respectively. Patients who did not have therapy initiated by 90 days after discharge had a low probability of later medication initiation. Persistence of treatment was high once initiated but treatment dosages were below recommended targets and, with the exception of carvedilol, were generally not increased after discharge [22].

Implantable Cardioverter Defibrillator and Cardiac Resynchronization Therapy

Hospitalization allows for consultation with an electrophysiologist for evaluation for implantable cardioverter defibrillator (ICD) and/or cardiac resynchronization (CRT) therapy [13, 23]. Patients with HFrEF should be screened for ICD therapy for primary prevention of sudden cardiac arrest. ICD therapy is indicated in: patients with nonischemic dilated cardiomyopathy, NYHA FC II or III symptoms and an LVEF ≤ 35%; patients with an LVEF ≤ 35% due to prior MI who are at least 40 days post-MI and have NYHA FC II-III symptoms; patients with LV dysfunction due to prior MI who are at least 40 days post-MI, have an LVEF ≤ 30%, and are NYHA FC I; and patients with nonsustained VT due to prior MI, LVEF ≤ 40%, and inducible VF or sustained VT at electrophysiology study. Ideally, device implantation should be delayed until patients are receiving optimal medical therapy, are no longer volume overloaded and are hemodynamically stable. The benefit of implanting a primary prevention ICD during hospitalization for ADHF has not been evaluated [24–26].

Approximately 40% of patients with HFrEF hospitalized for ADHF have a wide QRS complex. Cardiac resynchronization therapy may improve symptoms and survival in patients who have LVEF ≤ 35%, sinus rhythm, LBBB with a QRS duration ≥150 ms, and NYHA class II, III, or ambulatory IV symptoms on GDMT. CRT should be considered after discharge if the patient remains symptomatic despite appropriate GDMT [26–31].

Discharge Planning

The optimal timing for hospital discharge has not been prospectively evaluated. In general, patients should have resolution of heart failure symptoms at rest and with minimal activity; should be hemodynamically stable without lightheadedness at rest or with activity; should have stable kidney and liver function; should have normal electrolytes; should be on optimal GDMT; should have the cause of heart failure established; should have conditions/precipitating factors that worsen heart failure identified and corrected; and should have volume status as normal as possible [32, 33]. Patients with atrial fibrillation should have a controlled ventricular response. Hypertension should be well controlled.

In general, patients should be observed for 24 h after the transition from intravenous to oral diuretics. Patients may become congested again during this period. It is also possible that, with better GDMT and resolution of congestion, the dose of oral diuretic will be overestimated based on the preadmission or intravenous dose and will need to be decreased prior to discharge. Patients who have been treated with parenteral vasodilator or inotropic therapy should be observed for at least 24 h after these medications are stopped to insure that the patient is clinically stable, does not develop recurrent findings of hypoperfusion, is not hypotensive, and remains diuretic responsive and euvolemic.

Discharge criteria from the HFSA 2010 Comprehensive Heart Failure Practice Guidelines are summarized in Table 14.1 [34].

The transition from the inpatient to the outpatient setting is a vulnerable time for patients who have been hospitalized for ADHF. Hospitalization for heart failure may reflect an important change in cardiac function and pathophysiology and may indicate that the trajectory of the patient's underlying disease has changed. Patients are frequently discharged on a medical regimen that is different

Table 14.1 Discharge criteria for patients hospitalized for ADHF

Recommended for all HF patients	Exacerbating factors addressed
	Near optimal volume status observed
	Transition from intravenous to oral diuretic successfully completed
	Patient and family education completed, including clear discharge instructions
	LVEF documented
	Smoking cessation counseling initiated
	Near optimal pharmacologic therapy achieved, including ACE inhibitor and beta blocker (for patients with reduced LVEF), or intolerance documented (Sections 7 and 11)
	Follow-up clinic visit scheduled, usually for 7–10 days
Should be considered for patients with advanced HF or recurrent admissions for HF	Oral medication regimen stable for 24 h
	No intravenous vasodilator or inotropic agent for 24 h
	Ambulation before discharge to assess functional capacity after therapy
	Plans for post-discharge management (scale present in home, visiting nurse or telephone follow up generally no longer than 3 days after discharge)
	Referral for disease management, if available

Reprinted with permission from Lindenfeld et al. [13]

from and more complex than their regimen on admission. Patients are also discharged at a time when vital signs, volume status, renal function, appetite, salt and water intake, and the absorption, metabolism and effect of medications are changing. In addition, the majority of patients with heart failure have multiple comorbidities that are associated with an increased risk of mortality and preventable hospitalization and that are frequently not addressed during the ADHF hospitalization [35].

Important components of discharge planning are reviewed below [33, 36]:

Patient Education

The education of patients, family members and care-providers is an essential component of discharge planning. Patients should be educated about:

1. The dose, frequency and potential side effects of each medication; patients should be able to identify their medications and understand the reason for taking each medication; patients should receive explicit instructions about medication adjustment.
2. Warning signs and symptoms of worsening heart failure
3. Self-management skills including monitoring daily weights, controlling sodium intake, and monitoring blood pressure
4. Recommended level of activity
5. Clear guidelines for reporting signs and symptoms of heart failure, change in weight, and abnormal blood pressure to the appropriate care provider
6. Factors that may aggravate heart failure
7. Follow up in anticoagulation clinic in patients taking warfarin

In a randomized controlled trial of 223 patients hospitalized with ADHF, the addition of a 60 min one-on-one teaching session with a nurse educator to the standard discharge process resulted in fewer days hospitalized or death within the first 180 days after discharge, a lower risk of rehospitalization or death, fewer heart failure hospitalizations, increased self-care measures and a reduced cost of care [37]. In a smaller study, patients hospitalized for ADHF were randomized to an in-hospital educational program conducted by a multidisciplinary team (nurse or educator and a pharmacist) or standard care. Patients randomized to the educational program showed higher knowledge scores at discharge, an improvement in quality of life measured by the MLWHF Questionnaire and trends toward better compliance with ACEI and β-blocker therapy [38].

Discharge on GDMT

Insuring that patients are discharged on appropriate heart failure medications reduces mortality and rehospitalization. An analysis from the National Heart Care Project (an initiative by the Centers for Medicare & Medicaid Services designed to improve the quality of care for Medicare beneficiaries hospitalized with heart failure) looked at 17,456 patients age ≥65 years who had systolic dysfunction and no contraindication to ACEI or ARB who survived hospitalization for heart failure. ACEI were prescribed to only 68% of this ideal cohort. 78% of patients were prescribed either an ACEI or ARB. ACEI prescription was associated with a lower risk-adjusted 1-year mortality rate (HR 0.86) [39].

The relationship between the five ACC/AHA performance measures for patients hospitalized with heart failure (discharge instructions, evaluation of left ventricular systolic function, ACEI or ARB for LV systolic dysfunction, adult smoking cessation counseling and anticoagulation at discharge for atrial fibrillation) and sixty- to ninety-day mortality and combined mortality/rehospitalization rates were evaluated in 5791 patients in the Follow-up Cohort in the OPTIMIZE-HF registry [40]. None of the 5 measures was significantly associated with risk-adjusted 60–90 day post-discharge mortality using multivariable and propensity-adjusted analysis. ACEI or ARB use at discharge was associated with a significant decrease in risk-adjusted 60–90 day mortality or rehospitalization (HR 0.51). Beta-blocker use at discharge, which was also evaluated, was associated with a significant reduction in 60–90 day mortality [HR 0.48] and combined mortality or rehospitalization (HR 0.73).

A hospital based discharge medication program was initiated by Intermountain Health Care, a non-profit integrated health system including 20 hospitals that serves ~60% of the population of Utah and southern Idaho. The intent of this program was to insure that appropriate medications for secondary prevention were prescribed at discharge to all patients hospitalized for acute myocardial infarction, coronary heart disease, heart failure or atrial fibrillation. The measure for patients with HF was the prescription for an ACEI (or ARB if intolerant) at discharge. The proportion of HF patients who received a prescription for ACEI or ARB increased from ~64% before the initiation of the program to >90% after. This was associated with statistically significant reductions in 30 day and 1 year mortality (HR of 0.76 and 0.77, respectively) and 30 day and 1 year readmission (HR of 0.84 and 0.91, respectively) [41].

Comorbidities

Addressing the long-term management of common comorbid conditions should be part of transitional care planning [35, 36]. Community acquired pneumonia, influenza and other respiratory infections are among the most common precipitants of hospitalization for ADHF [42, 43]. Influenza and pneumococcal vaccination remain significantly underutilized in heart failure patients. The prevalence of vaccination varies widely by region and country from 22% to 37% for influenza vaccine and 1% to 22% for pneumococcal vaccine [44–46]. Patients hospitalized for ADHF should have their immunization status for influenza and pneumococcal disease reviewed and updated [47–49].

Patient Safety

Systems of care that insure patient safety should be adopted by all hospitals. This includes the adoption of "Safe Practices" endorsed by the National Quality Forum [50]. This document emphasizes the importance of accurate and timely communication of clinical information among patient caregivers, medication reconciliation, and the important components of safe discharge practices.

Written Discharge Instructions and Discharge Summary

All patients should be provided with written discharge instructions that address: discharge medications, activity level, diet, weight monitoring, follow-up appointments and what to do if symptoms worsen. In addition, clear and specific care information should be transmitted in a timely manner from the cardiologist to all of the patient's current health care providers and should address new medication initiation and dose up-titration, adverse effects of new medications, need for laboratory monitoring, and follow up plan [36, 51].

Post-Discharge Follow Up

There is significant variation among institutions with respect to time from discharge to physician follow up [52]. The ACCF/AHA guidelines recommend scheduling an early follow-up visit within 7–14 days and an early telephone follow-up within 3 days of hospital discharge [33] The HFSA practice guidelines recommend a follow-up clinic visit in 7–10 days after hospital discharge [34].

Before discharge, at the first post-discharge visit and at all subsequent visits, the following should be addressed: the initiation, titration and optimization of GDMT; assessment of vital signs, volume status and systemic perfusion; assessment of electrolytes and renal function; screening for common causes of worsening heart failure; and reinforcement of HF education including medication adherence and self-monitoring [53].

Multidisciplinary Disease Management Programs

The ACCF/AHA, HFSA, Canadian Cardiovascular Society and ESC guidelines endorse the use of multidisciplinary heart failure disease management programs (DMP) for patients discharged after hospitalization for ADHF, especially those at high risk for hospital readmission [33, 34, 36, 54]. These programs generally include comprehensive discharge planning plus post-discharge support. The ESC Guidelines recommend that the key characteristics of a heart failure DMP include [54]:

1. Using a team approach
2. Providing inpatient and outpatient services
3. Discharge planning, education and counseling strategies which promote self-care
4. Ongoing optimization of medical therapy
5. Prescription of a flexible diuretic regimen
6. Close attention to clinical deterioration
7. Vigilant follow-up and enhanced access to care.

Multiple meta-analyses of DMPs have confirmed that these programs reduce all-cause mortality at 12 months, reduce HF-related readmissions at 12 months and improve quality of life [55–58]. Yu and colleagues compared randomized controlled clinical trials of DMPs that were and were not effective in improving discharge outcomes in an effort to identify the essential characteristics of DMPs that resulted in improved outcomes [57]. They concluded that to be effective, DMPs should be multifaceted and should include: an in-hospital phase of care; intensive patient education; self-care supportive strategies; optimization of GDMT; and ongoing surveillance for and management of clinical deterioration. Another meta-analysis suggested that DMPs that employ case management interventions where patients are intensively monitored by telephone calls and home visits (usually by a specialist nurse), were especially effective in improving outcomes [58]. Strategies that employ follow-up by a specialized multidisciplinary team are also especially effective [55].

There has been increasing interest in structured telephone support (STS) and especially in home telemonitoring (TM). STS is monitoring and/or self-care management delivered using simple telephone technology. Home telemonitoring is a form of non-invasive, remote patient monitoring that involves the use of electronic devices and telecommunication technologies (e.g., monitoring devices, hand-held or wearable technologies, and intelligent sensors) for the digital transmission of physiologic and other disease-related data from the patient's home to a health care center providing care and clinical feedback. Several meta-analyses have demonstrated that STS reduces HF-related hospitalizations and probably all-cause mortality while TM reduces HF-related hospitalizations and all-cause mortality [59–61]. Both interventions improve quality of life, functional class, patient-knowledge and self-care [59].

A comprehensive systematic review and meta-analysis of transitional care interventions to prevent readmissions for people hospitalized with heart failure contracted by the Agency for Healthcare Research and Quality was recently published [62]. This analysis found that a high-intensity home-visiting program reduced all-cause readmission and the composite of all-cause readmission or death at 30 days and 3–6 months and decreased HF-specific readmission over 3–6 months. Multi-disciplinary HF (MDS-HF) clinic interventions reduced all-cause readmission. STS interventions reduced HF-specific readmission but not all cause readmission. Home-visiting programs, MDS-HF clinics, and STS interventions reduced mortality. Neither telemonitoring nor nurse-led clinic interventions reduced readmission or mortality.

Palliative Care

The ACCF/AHA and Canadian Cardiovascular Society (CCS) endorse early involvement of palliative care, especially in patients with advanced heart failure [33, 63, 64]. Palliative care needs to be distinguished from hospice. Palliative care is specialized multidisciplinary care that focuses on improving the quality of life for people of any age who are living with any serious illness. Hospice is a system of interdisciplinary care that is focused on improving quality of life and relieving suffering in the dying patient in the last months of life [65]. Palliative care should be considered in all patients with advanced heart failure to help identify and manage physical, psychological, and spiritual issues, to assist with decisions concerning advanced heart failure therapies, and to help with advance and end-of-life directives. Palliative care should be considered for many patients hospitalized with ADHF and should not be reserved for only patients at the end of life.

Risk for Rehospitalization

Transitional care is especially important in patients at high risk for rehospitalization. This includes patients with advanced age, previous hospitalizations for heart failure, multiple concomitant comorbidities, limited social support, frailty, cognitive and functional impairment or depression [66, 67]. A review of 26 unique readmission risk prediction models found that they performed poorly in discriminating which patients were at risk for rehospitalization [68]. Data from the EVEREST trial suggests that findings of persistent congestion identified a population at high risk for readmission [69]. Cognitive impairment measured by the Mini Cog exam in patients hospitalized for ADHF was found to be strongly associated with the composite end-point of rehospitalization or mortality (HR = 1.90) [70]. Cognitive impairment was identified as the most important predictor of post-discharge outcomes among 55 variables analyzed.

Other Issues

Treatment Based on Systolic Blood Pressure

Current practice guidelines emphasize the use of parenteral loop diuretics in the initial treatment of ADHF. Several expert panels have suggested that initial blood pressure be integrated into the initial treatment paradigm [71–73]. There is data that suggests that volume redistribution rather than volume overload causes acute decompensation in patients with ADHF who present with hypertension. In some of these patients, an acute increase in systemic vascular resistance results in an acute reduction in stroke volume and an acute elevation in PCWP with the rapid development of dyspnea with or without flash pulmonary edema. These patients generally do not have gradually progressive symptoms prior to hospitalization and have less evidence of edema and systemic venous congestion on presentation [74–76]. Mobilization of venous fluid from the splanchnic circulation may also play a role in these patients [77].

A consensus document from the Society of Academic Emergency Medicine /HFSA Acute Heart Failure Working Group has proposed that presenting systolic blood pressure be incorporated into the initial treatment paradigm by dividing patients into three groups: (1) hypertensive (SBP > 140 mmHg); (2) normotensive (SBP 100–140 mmHg); and (3) hypotensive (SBP < 100 mmHg). Patients in the hypertensive group would be treated with low dose diuretics and higher dose vasodilators. Patients in the normotensive group would be treated with diuretics and moderate dose vasodilators. Patients in the hypotensive group would be treated with diuretics and inotropes as needed [72]. There have been no prospective randomized trials that have evaluated a treatment strategy based on initial systolic blood pressure but several reports suggest that performing a randomized trial evaluating this approach is feasible [78–80].

Improving Survival After Hospitalization for ADHF

Hospitalization for ADHF is an event that identifies a patient at high risk for dying in the next year. In patients with chronic heart failure, HF hospitalization is a marker of disease progression and probably reflects a change in the trajectory of the underlying heart disease. A retrospective analysis from the Candesartan in Heart failure: Assessment of reduction in Mortality and morbidity (CHARM) trials assessed the risk after discharge from a first hospitalization for HF compared to patients who were not hospitalized for HF using time-updated Cox proportional-hazards models [81]. After adjustment for predictors of death, mortality rate was found to be increased after HF hospitalization with a HR of 3.15. Longer duration of hospitalization and repeat hospitalization increased the risk of dying. A retrospective analysis from the Digitalis Investigation Group (DIG) trial assessed the effect of incident HF hospitalization on subsequent mortality compared with no HF hospitalization in a propensity matched population [82]. Using matched Cox regression analysis, patients in the HF hospitalization group had a significantly increased risk of subsequent mortality compared with the no HF hospitalization group with a HR of 2.49. The HR for CV and HF mortality were 2.88 and 5.22, respectively. An analysis using health care utilization databases from British Columbia confirmed that the number of HF hospitalizations is a strong predictor of mortality in community HF patients with median survivals after the first, second, third and fourth hospitalizations of 2.4, 1.4, 1.0, and 0.6 years, respectively [83].

A number of clinical trials of newer medications that have attempted to show an impact on post-discharge outcomes have largely been negative. Agents that have been studied and shown to be ineffective include milrinone [84], nesiritide [85], the selective vasopressin (V_2) receptor antagonist tolvaptan [86, 87], levosimendan [88], the direct renin inhibitor aliskerin [89], the adenosine A_1 receptor antagonist rolofylline [90], and the endothelin receptor antagonist tezosentan [91]. There is substantial data that discharge on an ACEI and a β-blocker improves survival and decreases hospitalization [39–41, 92–94].

The Prospective Comparison of ARNI [Angiotensin Receptor–Neprilysin Inhibitor] with ACEI [Angiotensin-Converting–Enzyme Inhibitor] to Determine Impact on Global Mortality and Morbidity in Heart Failure (PARADIGM-HF) Trial randomized 8442 patients with NYHA FC II, III or IV heart failure to receive a combination of valsartan and the neprilysin inhibitor sacubitril or enalapril [95–97]. The primary end-point of the trial was the composite of cardiovascular death and heart failure hospitalization. Neprilysin is a neutral endopeptidase inhibitor that degrades several endogenous vasoactive peptides including natriuretic peptides, bradykinin and adrenomedullin. Sacubitril inhibits neprilysin (but not ACE or aminopeptidase P) and increases the levels of natriuretic peptides, bradykinin and adrenomedullin. In PARADIGM-HF, when compared with enalapril, the combination of valsartan and sacubitril reduced the primary end-point by 20%. Death from any cause was reduced by 16%, cardiovascular death by 20%, and HF hospitalization by 21%. Symptoms and physical limitations of heart failure were decreased. This combination was well tolerated with lower proportions of hyperkalemia, renal impairment and cough compared with enalapril.

This study was not conducted with patients hospitalized for ADHF. The combination has been approved by the FDA for use in patients with chronic heart failure (NYHA Class II-IV) and reduced ejection fraction to reduce the risk of cardiovascular death and hospitalization for heart failure in place of ACEI or ARB. The combination is marketed as Entresto. There has not been a consensus document that addresses whether patients with ADHF should be started on Entresto instead of ACEI or ARB or switched from ACEI or ARB to Entresto during HF hospitalization.

Ongoing Drug Development

A number of new drugs with novel mechanisms of action are being evaluated in ongoing clinical trials in patients with ADHF [98, 99].

Relaxin/Serelaxin

Relaxin is a naturally occurring vasoactive peptide hormone that is produced by the placenta and corpus luteum and also by the failing myocardium. It acts on a G-protein coupled receptor, RXFP1, which is abundantly expressed in the cardiovascular, renal, and reproductive systems. Activation of RXFPI increases the production of cAMP with a resulting increase in nitric oxide production. In addition, relaxin has anti-inflammatory and anti-fibrotic effects and causes upregulation of vascular matrix metalloproteinase-2 activity all of which result in vasodilation and increased vessel compliance [98–100].

In the Preliminary study of RELAXin in Acute Heart Failure (Pre-RELAX-AHF), 234 patients with acute heart failure, evidence of congestion on CXR, elevated BNP or NT-BNP, systolic blood pressure >125 mmHg, and mild-moderate renal insufficiency were treated with standard care and randomized to a 48-h infusion of placebo or one of four doses of relaxin [101]. When compared to placebo, treatment with relaxin was associated with dyspnea improvement at 6, 12, and 24 h by Likert scale and through day 14 by visual analogue scale. In addition, patients treated with relaxin had a shorter length of stay, greater days alive and out of the hospital, and reduced risk of cardiovascular death or HF readmission.

The RELAXin in Acute Heart Failure (RELAX-AHF) Trial randomized 1161 patients with the same clinical characteristics as Pre-RELAX-AHF to receive standard care plus a 48-h infusion of placebo or serelaxin 30 mcg/kg per day [102]. Serelaxin is recombinant human relaxin-2. Serelaxin is identical in structure to naturally occurring relaxin and is formulated as a sterile solution for infusion. The study had two primary end-points that evaluated dyspnea improvement. Serelaxin improved the change in the visual analogue scale area under the curve (VAS AUC) from baseline to day 5. Serelaxin had no significant effect on the proportion of patients with moderate or marked dyspnea improvement measured by Likert scale during the first 24 h. Serelaxin had no effect on cardiovascular death or HF readmission at 60 days or days alive and out of the hospital at 60 days. Treatment with serelaxin was associated with fewer deaths at 180 days. Several phase three trials of serelaxin are ongoing.

Ularitide

Urodilatin is a natriuretic peptide that is synthesized and secreted by distal renal tubular cells. Following intraluminal secretion, it binds to NPR-A receptors in the inner medullary collecting duct regulating renal sodium resorption and water homeostasis via cGMP-dependent signal transduction. Intravenous urodilatin increases diuresis and natriuresis and reduces pulmonary capillary wedge pressure (PCWP) and systemic vascular resistance [98, 99, 103].

Ularitide is a synthetically derived form of urodilatin. The SIRIUS II trial was a phase 2, randomized, double-blind, placebo controlled, dose-finding study in 221 patients with acute decompensation of chronic heart failure with dyspnea at rest or with minimal activity, cardiac index ≤2.5 L/min/m^2, and pulmonary capillary wedge pressure ≥18 mmHg. Patients received standard care and were randomized to a 24-h infusion of placebo or one of three doses of ularitide. At 6 h, patients treated with ularitide demonstrated a significant decrease in PCWP, improved dyspnea score, decreased systemic vascular resistance and increased cardiac index [104].The Efficacy and Safety of Ularitide for the Treatment of Acute Decompensated Heart Failure (TRUE-AHF) is an ongoing phase 3 trial designed to assess the effect of a 48-h continuous IV infusion of ularitide (15 ng/kg/min) versus placebo on the clinical status of patients with acute decompensated heart failure [43].

Istaroxime

Istaroxime is a novel steroidal intravenous inotropic agent unrelated to cardiac glycosides. The drug has unique inotropic/lusitropic properties [42, 98, 105]. Istaroxime inhibits Na^+/K^+ ATPase and stimulates sarcoplasmic reticulum Ca^{2+}adenosine triphosphatase isoform 2a. This affects cytosolic accumulation of calcium during systole resulting in an inotropic response and rapid sequestration of calcium during diastole resulting in a lusitropic response.

The Hemodynamic, Echocardiographic and Neurohormonal Effects of Istaroxime, a Novel Inotropic Agent: A Randomized Controlled Trial in Patients with Heart Failure (HORIZON-HF) trial randomized 121 patients with acute decompensated heart failure and LVEF $\leq 35\%$ on standard heart failure therapy to a 6-h infusion of placebo or one of three doses of istaroxime [106]. Patients underwent pulmonary artery catheterization within 48 h of admission and prior to randomization. Comprehensive 2-dimensional, Doppler, and tissue Doppler echocardiography were performed immediately before and within the last 30 min of study drug infusion. The primary end-point of the trial was change in PCWP from baseline compared to placebo after the 6-h infusion. Istaroxime significantly reduced PCWP, left ventricular end-diastolic pressure and heart rate and increased systolic blood pressure and cardiac index. There were no changes in neurohormones, renal function or troponin I. In addition, istaroxime improved systolic and diastolic function by echo parameters with evidence of increased contractility and decreased diastolic stiffness.

Omecamtiv Mecarbil (OM)

Omecamtiv Mecarbil is a small-molecule, cardiac-selective myosin activator. OM increases the number of myosin heads interacting with actin resulting in the generation of greater contractile force. OM improves myocardial contractility by prolonging systolic ejection time without changing myocardial oxygen consumption, myocyte calcium levels or the rate of left ventricular pressure development (LV dP/dt). In contrast, dobutamine increases LV dP/dt, decreases systolic ejection time, and increases myocardial oxygen consumption [98, 99, 106]. In healthy men, OM infusion resulted in dose-related increases in systolic ejection time, associated with increases in stroke volume, fractional shortening, and ejection fraction without changes in diastolic function [13]. In the phase II Acute Treatment with Omecamtiv Mecarbil to Increase Contractility in Acute Heart Failure (ATOMIC-AHF) study, patients admitted with acute heart failure, LVEF $\leq 40\%$, dyspnea and elevated natriuretic peptides were randomized to receive a 48-h infusion of placebo or one of three doses of OM [107]. The primary end-point was dyspnea relief at 6, 24 and 48 h using a patient-reported 7-level Likert scale. OM did not improve the primary endpoint. There were plasma concentration-related increases in left ventricular systolic ejection time ($p < 0.0001$) and decreases in end-systolic dimension ($p < 0.05$).

The Chronic Oral Study of Myosin Activation to Increase Contractility in Heart Failure (COSMIC-HF) trial is multicenter, Phase 2 trial designed to evaluate an oral modified release formulation of OM in chronic heart failure patients with reduced ejection fraction [108]. The trial consists of two parts, a dose escalation phase and a larger and longer expansion phase. The primary end-points for the expansion phase are to assess the maximum and pre-dose plasma concentration of OM. The secondary end-points are to assess changes from baseline in systolic ejection time, stroke volume, left ventricular end-systolic diameter, left ventricular end-diastolic diameter, heart rate and N-terminal pro-brain natriuretic peptide at week 20, as well as the safety and tolerability of OM including incidence of adverse events from baseline to week 24.

Conclusions

Hospitalization for ADHF identifies a patient at increased risk for dying in the next year. Initiation and optimization of guideline directed medical therapy is an important component of treatment of the hospitalized patient and to date, the only pharmacologic intervention that has been demonstrated to decrease post-discharge mortality and HF hospitalization.

Careful discharge planning is an important component of care in the patient hospitalized with ADHF. Patient education should address the dose, frequency and potential side effects of each medication, self-management skills, and guidelines for reporting signs and symptoms of worsening heart failure. All patients should be provided with written discharge instructions. Multidisciplinary heart failure disease management programs appear to be helpful in improving outcomes, especially in patients at high risk for hospital readmission.

References

1. Taylor AL, Ziesche S, Yancy C, Carson P, D'Agostino R Jr, Ferdinand K, et al. African-American Heart Failure Trial Investigators. Combination of isosorbide dinitrate and hydralazine in blacks with heart failure. N Engl J Med. 2004;351(20):2049–57. Epub 2004 Nov 8.
2. Effect of enalapril on survival in patients with reduced left ventricular ejection fractions and congestive heart failure. The SOLVD Investigators. N Engl J Med. 1991;325(5):293–302.
3. Effects of enalapril on mortality in severe congestive heart failure. Results of the Cooperative North Scandinavian Enalapril Survival Study (CONSENSUS). The CONSENSUS Trial Study Group. N Engl J Med. 1987;316(23):1429–35.
4. Heran BS, Musini VM, Bassett K, Taylor RS, Wright JM. Angiotensin receptor blockers for heart failure. Cochrane Database Syst Rev. 2012;(4):CD003040. https://doi.org/10.1002/14651858.CD003040.pub2.
5. Granger CB, McMurray JJ, Yusuf S, Held P, Michelson EL, Olofsson B. CHARM Investigators and Committees, et al. Effects of candesartan in patients with chronic heart failure and reduced left-ventricular systolic function intolerant to angiotensin-converting-enzyme inhibitors: the CHARM-Alternative trial. Lancet. 2003;362(9386):772–6. CrossRef PubMed.
6. Cohn JN, Tognoni G. Valsartan Heart Failure Trial Investigators. A randomized trial of the angiotensin-receptor blocker valsartan in chronic heart failure. N Engl J Med. 2001;345(23):1667–75. CrossRef PubMed.
7. Packer M, Coats AJ, Fowler MB, Katus HA, Krum H, Mohacsi P, Carvedilol Prospective Randomized Cumulative Survival Study Group, et al. Effect of carvedilol on survival in severe chronic heart failure. N Engl J Med. 2001;344(22):1651–8. CrossRef PubMed.
8. Hjalmarson A, Goldstein S, Fagerberg B, Wedel H, Waagstein F, Kjekshus J, et al. Effects of controlled-release metoprolol on total mortality, hospitalizations, and well-being in patients with heart failure: the Metoprolol CR/XL Randomized Intervention Trial in congestive heart failure (MERIT-HF). MERIT-HF Study Group. JAMA. 2000;283(10):1295–302.
9. The Cardiac Insufficiency Bisoprolol Study II (CIBIS-II): a randomised trial. Lancet. 1999;353(9146):9–13.
10. Pitt B, Remme W, Zannad F, Neaton J, Martinez F, Roniker B, et al. Eplerenone Post-Acute Myocardial Infarction Heart Failure Efficacy and Survival Study Investigators. Eplerenone, a selective aldosterone blocker, in patients with left ventricular dysfunction after myocardial infarction. N Engl J Med. 2003;348(14):1309–21. Epub 2003 Mar 31.
11. Pitt B, White H, Nicolau J, Martinez F, Gheorghiade M, Aschermann M, et al. EPHESUS Investigators. Eplerenone reduces mortality 30 days after randomization following acute myocardial infarction in patients with left ventricular systolic dysfunction and heart failure. J Am Coll Cardiol. 2005;46(3):425–31. CrossRef PubMed.
12. Yancy CW, Jessup M, Bozkurt B, Butler J, Casey DE Jr, Drazner MH, et al. American College of Cardiology Foundation/American Heart Association Task Force on Practice Guidelines. 2013 ACCF/AHA guideline for the management of heart failure: a report of the American College of Cardiology Foundation/American Heart Association Task Force on practice guidelines. Circulation. 2013;128(16):e240–327. https://doi.org/10.1161/CIR.0b013e31829e8776. Epub 2013 Jun 5.
13. Lindenfeld J, Albert NM, Boehmer JP, Collins SP, Ezekowitz JA, Givertz MM, et al. Heart Failure Society of America, HFSA 2010 comprehensive heart failure practice guideline. Section 12: evaluation and management of patients with acute decompensated heart failure. J Card Fail. 2010;16(6):e131–56. https://doi.org/10.1016/j.cardfail.2010.04.004.
14. Collins SP, Lindsell CJ, Storrow AB, Abraham WT. ADHERE Scientific Advisory Committee, Investigators and Study Group. Prevalence of negative chest radiography results in the emergency department patient with decompensated heart failure. Ann Emerg Med. 2006;47(1):13–8. Epub 2005 Jun 20.
15. Metra M, Torp-Pedersen C, Cleland JG, Di Lenarda A, Komajda M, Remme WJ, COMET investigators, et al. Should beta-blocker therapy be reduced or withdrawn after an episode of decompensated heart

failure? Results from COMET. Eur J Heart Fail. 2007;9(9):901–9. Epub 2007 Jun 19.
16. Butler J, Young JB, Abraham WT, Bourge RC, Adams KF Jr, Clare R, O'Connor C. ESCAPE Investigators. Beta-blocker use and outcomes among hospitalized heart failure patients. J Am Coll Cardiol. 2006;47(12):2462–9. CrossRef PubMed.
17. Fonarow GC, Abraham WT, Albert NM, Stough WG, Gheorghiade M, Greenberg BH, et al. OPTIMIZE-HF Investigators and Coordinators. Influence of beta-blocker continuation or withdrawal on outcomes in patients hospitalized with heart failure: findings from the OPTIMIZE-HF program. J Am Coll Cardiol. 2008;52(3):190–9. https://doi.org/10.1016/j.jacc.2008.03.048. CrossRef PubMed.
18. Gattis WA, O'Connor CM, Gallup DS, Hasselblad V, Gheorghiade M. IMPACT-HF Investigators and Coordinators. Predischarge initiation of carvedilol in patients hospitalized for decompensated heart failure: results of the Initiation Management Predischarge: Process for Assessment of Carvedilol Therapy in Heart Failure (IMPACT-HF) trial. J Am Coll Cardiol. 2004;43(9):1534–41.
19. Fonarow GC, Abraham WT, Albert NM, Stough WG, Gheorghiade M, Greenberg BH, et al. Dosing of beta-blocker therapy before, during, and after hospitalization for heart failure (from Organized Program to Initiate Lifesaving Treatment in Hospitalized Patients with Heart Failure). Am J Cardiol. 2008;102(11):1524–9. https://doi.org/10.1016/j.amjcard.2008.07.045. Epub 2008 Sep 6.
20. Albert NM, Yancy CW, Liang L, Zhao X, Hernandez AF, Peterson ED, et al. Use of aldosterone antagonists in heart failure. JAMA. 2009;302(15):1658–65. https://doi.org/10.1001/jama.2009.1493. CrossRef PubMed.
21. Golwala HB, Thadani U, Liang L, Stavrakis S, Butler J, Yancy CW, et al. Use of hydralazine-isosorbide dinitrate combination in African American and other race/ethnic group patients with heart failure and reduced left ventricular ejection fraction. J Am Heart Assoc. 2013;2(4):e000214. https://doi.org/10.1161/JAHA.113.000214. CrossRef PubMed PubMedCentral.
22. Gislason GH, Rasmussen JN, Abildstrom SZ, Schramm TK, Hansen ML, Buch P, et al. Persistent use of evidence-based pharmacotherapy in heart failure is associated with improved outcomes. Circulation. 2007;116(7):737–44. Epub 2007 Jul 23.
23. Michel T, Hoffman BB. Chapter 27. Treatment of myocardial ischemia and hypertension. In: Brunton LL, Chabner BA, Knollmann BC, editors. Goodman & Gilman's the pharmacological basis of therapeutics12. New York: McGraw-Hill; 2011. http://accessmedicine.mhmedical.com/content.aspx?bookid=374&Sectionid=41266234. Accessed 04 Aug 2015.
24. Moss AJ, Zareba W, Hall WJ, Klein H, Wilber DJ, Cannom DS, et al. Multicenter Automatic Defibrillator Implantation Trial II Investigators. Prophylactic implantation of a defibrillator in patients with myocardial infarction and reduced ejection fraction. N Engl J Med. 2002;346(12):877–83. Epub 2002 Mar 19.
25. Bardy GH, Lee KL, Mark DB, Poole JE, Packer DL, Boineau R, et al. Sudden Cardiac Death in Heart Failure Trial (SCD-HeFT) Investigators. Amiodarone or an implantable cardioverter-defibrillator for congestive heart failure. N Engl J Med. 2005;352(3):225–37. CrossRef PubMed.
26. Epstein AE, DiMarco JP, Ellenbogen KA, Estes NA , Freedman RA, et al. American College of Cardiology Foundation; American Heart Association Task Force on Practice Guidelines; Heart Rhythm Society.2012 ACCF/AHA/HRS focused update incorporated into the ACCF/AHA/HRS 2008 guidelines for device-based therapy of cardiac rhythm abnormalities: a report of the American College of Cardiology Foundation/American Heart Association Task Force on Practice Guidelines and the Heart Rhythm Society. Circulation. 2013;127(3):e283–352. https://doi.org/10.1161/CIR.0b013e318276ce9b. Epub 2012 Dec 19.
27. Bristow MR, Saxon LA, Boehmer J, Krueger S, Kass DA, De Marco T, et al. Comparison of Medical Therapy, Pacing, and Defibrillation in Heart Failure (COMPANION) Investigators. Cardiac-resynchronization therapy with or without an implantable defibrillator in advanced chronic heart failure. N Engl J Med. 2004;350(21):2140–50. CrossRef PubMed.
28. Cleland JG, Daubert JC, Erdmann E, Freemantle N, Gras D, Kappenberger L, Tavazzi L. Cardiac Resynchronization-Heart Failure (CARE-HF) Study Investigators. The effect of cardiac resynchronization on morbidity and mortality in heart failure. N Engl J Med. 2005;352(15):1539–49. Epub 2005 Mar 7.
29. Moss AJ, Hall WJ, Cannom DS, Klein H, Brown MW, Daubert JP, et al. MADIT-CRT Trial Investigators. Cardiac-resynchronization therapy for the prevention of heart-failure events. N Engl J Med. 2009;361(14):1329–38. https://doi.org/10.1056/NEJMoa0906431. Epub 2009 Sep 1.
30. Tang AS, Wells GA, Talajic M, Arnold MO, Sheldon R, Connolly S, Resynchronization-Defibrillation for Ambulatory Heart Failure Trial Investigators, et al. Cardiac-resynchronization therapy for mild-to-moderate heart failure. N Engl J Med. 2010;363(25):2385–95. https://doi.org/10.1056/NEJMoa1009540. Epub 2010 Nov 14.
31. Linde C, Abraham WT, Gold MR, St John Sutton M, Ghio S, Daubert C. REVERSE (REsynchronization reVErses Remodeling in Systolic left vEntricular dysfunction) Study Group. Randomized trial of cardiac resynchronization in mildly symptomatic heart failure patients and in asymptomatic patients with left ventricular dysfunction and pre-

vious heart failure symptoms. J Am Coll Cardiol. 2008;52(23):1834–43. https://doi.org/10.1016/j.jacc.2008.08.027. Epub 2008 Nov 7.
32. Go AS, Mozaffarian D, Roger VL, Benjamin EJ, Berry JD, Blaha MJ, et al. American Heart Association Statistics Committee and Stroke Statistics Subcommittee. Heart disease and stroke statistics—2014 update: a report from the American Heart Association. Circulation. 2014;129(3):e28–e292. https://doi.org/10.1161/01.cir.0000441139.02102.80. Epub 2013 Dec 18.
33. Dickstein K, Cohen-Solal A, Filippatos G, McMurray JJ, Ponikowski P, Poole-Wilson PA, et al. ESC Committee for practice guidelines (CPG). ESC guidelines for the diagnosis and treatment of acute and chronic heart failure 2008: the Task Force for the Diagnosis and Treatment of Acute and Chronic Heart Failure 2008 of the European Society of Cardiology. Developed in collaboration with the Heart Failure Association of the ESC (HFA) and endorsed by the European Society of Intensive Care Medicine (ESICM). Eur Heart J. 2008;29(19):2388–442. https://doi.org/10.1093/eurheartj/ehn309. Epub 2008 Sep 17.
34. National 2012. Heart Lung and Blood Institute. People Science Health. What is heart failure?. Available from: http://www.nhlbi.nih.gov/health/health-topics/topics/hf/. Accessed Feb 2012.
35. Hall MJ, DeFrances CJ, Williams SN, et al. National hospital discharge survey: 2007 summary. National health statistics reports; no 29. National Center for Health Statistics: Hyattsville; 2010. Available from: http://www.cdc.gov/nchs/data/nhsr/nhsr029.pdf.
36. Gheorghiade M, Pang PS. Acute heart failure syndromes. J Am Coll Cardiol. 2009;53(7):557–73. https://doi.org/10.1016/j.jacc.2008.10.041. CrossRef PubMed.
37. Gheorghiade M, Zannad F, Sopko G, Klein L, Piña IL, Konstam MA, et al. International Working Group on Acute Heart Failure Syndromes. Acute heart failure syndromes: current state and framework for future research. Circulation. 2005;112(25):3958–68. CrossRef PubMed.
38. Fang J, Mensah GA, Croft JB, Keenan NL. Heart failure-related hospitalization in the U.S., 1979 to 2004. J Am Coll Cardiol. 2008;52(6):428–34. https://doi.org/10.1016/j.jacc.2008.03.061. CrossRef PubMed.
39. Chen J, Normand SL, Wang Y, Krumholz HM. National and regional trends in heart failure hospitalization and mortality rates for Medicare beneficiaries, 1998-2008. JAMA. 2011;306(15):1669–78. https://doi.org/10.1001/jama.2011.1474. CrossRef PubMed PubMedCentral.
40. Fonarow GC, Abraham WT, Albert NM, Gattis WA, Gheorghiade M, Greenberg B, et al. Organized Program to Initiate Lifesaving Treatment in Hospitalized Patients with Heart Failure (OPTIMIZE-HF): rationale and design. Am Heart J. 2004;148(1):43–51. CrossRef PubMed.
41. Adams KF, Fonarow GC, Emerman CL, LeJemtel TH, Costanzo MR, Abraham WT, ADHERE Scientific Advisory Committee and Investigators, et al. Characteristics and outcomes of patients hospitalized for heart failure in the United States: rationale, design, and preliminary observations from the first 100,000 cases in the Acute Decompensated Heart Failure National Registry (ADHERE). Am Heart J. 2005;149(2):209–16. CrossRef PubMed.
42. Fonarow GC, Heywood JT, Heidenreich PA, Lopatin M, Yancy CW. ADHERE Scientific Advisory Committee and Investigators. Temporal trends in clinical characteristics, treatments, and outcomes for heart failure hospitalizations, 2002 to 2004: findings from Acute Decompensated Heart Failure National Registry (ADHERE). Am Heart J. 2007;153(6):1021–8. CrossRef PubMed.
43. Fonarow GC, Corday E. ADHERE Scientific Advisory Committee. Overview of acutely decompensated congestive heart failure (ADHF): a report from the ADHERE registry. Heart Fail Rev. 2004;9(3):179–85. CrossRef PubMed.
44. Cleland JG, Swedberg K, Cohen-Solal A, Cosin-Aguilar J, Dietz R, Follath F, et al. The Euro Heart Failure Survey of the EUROHEART survey programme. A survey on the quality of care among patients with heart failure in Europe. The Study Group on Diagnosis of the Working Group on Heart Failure of the European Society of Cardiology. The Medicines Evaluation Group Centre for Health Economics University of York. Eur J Heart Fail. 2000;2(2):123–32. CrossRef PubMed.
45. Cleland JG, Swedberg K, Follath F, Komajda M, Cohen-Solal A, Aguilar JC, et al. Study Group on Diagnosis of the Working Group on Heart Failure of the European Society of Cardiology. The EuroHeart Failure survey programme-- a survey on the quality of care among patients with heart failure in Europe. Part 1: patient characteristics and diagnosis. Eur Heart J. 2003;24(5):442–63. CrossRef PubMed.
46. Komajda M, Follath F, Swedberg K, Cleland J, Aguilar JC, Cohen-Solal A, et al. Study Group on Diagnosis of the Working Group on Heart Failure of the European Society of Cardiology. The EuroHeart Failure Survey programme--a survey on the quality of care among patients with heart failure in Europe. Part 2: treatment. Eur Heart J. 2003;24(5):464–74. CrossRef PubMed.
47. Nieminen MS, Brutsaert D, Dickstein K, Drexler H, Follath F, Harjola VP, et al. EuroHeart Survey Investigators; Heart Failure Association, European Society of Cardiology. EuroHeart Failure Survey II (EHFS II): a survey on hospitalized acute heart failure patients: description of population. Eur Heart J. 2006;27(22):2725–36. Epub 2006 Sep 25.

48. Fonarow GC, Abraham WT, Albert NM, Stough WG, Gheorghiade M, Greenberg BH, OPTIMIZE-HF Investigators and Hospitals, et al. Age- and gender-related differences in quality of care and outcomes of patients hospitalized with heart failure (from OPTIMIZE-HF). Am J Cardiol. 2009;104(1):107–15. https://doi.org/10.1016/j.amjcard.2009.02.057. CrossRef PubMed.
49. Gheorghiade M, Abraham WT, Albert NM, Greenberg BH, O'Connor CM, She L, et al. OPTIMIZE-HF Investigators and Coordinators. Systolic blood pressure at admission, clinical characteristics, and outcomes in patients hospitalized with acute heart failure. JAMA. 2006;296(18):2217–26. CrossRef PubMed.
50. Yancy CW, Lopatin M, Stevenson LW, De Marco T, Fonarow GC. ADHERE Scientific Advisory Committee and Investigators. Clinical presentation, management, and in-hospital outcomes of patients admitted with acute decompensated heart failure with preserved systolic function: a report from the Acute Decompensated Heart Failure National Registry (ADHERE) Database. J Am Coll Cardiol. 2006;47(1):76–84. PubMed PMID 16386668. CrossRef PubMed.
51. Fonarow GC, Stough WG, Abraham WT, Albert NM, Gheorghiade M, Greenberg BH, OPTIMIZE-HF Investigators and Hospitals, et al. Characteristics, treatments, and outcomes of patients with preserved systolic function hospitalized for heart failure: a report from the OPTIMIZE-HF Registry. J Am Coll Cardiol. 2007;50(8):768–77. PubMed PMID 17707182. CrossRef PubMed.
52. Lenzen MJ, Scholte OP, Reimer WJ, Boersma E, Vantrimpont PJ, Follath F, Swedberg K, et al. Differences between patients with a preserved and a depressed left ventricular function: a report from the EuroHeart Failure Survey. Eur Heart J. 2004;25(14):1214–20. CrossRef PubMed.
53. Grady KL, Dracup K, Kennedy G, Moser DK, Piano M, Stevenson LW, et al. Team management of patients with heart failure: a statement for healthcare professionals from The Cardiovascular Nursing Council of the American Heart Association. Circulation. 2000;102(19):2443–56. PubMed PMID 11067802. CrossRef PubMed.
54. Yancy CW, Abraham WT, Albert NM, Clare R, Stough WG, Gheorghiade M, et al. Quality of care of and outcomes for African Americans hospitalized with heart failure: findings from the OPTIMIZE-HF (Organized Program to Initiate Lifesaving Treatment in Hospitalized Patients With Heart Failure) registry. J Am Coll Cardiol. 2008;51(17):1675–84. https://doi.org/10.1016/j.jacc.2008.01.028. CrossRef PubMed.
55. Jencks SF, Williams MV, Coleman EA. Rehospitalizations among patients in the Medicare fee-for-service program. N Engl J Med. 2009;360(14):1418–28. https://doi.org/10.1056/NEJMsa0803563. CrossRef PubMed.
56. Heidenreich PA, Sahay A, Kapoor JR, Pham MX, Massie B. Divergent trends in survival and readmission following a hospitalization for heart failure in the Veterans Affairs health care system 2002 to 2006. J Am Coll Cardiol. 2010;56(5):362–8. https://doi.org/10.1016/j.jacc.2010.02.053. CrossRef PubMed.
57. Bueno H, Ross JS, Wang Y, Chen J, Vidán MT, Normand SL, et al. Trends in length of stay and short-term outcomes among Medicare patients hospitalized for heart failure, 1993-2006. JAMA. 2010;303(21):2141–7. https://doi.org/10.1001/jama.2010.748. CrossRef PubMed PubMedCentral.
58. Tuppin P, Cuerq A, de Peretti C, Fagot-Campagna A, Danchin N, Juillière Y, et al. Two-year outcome of patients after a first hospitalization for heart failure: a national observational study. Arch Cardiovasc Dis. 2014;107(3):158–68. https://doi.org/10.1016/j.acvd.2014.01.012. Epub 2014 Mar 21.
59. Jessup M, Abraham WT, Casey DE, Feldman AM, Francis GS, Ganiats TG, et al. 2009 focused update: ACCF/AHA Guidelines for the Diagnosis and Management of Heart Failure in Adults: a report of the American College of Cardiology Foundation/American Heart Association Task Force on Practice Guidelines: developed in collaboration with the International Society for Heart and Lung Transplantation. Circulation. 2009;119(14):1977–2016. https://doi.org/10.1161/CIRCULATIONAHA.109.192064. Epub 2009 Mar 26.
60. Kaul P, Ezekowitz JA, Armstrong PW, Leung BK, Savu A, Welsh RC, et al. Incidence of heart failure and mortality after acute coronary syndromes. Am Heart J. 2013;165(3):379–85. https://doi.org/10.1016/j.ahj.2012.12.005. Epub 2013 Jan 22.
61. Steg PG, Dabbous OH, Feldman LJ, Cohen-Solal A, Aumont MC, López-Sendón J. Global Registry of Acute Coronary Events Investigators. et al. Determinants and prognostic impact of heart failure complicating acute coronary syndromes: observations from the Global Registry of Acute Coronary Events (GRACE). Circulation. 2004;109(4):494–9. Epub 2004 Jan 26.
62. Weintraub NL, Collins SP, Pang PS, Levy PD, Anderson AS, Arslanian-Engoren C, American Heart Association Council on Clinical Cardiology and Council on Cardiopulmonary, Critical Care, Perioperative and Resuscitation, et al. Acute heart failure syndromes: emergency department presentation, treatment, and disposition: current approaches and future aims: a scientific statement from the American Heart Association. Circulation. 2010;122(19):1975–96. https://doi.org/10.1161/CIR.0b013e3181f9a223. Epub 2010 Oct 11.
63. Campbell RT, Jhund PS, Castagno D, Hawkins NM, Petrie MC, McMurray J. What have we

learned about patients with heart failure and preserved ejection fraction from DIG-PEF, CHARM-preserved, and I-PRESERVE? J Am Coll Cardiol. 2012;60(23):2349–56. https://doi.org/10.1016/j.jacc.2012.04.064. Epub 2012 Nov 7.
64. Clark AL, Cleland JG. Causes and treatment of oedema in patients with heart failure. Nat Rev Cardiol. 2013;10(3):156–70. https://doi.org/10.1038/nrcardio.2012.191. Epub 2013 Jan 15.
65. ter Maaten JM, Valente MA, Damman K, Hillege HL, Navis G, Voors AA. Diuretic response in acute heart failure-pathophysiology, evaluation, and therapy. Nat Rev Cardiol. 2015;12(3):184–92. https://doi.org/10.1038/nrcardio.2014.215. Epub 2015 Jan 6.
66. Ronco C, Cicoira M, McCullough PA. Cardiorenal syndrome type 1: pathophysiological crosstalk leading to combined heart and kidney dysfunction in the setting of acutely decompensated heart failure. J Am Coll Cardiol. 2012;60(12):1031–42. https://doi.org/10.1016/j.jacc.2012.01.077. Epub 2012 Jul 25.
67. Gehlbach BK, Geppert E. The pulmonary manifestations of left heart failure. Chest. 2004;125(2):669–82. CrossRef PubMed.
68. Guazzi M. Alveolar gas diffusion abnormalities in heart failure. J Card Fail. 2008;14(8):695–702. https://doi.org/10.1016/j.cardfail.2008.06.004. Epub 2008 Jul 18.
69. Uhley HN, Leeds SE, Sampson JJ, Friedman M. Role of pulmonary lymphatics in chronic pulmonary edema. Circ Res. 1962;11:966–70. CrossRef PubMed.
70. Mackersie RC, Christensen J, Lewis FR. The role of pulmonary lymphatics in the clearance of hydrostatic pulmonary edema. J Surg Res. 1987;43(6):495–504. CrossRef PubMed.
71. Hochberg I, Abassi Z, Azzam ZS. Patterns of alveolar fluid clearance in heart failure. Int J Cardiol. 2008;130(2):125–30. https://doi.org/10.1016/j.ijcard.2008.03.015. Epub 2008 Jun 24.
72. Guazzi M, Phillips SA, Arena R, Lavie CJ. Endothelial dysfunction and lung capillary injury in cardiovascular diseases. Prog Cardiovasc Dis. 2015;57(5):454–62. https://doi.org/10.1016/j.pcad.2014.11.003. Epub 2014 Nov 12.
73. Chaudhry S, Wang Y, Concato J, Gill TM, Krumholz HM. Patterns of weight change preceding hospitalization for heart failure. Circulation. 2007;116(14):1549–54. Epub 2007 Sep 10.
74. Adamson PB, Magalski A, Braunschweig F, Böhm M, Reynolds D, Steinhaus D, et al. Ongoing right ventricular hemodynamics in heart failure: clinical value of measurements derived from an implantable monitoring system. J Am Coll Cardiol. 2003;41(4):565–71. CrossRef PubMed.
75. Ohlsson A, Steinhaus D, Kjellström B, Ryden L, Bennett T. Central hemodynamic responses during serial exercise tests in heart failure patients using implantable hemodynamic monitors. Eur J Heart Fail. 2003;5(3):253–9. CrossRef PubMed.
76. Adamson PB, Kjellström B, Braunschweig F, Magalski A, Linde C, Kolodiezj A, et al. Ambulatory hemodynamic monitoring from an implanted device: components of continuous 24-hour pressures that correlate to supine resting conditions and acute right heart catheterization. Congest Heart Fail. 2006;12(1):14–9. CrossRef PubMed.
77. Aaron MF, Aranda JM, Renlund DG, Fonarow GC, Feldman DS, Cho YK, et al. The effect of postural changes on intracardiac filling pressures[abstract]. J Card Fail. 2008;14:S28.
78. Zile MR, Bennett TD, St John Sutton M, Cho YK, Adamson PB, Aaron MF, et al. Transition from chronic compensated to acute decompensated heart failure: pathophysiological insights obtained from continuous monitoring of intracardiac pressures. Circulation. 2008;118(14):1433–41. https://doi.org/10.1161/CIRCULATIONAHA.108.783910. Epub 2008 Sep 15.
79. Zile MR, Adamson PB, Cho YK, Bennett TD, Bourge RC, Aaron MF, et al. Hemodynamic factors associated with acute decompensated heart failure: part 1 – insights into pathophysiology. J Card Fail. 2011;17(4):282–91. https://doi.org/10.1016/j.cardfail.2011.01.010. Epub 2011 Feb 26.
80. Milo-Cotter O, Adams KF, O'Connor CM, Uriel N, Kaluski E, Felker GM, et al. Acute heart failure associated with high admission blood pressure--a distinct vascular disorder? Eur J Heart Fail. 2007;9(2):178–83. Epub 2006 Jul 31.
81. Cotter G, Moshkovitz Y, Milovanov O, Salah A, Blatt A, Krakover R, et al. Acute heart failure: a novel approach to its pathogenesis and treatment. Eur J Heart Fail. 2002;4(3):227–34. CrossRef PubMed.
82. Kaluski E, Kobrin I, Zimlichman R, Marmor A, Krakov O, Milo O, et al. RITZ-5: randomized intravenous TeZosentan (an endothelin-A/B antagonist) for the treatment of pulmonary edema: a prospective, multicenter, double-blind, placebo-controlled study. J Am Coll Cardiol. 2003;41(2):204–10. CrossRef PubMed.
83. Mebazaa A, Pang PS, Tavares M, Collins SP, Storrow AB, Laribi S, et al. The impact of early standard therapy on dyspnoea in patients with acute heart failure: the URGENT-dyspnoea study. Eur Heart J. 2010;31(7):832–41. https://doi.org/10.1093/eurheartj/ehp458. Epub 2009 Nov 11.
84. Balmain S, Padmanabhan N, Ferrell WR, Morton JJ, McMurray JJ. Differences in arterial compliance, microvascular function and venous capacitance between patients with heart failure and either preserved or reduced left ventricular systolic function. Eur J Heart Fail. 2007;9(9):865–71. Epub 2007 Jul 19.

85. Cotter G, Metra M, Milo-Cotter O, Dittrich HC, Gheorghiade M. Fluid overload in acute heart failure--re-distribution and other mechanisms beyond fluid accumulation. Eur J Heart Fail. 2008;10(2):165–9. https://doi.org/10.1016/j.ejheart.2008.01.007. CrossRef PubMed.
86. Cotter G, Felker GM, Adams KF, Milo-Cotter O, O'Connor CM. The pathophysiology of acute heart failure--is it all about fluid accumulation? Am Heart J. 2008;155(1):9–18. CrossRef PubMed.
87. Felker GM, Leimberger JD, Califf RM, Cuffe MS, Massie BM, Adams KF Jr, et al. Risk stratification after hospitalization for decompensated heart failure. J Card Fail. 2004;10(6):460–6. CrossRef PubMed.
88. Fonarow GC, Adams KF Jr, Abraham WT, Yancy CW. ADHERE Scientific Advisory Committee, Study Group, and Investigators, Boscardin WJ. Risk stratification for in-hospital mortality in acutely decompensated heart failure: classification and regression tree analysis. JAMA. 2005;293(5):572–80. CrossRef PubMed.
89. Lee DS, Austin PC, Rouleau JL, Liu PP, Naimark D, Tu JV. Predicting mortality among patients hospitalized for heart failure: derivation and validation of a clinical model. JAMA. 2003;290(19):2581–7. CrossRef PubMed.
90. Collins S, Storrow AB, Kirk JD, Pang PS, Diercks DB, Gheorghiade M. Beyond pulmonary edema: diagnostic, risk stratification, and treatment challenges of acute heart failure management in the emergency department. Ann Emerg Med. 2008;51(1):45–57. Epub 2007 Sep 14.
91. Collins S, Storrow AB, Albert NM, Butler J, Ezekowitz J, Felker GM. SAEM/HFSA Acute Heart Failure Working Group. et al. Early management of patients with acute heart failure: state of the art and future directions. A consensus document from the society for academic emergency medicine/heart failure society of America acute heart failure working group. J Card Fail. 2015;21(1):27–43. https://doi.org/10.1016/j.cardfail.2014.07.003. Epub 2014 Jul 18.
92. Stevenson LW, Perloff JK. The limited reliability of physical signs for estimating hemodynamics in chronic heart failure. JAMA. 1989;261(6):884–8. PubMed PMID 2913385. CrossRef PubMed.
93. Kay JM, Edwards FR. Ultrastructure of the alveolar-capillary wall in mitral stenosis. Pathobiology. 1973;111(4):239–45.
94. Kingsbury MP, Huang W, Donnelly JL, Jackson E, Needham E, Turner MA, Sheridan DJ. Structural remodelling of lungs in chronic heart failure. Basic Res Cardiol. 2003;98(5):295–303. Epub 2003 May 16.
95. Huang W, Kingsbury MP, Turner MA, Donnelly JL, Flores NA, Sheridan DJ. Capillary filtration is reduced in lungs adapted to chronic heart failure: morphological and haemodynamic correlates. Cardiovasc Res. 2001;49(1):207–17. CrossRef PubMed.
96. Davies SW, Bailey J, Keegan J, Balcon R, Rudd RM, Lipkin DP. Reduced pulmonary microvascular permeability in severe chronic left heart failure. Am Heart J. 1992;124(1):137–42. CrossRef PubMed.
97. Rossi JS, Flaherty JD, Fonarow GC, Nunez E, Gattis Stough W, Abraham WT, et al. Influence of coronary artery disease and coronary revascularization status on outcomes in patients with acute heart failure syndromes: a report from OPTIMIZE-HF (Organized Program to Initiate Lifesaving Treatment in Hospitalized Patients with Heart Failure). Eur J Heart Fail. 2008;10(12):1215–23. https://doi.org/10.1016/j.ejheart.2008.09.009. Epub 2008 Nov 8.
98. Flaherty JD, Bax JJ, De Luca L, Rossi JS, Davidson CJ, Filippatos G, Acute Heart Failure Syndromes International Working Group, et al. Acute heart failure syndromes in patients with coronary artery disease early assessment and treatment. J Am Coll Cardiol. 2009;53(3):254–63. PubMed PMID 19147042. CrossRef PubMed.
99. Thygesen K, Alpert JS, White HD, Joint ESC/ACCF/AHA/WHF Task Force for the Redefinition of Myocardial Infarction, Jaffe AS, Apple FS, Galvani M, Katus HA, Newby LK, Ravkilde J, et al. Universal definition of myocardial infarction. Circulation. 2007;116(22):2634–53. Epub 2007 Oct 19
100. Kociol RD, Pang PS, Gheorghiade M, Fonarow GC, O'Connor CM, Felker GM. Troponin elevation in heart failure prevalence, mechanisms, and clinical implications. J Am Coll Cardiol. 2010;56(14):1071–8. https://doi.org/10.1016/j.jacc.2010.06.016. CrossRef PubMed.
101. Peacock WF 4th, De Marco T, Fonarow GC, Diercks D, Wynne J, Apple FS, Investigators ADHERE, Wu AH. Cardiac troponin and outcome in acute heart failure. N Engl J Med. 2008;358(20):2117–26. https://doi.org/10.1056/NEJMoa0706824. PMID: 18480204 [PubMed - indexed for MEDLINE] CrossRef PubMed.
102. You JJ, Austin PC, Alter DA, Ko DT, Tu JV. Relation between cardiac troponin I and mortality in acute decompensated heart failure. Am Heart J. 2007;153(4):462–70. CrossRef PubMed.
103. Cleland JG, Pennell DJ, Ray SG, Coats AJ, Macfarlane PW, Murray GD. Carvedilol hibernating reversible ischaemia trial: marker of success investigators, et al. Myocardial viability as a determinant of the ejection fraction response to carvedilol in patients with heart failure (CHRISTMAS trial): randomised controlled trial. Lancet. 2003;362(9377):14–21. CrossRef PubMed.
104. Beohar N, Erdogan AK, Lee DC, Sabbah HN, Kern MJ, Teerlink J, et al. Acute heart failure syndromes and coronary perfusion. J Am Coll Cardiol. 2008;52(1):13–6. https://doi.org/10.1016/j.jacc.2008.03.037. CrossRef PubMed.

105. Drazner MH, Hellkamp AS, Leier CV, Shah MR, Miller LW, Russell SD, et al. Value of clinician assessment of hemodynamics in advanced heart failure: the ESCAPE trial. Circ Heart Fail. 2008;1(3):170–7. https://doi.org/10.1161/CIRCHEARTFAILURE.108.769778. CrossRef PubMed PubMedCentral.
106. Ely JW, Osheroff JA, Chambliss ML, Ebell MH. Approach to leg edema of unclear etiology. J Am Board Fam Med. 2006;19(2):148–60. CrossRef PubMed.
107. Leier CV, Silver MA, Massie BM, Young JB, Fowler MB, Ventura HO, Hershberger RE. Nuggets, pearls, and vignettes of master heart failure clinicians. Part 1--the medical history. Congest Heart Fail. 2001;7(5):245–9. CrossRef PubMed.
108. Payvar S, Spertus JA, Miller AB, Casscells SW, Pang PS, Zannad F. Efficacy of Vasopressin Antagonism in Heart Failure Outcome Study with Tolvaptan (EVEREST) Investigators. et al. Association of low body temperature and poor outcomes in patients admitted with worsening heart failure: a substudy of the Efficacy of Vasopressin Antagonism in Heart Failure Outcome Study with Tolvaptan (EVEREST) trial. Eur J Heart Fail. 2013;15(12):1382–9. https://doi.org/10.1093/eurjhf/hft113. Epub 2013 Jul 15

15 Guideline Directed Medical Therapy and How to Get There

Sawan Dutta, Yevgeniy Brailovsky, and Indranee Rajapreyar

Introduction

The pharmacologic treatment of Stage C heart failure with reduced ejection fraction (HFrEF) is well established through a number of clinical trials over the past few decades. The foundation of therapy is based on the four pillars of guideline directed medical therapy (GDMT): (1) angiotensin receptor-neprilysin inhibitors (ARNi)/angiotensin converting enzyme inhibitors (ACEi)/angiotensin receptor blockers (ARB), (2) beta blockers (BB), (3) mineralocorticoid receptor antagonists (MRA), and (4) sodium-glucose cotransporter-2 inhibitors (SGLT2i). The use of all four drug classes is estimated to reduce all-cause mortality in HFrEF by 73% compared with no treatment [1]. In addition, cross-trial analysis shows that survival is improved by 6.3 years (in a 55-year-old patient) with quadruple therapy compared to the two drug conventional therapy (ACEi/ARB and BB) [2]. Despite the benefits of GDMT, the integration and up-titration to target doses of these therapies remain insufficient. Prior to the approval of SGLT2i, the CHAMP-HF study of 150 primary care and cardiology practices determined that only 1% of patients were receiving target doses of triple therapy with ARNi/ACEi/ARB, BB, and MRA [3]. After an episode of acute decompensated heart failure, rapid uptitration of GDMT to target doses with frequent follow up visits decreased hospitalizations and improved survival and quality of life [4]. Here we discuss the pivotal trials supporting GDMT and the optimal way to integrate its use in clinical practice.

S. Dutta (✉)
Thomas Jefferson University Hospital, Philadelphia, PA, USA

Y. Brailovsky
Division of Cardiology, Columbia University, New York, NY, USA

I. Rajapreyar
Tufts Medical Center, Boston, MA, USA

Pillars of Guideline Directed Medical Therapy

The timeline of the key trials establishing the pharmacological treatment of HFrEF is shown in Fig. 15.1. Each of these clinical studies are organized based on their pharmaceutical class and are discussed in the following sections.

RAAS Inhibitors (ARNi/ACEi/ARB)

Class 1A Recommendation: In patients with HFrEF and NYHA class II-IV symptoms, the use of ARNi is recommended to reduce morbidity and mortality. If intolerant to ARNi, the use of ACEi is recommended. If intolerant to both, the use of ARB is recommended [5].

ACEi and ARB were part of the initial therapeutic class that showed mortality benefit in HFrEF. Enalapril, the ACEi evaluated in the

H. J. Eisen (ed.), *Heart Failure I*, https://doi.org/10.1007/978-3-032-12626-9_15

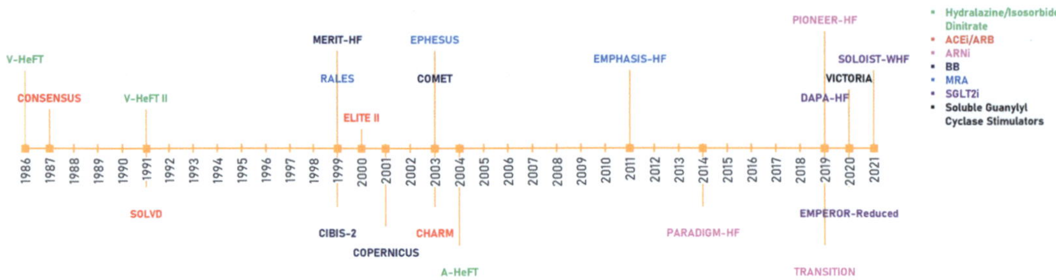

Fig. 15.1 Timeline of key trials for HFrEF medical therapy and organized by pharmaceutical class

SOLVD trial on minimal background betablocker therapy (8%) reduced all- cause mortality by 16%. The burden of hospitalizations for cardiovascular causes, although lower in the enalapril group, was still more than 50% [6]. Median survival in the enalapril group in the long-term follow of the SOLVD study was still low at 5.5 years with approximately only 20% survival at the end of 12-year follow up [7].

In HFrEF patients with age > 60 years, losartan was not superior to captopril in improving survival [8]. Valsartan did not improve survival but reduced hospitalizations in patients with HFrEF [9]. Candesartan at a dose of 32 mg once daily reduced cardiovascular death and hospitalization by 30% in patients intolerant to ACEi [10]. Meta-analysis did not show significant benefit of ARB compared to placebo or ACEi in reducing mortality [11]. Hence the use of ARB is recommended in patients intolerant to ACEi due to its variable effects on mortality.

Renin angiotensin aldosterone system inhibition with combination of ARB and neprilysin inhibitor (sacubitril-valsartan) to increase the activity of natriuretic peptides and other vasoactive peptides was evaluated in the PARADIGM-HF and PIONEER-HF trials (Table 15.1). Sacubitril-valsartan reduced the risk of death from cardiovascular causes or first hospitalization for worsening heart failure by 20% when compared to placebo in patients with NYHA class II or III HFrEF and a background therapy of beta-blocker in approximately 93% of patients [12]. In patients admitted with acute decompensated HFrEF, sacubitril-valsartan decreased natriuretic peptides (NT-ProBNP) levels and significantly reduced cardiovascular death or rehospitalization for HF when compared to enalapril with a short-follow up of 8 weeks [13].

Beta-Blockers

Class 1A Recommendation: In patients with current or prior symptomatic HFrEF, use of 1 of 3 beta blockers (bisoprolol, carvedilol, sustained-release metoprolol succinate) is recommended to reduce mortality and hospitalizations [5].

Beta blockers emerged as the second pillar of GDMT, as their use was beneficial to reduce the overactivation of the sympathetic nervous system in heart failure. As outlined in the clinical trials in Table 15.2, the use of one of three beta blockers, in addition to RAAS inhibition, reduces mortality and risk of hospitalization in HFrEF. Beta blockers have the strongest survival benefit and LV reverse remodeling; hence, the goal should be to titrate to target doses studied in clinical trials. The benefits of carvedilol in improving left ventricular ejection and survival was dose-dependent [15]. The optimal initiation of beta-blockers should be once euvolemia is achieved in patients with HFrEF.

Table 15.1 Summary of key trials with Angiotensin Receptor-Neprilysin Inhibitors

Trial	Clinical question	Design	Population	Main outcomes
Prospective Comparison of ARNI with ACEI to Determine Impact on Global Mortality and Morbidity in Heart Failure (PARADIGM-HF) [12]	Whether sacubitril-valsartan (ARNi) was superior to enalapril in reducing morbidity and mortality in chronic HFrEF	Multicenter, prospective, randomized, comparative trial	Age > 18, NYHA class II-IV with LVEF < 40% (later updated to <35%), BNP > 150 or NT-proBNP > 600, or HF hospitalization within last 12 months, and on stable BB and ACEi/ARB therapy 4 weeks prior	Sacubitril-valsartan (ARNi) use compared to enalapril (ACEi) alone in HF, reduced risks of cardiovascular death and HF hospitalization by 20% and all-cause mortality by 16%
Comparison of Sacubitril–Valsartan versus Enalapril on Effect on NT-proBNP in Patients Stabilized from an Acute Heart Failure Episode (PIONEER—HF) [13]	Efficacy and safety of the initiation of sacubitril–valsartan vs. enalapril, after hemodynamic stabilization among patients who were hospitalized for acute decompensated heart failure	Multicenter, double-blind, randomized, active-controlled trial	Age > 18, with symptomatic acute decompensated heart failure, LVEF < 40%, NT-proBNP > 1600 or BNP > 400, and enrolled between 24 hours and 10 days after presentation	In patients hospitalized with acute decompensated heart failure, initiation of sacubitril–valsartan resulted in greater reduction in NT-proBNP compared to enalapril (−46.7% vs. −25.3%), without significantly different rates of adverse effects
TRANSITION: Pre-discharge and posT-discharge tReatment Initiation With Sacubitril-Valsartan in heArt Failure patieNtS With Reduced ejectIon-fracTion hospItalized for an Acute decOmpensation eveNt [14]	Assess tolerability and optimal time point for initiation of sacubitril-valsartan in patients stabilized after acute decompensated HF	Multicenter, randomized, open-label, parallel-group trial	Age > 18, hospitalized for ADHF and stabilized >24 hours, with NYHA class II-IV and LVEF < 40%, and on any dose of ACEi/ARB	Initiation of sacubitril-valsartan in patients with HFrEF after stabilization from an ADHF event, either in hospital or shortly after discharge, is feasible with about half of the patients achieving target dose within 10 weeks

Mineralocorticoid Receptor Antagonists

Class 1A Recommendation: In patients with HFrEF and NYHA class II to IV symptoms, an MRA (spironolactone or eplerenone) is recommended to reduce morbidity and mortality (if eGFR > 30 mL/min/1.73m² and serum potassium < 5 mEq/L [5].

The RALES and EMPHASIS-HF trials both showed the benefit of two mineralocorticoid receptor antagonists (spironolactone and eplerenone) in reducing mortality and morbidity in HFrEF (Table 15.3). Notably, this benefit was only studied in patients with baseline creatinine <2.5 mg/dL and potassium <5 mEq/L. Furthermore, the EPHESUS trial showed the survival benefit of eplerenone in the acute post MI period with LVEF < 40%. All-cause mortality was reduced in the spironolactone group by 30% and reduction was attributed to reduction in worsening heart failure and sudden cardiac death. Beta-blocker use was only 15% in the spironolactone group [20]. Patients enrolled in the EMPHASIS-HF trial receiving eplerenone also experienced a 37% reduction in death from cardiovascular cause or hospitalization for heart failure with 87% use of background beta-blocker therapy [21].

Sodium-Glucose-Cotransporter-2 Inhibitors

Class IA Recommendation: In patients with symptomatic chronic HFrEF, SGLT2i are recom-

Table 15.2 Summary of key trials with Beta Blockers

Trial	Clinical question	Design	Population	Main outcomes
Cardiac Insufficiency Bisoprolol Study II [16] (CIBIS II)	Efficiency of bisoprolol in decreasing all-cause mortality in chronic heart failure	Double-blind randomized placebo-controlled trial	Symptomatic NYHA Class III-IV with LVEF < 35% and receiving treatment with diuretics and ACEi (if intolerant, other vasodilators allowed)	34% relative risk reduction in all-cause mortality and sudden death with bisoprolol vs. placebo, in addition to standard therapy for HF
Metoprolol CR/XL Randomized Intervention Trial in Congestive Heart Failure [17] (MERIT-HF)	Effects of controlled-release/extended-release metoprolol succinate on mortality, hospitalization, symptoms, and quality of life in patients with heart failure	Randomized, double-blind controlled trial with a single-blind, 2 week placebo run-in period	Symptomatic NYHA Class II-IV with LVEF < 40% and receiving treatment with diuretics and ACEi ((if intolerant, other vasodilators allowed)	Metoprolol CR/XL use resulted in 34% reduction in all-cause mortality compared to placebo
Carvedilol Prospective Randomized Cumulative Survival [18] (COPERNICUS)	Effect of carvedilol on morbidity of patients with severe chronic heart failure	Double-blind, parallel-group, randomized, placebo-controlled trial	Dyspnea or fatigue at rest or on minimal exertion (NYHA Class III-IV) with LVEF < 25% and receiving treatment with diuretic and ACEi/ARB	Carvedilol reduced annual mortality by 35% and combined risk of death or HF hospitalization by 31% when compared to placebo
Comparison of carvedilol and metoprolol on clinical outcomes in patients with chronic heart failure in the Carvedilol Or Metoprolol European Trial [19] (COMET)	Compare the effects of carvedilol and metoprolol on mortality and morbidity in patients with mild to severe chronic heart failure	Multicenter, randomized, double-blind, parallel-group trial	Symptomatic NYHA Class II-IV with LVEF < 35%, treatment with diuretics and ACEi, and cardiovascular-related admission in prior 2 years	Carvedilol reduced all-cause mortality by 17% compared to metoprolol tartrate (34% vs. 40%)

mended to reduce hospitalization for HF and cardiovascular mortality, irrespective of presence of diabetes [5].

Sodium-glucose-contransporter-2 inhibitors became a part of GDMT due to additive benefits in patients with HFrEF. The DAPA-HF and EMPEROR-Reduced showed the reduction in mortality and risk of hospitalization with the use of dapagliflozin or empagliflozin in addition to standard therapy regardless of the presence of diabetes (Table 15.4). The other beneficial aspect of SGLT2i is the starting and target dose are equivalent, meaning further dose titration is not needed. When considering patients with type 2 diabetes and symptomatic heart failure (reduced and preserved), the SOLOIST-WHF trial showed that the SGLT1/2 inhibitor sotagliflozin significantly reduced cardiovascular death and risk of hospitalization [23]. Patients with type 1 diabetes, chronic kidney disease with reduced eGFR <30 ml/min/1.73 m^2 in the DAPA- HF and <20 ml/min/1.73 m^2 in the EMPEROR-Reduced trial were excluded from the SGLT2i trials. There is risk for genital yeast infections and euglycemic ketoacidosis with the use of SGLT2i [24] (EMPEROR-Reduced).

Table 15.3 Summary of key trials with Mineralocorticoid Receptor Antagonists

Trial	Clinical question	Design	Population	Main outcomes
Randomized Aldactone Evaluation Study [20] (RALES)	Effect of spironolactone on morbidity and mortality in patients with severe heart failure	Multicenter, double-blinded, parallel-group, randomized, placebo-controlled trial	NYHA Class III or IV with LVEF < 35% and receiving treatment with loop diuretic and ACEi	Spironolactone reduces risk of all-cause mortality by 30% compared to placebo
Eplerenone in Mild Patients Hospitalization and Survival Study in Heart Failure [21] (EMPHASIS-HF)	Effect of eplerenone on clinical outcomes in patients with systolic heart failure and mild symptoms	Randomized, double-blind, prospective, superiority, placebo-controlled trial	Age > 55, NYHA class II with LVEF < 30% (or LVEF 30–35% with QRS duration > 120), treatment with ACEi/ARB and BB (unless contraindicated) and CV hospitalization in prior 6 months or BNP > 250 pg/mL or pro-BNP > 500 pg/mL (men) or pro-BNP > 750 pg/mL (women)	Eplerenone reduced the risk of death and hospitalization by 37% among patients with systolic heart failure and mild symptoms compared to placebo
Eplerenone Post–Acute Myocardial Infarction Heart Failure Efficacy and Survival Study [22] (EPHESUS)	Efficacy of eplerenone on mortality and hospitalization in patients with acute MI complicated by LV dysfunction and heart failure	Multicenter, international, randomized, double-blind, placebo-controlled trial	Symptomatic (or diabetic without symptoms) heart failure with LVEF < 40% and MI in prior 3–14 days	Eplerenone reduced all-cause mortality by 15% among patients with acute MI complicated by LV dysfunction compared to placebo

Table 15.4 Summary of key trials with SGLT-2 Inhibitors

Trial	Clinical question	Design	Population	Main outcomes
DAPA-HF [25] (Dapagliflozin and Prevention of Adverse Outcomes in Heart Failure)	Efficacy and safety of dapagliflozin in patients with heart failure and a reduced ejection fraction, regardless of the presence or absence of diabetes	Multicenter, double-blind, parallel-group, randomized, controlled trial	Age > 18, NYHA class II-IV with LVEF < 40%, NT-proBNP level > 600 (or > 400 if HF hospitalization in last 12 months or > 900 if baseline afib/flutter) and receiving standardized device (ICD and/or CRT) and drug therapy (ACEi/ ARB/ARNI and BB, unless contraindicated)	In patients with HFrEF, regardless of presence of diabetes, dapagliflozin reduced the relative risk of worsening HF and death from cardiovascular cause by 26% compared to placebo (16.3% vs. 21.2%)
Empagliflozin Outcome Trial in Patients with Chronic Heart Failure and a Reduced Ejection Fraction [24] (EMPEROR-Reduced)	Efficacy of empagliflozin in patients with heart failure with reduced ejection fraction, regardless of presence or absence of diabetes	Multinational, multicenter, double-blind, parallel-group, randomized, controlled trial	Age > 18, NYHA class II-IV with LVEF < 40%, HF hospitalization within last 12 months or NT-proBNP > 600 (EF < 30%) or NT-proBNP > 1000 (EF 31–35%) or NT-proBNP > 2500 (EF 36–40%) or double the NT-proBNP cut offs in patients with Afib and on standard device and drug therapy	In patients with HFrEF, regardless of presence of diabetes, empagliflozin reduced relative risk of cardiovascular death or hospitalization by 25% compared to placebo (19.4% vs. 24.7%)

Additional Medical Therapy Considerations

Hydralazine and Isosorbide Dinitrate

Class IA Recommendation: For patients who self-identify as African American with NYHA class III-IV HFrEF, who are receiving optimal medical therapy, the combination of hydralazine and isosorbide dinitrate is recommended to improve symptoms and reduce mortality and morbidity [5].

Class IIB Recommendation: In patient with current or previous symptomatic HFrEF, who cannot tolerate first-line RAAS inhibition because of drug intolerance or renal insufficiency, a combination of hydralazine and isosorbide dinitrate might be considered to reduce morbidity and mortality [5].

Prior to the standard use of ACEi and BB, the V-HeFT trial showed that there was a trend towards survival benefit in the use of hydralazine and isosorbide dinitrate in self-identified African American patients with symptomatic systolic heart failure compared to placebo. This finding led to the A-HeFT trial which specifically evaluated African American patients with NYHA Class III-IV heart failure (Table 15.5). In addition to standard medical therapy, the addition of hydralazine and isosorbide dinitrate resulted in 39% reduction in all-cause mortality and 33% reduction in first HF hospitalization [26].

Soluble Guanylyl Cyclase Stimulators

Class IIB Recommendation: In select high-risk HFrEF patients on GDMT with recent worsening HF, an oral soluble guanylate cyclase stimulator

Table 15.5 Summary of key trials with Hydralazine and Isosorbide Dinitrate

Trial	Clinical question	Design	Population	Main outcomes
Vasodilator Heart Failure Trial [27] (V-HeFT)	In patients with dilated cardiomyopathy and systolic heart failure, does vasodilator therapy with hydralazine/isosorbide dinitrate confer a survival benefit compared to prazosin or placebo?	Multicenter, double-blind, parallel group, randomized, placebo-controlled trial	Age 18–75, dilated cardiomyopathy, reduced exercise tolerance	Reduction in mortality was 38% after 1 year with hydralazine/isosorbide dinitrate. No significant difference in mortality between the three groups. Trend towards survival improvement and significant improvement in LVEF with hydralazine/isosorbide dinitrate
Vasodilator Heart Failure Trial [28] (V-HeFT) II	Comparison of enalapril to hydralazine/isosorbide dinitrate in HFrEF survival	Multicenter, randomized, intention to treat	Men age 18–75, reduced exercise tolerance, cardiac dysfunction, and on stable diuretic and digoxin therapy	Two-year mortality was lower with enalapril compared to hydralazine/isosorbide dinitrate (18% vs. 25%)
African American Heart Failure Trial [26] (A-HeFT)	Among self-identified African Americans with HFrEF, does hydralazine/isosorbide dinitrate improve survival compared to placebo	Multicenter, double-blinded, parallel-group, randomized, placebo-controlled trial	Age > 18, self identified as African American, NYHA Class III-IV on standard HF therapy with evidence of LV dysfunction within last 6 months	In addition to standard therapy, hydralazine/isosorbide dinitrate was associated with 39% reduction in all-cause mortality and 33% reduction in first HF hospitalization in African American patients compared to placebo

Table 15.6 Summary of key trials with Hydralazine and Isosorbide Dinitrate

Trial	Clinical question	Design	Population	Main outcomes
Vericiguat Global Study in Subjects with Heart Failure with Reduced Ejection Fraction [29] (VICTORIA)	Comparison of vericiguat to placebo in patients with high-risk HFrEF	Phase 3, randomized, double-blind, placebo-controlled trial	Age > 18, NYHA Class II-IV with LVEF < 45% within last 12 months on GDMT, and BNP > 300 or NT-proBNP > 1000 (BNP > 500 or NT-proBNP > 1600 in afib) and recent HF hospitalization or IV diuretic use	Incidence of death from cardiovascular causes or HF hospitalization was lower with vericiguat compared to placebo (35.5% vs. 38.8%)

(vericiguat) may be considered to reduce HF hospitalization and cardiovascular death [5].

Endothelial dysfunction in HF results in reduction of cGMP and nitric oxide production. The benefit of soluble guanylyl cyclase stimulators (vericiguat) therapy is to stimulate cGMP production resulting in improvement in endothelial cell function and decrease in cardiac remodeling. In patients with chronic HFrEF with recent hospitalization, the VICTORIA trial showed vericiguat to be beneficial to reduce the incidence of HF death or hospitalization in addition to standard therapy in compared to placebo (Table 15.6).

Pathway for Therapy Initiation and Optimization

Conventional sequencing for establishing GDMT involves a sequential step-wise approach: (1) start with ACEi/ARB, (2) add BB, (3) add MRA, (4) switch ACEi/ARB to ARNi, (5) add SGLT2i. With this method, each medication is titrated to its target dose before adding additional therapy, which results in a significant delay of 6–12 months before reaching goal therapy. The consensus practice guidelines across the different cardiology societies are summarized in Table 15.7.

In addition to the introduction of four pillars in each patient, the goal should also include uptitration of medications to their goal therapeutic targets. A study by Shen et al., modeled rapid up-titration vs. conventional titration using data from 5 trials: SOLVD, MERIT-HF, EMPHASIS-HF, PARADIGM-HF, DAPA-HF. They found that in comparison to the conventional approach, an accelerated approach prevented at least 14 deaths and greater than three times the amount of heart failure hospitalizations [33]. In addition, the STRONG-HF randomized clinical trial showed that in patients hospitalized with acute decompensated heart failure, rapid titration of GDMT to goal (excluding SGLT2i) within 2 weeks of discharge and close follow-up reduced the risk of 180-day all-cause death or heart failure readmission compared to usual care [4].

There are different approaches to achieve this rapid therapy initiation and optimization, which are outlined in the Table 15.8.

Utilizing the rapid therapy initiation approach is the most effective way to ensure patients are efficiently started on the four pillars of GDMT to reduce the risk of mortality and rehospitalization. The recommended initiation doses and target doses are outlined in Tables 15.9, 15.10, 15.11 and 15.12. Although there is no consensus on how to achieve this rapid initiation, based off the data from clinical trials and the proposed approaches, we recommend the proposal outlined in Fig. 15.2.

Table 15.7 Summary of societal guidelines for GDMT optimization

Society	Approach
2021 European Society of Cardiology [30]	Start triad of ACEi/ARNI, BB and MRA Titrate triad to target dose Add SGLT2i
2021 ACC Expert Consensus Pathway [31]	Start with BB and ARNI/ACEI/ARB Add MRA and monitor electrolytes Add SGL2i for NYHA class II-IV Titrate medications to maximally tolerated dose Timeline: adjustment of medications every 2 weeks to achieve target GDMT within 3–6 months of initial diagnosis
2021 Canadian Cardiovascular Society [32]	Treat with 4 pillars of GDMT Optimize dose by 3–6 months after initial diagnosis No consensus on titration/initiation but may consider in-parallel vs. strict sequential approach

Table 15.8 Summary of approaches for rapid therapy initiation

Proposal	Approach	Timeline
Packer and McMurray [34]	1. Start BB + SGLT2i 2. Add ARNi 3. Add MRA	Initiation: 4 weeks Titration: as tolerated
Greene et al. [35]	Initiate 4 pillars at low doses	Initiation: 1 week Titration: 1 month
Miller et al. [36]	1. Initiate a med from each cluster: Cluster A (diuretic and SGLT2i) Cluster B (ARNi and MRA) Cluster C (BB and SNI) 2. After 1–2 weeks, add second cluster B medication 3. Initiate or up-titrate up to 3 meds per visit	Initiation: 3–6 weeks Titration: 12 weeks
Rosano et al. [37]	Personalized based on hemodynamic profile and renal function: 9 Different profiles based on HR, BP, CKD, and Afib	Initiation and titration based off patient profile and response to tolerated doses

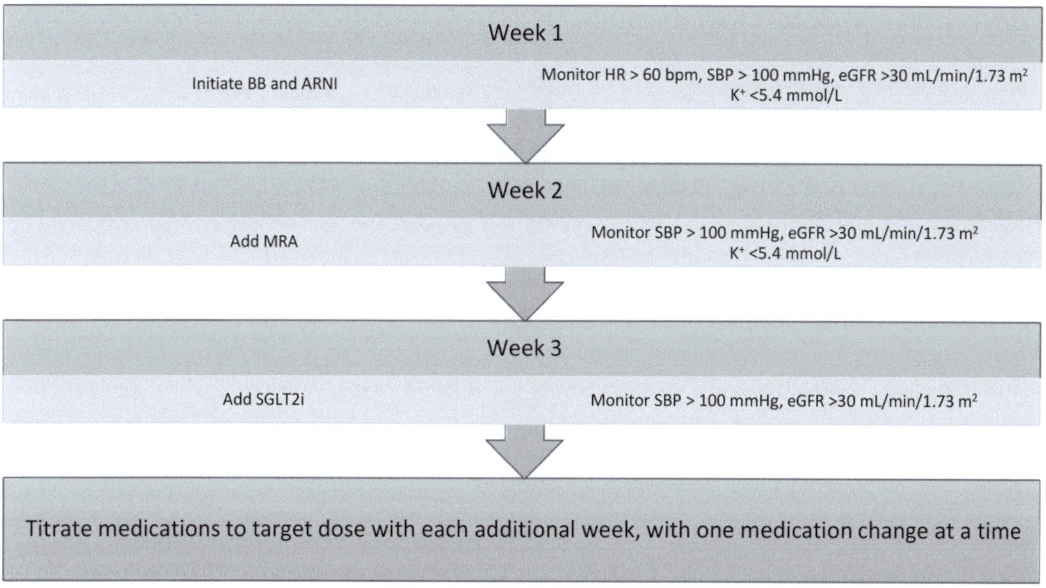

Fig. 15.2 Proposed initiation and titration of GDMT in HFrEF

Recommended Initial and Target Dosing of GDMT [5]

Table 15.9 RAAS inhibitor dosing

ARNI	**Initial dose**	**Target dose**
Sacubitril-Valsartan	49 mg Sacubitril—51 mg valsartan BID (can initiate at lower dose 24–26 mg)	97 mg sacubitril—103 mg valsartan BID
ACEi	**Initial dose**	**Target dose**
Captopril	6.25 mg TID	50 mg TID
Enalapril	2.5 mg BID	10–20 mg BID
Fosinopril	5–10 mg daily	40 mg daily
Lisinopril	2.5–5 mg daily	20–40 mg daily
Perindopril	2 mg daily	8–16 mg daily
Quinapril	5 mg BID	20 mg BID
Ramipril	1.25–2.5 mg daily	10 mg daily
Transdolapril	1 mg daily	4 mg daily
ARB	**Initial dose**	**Target dose**
Candesartan	4–8 mg daily	32 mg daily
Losartan	25–50 mg daily	50–150 mg daily
Valsartan	20–40 mg daily	160 mg BID

Table 15.10 Beta blocker dosing

Name	Initial dose	Target dose
Bisoprolol	1.25 mg daily	10 mg daily
Carvedilol	3.125 mg daily	25–50 mg BID
Carvedilol CR	10 mg daily	80 mg daily
Metoprolol Succinate ER	12.5–25 mg daily	200 mg daily

Table 15.11 MRA dosing

Name	Initial dose	Target dose
Spironolactone	12.5–25 mg daily	25–50 mg daily
Eplerenone	25 mg daily	50 mg daily

Table 15.12 SGLT2i dosing

Name	Initial dose	Target dose
Dapagliflozin	10 mg daily	10 mg daily
Empagliflozin	10 mg daily	10 mg daily

Conclusion and Recommendations

The foundation of therapy for Stage C heart failure is based on multiple clinical trials over the last few decades which have established the four pillars of guideline directed medical therapy. Appropriate use and titration of all four pillars in combination has significant improvements in all cause mortality in heart failure. Despite this benefit, this combination therapy is still underutilized. Recognizing that there are many limitations in starting these medications, the recommendation is that physicians initiate and rapidly uptitrate the four pillars to their target doses to provide the greatest survival benefits to their patients with HFrEF.

Disclosures The authors have nothing to disclose.

Funding There was no funding to report.

References

1. Bassi NS, Ziaeian B, Yancy CW, Fonarow GC. Association of optimal implementation of sodium-glucose cotransporter 2 inhibitor therapy with outcome for patients with heart failure. JAMA Cardiol. 2020;5(8):948–51. https://doi.org/10.1001/jamacardio.2020.0898.
2. Vaduganathan M, Claggett BL, Jhund PS, et al. Estimating lifetime benefits of comprehensive disease-modifying pharmacological therapies in patients with heart failure with reduced ejection fraction: a comparative analysis of three randomised controlled trials. Lancet. 2020;396(10244):121–8. https://doi.org/10.1016/s0140-6736(20)30748-0.
3. Greene SJ, Butler J, Albert NM, et al. Medical therapy for heart failure with reduced ejection fraction: the CHAMP-HF registry. J Am Coll Cardiol. 2018;72(4):351–66. https://doi.org/10.1016/j.jacc.2018.04.070.
4. Mebazaa A, Davison B, Chioncel O, et al. Safety, tolerability and efficacy of up-titration of guideline-directed medical therapies for acute heart failure (STRONG-HF): a multinational, open-label, randomised, trial. Lancet. 2022;400(10367):1938–52. https://doi.org/10.1016/s0140-6736(22)02076-1.
5. 2022 AHA/ACC/HFSA Guideline for the Management of Heart Failure. J Card Fail. 2022;28(5):e1–e167. https://doi.org/10.1016/j.cardfail.2022.02.010.
6. Yusuf S, Pitt B, Davis CE, Hood WB, Cohn JN. Effect of enalapril on survival in patients with reduced left ventricular ejection fractions and congestive heart failure. N Engl J Med. 1991;325(5):293–302. https://doi.org/10.1056/nejm199108013250501.
7. Jong P, Yusuf S, Rousseau MF, Ahn SA, Bangdiwala SI. Effect of enalapril on 12-year survival and life expectancy in patients with left ventricular systolic dysfunction: a follow-up study. Lancet. 2003;361(9372):1843–8. https://doi.org/10.1016/s0140-6736(03)13501-5.
8. Pitt B, Poole-Wilson PA, Segal R, et al. Effect of losartan compared with captopril on mortality in patients with symptomatic heart failure: randomised trial--the Losartan Heart Failure Survival Study ELITE II. Lancet. 2000;355(9215):1582–7. https://doi.org/10.1016/s0140-6736(00)02213-3.
9. Cohn JN, Tognoni G. A randomized trial of the angiotensin-receptor blocker valsartan in chronic heart failure. N Engl J Med. 2001;345(23):1667–75. https://doi.org/10.1056/NEJMoa010713.
10. Pfeffer MA, Swedberg K, Granger CB, et al. Effects of candesartan on mortality and morbidity in patients with chronic heart failure: the CHARM-overall programme. Lancet. 2003;362(9386):759–66. https://doi.org/10.1016/s0140-6736(03)14282-1.
11. Jong P, Demers C, McKelvie RS, Liu PP. Angiotensin receptor blockers in heart failure: meta-analysis of randomized controlled trials. J Am Coll Cardiol. 2002;39(3):463–70. https://doi.org/10.1016/S0735-1097(01)01775-2.
12. McMurray JJ, Packer M, Desai AS, et al. Angiotensin-neprilysin inhibition versus enalapril in heart failure. N Engl J Med. 2014;371(11):993–1004. https://doi.org/10.1056/NEJMoa1409077.
13. Velazquez EJ, Morrow DA, DeVore AD, et al. Angiotensin-Neprilysin inhibition in acute decompensated heart failure. N Engl J Med. 2019;380(6):539–48. https://doi.org/10.1056/NEJMoa1812851.
14. Wachter R, Senni M, Belohlavek J, et al. Initiation of sacubitril/valsartan in haemodynamically stabilised heart failure patients in hospital or early after discharge: primary results of the randomised TRANSITION study. Eur J Heart Fail. 2019;21(8):998–1007. https://doi.org/10.1002/ejhf.1498.
15. Bristow MR, Gilbert EM, Abraham WT, et al. Carvedilol produces dose-related improvements in left ventricular function and survival in subjects with chronic heart failure. Circulation. 1996;94(11):2807–16. https://doi.org/10.1161/01.CIR.94.11.2807.
16. The Cardiac Insufficiency Bisoprolol Study II (CIBIS-II): a randomised trial. Lancet. 1999;353(9146):9–13. https://doi.org/10.1016/S0140-6736(98)11181-9.
17. Effect of metoprolol CR/XL in chronic heart failure: metoprolol CR/XL randomised intervention trial in-congestive heart failure (MERIT-HF). Lancet.

1999;353(9169):2001–7. https://doi.org/10.1016/S0140-6736(99)04440-2.

18. Packer M, Fowler MB, Roecker EB, et al. Effect of carvedilol on the morbidity of patients with severe chronic heart failure. Circulation. 2002;106(17):2194–9. https://doi.org/10.1161/01.CIR.0000035653.72855.BF.
19. Poole-Wilson PA, Swedberg K, Cleland JGF, et al. Comparison of carvedilol and metoprolol on clinical outcomes in patients with chronic heart failure in the Carvedilol Or Metoprolol European Trial (COMET): randomised controlled trial. Lancet. 2003;362(9377):7–13. https://doi.org/10.1016/S0140-6736(03)13800-7.
20. Pitt B, Zannad F, Remme WJ, et al. The effect of spironolactone on morbidity and mortality in patients with severe heart failure. N Engl J Med. 1999;341(10):709–17. https://doi.org/10.1056/nejm199909023411001.
21. Zannad F, McMurray JJV, Krum H, et al. Eplerenone in patients with systolic heart failure and mild symptoms. N Engl J Med. 2010;364(1):11–21. https://doi.org/10.1056/NEJMoa1009492.
22. Pitt B, Remme W, Zannad F, et al. Eplerenone, a selective aldosterone blocker, in patients with left ventricular dysfunction after myocardial infarction. N Engl J Med. 2003;348(14):1309–21. https://doi.org/10.1056/NEJMoa030207.
23. Bhatt DL, Szarek M, Steg PG, et al. Sotagliflozin in patients with diabetes and recent worsening heart failure. N Engl J Med. 2021;384(2):117–28. https://doi.org/10.1056/NEJMoa2030183.
24. Packer M, Anker SD, Butler J, et al. Cardiovascular and renal outcomes with empagliflozin in heart failure. N Engl J Med. 2020;383(15):1413–24. https://doi.org/10.1056/NEJMoa2022190.
25. McMurray JJV, Solomon SD, Inzucchi SE, et al. Dapagliflozin in patients with heart failure and reduced ejection fraction. N Engl J Med. 2019;381(21):1995–2008. https://doi.org/10.1056/NEJMoa1911303.
26. Taylor AL, Ziesche S, Yancy C, et al. Combination of isosorbide dinitrate and hydralazine in blacks with heart failure. N Engl J Med. 2004;351(20):2049–57. https://doi.org/10.1056/NEJMoa042934.
27. Cohn JN, Archibald DG, Ziesche S, et al. Effect of vasodilator therapy on mortality in chronic congestive heart failure. N Engl J Med. 1986;314(24):1547–52. https://doi.org/10.1056/nejm198606123142404.
28. Cohn JN, Johnson G, Ziesche S, et al. A comparison of enalapril with hydralazine–isosorbide dinitrate in the treatment of chronic congestive heart failure. N Engl J Med. 1991;325(5):303–10. https://doi.org/10.1056/nejm199108013250502.
29. Armstrong PW, Pieske B, Anstrom KJ, et al. Vericiguat in patients with heart failure and reduced ejection fraction. N Engl J Med. 2020;382(20):1883–93. https://doi.org/10.1056/NEJMoa1915928.
30. McDonagh TA, Metra M, Adamo M, et al. 2021 ESC guidelines for the diagnosis and treatment of acute and chronic heart failure: developed by the task force for the diagnosis and treatment of acute and chronic heart failure of the European Society of Cardiology (ESC) with the special contribution of the Heart Failure Association (HFA) of the ESC. Eur Heart J. 2021;42(36):3599–726. https://doi.org/10.1093/eurheartj/ehab368.
31. Maddox TM, Januzzi JL Jr, Allen LA, et al. 2021 update to the 2017 ACC expert consensus decision pathway for optimization of heart failure treatment: answers to 10 pivotal issues about heart failure with reduced ejection fraction: a report of the American College of Cardiology Solution Set Oversight Committee. J Am Coll Cardiol. 2021;77(6):772–810. https://doi.org/10.1016/j.jacc.2020.11.022.
32. McDonald M, Virani S, Chan M, et al. CCS/CHFS heart failure guidelines update: defining a new pharmacologic standard of care for heart failure with reduced ejection fraction. Can J Cardiol. 2021;37(4):531–46. https://doi.org/10.1016/j.cjca.2021.01.017.
33. Shen L, Jhund PS, Docherty KF, et al. Accelerated and personalized therapy for heart failure with reduced ejection fraction. Eur Heart J. 2022;43(27):2573–87. https://doi.org/10.1093/eurheartj/ehac210.
34. Packer M, McMurray JJV. Rapid evidence-based sequencing of foundational drugs for heart failure and a reduced ejection fraction. Eur J Heart Fail. 2021;23(6):882–94. https://doi.org/10.1002/ejhf.2149.
35. Greene SJ, Butler J, Fonarow GC. Simultaneous or rapid sequence initiation of quadruple medical therapy for heart failure—optimizing therapy with the need for speed. JAMA Cardiol. 2021;6(7):743–4. https://doi.org/10.1001/jamacardio.2021.0496.
36. Miller RJH, Howlett JG, Fine NM. A novel approach to medical management of heart failure with reduced ejection fraction. Can J Cardiol. 2021;37(4):632–43. https://doi.org/10.1016/j.cjca.2020.12.028.
37. Rosano GMC, Moura B, Metra M, et al. Patient profiling in heart failure for tailoring medical therapy. A consensus document of the Heart Failure Association of the European Society of Cardiology. Eur J Heart Fail. 2021;23(6):872–81. https://doi.org/10.1002/ejhf.2206.

16 Group 2 Pulmonary Hypertension: PH Due to Left Heart Disease

Tirth A. Patel and Howard J. Eisen

Introduction and Epidemiology

Pulmonary hypertension (PH) is defined by elevated mean pulmonary artery pressure (mPAP) >20 mmHg at rest. The definition of pulmonary hypertension was revised in 2018 at 6th World Symposium of Pulmonary Hypertension (WSPH). Based on WHO classification Group 2 pulmonary hypertension is related to left sided heart disease is defined by mPAP >20 mmHg and pulmonary capillary wedge pressure (PCWP) >15 mmHg during right heart catheterization [1–3]. It is the most common form of PH in the United States and is associated with significantly increased morbidity and mortality. The presence of left heart disease with PH is linked to worse exercise tolerance, higher rates of hospitalization, and reduced survival compared to patients with left heart disease without PH.

Classification and Subtypes

The sixth World Symposium on Pulmonary Hypertension (WSPH) in 2018 revised the hemodynamic definitions of pulmonary hypertension (PH) to improve early detection and prognostication. The threshold for mean pulmonary arterial pressure (mPAP) was lowered from ≥25 mmHg to >20 mmHg [1]. This change is based on normative data showing that the upper limit of normal mPAP is approximately 20 mmHg, and that mPAP >20 mmHg is associated with increased mortality and risk of pulmonary vascular disease, even in the 21–24 mmHg range. Post-capillary PH (Group 2 PH) is subdivided into Isolated post-capillary PH (Ipc-PH) and combined pre- and post-capillary PH (Cpc-PH) [4].

Subtypes	Hemodynamics
Ipc-PH	mPAP > 20 mmHg, PCWP > 15 mmHg, PVR ≤ 2 WU
Cpc-PH	mPAP > 20 mmHg, PCWP > 15 mmHg, PVR > 2 WU

It is important to distinguish between two subtypes, as based on the American Heart association, when Cpc-PH is observed in patients with heart failure, it is associated with increased mortality compared to Ipc-PH [5]. It may reflect impact of advanced pulmonary vascular remodeling. The rationale for these changes includes data showing that even mild elevations in mPAP and PVR are linked to increased morbidity and mortality, and that earlier identification may allow for more timely intervention [6]. The WSPH also recommended considering additional hemodynamic markers—such as diastolic pressure gradient (DPG), transpulmonary gradient (TPG), and pulmonary arterial compliance—for prognostica-

T. A. Patel
Department of Cardiology, Thomas Jefferson University Hospital, Philadelphia, PA, USA
e-mail: tirth.patel@jefferson.edu

H. J. Eisen (✉)
Division of Cardiology, Thomas Jefferson University, Philadelphia, PA, USA
e-mail: howard.eisen@jefferson.edu

H. J. Eisen (ed.), *Heart Failure I*, https://doi.org/10.1007/978-3-032-12626-9_16

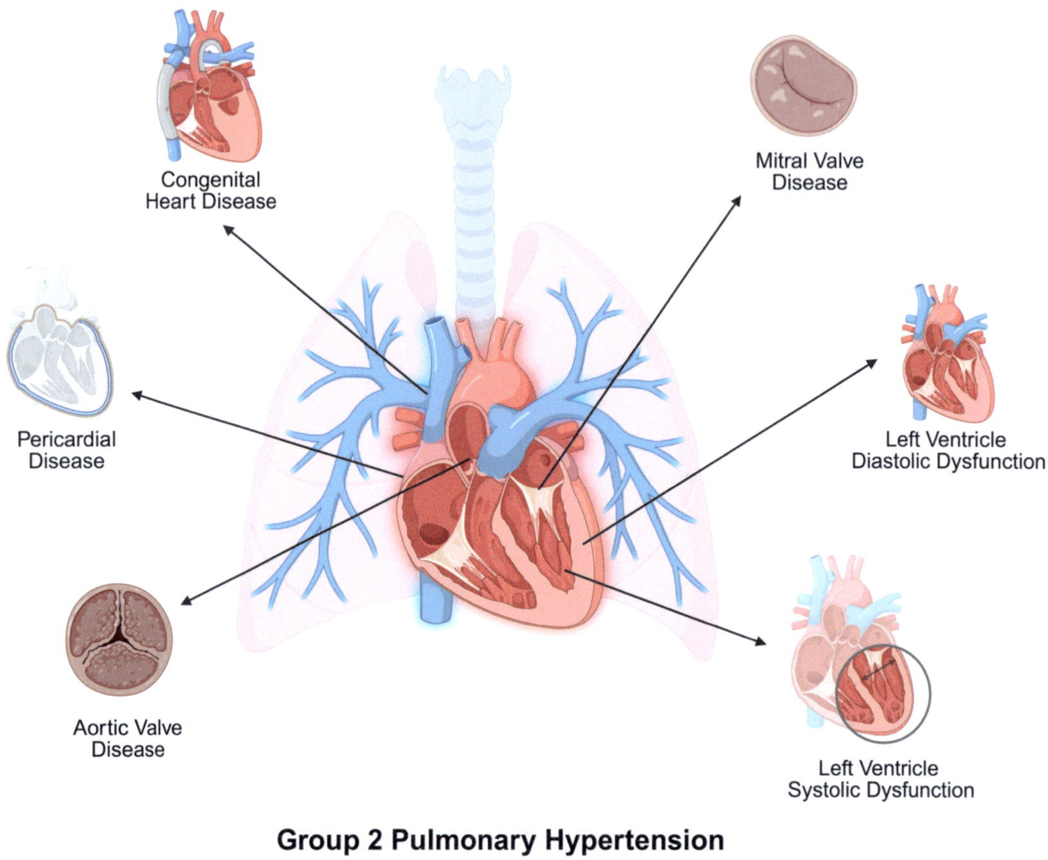

Fig. 16.1 Etiology of Group 2 pulmonary hypertension. (Created in BioRender. Patel, T. (2025) https://BioRender.com/v79ytxe)

tion, especially in PH due to left heart disease, although these are not required for the primary definition (Fig. 16.1).

Etiology and Pathophysiology

Group 2 PH can be related to left ventricular systolic dysfunction (Heart failure with reduced ejection fraction—HFrEF), left ventricular diastolic dysfunction (Heart failure with preserved ejection fraction—HFpEF), left heart related valvular disorders i.e. mitral stenosis, mitral regurgitation, aortic stenosis, aortic regurgitation or congenital heart disease. It involves a sequence of hemodynamic and structural changes in the pulmonary circulation. Long standing increased in left atrial pressure leads to passive increase in pulmonary venous pressure. This causes vasoconstriction in pulmonary capillaries leading to PH. At histopathological level, there is a scarcity of data in patients with group 2 PH compared to group 1 PH. One small study looking at histopathology found evidence of more prominent intimal thickening of pulmonary veins compared to pulmonary arteries. Venous remodeling was co-relating with severity of pulmonary hypertension [7]. In Ipc-PH, persistently elevated left sided atrial or ventricular filling pressure is primary hemodynamic insult leading to PH. This causes increased pulmonary venous and capillary pressure leading to increase in mPAP without increasing PVR. Pulmonary vasculature remains largely un-remodeled and right ventricular afterload is related to elevated left sided filling pressure [8–11]. Whereas in patients with Cpc-PH, there is further development of pulmonary vascular disease due to vasoconstriction and abnormal remodeling of pulmonary vasculature [12]. This

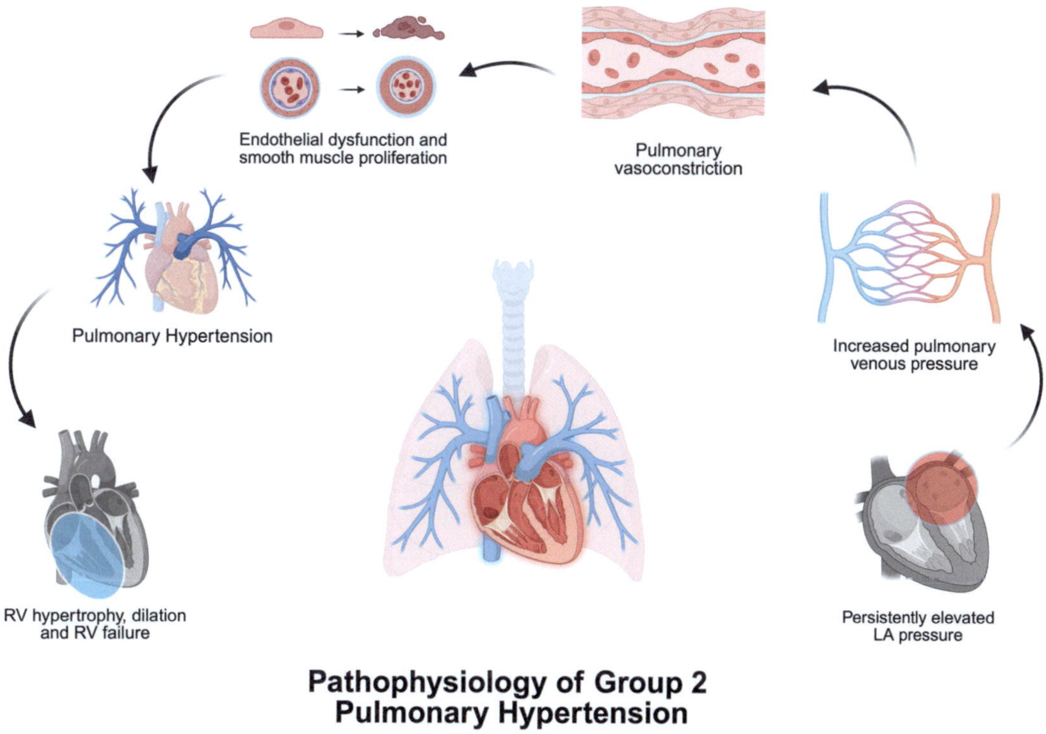

Fig. 16.2 Pathophysiology of Group 2 pulmonary hypertension. (Created in BioRender. Patel, T. (2025) https://BioRender.com/88ihlcs)

leads to endothelial dysfunction, smooth muscle cell proliferation, vasoconstriction and fibrosis [13]. This leads to increased PVR, and it adds pre-capillary component to PH. The elevation in mPAP is out of proportion to increased left sided filling pressure [14]. This long-standing elevated after-load causes right ventricle hypertrophy, dilation and subsequent right ventricle failure [15]. In patients with end stage bi-ventricular failure mPAP may drop significantly without marked change in PVR related to decreased RV stroke volume. Based on some studies there is a signal towards genetic predisposition causing Cpc-PH [16]. Central or obstructive sleep apnea may exacerbate PH from hypoxemia. Progression of Ipc-PH to Cpc-PH is associated with marked worsening of symptoms, impaired exercise capacity and increased mortality [6]. It is mainly related to decreased compliance of pulmonary vasculature and worsening of right ventricular function related to right ventricular-pulmonary artery uncoupling (Fig. 16.2).

Clinical Presentation

The symptoms and signs of pulmonary hypertension due to Group 2 pulmonary hypertension are generally nonspecific and overlap with those of underlying heart failure. The most common symptoms are exertional dyspnea and fatigue. Other symptoms include orthopnea, paroxysmal nocturnal dyspnea, lower extremity edema. In very advanced cases patients may present with syncope or chest discomfort. These symptoms reflect both elevated left-sided filling pressures and, in more advanced disease, right ventricular dysfunction and impaired cardiac output [6, 9, 11, 17, 18].

On physical examination, patients mainly present with signs of right sided heart failure. It includes elevated jugular venous pressure, peripheral edema, hepatic congestion and ascites. A loud P2 (accentuated pulmonary component of the second heart sound), right ventricular heave, and tricuspid regurgitation murmur may be present, especially in CpcPH, where pulmonary vascular resistance is elevated and right ventricular dysfunction is more pronounced as discussed above [6, 13].

In IpcPH, symptoms and signs are often dominated by left-sided heart failure, and it has less prominent findings of right-sided findings. Patients with CpcPH are more likely to exhibit severe exercise intolerance abd pronounced right heart failure signs. Sometimes patients often have worsening hypoxia and reduced exercise capacity. It suggests impaired oxygen delivery and gas exchange. The presence of CpcPH is associated with more severe right ventricular dysfunction and a worse prognosis compared to IpcPH [13].

Diagnostic Approach

The recommended diagnostic approach for Group 2 pulmonary hypertension begins with noninvasive assessment which includes blood work, echocardiogram and advanced imaging. It is usually confirmed by invasive hemodynamic evaluation i.e. right heart catheterization (RHC).

Echocardiography is the primary screening tool to estimate pulmonary artery systolic pressure, assess left ventricular systolic and diastolic function, and identify left-sided valvular disease [19]. It also evaluates right ventricular size and function and can help distinguish Group 2 PH from other etiologies by identifying features of left heart disease [20]. Biomarkers like Natriuretic peptides (BNP, NT-proBNP) are often elevated in left heart disease and support the diagnosis of heart failure but are not specific for PH etiology [9]. Cardiac MRI or CT may be considered in select cases for further anatomical and functional assessment, particularly when echocardiographic windows are suboptimal or when additional structural information is needed. Invasive hemodynamic evaluation with RHC is required for definitive diagnosis and classification of pulmonary hypertension [19]. It helps to define the subtype of group 2 PH by defining the pulmonary vascular resistance (PVR), PCWP and mPAP [9]. As discussed above in patients with group 2 PH has mPAP >20 mmHg, PCWP >15 mmHg. PVR further classifies it into two subtypes based on PVR. Accurate measurement of PCWP is critical to differentiate. Transducer must be at zero level. It is usually at the level of midthoracic or halfway between anterior sternum and bed surface in supine position. It aligns with left atrium [21]. PCWP should be measured at the end of expiration. If there is fluctuation in PCWP then mean of 3 readings should be obtained. Several factors can affect the measurement of PCWP and hence the diagnosis of PH [22]. In patients whom reliable PCWP cannot be assessed left ventricular end-diastolic pressure (LVEDP) may be used. In patient with borderline hemodynamics or suspected HFpEF, a special consideration should be given to fluid challenge or exercise testing during RHC to unmask underlying post-capillary PH. Vasoreactivity testing is not routinely recommended in Group 2 PH [19]. Accurate hemodynamic assessment is critical to distinguish Group 2 PH from Group 1 PAH, as management strategies differ substantially.

Management Strategies

Primary management of Group 2 PH is based upon underlying etiology. It focuses on optimizing hemodynamics, as this form of PH is due to a consequence of elevated left-sided filling pressures, with or without evidence of secondary pulmonary vascular remodeling [10, 22].

Guideline-directed medical therapy for the underlying left heart disease is the cornerstone of management. For patients who has evidence of volume overload, aggressive diuretics improves symptoms of dyspnea by controlling congestion. There is strong evidence suggesting use of ACE inhibitors [23] or ARBs, [24] beta-blockers, [25] mineralocorticoid receptor antagonists, [26] SGLT2 inhibitors, [27] and sacubitril/valsartan, [28] tailored to the specific heart failure phenotype (HFrEF or HFpEF), in reducing re-hospitalization, mortality and/or improvement in quality of life [29, 30]. It is also important to manage comorbidities such as sleep apnea, obesity to further optimize state of hypoxemia and inflammation respectively. GLP-1RA has shown significant impact by promoting weight loss and reducing the state of inflammation related to obesity in various subset of population [31]. In patients with significant mitral valve disease or aortic valve disease, timely surgical or percutaneous intervention is indicated to relieve left-sided pressure overload which may reduce pulmonary pressures [29, 30]. For refractory or advanced cases related to group 2 PH, early referral to advanced heart failure centers is recommended for consideration of advanced therapies, including mechanical circulatory support or heart transplantation.

Pulmonary arterial hypertension (PAH) targeting agents like endothelin receptor antagonists, prostanoids, phosphodiesterase-5 inhibitors, and soluble guanylate cyclase stimulators are not recommended to be used routinely in Group 2 PH. There are several randomized trials and systematic reviews, which have shown no clinically significant benefit. In some cases, their use is associated with potential harm related to increased risk of pulmonary edema or fluid retention. There is very limited evidence suggesting use of sildenafil or riociguat in group 2 PH patients. It may improve hemodynamics or exercise capacity in select patients with combined pre- and post-capillary PH (CpcPH), but these findings are not robust enough to support routine use, and such therapy should only be considered in highly selected cases with close monitoring for adverse effects. The risk of precipitating pulmonary edema is particularly high in patients with elevated left-sided filling pressures [9, 22, 32, 33].

There are emerging and device-based therapies under investigation. Pulmonary artery pressure sensors (e.g., CardioMEMS) have demonstrated utility in selected heart failure patients by enabling remote hemodynamic monitoring and guiding therapy adjustments, which may help reduce pulmonary pressures and hospitalizations. Interatrial shunt devices designed to decompress the left atrium are being studied, but their safety and efficacy remain uncertain, especially in patients with even mild elevations in PVR, where they may worsen right heart failure. In advanced or refractory cases, left ventricular assist devices (LVADs) can reduce left-sided pressures and may facilitate reverse remodeling of the pulmonary vasculature. In some cases, LVADs are combined with pulmonary vasodilators to optimize PVR prior to heart transplantation. Enrollment in clinical trials is encouraged for patients with persistent PH despite optimal management, particularly those with CpcPH [29, 30, 33].

There is scope for further research. It will be helpful to identify subgroups of group 2 PH that can benefit from targeted therapies, assessing long-term safety and efficacy of device-based interventions. The management of pediatric patients with Group 2 PH also needs to more research. So overall current consensus emphasizes that the mainstay of therapy for Group 2 PH is optimal management of the underlying left heart disease and PAH-targeted therapies reserved only for select cases [8, 22, 33].

Prognosis and Outcomes

Prognosis is particularly poor in patients with the combined pre- and post-capillary PH (CpcPH) phenotype. Even mild elevations in PVR (>2 WU) confer increased risk.

The American Heart Association states that CpcPH is observed in approximately 12% of heart failure patients and is associated with increased mortality compared to IpcPH [6]. CpcPH is associated with higher rates of right ventricular dysfunction, heart failure hospitalizations, and all-cause mortality [4, 18, 34, 35]. In large cohorts, CpcPH patients found to have increased two-fold risk of adverse cardiac events compared to IpcPH. It holds true even after adjustment for confounders. This holds true across different etiologies, including heart failure (both HFrEF and HFpEF), valvular disease, and congenital left-sided lesions [22].

Group 2 PH can impact quality of life, functional status, and the risk of progression to right heart failure. Management should focus on optimizing therapy for the underlying left heart disease as discussed above because pulmonary arterial hypertension-targeted therapies have not demonstrated benefit yet and may be harmful in this population.

Key prognostic markers in this population include PVR, diastolic pressure gradient (DPG), pulmonary arterial compliance, and natriuretic peptide levels (e.g., NT-proBNP). Elevated PVR and DPG are strongly associated with right ventricular dysfunction and poor outcomes. Reduced pulmonary arterial compliance and elevated NT-proBNP independently predict mortality. The presence of CpcPH, right ventricular dysfunction, and persistent elevation of these hemodynamic markers identify patients at highest risk [3, 6].

Future Directions and Research

There are gaps in evidence related to the optimal management of patients with persistent PH after successful valvular intervention. There are also uncertainties regarding the role of device-based therapies and understanding which subgroups of Group 2 PH will benefit from novel treatments. Ongoing research is needed to clarify these issues so that we can improve long-term outcomes in high-risk population.

Major emphasis should be given to refine clinical phenotypes, especially distinguishing between IpcPH and CpcPH. Developing a staging systems may help to better capture disease progression and therapeutic windows. This includes individualized hemodynamic assessment to recognise unique subtypes such as PH in hypertrophic or amyloid cardiomyopathy and PH associated with specific valvular disease [3, 35]. There are multiple ongoing research looking in to molecular pathways that are involved in pulmonary vascular remodeling, fibrosis, oxidative stress, and metabolic dysfunction. Identifying these pathways and finding targets to reverse or modify these can be a potential therapeutic targets. Current and recent clinical trials are evaluating agents such as soluble guanylate cyclase stimulators (e.g., vericiguat, riociguat), phosphodiesterase-5 inhibitors (e.g., sildenafil), and prostanoids (e.g., treprostinil), particularly in pediatric and advanced heart failure populations. However, pulmonary vasodilators remain investigational due to the risk of worsening left-sided congestion due to pulmonary edema. It has also not shown consistent benefit in adults as discussed above [33, 35, 36]. Device-based strategies to monitor pulmonary artery pressure monitoring in seated position like Cordella™ PA Sensor System [37] and interventional strategies like interatrial or coronary sinus shunt devices to optimize hemodynamics and reduce left atrial pressure are ongoing [38]. These approaches are being tested in select patient populations, but safety concerns and identifying right patient population still needs further investigation. Methodological innovations have helped to identify need for pragmatic clinical trial designs, next-generation analytics, and broader inclusion of left heart disease patients in research to address the heterogeneity of Group 2 PH and to identify subgroups most likely to benefit from novel interventions [33]. The American Heart Association highlights the need for dedicated studies of pulmonary vasodilators and device-based therapies in children with Group 2 PH, as current evidence is limited and safety profiles are not well established.

Overall, the field is moving toward individualized, phenotype-driven approaches, with ongoing trials and translational research aimed at identifying safe and effective therapies for high-risk subgroups within Group 2 PH.

References

1. Simonneau G, Montani D, Celermajer DS, et al. Haemodynamic definitions and updated clinical classification of pulmonary hypertension. Eur Respir J. 2019;53(1):1801913. https://doi.org/10.1183/13993003.01913-2018. Published 2019 Jan 24.
2. Brusca SB, Zou Y, Elinoff JM. How low should we go? Potential benefits and ramifications of the pulmonary hypertension hemodynamic definitions proposed by the 6th World Symposium. Curr Opin Pulm Med. 2020;26(5):384–90. https://doi.org/10.1097/MCP.0000000000000699.
3. Maron BA. Revised definition of pulmonary hypertension and approach to management: a clinical primer. J Am Heart Assoc. 2023;12(8):e029024. https://doi.org/10.1161/JAHA.122.029024.

4. Caravita S, Faini A, Carolino D'Araujo S, et al. Clinical phenotypes and outcomes of pulmonary hypertension due to left heart disease: role of the pre-capillary component. PLoS One. 2018;13(6):e0199164. https://doi.org/10.1371/journal.pone.0199164. Published 2018 Jun 19.
5. Kovacs G, Bartolome S, Denton CP, et al. Definition, classification and diagnosis of pulmonary hypertension. Eur Respir J. 2024;64(4):2401324. https://doi.org/10.1183/13993003.01324-2024. Published 2024 Oct 31
6. Konstam MA, Kiernan MS, Bernstein D, et al. Evaluation and management of right-sided heart failure: a scientific statement from the American Heart Association. Circulation. 2018;137(20):e578–622. https://doi.org/10.1161/CIR.0000000000000560.
7. Fayyaz AU, Edwards WD, Maleszewski JJ, et al. Global pulmonary vascular remodeling in pulmonary hypertension associated with heart failure and preserved or reduced ejection fraction. Circulation. 2018;137(17):1796–810. https://doi.org/10.1161/CIRCULATIONAHA.117.031608.
8. Ltaief Z, Yerly P, Liaudet L. Pulmonary hypertension in left heart diseases: pathophysiology, hemodynamic assessment and therapeutic management. Int J Mol Sci. 2023;24(12):9971. https://doi.org/10.3390/ijms24129971. Published 2023 Jun 9.
9. Al-Omary MS, Sugito S, Boyle AJ, Sverdlov AL, Collins NJ. Pulmonary hypertension due to left heart disease: diagnosis, pathophysiology, and therapy. Hypertension. 2020;75(6):1397–408. https://doi.org/10.1161/HYPERTENSIONAHA.119.14330.
10. Riley JM, Fradin JJ, Russ DH, Warner ED, Brailovsky Y, Rajapreyar I. Post-capillary pulmonary hypertension: clinical review. J Clin Med. 2024;13(2):625. https://doi.org/10.3390/jcm13020625. Published 2024 Jan 22
11. van de Veerdonk MC, Roosma L, Trip P, et al. Clinical-imaging-pathological correlation in pulmonary hypertension associated with left heart disease. Eur Respir Rev. 2024;33(171):230144. https://doi.org/10.1183/16000617.0144-2023. Published 2024 Feb 28
12. Huston JH, Shah SJ. Understanding the pathobiology of pulmonary hypertension due to left heart disease. Circ Res. 2022;130(9):1382–403. https://doi.org/10.1161/CIRCRESAHA.122.319967.
13. Omote K, Sorimachi H, Obokata M, et al. Pulmonary vascular disease in pulmonary hypertension due to left heart disease: pathophysiologic implications. Eur Heart J. 2022;43(36):3417–31. https://doi.org/10.1093/eurheartj/ehac184.
14. Hsu S, Houston BA, Tampakakis E, et al. Right ventricular functional reserve in pulmonary arterial hypertension. Circulation. 2016;133(24):2413–22. https://doi.org/10.1161/CIRCULATIONAHA.116.022082.
15. Melenovsky V, Hwang SJ, Lin G, Redfield MM, Borlaug BA. Right heart dysfunction in heart failure with preserved ejection fraction. Eur Heart J. 2014;35(48):3452–62. https://doi.org/10.1093/eurheartj/ehu193.
16. Assad TR, Hemnes AR, Larkin EK, et al. Clinical and biological insights into combined post- and pre-capillary pulmonary hypertension. J Am Coll Cardiol. 2016;68(23):2525–36. https://doi.org/10.1016/j.jacc.2016.09.942.
17. Inampudi C, Silverman D, Simon MA, et al. Pulmonary hypertension in the context of heart failure with preserved ejection fraction. Chest. 2021;160(6):2232–46. https://doi.org/10.1016/j.chest.2021.08.039.
18. Lee F, Mielniczuk LM. Pulmonary hypertension due to left heart disease-a practical approach to diagnosis and management. Can J Cardiol. 2021;37(4):572–84. https://doi.org/10.1016/j.cjca.2020.11.003.
19. Charalampopoulos A, Lewis R, Hickey P, et al. Pathophysiology and diagnosis of pulmonary hypertension due to left heart disease. Front Med (Lausanne). 2018;5:174. https://doi.org/10.3389/fmed.2018.00174. Published 2018 Jun 6
20. Maeder MT, Schoch OD, Kleiner R, Joerg L, Weilenmann D, Swiss Society For Pulmonary Hypertension. Pulmonary hypertension associated with left-sided heart disease. Swiss Med Wkly. 2017;147:w14395. https://doi.org/10.57187/smw.2017.14395. Published 2017 Jan 17.
21. Kovacs G, Avian A, Pienn M, Naeije R, Olschewski H. Reading pulmonary vascular pressure tracings. How to handle the problems of zero leveling and respiratory swings. Am J Respir Crit Care Med. 2014;190(3):252–7. https://doi.org/10.1164/rccm.201402-0269PP.
22. Maron BA, Bortman G, De Marco T, et al. Pulmonary hypertension associated with left heart disease. Eur Respir J. 2024;64(4):2401344. https://doi.org/10.1183/13993003.01344-2024. Published 2024 Oct 31
23. Packer M, Poole-Wilson PA, Armstrong PW, et al. Comparative effects of low and high doses of the angiotensin-converting enzyme inhibitor, lisinopril, on morbidity and mortality in chronic heart failure. ATLAS Study Group Circ. 1999;100(23):2312–8. https://doi.org/10.1161/01.cir.100.23.2312.
24. Willenheimer R. Angiotensin receptor blockers in heart failure after the ELITE II trial. Curr Control Trials Cardiovasc Med. 2000;1(2):79–82. https://doi.org/10.1186/cvm-1-2-079. PMID: 11714415; PMCID: PMC59604.
25. Eichhorn EJ, Bristow MR. The carvedilol prospective randomized cumulative survival (COPERNICUS) trial. Curr Control Trials Cardiovasc Med. 2001;2(1):20–3. https://doi.org/10.1186/cvm-2-1-020. PMID: 11806769; PMCID: PMC59648.
26. Pitt B, Zannad F, Remme WJ, et al. The effect of spironolactone on morbidity and mortality in patients with severe heart failure. Randomized Aldactone Evaluation Study Investigators. N Engl J Med. 1999;341(10):709–17. https://doi.org/10.1056/NEJM199909023411001.

27. Talha KM, Anker SD, Butler J. SGLT-2 Inhibitors in heart failure: a review of current evidence. Int J Heart Fail. 2023;5(2):82–90. https://doi.org/10.36628/ijhf.2022.0030. PMID: 37180562; PMCID: PMC10172076.
28. Gronda E, Vanoli E, Iacoviello M. The PARAGON-HF trial: the sacubitril/valsartan in heart failure with preserved ejection fraction. Eur Heart J Suppl. 2020;22(Suppl L):L77–81. https://doi.org/10.1093/eurheartj/suaa140. PMID: 33727901; PMCID: PMC7944492.
29. Frantz RP. Group 2 pulmonary hypertension: from diagnosis to treatment. Curr Opin Pulm Med. 2023;29(5):391–8. https://doi.org/10.1097/MCP.0000000000001002.
30. Kennedy JLW, Mihalek AD. Update in approaches to pulmonary hypertension because of left heart disease. Curr Opin Pulm Med. 2022;28(5):337–42. https://doi.org/10.1097/MCP.0000000000000891.
31. Waqas SA, Sohail MU, Saad M, et al. Efficacy of GLP-1 receptor agonists in patients with heart failure and mildly reduced or preserved ejection fraction: a systematic review and meta-analysis. J Card Fail. 2025; https://doi.org/10.1016/j.cardfail.2025.01.022. Published online February 22 2025.
32. Kido K, Coons JC. Efficacy and safety of the use of pulmonary arterial hypertension pharmacotherapy in patients with pulmonary hypertension secondary to left heart disease: a systematic review. Pharmacotherapy. 2019;39(9):929–45. https://doi.org/10.1002/phar.2314.
33. Hopper RK, Hansmann G, Hollander SA, et al. Clinical management and transplant considerations in pediatric pulmonary hypertension due to left heart disease: a scientific statement from the American Heart Association. Circ Heart Fail. 2025;18(1):e000086. https://doi.org/10.1161/HHF.0000000000000086.
34. Ibe T, Wada H, Sakakura K, et al. Combined pre- and post-capillary pulmonary hypertension: the clinical implications for patients with heart failure. PLoS One. 2021;16(3):e0247987. https://doi.org/10.1371/journal.pone.0247987. Published 2021 Mar 2
35. Awada C, Boucherat O, Provencher S, Bonnet S, Potus F. The future of group 2 pulmonary hypertension: exploring clinical trials and therapeutic targets. Vasc Pharmacol. 2023;151:107180. https://doi.org/10.1016/j.vph.2023.107180.
36. Lteif C, Ataya A, Duarte JD. Therapeutic challenges and emerging treatment targets for pulmonary hypertension in left heart disease. J Am Heart Assoc. 2021;10(11):e020633. https://doi.org/10.1161/JAHA.120.020633.
37. Guichard JL, Bonno EL, Nassif ME, et al. Seated pulmonary artery pressure monitoring in patients with heart failure: results of the PROACTIVE-HF Trial. JACC Heart Fail. 2024;12(11):1879–93. https://doi.org/10.1016/j.jchf.2024.05.017.
38. Stone GW, Lindenfeld J, Rodés-Cabau J, et al. Interatrial shunt treatment for heart failure: the randomized RELIEVE-HF Trial. Circulation. 2024;150(24):1931–43. https://doi.org/10.1161/CIRCULATIONAHA.124.070870.

Cardiac Amyloidosis

17

Chukwuemezie Kamanu, Sawan Dutta,
Avish Patel, and Yevgeniy Brailovsky

Introduction

Amyloidosis describes a group of diseases characterized by the tissue deposition of amyloid fibrils—misfolded proteins or protein fragments that have aggregated and stabilized in primarily beta-pleated sheet configuration. This can disrupt the tissue structure and subsequently alter organ function [1].

Infiltration of the myocardium by amyloid fibrils leads to restrictive cardiomyopathy and heart failure, known as Amyloid Cardiomyopathy [2]. This progressive loss of function disrupts the cardiac conduction system, increasing the risk of arrhythmias [3]. Cardiac amyloidosis is primarily caused by two major subtypes: light chain (AL) amyloidosis and transthyretin (ATTR) amyloidosis, which account for over 95% of the cardiac amyloidosis cases. ATTR amyloidosis can be further characterized into wild type (ATTRwt) and variant type (ATTRv). AA amyloidosis is another form of the disease associated with chronic inflammatory conditions. This is a rare cause of cardiac amyloidosis. Cardiac amyloidosis remains underdiagnosed. There have been substantial recent advances in disease modifying therapeutics, with associated improvement in morbidity and mortality. As such, there is a renewed interest in improved screening techniques, non-invasive diagnostic strategies, and earlier identification of disease [1, 4]. In this review we aim to explore the epidemiology of amyloidosis, pathophysiology, diagnostic strategies, and advancements in therapeutic targets.

C. Kamanu · S. Dutta · A. Patel
Department of Internal Medicine, Thomas Jefferson University Hospital, Philadelphia, PA, USA
e-mail: Chukwuemezie.Kamanu@jefferson.edu; sawan.dutta@jefferson.edu; Avish.Patel@jefferson.edu

Y. Brailovsky (✉)
Division of Cardiology, Columbia University, New York, NY, USA
e-mail: yevgeniy.brailovsky@jefferson.edu

H. J. Eisen (ed.), *Heart Failure I*, https://doi.org/10.1007/978-3-032-12626-9_17

Nomenclature

The Nomenclature for amyloidosis was made by the Nomenclature Committee of the International Society of Amyloidosis (ISA). They based the system on the biochemical makeup of the specific amyloid fibril protein involved in each subtype [5, 6]. Each type of amyloidosis is named starting with the prefix "A" and then the abbreviation of the specific precursor protein involved. For example, the serum amyloid A protein causes AA amyloidosis, immunoglobulin light chains cause AL amyloidosis, and the transthyretin protein causes ATTR amyloidosis [6]. ATTR has two types, the wild-type known as "ATTRwt" and the variant-type "ATTRv" named based on the genetics of the transthyretin protein [7]. Notably, ATTRwt, used to be called "senile amyloidosis", but that has fallen out of favor. Similarly, ATTRv used to be called hereditary ATTR.

The abbreviations for cardiomyopathies associated with amyloidosis are AL-CM for AL amyloid cardiomyopathy and ATTR-CM for ATTR amyloid cardiomyopathy. These are the typical nomenclature used when mentioning the clinical impact of each type of amyloidosis on the heart. Classification is crucial as specific management strategies differ based the type of amyloid protein and organ involvement.

Epidemiology

Incidence and prevalence varies widely among different forms of cardiac amyloidosis.

ATTRwt is more prevalent in older adults diagnosed in the 8th or 9th decade but can also be seen as early as 5th decade [8]. ATTR exhibits male predominance compared to AL [8]. Notably, ATTRwt primarily affects the heart [1, 9].

There are over 120 TTR gene mutations that can lead to ATTRv with substantial geographical variation. Approximately 3–4% of African American population carries a TTR gene mutation (Val122Ile), which increases their risk of cardiac amyloidosis [10]. Distinct mutations can influence age of onset and organ-specific involvement. Certain regions such as Portugal, Sweden, and Japan also carry higher frequency of certain mutations [10].

Cardiac involvement specifically in relation to ATTR has been associated with the Ile68Leu and Leu111Met mutations [11]. The V122I mutation is the most frequent in the US, affecting 3–3.5% of African Americans [12]. In contrast, the Val30Met variant is the most prevalent form of ATTR in Europe [11]. Endemic populations in Portugal, Brazil, and Japan with early-onset Val30Met disease typically present with a neurological phenotype, with frequent disease onset occurring in the thirties and forties [11].

Incidence

Amyloidosis diagnosis is likely increasing due to improved techniques and heightened awareness. A report from the United States suggests an annual incidence of AL at approximately 12 cases per million population [13]. This translates to an incidence of about 2500 to 5000 cases of AL in the United States per year [14].

Limited data hinders accurate national estimates. Incidence data from France (2011–2019) suggests a rise in ATTR cardiomyopathy (0.6–3.6 per 100,000 person-years), mirroring the potential trend in the US with improved diagnostics [15]. ATTRv is rarer than AL amyloidosis, with a typical onset in the 6th decade. ATTRwt, often undiagnosed, was found in 25% of elderly males in one autopsy study [9]. Overall cardiac amyloidosis incidence in the US (2000–2012) was 36.5 per 100,000 person-years [16], with a rise observed in older adults and African Americans, likely due to a combination of AL and ATTR types [9].

Prevalence

Improved diagnostics and heightened awareness likely contribute to the increasing prevalence of amyloidosis [17]. AL prevalence is estimated at 1:25,000 [18] with 30,000–45,000 cases in the

US [13]. In contrast, ATTR prevalence is higher (155–191 cases/million for ATTRwt and 5.2 cases/million for ATTRv Prevalence also increased with age with most patients diagnosed over 60 and ATTRwt predominantly affecting males [13, 19].

Historical Outcomes

AL generally carries a worse prognosis than ATTR with a median survival is significantly lower for AL (1-year: 43.3%, 3-year: 40.4%, 5-year: 35.4%) compared to ATTR (1-year: 85.1%, 3-year:57.3%, 5-year: 31.4%) [20]. Unadjusted 5-year mortality rates are also higher for AL cardiac amyloidosis (65%) compared to ATTR cardiac amyloidosis (44%) [20].

Within ATTR, the wild type is more common in older patients with overall better prognosis than the hereditary form [12]. The median survival in the ATTRwt is 3–6 years since the time of diagnosis. Outcomes are worse in relation to factors such as elevated N-terminal-pro-B-type natriuretic peptide, troponin T levels, and pericardial effusions [21].

ATTRwt has a better prognosis than ATTRv (median survival 3–6 years) [12, 22]. Untreated ATTR rapidly progresses to heart failure, conduction abnormalities, and arrhythmias, with cardiac complications being the leading cause of death [10, 12]. The Val122Ile mutation is associated with a median survival of 2.5 years if left untreated [23]. Other variant mutations fare better (median survival 5.8 years) [12, 21].

The median survival for AL is about 6 months with cardiac involvement [21, 24]. Fortunately, advancements in treatment have significantly improved outcomes, with some patients now living over 10 years [25, 26]. The degree of cardiac involvement remains a key prognostic factor. Compared to AL, ATTR is generally associated with a better prognosis due to more indolent course and emergence of disease-modifying therapies [27].

Select patients with cardiac amyloidosis may benefit from heart transplantation. Post-transplantation outcomes are better with patients with ATTR amyloidosis when compared with AL. After heart transplant, 1 year survival rate is 83% for AL patients in comparison to 94% for ATTR [28]. Historically, post heart transplant outcomes have been substantially worse for patients with amyloidosis as compared to other forms of cardiomyopathy, but in recent years, this gap has closed and now associated with similar outcomes [29]. Overall median survival after heart transplant for patients with Amyloid related cardiomyopathy improved to 10.2 years [30].

Pathophysiology

The pathophysiology of amyloidosis impact on the tissues is caused by extracellular deposition of the protein fibrils [14]. The proteins misfold, aggregate, and deposit as fibrils made of amyloid protein leading to altered tissue architecture and subsequent organ involvement [14]. While the impact of amyloid tissue deposition in the tissues may be similar, the exact pathophysiology varies drastically between different forms of amyloidosis (Fig. 17.1).

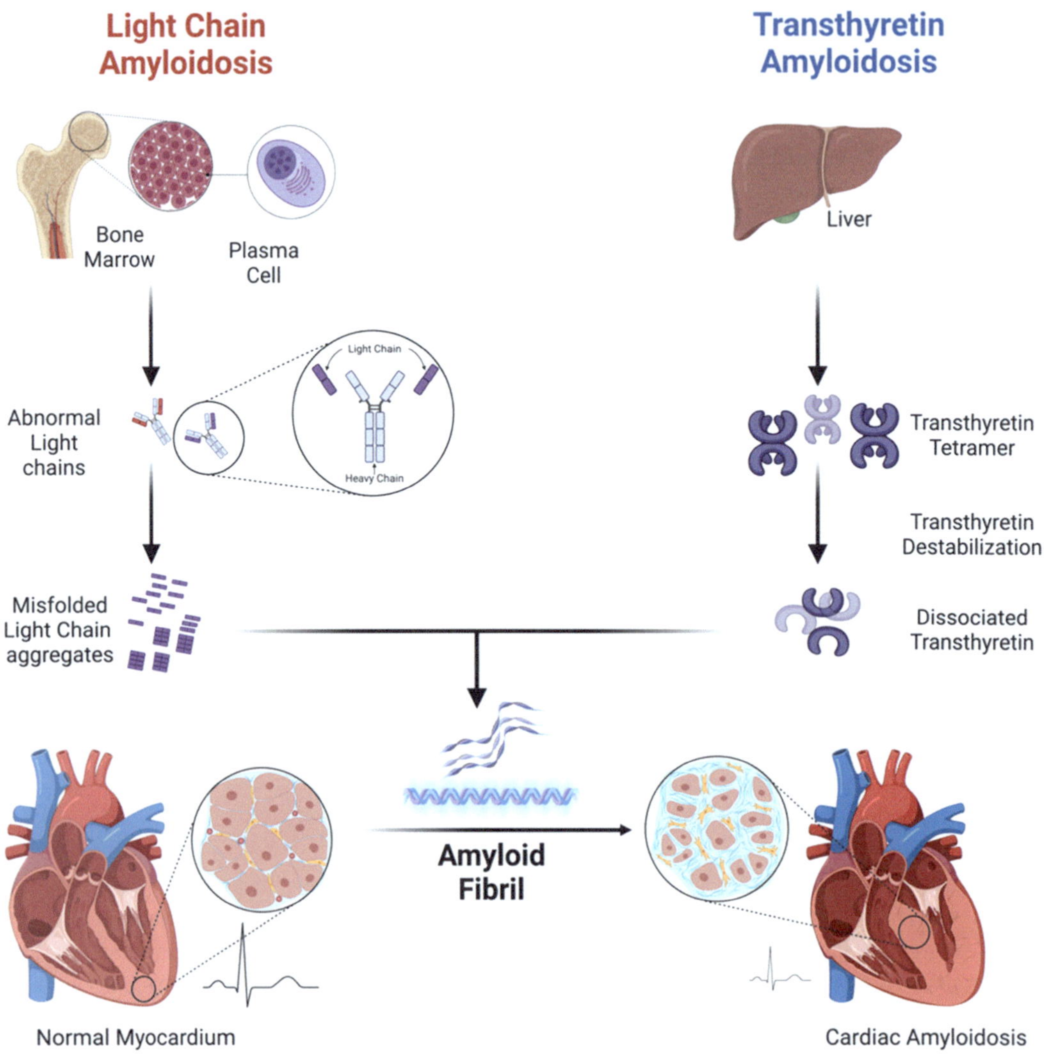

Fig. 17.1 Pathophysiology of light chain and transthyretin amyloidosis. (Figure created with BioRender.com)

AL

AL is caused by deposits of misfolded monoclonal immunoglobulin light chains. This is a systemic disorder involving extracellular deposition of these fibrils [12, 21]. The monoclonal light chains are made from small B-cell clones which are usually plasma cells in the bone marrow. The plasma cells secrete the monoclonal free light chains that lead to fibril formation [31].

Misfolded light chain immunoglobulins aggregate into amyloid fibrils [32]. The fibrils deposit in organs like the heart, kidney, liver, nerves, and others [31, 32]. The deposits disrupt organ structure and function, leading to clinical signs and symptoms [31, 32]. Additionally, light chains directly impact organ function through oxidative stress and cell death pathways [33].

These mechanisms often lead to multiorgan involvement with heart involvement in over 50% of cases. The syndrome leads to restrictive cardiomyopathy and arrhythmias with cardiac involvement, kidney injury and nephrotic syndrome with renal involvement, and peripheral neuropathy with nerve involvement [32].

ATTR

The transthyretin protein is made in the liver with a function to transport thyroid hormone and retinol. Transthyretin is homotetrameric protein, which gets destabilized due to either genetic mutations (ATTRv) or intrinsic factors associated with aging (ATTRwt) [34].

Destabilization leads to dissociation from tetramers into unstable monomers and is a rate limiting step in amyloid fibril formation. These misfolded monomers aggregate to form protofibrils and ultimately amyloid fibrils. Factors like pH, proteolytic cleavage, and pre-existing amyloid seeds can influence this process and accelerate fibril formation [35].

ATTR also involves protein deposition and infiltration into organs that phenotipically may present similarly to AL. ATTR mainly involves the heart, peripheral and autonomic systems, but can also have other organ involvement [12].

ATTRv amyloidosis can be caused by >100 mutations in the TTR gene. The mutations increase the probability of TTR protein to misfold and aggregate into amyloid fibrils [12, 36]. The variant type has an autosomal dominant pattern of inheritance. On the other hand, ATTRwt does not have any clear genetic influence and exact pathophysiology is unclear [10, 37].

Clinical Presentation

Cardiac amyloidosis, regardless of its type (AL or ATTR), usually present as a heart failure syndrome due to restrictive cardiomyopathy. This can manifest clinically with peripheral edema, jugular vein distention, ascites, dyspnea, orthopnea, fatigue, and hepatic congestion. Beyond heart failure symptoms, amyloid deposition can disrupt the heart's conduction system, leading to arrhythmias [7]. Cardiac tachy- and brady-arrhythmias are often poorly tolerated due to restrictive nature of cardiomyopathy and patients can present with cardiogenic shock as the initial clinical presentation [38].

While both AL and ATTR share some clinical features, there are subtle differences. AL commonly presents with additional manifestations like nephrotic syndrome, macroglossia, purpura on the eyelids [39]. In contrast, ATTR often involves peripheral neuropathy, spinal stenosis and bicep tendon rupture. Notably, ATTRwt typically affects older adults, who frequently present with new-onset heart failure and commonly atrial arrhythmias [7].

The non-specific nature of symptoms like dyspnea, fatigue, and edema can easily lead to misdiagnosis as another form of heart failure. The wide variability of signs and symptoms across patients makes early detection challenging [7]. A high index of clinical suspicion is crucial for timely workup of suspected amyloidosis, particularly in patients with new-onset heart failure. Because of these diagnostic complexities, the following section will explore specific tools and strategies for diagnosing amyloidosis.

At Risk Populations

Recognition of the clinical characteristics associated with cardiac amyloidosis is essential for diagnosis at early stages of heart disease. A study at the UK National Amyloidosis Center showed that patients used hospital services a median of 17 times during the 3 years prior to diagnosis with ATTR [12]. To mitigate this delay, appropriate identification of at-risk populations is necessary. The recommendations by cardiology societies on when to suspect amyloidosis are outlined in Table 17.1.

Patients often present with symptoms of heart failure and are underdiagnosed despite the fact that approximately 13% of cases of heart failure with preserved ejection fraction (HFpEF) are likely due to ATTR amyloidosis [40]. In addition, in patients with aortic stenosis (AS) up to 15% of patients and 30% of the subset with low-flow low-gradient AS have cardiac amyloidosis [41]. Certain extra cardiac manifestations also should prompt consideration for cardiac amyloidosis. Approximately 10–16% of patients with carpal tunnel have tenosynovial amyloid deposits and about 20% of men >70 yo develop cardiac amyloid 9 years after carpal tunnel surgery [42]. For patients with spinal stenosis undergoing surgery, 13–21% have TTR deposits in ligamentum flavum [43, 44]. Bicep Tendon Rupture occurs in ~33.3% of patients with ATTRwt and only 2.5% of patients with other causes of HF [45] (Fig. 17.2).

Table 17.1 The recommendations by cardiology societies on when to suspect amyloidosis

Society	Features to Suspect Amyloidosis
Canadian Cardiovascular Society 2020	Unexplained increased LV wall thickness Patient >60 years age with low-flow low-gradient AS and LVEF >40% Unexplained neuropathy and/or dysautonomia History of bilateral carpal tunnel syndrome
European Society of Cardiology 2021	Unexplained LVH HF with bilateral carpal tunnel syndrome, peripheral neuropathy, renal dysfunction Aortic stenosis with low-flow, low gradient AS, myocardial granular sparkling, abnormal GLS
American College of Cardiology 2023	Cardiac: increased LV wall thickness in the absence of hypertension or valvular heart disease, HF symptoms, diastolic dysfunction, AF, conduction system disease, elevated cardiac biomarkers Extracardiac: carpal tunnel syndrome, spinal stenosis, hip or knee replacement, prior shoulder surgery, proteinuria, or peripheral/autonomic neuropathy

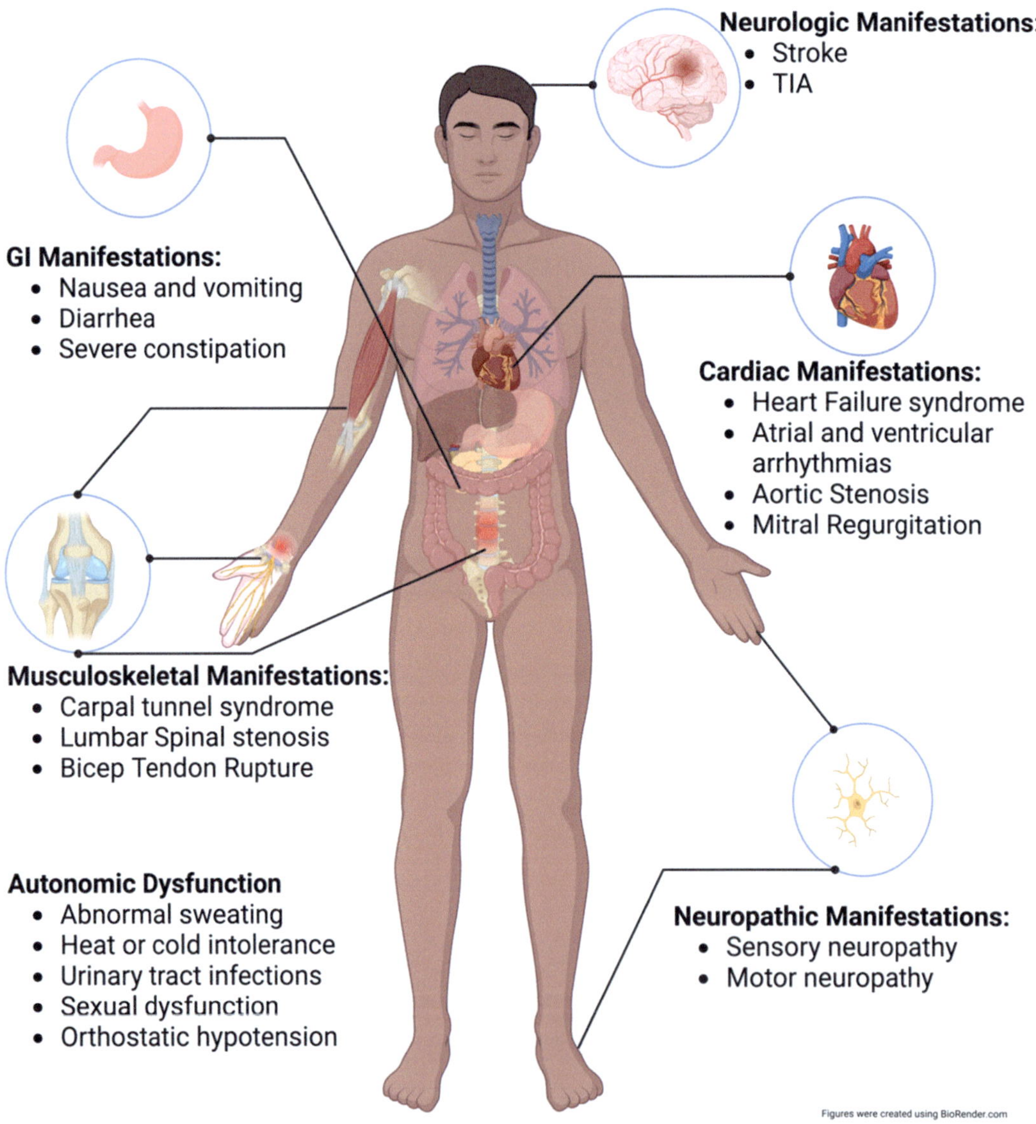

Fig. 17.2 Common cardiac and extra cardiac manifestations of systemic amyloidosis. (Figure created with BioRender.com)

Diagnosis

A combination of clinical, lab, electrocardiographic, and imaging findings help to suggest a need for diagnostic workup of cardiac amyloidosis. Lab findings often show persistent low-level troponin elevation and elevated B-type natriuretic peptide (BNP)/N-terminal proBNP but are nonspecific. Electrocardiogram (ECG) may classically show low and discordant QRS voltage for degree of increased LV wall thickness. However, low QRS voltage (defined as amplitude ≤ 5 mm in limb leads and 10 mm in precordial leads) may only be seen in about 30% of individuals with cardiac amyloidosis and prevalence may be higher later in disease progression [46]. Other ECG abnormalities such as atrial fibrillation, conduction system disease and pseudo-infarct pattern may be present. In ATTR, individuals are more likely to have a left bundle branch block (LBBB) or higher grade AV block [47].

Echocardiogram

Echocardiogram is often the initial step in diagnostic work up that may increase suspicion for cardiac amyloidosis. Typical features include increased biventricular myocardial wall thickness (especially in the absence of other causes of increased thickness), bi-atrial enlargement, diastolic dysfunction, sparkling appearance of the myocardium, and non-dilated LV. Systolic function is often preserved early in the disease course, but may decline as the disease progresses. Left ventricular longitudinal strain is often reduced with apical sparing giving the characteristic "cherry on top" appearance on strain imaging (apical strain to basal-mid average strain ration >1.1). Some have suggested few features on echocardiography that may help differentiate AL and ATTR amyloidosis. LV hypertrophy is typically symmetrical in AL and asymmetric with greater increase in LV and RV masses in ATTR amyloidosis [48]. Nonetheless, echocardiogram is insufficient to definitely rule in or rule out cardiac amyloidosis or differentiate different types with any degree of certainty and more definitive diagnostic strategies are necessary.

Cardiac Magnetic Resonance (CMR)

Cardiac magnetic resonance (CMR) imaging is beneficial for differentiating infiltrative processes and causes of increased wall thickness but cannot differentiate types of amyloid and is not sufficient for diagnosis alone. Characteristic findings are similar to echocardiography with restrictive physiology, diastolic dysfunction, bi-atrial enlargement, and increased myocardial mass and thickening. Gadolinium enhanced sequences typically show diffuse circumferential subendocardial late gadolinium enhancement and inability to null the myocardium. Due to extracellular deposition of amyloid, there is increased longitudinal relaxation time and extracellular volume fraction [49] which are highly sensitive.

Emerging Technologies—PET Imaging

Accurately quantifying cardiac amyloid burden has become increasingly important for understanding therapeutic efficacy and potentially facilitating earlier diagnosis and treatment of cardiac amyloidosis [50, 51]. Traditionally, assessment relies on indirect methods like TTE, CMR, and radionuclide scintigraphy [50].

More specific methods are evolving, including beta-amyloid-binding radiotracers employed in positron emission tomography (PET) that were initially developed for Alzheimer's disease [50, 51]. These radiotracers hold promise for cardiac amyloidosis by enabling direct detection of amyloid fibrils. F-florbetapir, for instance, demonstrates the ability to detect cardiac amyloid even in early stages, although with potentially lower myocardial uptake in ATTR-CM compared to AL-CM [50, 51]. A study investigated a novel radiotracer, I-evuzamitide, demonstrating significantly higher quantitative uptake in the left ventricle (LV) and right ventricle (RV) of participants with either AL-CM or ATTRwt-CM compared to controls [50]. Notably, I-evuzamitide might offer more accurate amyloid quantification in ATTRwt-CM than F-florbetapir [50]. While both F-florbetapir and I-evuzamitide show promise, neither has definitively proven the ability to differentiate between AL and ATTR types. Larger, multicenter studies are crucial to validate these findings and further evaluate the clinical utility of I-evuzamitide PET for early diagnosis and therapeutic monitoring in cardiac amyloidosis.

After initial workup revealing suspicion for cardiac amyloidosis, the first step should be a monoclonal protein screen to assess for plasma cell disorder. This can be done by laboratory testing for serum free light chain (sFLC), serum immunofixation (SIFE) and urine immunofixation (UIFE). A monoclonal protein test is positive if there is an abnormal serum kappa/lambda ratio of <0.26 or >1.65 in the absence of renal disease (normal K/L ratio in severe CKD is 0.54–3.30) or a monoclonal protein was detected on IFE. An elevated K/L ratio can be normal in CKD because healthy kidneys clear more kappa than lambda, while a low K/L ratio is never normal and may suggest a lambda monoclonal process. If a monoclonal protein process is detected, then biopsy of the affected organ is necessary. If no monoclonal protein is detected and sFLC ratio is normal, then Al can be excluded with 99% negative predictive value [34, 52].

If no monoclonal protein is detected and clinical suspicion of ATTR exists, then cardiac scintigraphy with technetium-based compounds (Tc-PYP) and nuclear SPECT is the next best diagnostic step. Grade 2 or 3 cardiac uptake greater than bone or bone to chest wall uptake ratio >1.5 at one-hour is consistent with ATTR [34]. Tc-PYP imaging must always be done with SPECT to confirm myocardial uptake and exclude the possibility of blood pool uptake resulting in false positive result [53]. Notably, AL has poor (10%) or no radioisotope uptake, but AL can result in false positive result, therefore PYP should not be used in patients with plasma cell dyscrasia. Genetic testing is required to distinguish ATTRv from ATTRwt (Fig. 17.3).

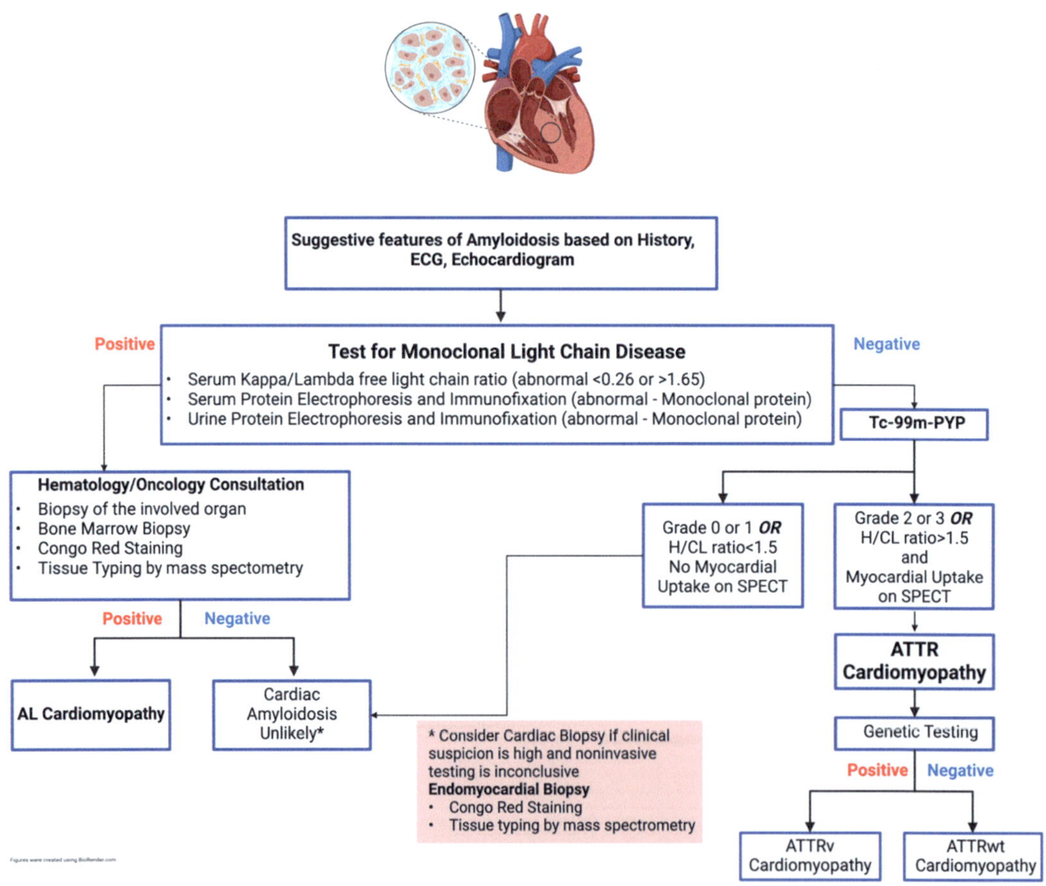

Fig. 17.3 Suggested flowdiagram for diagnosis of cardiac amyloidosis. (Figure created with BioRender.com)

Genetic Testing

Genetic testing and counseling are indicated in individuals with ATTR. There are greater than 100 variants. If a pathogenic or likely pathogenic variant of TTR is identified, first degree relatives should be screened. Evaluation is useful in determining treatment strategies that may be beneficial based on variant. Limitations of genetic testing are that TTR variants show incomplete penetrance and variable expressivity, and by an unclear mechanism, TTR is age dependent and often appears later in life [34].

Role of Tissue Biopsy in Diagnosis

The standard of evaluation includes tissue biopsy to demonstrate presence of amyloid, but endomyocardial biopsy is often not needed. When AL is suspected by the presence of monoclonal protein, biopsy of the involved organ is necessary for confirmative diagnosis. Abdominal fat pad is the least invasive and most common biopsy site but has variable sensitivity for diagnosis (Table 17.2). Endomyocardial biopsy is the gold standard for diagnosis and should be considered when there is a high clinical suspicion of cardiac amyloidosis with abnormal monoclonal protein by IFE and/or K/L ratio above the upper range of normal, high clinical suspicion of ATTR despite negative or equivocal PYP scan or if cardiac scintigraphy is unavailable [54].

Characteristic features on tissue biopsy include light pink amorphous extracellular material on hematoxylin and eosin stain. Amyloid tissue has affinity for Congo red stain and will appear salmon-pink color on light microscopy, while under polarized light the tissue will have pathognomonic apple-green birefringence. These features are common to all forms of amyloidosis and do not distinguish between specific types. All Congo Red positive specimens must be sent for tissue typing using mass spectrometry, which is the gold standard in identifying precise protein composition. Immunohistochemistry and immunofluorescence are antibody-based assays that are helpful in identifying specific types of amyloidosis, but are limited to Anti-TTR, anti-AA, anti-lambda, and anti-kappa antibodies [55].

Table 17.2 Options for biopsy site and their respective sensitivity and specificity to detect amyloidosis

Biopsy site	Diagnostic yield	Indication
Abdominal Fat Pad	Sensitivity is variable with 84% sensitivity for AL, 45% for ATTR variant, and 15% for ATTR wild-type. Sensitivity is also lower if presentation is earlier in disease course. A negative biopsy does not exclude AL or ATTR amyloidosis.	Multi-systemic disease
Bone Marrow	Sensitivity is estimated at 63%.	Detection of a monoclonal protein often prompts bone marrow biopsy to rule out multiple myeloma and assess for amyloid deposition
Endomyocardial biopsy	Sensitivity is estimated at 87–98%. Biopsy shows salmon-colored amyloid fibrils on 'congo-red' stain and 'apple-green' birefringence on electron microscopy.	A definitive diagnosis and subtyping of cardiac amyloidosis (CA) necessitates tissue biopsy, except in cases where a negative monoclonal protein assessment coincides with Grade 2–3 myocardial uptake, indicative of ATTR amyloidosis

Risk Stratification

ATTR

Accurate risk stratification in ATTR is crucial for guiding management and predicting outcomes. Current approaches incorporate clinical, imaging, biomarker, and functional data. Disease progression is typically assessed using a multi-domain framework encompassing clinical, laboratory, and imaging markers [36].

Biomarkers such as N-terminal pro-B-type natriuretic peptide (NT-proBNP) and troponin T are pivotal for risk stratification [36]. Several staging systems have been proposed. The Mayo Clinic system utilizes NT-proBNP and troponin T to categorize patients into stages using cut off values of NT-proBNP (3000 pg/ml) and troponin T (0.05 ng/ml). Patients are classified into three stages: Stage I (both biomarkers below cutoff), Stage II (one above), and Stage III (both above), with respective 4-year survival rates of 57%, 42%, and 18% [36]. The National Amyloidosis Centre (NAC) system incorporates NT-proBNP and estimated glomerular filtration rate (eGFR) [56]. Both systems demonstrate the prognostic value of these biomarkers.

A survival analysis was conducted to evaluate the association between the initiation or escalation of oral diuretic therapy at the 1-year follow-up and subsequent all-cause mortality. Results from both the NAC cohort and an external validation cohort demonstrated a consistent link between increased diuretic use and higher mortality rates [57]. This finding suggests that this association is robust across diverse clinical settings despite variations in treatment practices [57]. TTE and CMR are essential for assessing disease severity and progression. TTE parameters including left ventricular hypertrophy mitral annular plane systolic excursion and right ventricular free-wall strain are associated with adverse outcomes [58, 59]. CMR-derived measures, such as late gadolinium enhancement and extracellular volume fraction provide additional prognostic information [60].

Functional assessments, including cardiopulmonary exercise testing (CPET) and six-minute walk test (6MWT), offer valuable insights into disease progression and prognosis. Reduced peak oxygen uptake (pVO2) on CPET(<50% predicted) and decreased 6MWT < 350 m are independently associated with increased mortality [61, 62]. Incorporating peak oxygen uptake (pVO2) into risk assessment models for ATTR-CA patients significantly enhances the predictive power of biomarkers such as NT-proBNP and estimated glomerular filtration rate. This integration led to a 35% improvement in distinguishing between patients at different risk levels and reclassified 67% of patients experiencing major adverse cardiovascular events (MACE) into higher risk categories [62]. These functional measures can enhance risk stratification when combined with biomarker-based staging systems.

A comprehensive approach incorporating clinical, imaging, biomarker, and functional assessments is essential for accurate risk stratification in ATTR. Further research is needed to refine these models and identify novel prognostic markers.

AL

The severity of cardiac involvement stands as the most significant predictor of prognosis for individuals with AL amyloidosis [34] Clinicians often use the Mayo 2012 scoring system to assess this risk [25]. The Mayo 2012 model assigns one point for each of the following: elevated levels of troponin T (greater than or equal to 0.025 mg/L), N-terminal pro brain natriuretic peptide (NT-proBNP; greater than or equal to 1800 ng/L) or BNP greater than or equal to 400 ng/L, and a difference in serum free light chains (dFLC) greater than or equal to 180 mg/L. This scoring system is particularly helpful in identifying patients at very high risk of complications [25].

Treatment

AL

The mainstay of therapy for AL is centered around targeting plasma cell and thereby reducing the light chain burden. The most common treatment is the combination regimen: CyBorD (bortezomib, cyclophosphamide, and dexamethasone) [63]. The treatment landscape has undergone a significant shift with the incorporation of daratumumab alongside CyBorD as a first-line therapy, which has demonstrated superior outcomes with improved survival without major organ dysfunction or relapse compared to CyBorD alone [64] (Fig. 17.4).

Stem Cell Transplant

The use of autologous stem cell transplantation (ASCT) for AL has undergone significant transformation. While advancements in patient selection, and initial treatment regimens have occurred, only a limited number of patients qualify for ASCT.

The optimal timing and role of ASCT remain unclear due to the scarcity of large-scale clinical trials. An early randomized study demonstrated that a high-dose melphalan plus autologous stem-cell rescue was not superior to standard-dose melphalan plus dexamethasone [65].

Modern data suggests improved outcomes with stricter patient selection and better support-

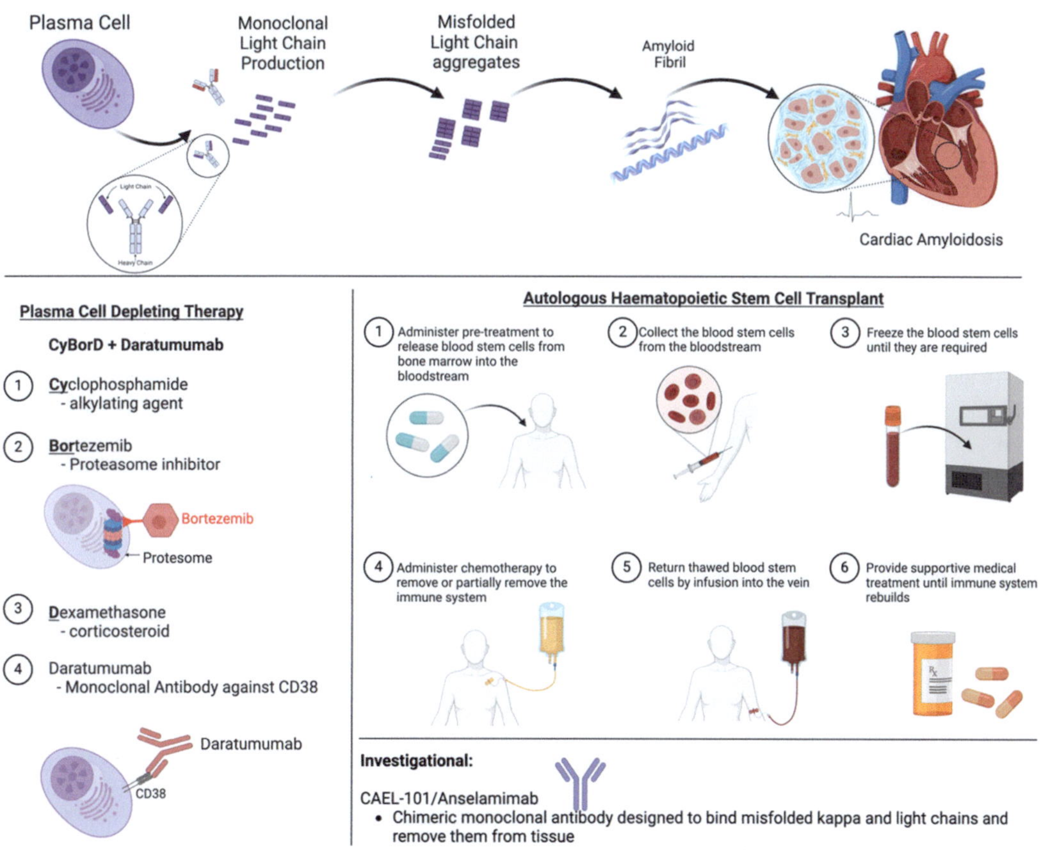

Fig. 17.4 Treatment strategies for light chain amyloidosis. (Figure created with BioRender.com)

ive care [66]. Despite advancements in multi-drug induction therapies, the risk-benefit profile of high-dose melphalan (HDM) with ASCT continues to evolve. ASCT is cautiously offered to younger patients with good performance status following a comprehensive evaluation. Patients without significant cardiac dysfunction as assessed by clinical status, ejection fraction, cardiac biomarkers (NT-ProBNP < 1800 pg/ml), and global longitudinal strain (GLS) are pioritized [67]. Additionally, patients with no history of hypotension requiring blood pressure support (systolic <90 mmHg) are considered. Only patients who achieve at least a very good partial response (VGPR) after induction therapy are considered for ASCT [67]. This selective approach ensures ASCT is offered to patients who are most likely to experience a successful outcome [67]. ASCT remains a valuable treatment option for select AL amyloidosis patients, but its use requires careful consideration of patient characteristics and ongoing research to determine its optimal application.

Evaluating a patient's response to AL amyloidosis treatment involves assessing both hematologic and organ-specific improvements. Hematologic response is measured by tracking reductions in clonal immunoglobulin levels in the serum and blood and serum free light chain levels [68]. Organ specific response is assessed by measuring organ specific biomarkers in the blood and urine. Achieving a deep hematologic response has been shown to translate into significant improvements in organ function and overall survival [69].

ATTR

Two primary treatment strategies have emerged as demonstrably effective for ATTR.

1. **Stabilizers**

   In ATTR, TTR tetramer dissociation into aggregation-prone monomers is a critical step. Small molecules that bind TTR's thyroxine sites stabilize the tetramer and hinder amyloid fibril formation [70]
2. **Silencers**

   These therapies aim to reduce the overall production of TTR protein by the liver, thereby limiting the substrate available for amyloid fibril formation [70].

In addition to these established approaches, several promising agents are in the early stages of development. These agents represent novel therapeutic avenues and include depleters, in vivo gene editing, extractors/degraders (Fig. 17.5).

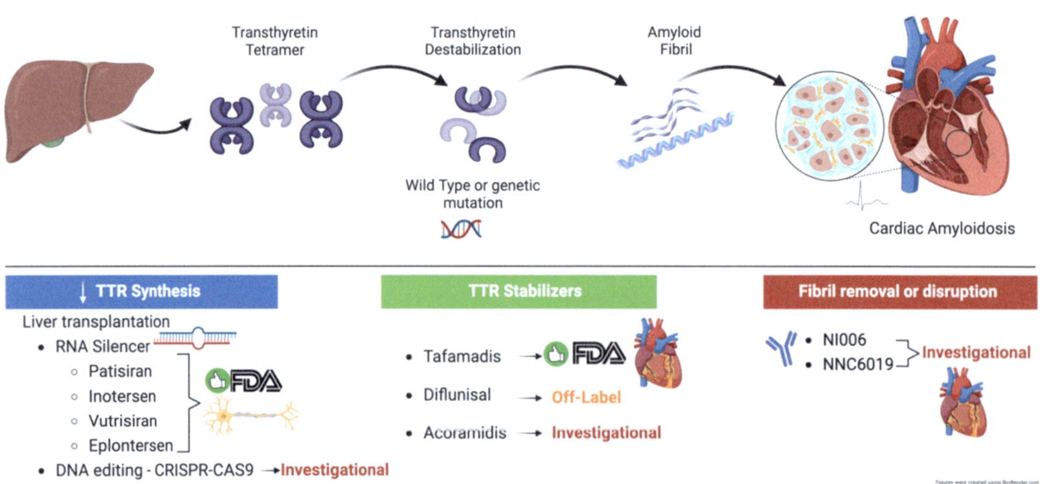

Fig. 17.5 Treatment strategies for transthyretin amyloidosis. (Figure created with BioRender.com)

Stabilizers

Tafamidis

Tafamidis is currently the sole FDA-approved therapy for ATTR-CM. This orally administered medication exerts its therapeutic effect by binding to the thyroxine binding site on TTR protein [71]. This stabilizes the TTR tetramer, hindering its dissociation into potentially harmful monomers [71].

The pivotal phase 3 ATTR-ACT trial provided the foundation for tafamidis FDA approval in ATTR-CM. This international, double-blind, placebo-controlled study enrolled patients with ATTRwt-CM or ATTRv-CM [72]. At the 30-month follow-up, tafamidis significantly reduced the primary composite endpoint, a composite of all-cause mortality and cardiovascular-related hospitalization [72]. The study suggested greater benefit for patients with NYHA class I-II symptoms as compared to NYHA class III at baseline. This underscores the importance of early diagnosis in ATTR-CM management.

Tafamidis also demonstrated improved functional capacity and quality of life with a slower decline in both 6-minute walk test distance and Kansas City Cardiomyopathy Questionnaire score [72].

Importantly, the trial did not identify any significant adverse events that occurred more frequently in the tafamidis arms compared to the placebo arm.

Acoramidis

Acoramidis (previously known as AG10) represents another promising oral medication for ATTR. Its mechanism of action involves forming hydrogen bonds with the TTR protein in a manner that closely resembles the hydrogen bonds established by the T119M protective TTR gene mutation [73]. The T119M mutation is a naturally occurring genetic variation associated with increased lifespan in carriers and is believed to exert its protective effect by promoting the stability of TTR tetramers, thereby preventing their dissociation and subsequent amyloid fibril formation. The ATTRibute-CM trial, a randomized clinical study, investigated the effectiveness of Acoramidis in patients with symptomatic ATTR cardiomyopathy (ATTR-CM). A total of 632 participants were enrolled and randomly assigned to receive either 800 mg of Acoramidis or a placebo, administered twice daily. The primary analysis employed a four-tiered hierarchical approach, evaluating outcomes in a specific order to account for multiple comparisons. These outcomes included: All-cause mortality, cardiovascular-related hospitalization, change in NT-proBNP levels from baseline and change in 6-minute walk test distance from baseline.

The results favored the acoramidis group compared to the placebo group based on the Finkelstein-Schoenfeld test (p-value <0.001). This finding translates to a win ratio of 1.8, suggesting a significant advantage for acoramidis (95% confidence interval: 1.4–2.2) [74].

The ATTRibute-CM trial provides compelling evidence for the efficacy of acoramidis in treating ATTR-CM [74]. At the time of writing this manuscript, Acoramidis was undergoing review by the FDA.

Diflusinal

Diflunisal is a non-steroidal anti-inflammatory drug (NSAID) which has emerged as a potential treatment for ATTR-CM due to its ability to stabilize the TTR [75]. While diflunisal offers a potential therapeutic strategy, it is important to acknowledge its associated adverse effects characteristic of other NSAIDs. These can include gastrointestinal bleeding, renal dysfunction, fluid retention and hypertension. However, the dosage used for ATTR-CM (250 mg twice daily) is lower compared to the dose used for its anti-inflammatory effects. This lower dose often translates to better tolerability for patients [71, 75].

For patients receiving diflunisal for ATTR-CM, regular monitoring of renal function, heart failure symptoms, gastrointestinal bleeding is crucial to ensure patient safety [71, 75].

It is important to note that diflunisal is not currently approved by the FDA for the treatment of ATTR-CM and is considered an "off-label" use.

RNA Silencers

There are two main processes to achieve TTR protein silencing for ATTR treatment:

Antisense Oligonucleotides (ASOs): These single-stranded molecules distribute widely throughout the body following administration and bind to target mRNA, both extracellularly and intracellularly. Within the cell nucleus, ASOs recruit RNase H2, an enzyme that degrades the targeted mRNA, ultimately silencing TTR production [76].

Small Interfering RNA (siRNA): Double-stranded siRNA molecules consist of a sense strand and an antisense strand. Upon entering the cytoplasm, the antisense strand associates with Ago2 protein, forming a complex that binds to target mRNA. This RNA-induced silencing complex then degrades the mRNA, leading to TTR silencing [76].

Due to TTR's role in transporting retinol (vitamin A), patients receiving silencing therapy require supplementation with Vitamin A. RNA silencers have shown lots of promise in clinical trials for ATTR cardiomyopathy but have not yet been approved for cardiomyopathy.

Inotersen, a modified antisense oligonucleotide, reduces transthyretin production in the liver by degrading its mRNA. In the NEURO-TTR trial, inotersen significantly improved neuropathy scores (mNIS+7) compared to placebo in patients with hereditary transthyretin amyloidosis with polyneuropathy (n = 172, 2:1 randomization). Notably, Inotersen was associatged with thrombocytopenia (3%) and glomerulonephritis (3%). Importantly, Inotersen treatment did not affect key measures of cardiac function (left ventricular wall thickness and global longitudinal strain) in either the entire study population or subgroups with evidence of amyloid cardiomyopathy. This trial led to the FDA approval of inotersen for hereditary transthyretin amyloidosis with polyneuropathy [77]. Despite FDA approval for ATTRv polyneuropathy, Inotersen is not under investigation for ATTR-CM due to newer ASOs with improved safety profiles [70].

Patisiran, a small interfering RNA (siRNA) encapsulated in lipid nanoparticles, targets transthyretin mRNA in the liver, reducing production of TTR. The APOLLO trial investigated patisiran's efficacy in patients with ATTR familial amyloid polyneuropathies. In this 2:1 randomized trial (n = 225), patisiran treatment halted or reversed neuropathy progression at 18 months [78]. Notably, in a pre-defined subgroup with evidence of cardiac involvement (n = 126), patisiran improved cardiac parameters including reduced left ventricular wall thickness, improved global longitudinal strain, and lowered NT-proBNP levels. A post-hoc analysis of APOLLO suggested a significant reduction in cardiac hospitalizations and mortality with patisiran [79].

The APOLLO-B trial further explored patisiran's effects on cardiomyopathy. This phase 3 study enrolled 356 patients with ATTR-CM (excluding NYHA class IV) and randomized them 1:1 to patisiran or placebo. The primary outcome, a 6-minute walk test (6MWT) distance change at 12 months, showed a significantly greater improvement in the patisiran group. These findings suggest patisiran's potential to improve quality of life in patients with ATTR-CM [80]. Unfortunately, due to its modest effect, Patisiran was not approved by the FDA for ATTR-CM.

Vutrisiran, a new-generation RNA interference (RNAi) therapy targeting transthyretin, offers distinct advantages over patisiran. Notably, vutrisiran is administered subcutaneously every 3 months, compared to patisiran's intravenous dosing every 3 weeks. The HELIOS-A trial, a phase 3, global, open-label study, evaluated vutrisiran's efficacy and safety on neuropathy outcomes compared to an external placebo group. Vutrisiran treatment demonstrated rapid (within 3 weeks) and sustained reductions in serum transthyretin (TTR) levels over 18 months [78]. Building on these promising findings, the HELIOS-B trial tested vutrisiran's efficacy in patients with cardiomyopathy associated with ATTRv or ATTRwt. HELIOS-B demonstrated a reduced risk of all cause mortality and recurrent cardiovascular events compared to placebo (HR 0.72; 95% CI, 0.56–0.93; P = 0.01) and improved functional capacity with less of a decline 6-minute walk distance and less of a decline in the KCCQ-OS score [81].

Eplontersen, a next-generation antisense oligonucleotide, targets transthyretin production in the liver. To enhance delivery to hepatocytes, the primary source of transthyretin, eplontersen is conjugated to a triantennary N-acetyl galactosamine (GalNAc) ligand. This GalNAc-conjugation significantly increases the potency of the antisense oligonucleotide, allowing for lower and potentially less frequent dosing [82]. In a study with healthy volunteers, subcutaneous administration of eplontersen (45 mg every 4 weeks for a total of 4 doses) achieved a substantial mean reduction of 86% in serum transthyretin concentration [83]. Eplontersen represents the latest advancement in RNA-targeting therapies for transthyretin amyloidosis. Eplontersen is currently approved for patients with ATTRv polyneuropathy. The CARDIO-TTRansform trial (NCT04136171), a pivotal multinational phase III randomized, double-blind, placebo-controlled trial which will assess the effectiveness of subcutaneous eplontersen administered every 4 weeks compared to a placebo in patients with ATTR-CM [84].

Emerging Therapies Undergoing Clinical Trials

CRISPR-Cas9

CRISPR-Cas9 technology offers a promising approach for treating ATTR. It works by targeting the DNA sequence responsible for producing TTR in hepatocytes, potentially halting the progression of the disease [85].

The CRISPR-Cas9 system has two key components: *Guide RNA* molecule guides the *Cas9* protein to the exact DNA sequence that needs to be edited. *Cas9* protein acts like a molecular scissor, cutting the target DNA at a specific location. Once the DNA is cut, the cell's natural repair mechanisms take over. This approach holds promise for ATTR, particularly the ATTRv, as it is a monogenic disease caused by a single gene mutation.

NTLA-2001 is a groundbreaking gene-editing treatment for transthyretin amyloidosis (ATTR) that utilizes the CRISPR-Cas9 system. NTLA-2001 utilizes lipid nanoparticle (LNP) targeted to the liver, which acts as a carrier for the guide RNA and the Human-codon-optimized messenger RNA (mRNA) encoding Cas9 protein from *Streptococcus pyogenes* [86]. Phase 1 study of NTLA-2001 involved six patients ATTRv amyloidosis with polyneuropathy. Within the first 28 days after single intravenous infusion of NTLA-2001, there was a significant and lasting reduction in TTR production [87].

Unlike current treatments like small interfering RNA (siRNA) and antisense oligonucleotides (ASO) that require frequent dosing, CRISPR-Cas9 offers the potential for a one-time treatment [88]. However, several key questions remain to be fully addressed before widespread clinical application such as long term clinical safety and off target editing [88]. The MAGNITUDE trial (NCT06128629) is a large-scale (n = 765) randomized, double-blind, placebo-controlled study assessing the safety and efficacy of a single 55 mg dose of NTLA-2001 in ATTR-CM patients. It will evaluate the effect of NTLA-2001 on a combined endpoint of cardiovascular death and related events.

Depleter Therapy

While advancements have been made in ATTR amyloidosis management, there remains a lack of therapies specifically designed to remove TTR amyloid deposits and reverse consequent cardiac dysfunction.

NI006

NI006, a recombinant human anti-ATTR monoclonal IgG1 antibody, represents a promising strategy. It selectively binds to amyloid conformations of ATTRwt and ATTRv, but not physiologically folded TTR. Preclinical studies suggest NI006 promotes ATTR depletion through antibody-mediated phagocytosis of fibrils and tissue deposit removal. After 4 months of treatment, higher total NI006 exposure correlated with lower cardiac tracer uptake on scintigraphy and reduced extracellular volume measured by cardiac MRI, compared to baseline values. Extended treatment up to 12 months appeared to further decrease these parameters. Conversely, placebo recipients displayed an apparent increase in cardiac tracer uptake and extracellular volume on MRI at the four-month mark. The use of N1006 did not have any adverse clinical events in the phase 1 trial [89].

The prevailing hypothesis suggests that mechanical impairment caused by amyloid deposits is the primary driver of cardiac dysfunction in ATTR cardiomyopathy, leading to increased ventricular stiffness and diastolic dysfunction. Therefore, reducing the amyloid deposit burden represents a logical therapeutic target for this condition [90, 91].

A currently ongoing Phase 3, randomized, double-blind, placebo-controlled, multicenter trial is evaluating the efficacy and safety of ALXN2220, an amyloid depleter, in adult participants with ATTR-CM. The primary objective is to assess the treatment's efficacy by comparing the ALXN2220 to placebo regarding a composite endpoint encompassing all-cause mortality and total cardiovascular clinical events. Results are anticipated within the next few years.

NNC6019

NNC6019 (formerly PRX004) is an investigational intravenous monoclonal antibody designed to target misfolded TTR amyloid deposits. It exhibits selective binding to these pathological forms, sparing native circulating TTR. This mechanism offers a potential therapeutic approach for clearing amyloid deposits within the myocardium [70].

A phase 1 clinical trial (NCT03336580) evaluated the safety and tolerability of NNC6019 in 21 patients diagnosed with ATTRv. The findings demonstrated a favorable safety profile with no reports of serious adverse events [92].

A currently ongoing phase 2 clinical trial (NCT05442047) is further investigating the efficacy of NNC6019 in ATTR. This randomized, placebo-controlled study employs a 2:1 allocation scheme, comparing NNC6019 with placebo. The primary outcome measures focus on functional capacity assessed by the 6-minute walk test (6MWT) and NT-proBNP levels. The results of this ongoing trial are anticipated to provide more definitive data on the efficacy of NNC6019 in managing ATTR (Fig. 17.6).

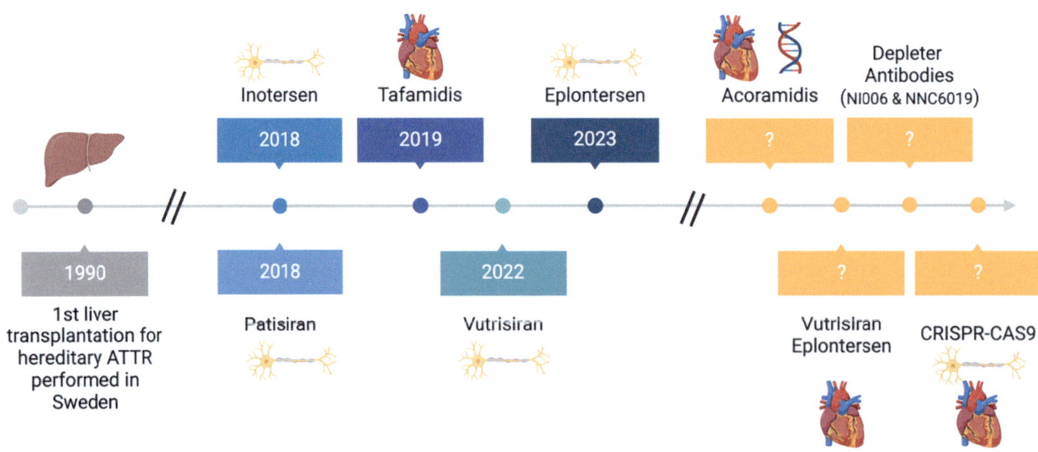

Fig. 17.6 Timeline of development of treatment strategies for transthyretin amyloidosis. (Figure created with BioRender.com)

Unanswered Questions

The emergence of various therapies for ATTR, like stabilizers and silencers, brings exciting possibilities but also highlights the need for better risk stratification. A key question is how to match the right therapy to the right patient. Will silencers, which target the production of the TTR protein, be more effective in the early stages of the disease before extensive amyloid deposits form? Conversely, would stabilizers, which prevent misfolding of the TTR protein, be more beneficial in later stages to manage existing deposits?

Another area of exploration is the potential of depleting therapies that directly remove circulating TTR protein. If approved, when would these therapies be most advantageous? Could they potentially halt or even reverse disease progression, particularly in later stages?

The ultimate goal of ATTR amyloidosis treatment would be complete disease reversal. With these new therapies, is this "holy grail" a realistic possibility? Can we eliminate the need for heart transplants altogether?

Furthermore, the discussion is shifting towards proactive management. Should CRISPR gene editing be considered for individuals with known TTR gene mutations, even before symptoms arise? This approach raises ethical and safety concerns that need careful consideration.

Could gene carriers benefit from preventive treatment with stabilizers or silencers? Prophylactic therapy has the potential to prevent the onset of clinical manifestations entirely.

As clinical trials progress and provide more data, we can expect a more personalized approach to ATTR amyloidosis treatment. This will allow clinicians to optimize treatment strategies for individual patients, leading to better outcomes.

Liver Transplant

Liver transplantation emerged as a definitive treatment for ATTRv in 1990 (Fig. 17.6). The underlying rationale for this intervention lies in the fact that the liver serves as the primary site of synthesis for transthyretin (TTR), the precursor protein involved in amyloid formation. By replacing the liver, the source of mutated TTR is eliminated, halting disease progression. Supporting this concept, orthotopic liver transplantation (OLT) leads to a rapid clearance of mutant TTR from the circulation [77]. The success of liver transplantation (LT) for transthyretin amyloidosis varies depending on individual patient characteristics. Several factors have been identified as positive prognostic indicators such as early stage disease, early onset disease (age < 50), V30M variant, short disease duration before transplant and absence of cardiac involvement [93].

The therapeutic benefit of LT may be limited due to the ongoing deposition of wild-type (wt) TTR. This residual protein can continue to form amyloid fibrils, leading to a progressive decline in both cardiac and neurological function after transplantation. Consequently, patients may experience a significant decline in quality of life (QOL) despite undergoing LT [94].

Furthermore, LT recipients require lifelong immunosuppressive therapy to prevent graft rejection. Immunospuppression carries its own set of risks. Additionally, patients face a mortality risk associated with the transplant procedure itself, with reported 1-year mortality rates ranging from 7% to 30% [95, 96].

A long-term retrospective study revealed that the primary causes of death within the first year post-LT were related to worsening amyloidosis [95, 96]. This can manifest as progression of pre-existing neuropathy or cardiac dysfunction. The emergence of novel pharmacotherapies for ATTRv has significantly altered the treatment landscape for this condition. These medications are now considered the first-line approach for managing the disease process. Consequently, liver transplantation (LT), previously a cornerstone therapy, is performed less frequently in the current clinical era. This shift reflects the potential of pharmacotherapies to slow disease progression, offering a less invasive and more efficacious treatment option for many patients.

Heart Transplant

The rapid strides made in ATTR therapies are counterbalanced by the relative paucity of recent advancements for patients with the most severe disease presentation: end-stage heart failure. Historically, cardiac transplantation for AL and ATTR was largely avoided due to prohibitively high rates of complications and mortality following the procedure [97]. The increased recognition of ATTR, coupled with the rapid development of plasma cell-directed therapies for AL, have significantly improved patient outcomes [98, 99]. Patients with cardiac-amyloidosis have multiple challenges for successful durable mechanical circulatory support (MCS), such as left ventricular assist devices (LVAD). Factors include: small ventiricular cavities leading to difficult inflow cannula placement, biventricular dysfunction leading to high risk for right venticular failure if LVAD is used alone and increased risk for infection for AL on active chemotherapy [100, 101]. Alternative management strategies beyond durable LVAD bridge to transplant are often necessary for end-stage cardiac amyloidosis. Temporary MCS devices, such as intra-aortic balloon pumps (IABP) or percutaneous microaxial pumps, represent a potential bridge to transplantation for select patients with cardiac amyloidosis [102].

The viability of cardiac transplantation for amyloidosis hinges on several critical considerations, with the specific amyloidosis subtype playing a significant role in determining candidacy and outcomes.

Management of ATTRv amyloidosis with mixed cardiomyopathy and neuropathy phenotype requires a nuanced approach based on genotype and therapeutic advancements. Cardiac transplantation alone may be insufficient for genotypes like V30M and T60A, which cause a mixed phenotype with both cardiomyopathy and neuropathy. In ATTRv, liver transplant's role is diminishing with effective therapies like patisiran, inotersen, vutrisiran, and eplontersen. For cardiac transplant, thorough neurological assessment, including assessment of autonomic function, are crucial [101].

Advanced age of patients with ATTR-wt often precludes cardiac transplantation as a viable treatment option [101, 103]. However, for pateints diagnosed at an earlier age with severe cardiac dysfunction and limited systemic involvement, heart transplantation may be a viable option.

AL necessitates thorough evaluation for extracardiac organ involvement due to its multisystemic nature. Pre-transplant, demonstration of an adequate response to light chain suppression is crucial, as progressive amyloid deposition remains a post-transplantation mortality risk [28, 101].

While cardiac transplantation in systemic amyloidosis presents distinct challenges, the past decade has witnessed remarkable progress. Rigorous patient selection and the advent of potent plasma cell-directed therapies pave the way for a future with improved outcomes in this complex patient population.

Multidisciplinary Approach

The multidisciplinary nature of amyloidosis care necessitates the designation of a lead clinician to facilitate coordinated management across specialties. Typically, cardiologists assume this role for patients with ATTR-CM, while hematologists often lead care for patients with AL-CM [104]. The successful implementation of a multidisciplinary model for amyloidosis can serve as a blueprint for managing other complex diseases. By identifying key triggers for specialist involvement, this approach could be adapted and operationalized for cardiac conditions with multisystem involvement [104].

Effective management of amyloidosis demands a multidisciplinary approach, with specialists playing crucial roles at key junctures. Hematologists are vital for interpreting monoclonal light chain tests to identify potential underlying plasma cell disorders. Collaboration with cardiothoracic surgeons and heart failure specialists is crucial in determining the eligibility and risks of advanced therapies like heart transplantation or mechanical circulatory support [104].

Neurologists play a key role in the multidisciplinary amyloidosis program. Substantial proportion of patients have neuropathic involvement, requiring specialized expertise for diagnosis and symptomatic management. Furthermore, at the time of writing this review, currently available RNA silencers are all approved for ATTRv associated polyneuropathy.

As heart failure in patients with cardiac amyloidosis progresses despite volume optimization, specialized care becomes essential. An amylodiosis center can tailor heart failure medications specifically for amyloidosis, potentially improving their effectiveness compared to standard regimens [105]. Multidisciplinary care is also essential as the severity of specific organ symptoms is crucial in determining a patient's candidacy for heart transplantation.

Historically challenging to diagnose due to its rapid progression and multisystem involvement, amyloidosis now benefits from powerful diagnostic tools and therapeutic advancements. This paves the way for improved patient outcomes and quality of life. A multidisciplinary care model fosters synchronized clinical management, ensuring timely and personalized care for this complex disease.

References

1. Ruberg FL, Berk JL. Transthyretin (TTR) cardiac amyloidosis. Circulation. 2012;126(10):1286–300. https://doi.org/10.1161/circulationaha.111.078915.
2. Fontana M, Ćorović A, Scully P, Moon JC. Myocardial amyloidosis: the exemplar interstitial disease. JACC Cardiovasc Imaging. 2019;12(11 Pt 2):2345–56. https://doi.org/10.1016/j.jcmg.2019.06.023.
3. Barbhaiya CR, Kumar S, Baldinger SH, et al. Electrophysiologic assessment of conduction abnormalities and atrial arrhythmias associated with amyloid cardiomyopathy. Heart Rhythm. 2016;13(2):383–90. https://doi.org/10.1016/j.hrthm.2015.09.016.
4. Varga C, Dorbala S, Lousada I, et al. The diagnostic challenges of cardiac amyloidosis: a practical approach to the two main types. Blood Rev. 2021;45:100720. https://doi.org/10.1016/j.blre.2020.100720.
5. Sipe J, Benson M, Buxbaum J, et al. Amyloid fibril protein nomenclature: 2012 recommendations from the Nomenclature Committee of the International Society of Amyloidosis. Amyloid. 2010;17:101–4. https://doi.org/10.3109/13506129.2010.526812.
6. Sipe JD, Benson MD, Buxbaum JN, et al. Amyloid fibril proteins and amyloidosis: chemical identification and clinical classification International Society of Amyloidosis 2016 Nomenclature Guidelines. Amyloid. 2016;23(4):209–13. https://doi.org/10.1080/13506129.2016.1257986.
7. Kittleson MM, Ruberg FL, Ambardekar AV, et al. 2023 ACC expert consensus decision pathway on comprehensive multidisciplinary care for the patient with Cardiac Amyloidosis. J Am Coll Cardiol. 2023;81(11):1076–126. https://doi.org/10.1016/j.jacc.2022.11.022.
8. Aimo A, Merlo M, Porcari A, et al. Redefining the epidemiology of cardiac amyloidosis. A systematic review and meta-analysis of screening studies. Eur J Heart Fail. 2022;24(12):2342–51. https://doi.org/10.1002/ejhf.2532.
9. Gilstrap LG, Dominici F, Wang Y, et al. Epidemiology of cardiac amyloidosis-associated heart failure hospitalizations among fee-for-service Medicare beneficiaries in the United States. Circ Heart Fail. 2019;12(6):e005407. https://doi.org/10.1161/circheartfailure.118.005407.
10. Ruberg FL, Grogan M, Hanna M, Kelly JW, Maurer MS. Transthyretin amyloid cardiomyopathy: JACC state-of-the-art review. J Am Coll Cardiol. 2019;73(22):2872–91. https://doi.org/10.1016/j.jacc.2019.04.003.
11. Yamamoto H, Yokochi T. Transthyretin cardiac amyloidosis: an update on diagnosis and treatment. ESC Heart Fail. 2019;6(6):1128–39. https://doi.org/10.1002/ehf2.12518.
12. Lane T, Fontana M, Martinez-Naharro A, et al. Natural history, quality of life, and outcome in cardiac Transthyretin Amyloidosis. Circulation. 2019;140(1):16–26. https://doi.org/10.1161/CIRCULATIONAHA.118.038169.
13. Gertz MA, Dispenzieri A. Systemic amyloidosis recognition, prognosis, and therapy: a systematic review. JAMA. 2020;324(1):79–89. https://doi.org/10.1001/jama.2020.5493.
14. Wechalekar AD, Gillmore JD, Hawkins PN. Systemic amyloidosis. Lancet. 2016;387(10038):2641–54. https://doi.org/10.1016/s0140-6736(15)01274-x.
15. Damy T, Bourel G, Slama M, et al. Incidence and survival of transthyretin amyloid cardiomyopathy from a French nationwide study of in- and out-patient databases. Orphanet J Rare Dis. 2023;18(1):345. https://doi.org/10.1186/s13023-023-02933-w.
16. Tanskanen M, Peuralinna T, Polvikoski T, et al. Senile systemic amyloidosis affects 25% of the very aged and associates with genetic variation in alpha2-macroglobulin and tau: a population-based autopsy study. Ann Med. 2008;40(3):232–9. https://doi.org/10.1080/07853890701842988.

17. Zampieri M, Nardi G, Del Monaco G, et al. Changes in the perceived epidemiology of amyloidosis: 20 year-experience from a Tertiary Referral Centre in Tuscany. Int J Cardiol. 2021;335:123–7. https://doi.org/10.1016/j.ijcard.2021.04.023.
18. Quock TP, Yan T, Chang E, Guthrie S, Broder MS. Epidemiology of AL amyloidosis: a real-world study using US claims data. Blood Adv. 2018;2(10):1046–53. https://doi.org/10.1182/bloodadvances.2018016402.
19. González-López E, Gagliardi C, Dominguez F, et al. Clinical characteristics of wild-type transthyretin cardiac amyloidosis: disproving myths. Eur Heart J. 2017;38(24):1895–904. https://doi.org/10.1093/eurheartj/ehx043.
20. Escher F, Senoner M, Doerler J, et al. When and how do patients with cardiac amyloidosis die? Clin Res Cardiol. 2020;109(1):78–88. https://doi.org/10.1007/s00392-019-01490-2.
21. Grogan M, Dispenzieri A, Gertz MA. Light-chain cardiac amyloidosis: strategies to promote early diagnosis and cardiac response. Heart. 2017;103(14):1065–72. https://doi.org/10.1136/heartjnl-2016-310704.
22. Quarta CC, Solomon SD, Uraizee I, et al. Left ventricular structure and function in transthyretin-related versus light-chain cardiac amyloidosis. Circulation. 2014;129(18):1840–9. https://doi.org/10.1161/CIRCULATIONAHA.113.006242.
23. Chacko L, Karia N, Venneri L, et al. Progression of echocardiographic parameters and prognosis in transthyretin cardiac amyloidosis. Eur J Heart Fail. 2022;24(9):1700–12. https://doi.org/10.1002/ejhf.2606.
24. Bozkurt B, Colvin M, Cook J, et al. Current diagnostic and treatment strategies for specific dilated cardiomyopathies: a Scientific Statement from the American Heart Association. Circulation. 2016;134(23):e579–646. https://doi.org/10.1161/CIR.0000000000000455.
25. Dispenzieri A, Gertz MA, Kyle RA, et al. Serum cardiac troponins and N-terminal pro-brain natriuretic peptide: a staging system for primary systemic amyloidosis. J Clin Oncol. 2004;22(18):3751–7. https://doi.org/10.1200/jco.2004.03.029.
26. Lilleness B, Ruberg FL, Mussinelli R, Doros G, Sanchorawala V. Development and validation of a survival staging system incorporating BNP in patients with light chain amyloidosis. Blood. 2019;133(3):215–23. https://doi.org/10.1182/blood-2018-06-858951.
27. Chan N, Teruya S, Mirabal A, et al. Temporal outcomes of patients diagnosed with transthyretin cardiac amyloidosis. J Card Fail. 2024; https://doi.org/10.1016/j.cardfail.2024.02.014.
28. Chen Q, Moriguchi J, Levine R, et al. Outcomes of heart transplantation in cardiac amyloidosis patients: a single center experience. Transplant Proc. 2021;53(1):329–34. https://doi.org/10.1016/j.transproceed.2020.08.020.
29. Griffin JM, Chiu L, Axsom KM, et al. United network for organ sharing outcomes after heart transplantation for al compared to ATTR cardiac amyloidosis. Clin Transpl. 2020;34(10):e14028. https://doi.org/10.1111/ctr.14028.
30. Ohiomoba RO, Youmans QR, Ezema A, et al. Cardiac transplantation outcomes in patients with amyloid cardiomyopathy. Am Heart J. 2021;236:13–21. https://doi.org/10.1016/j.ahj.2021.02.016.
31. Ikura H, Endo J, Kitakata H, Moriyama H, Sano M, Fukuda K. Molecular mechanism of pathogenesis and treatment strategies for AL amyloidosis. Int J Mol Sci. 2022;23(11):6336.
32. Desport E, Bridoux F, Sirac C, et al. Al amyloidosis. Orphanet J Rare Dis. 2012;7:54. https://doi.org/10.1186/1750-1172-7-54.
33. Shi J, Guan J, Jiang B, et al. Amyloidogenic light chains induce cardiomyocyte contractile dysfunction and apoptosis via a non-canonical p38alpha MAPK pathway. Proc Natl Acad Sci USA. 2010;107(9):4188–93. https://doi.org/10.1073/pnas.0912263107.
34. Kittleson MM, Maurer MS, Ambardekar AV, et al. Cardiac amyloidosis: evolving diagnosis and management: a scientific statement from the American Heart Association. Circulation. 2020;142(1):e7–e22. https://doi.org/10.1161/CIR.0000000000000792.
35. Criddle RS, Hansen LD, Woodfield BF, Tolley HD. Modeling transthyretin (TTR) amyloid diseases, from monomer to amyloid fibrils. PLoS One. 2024;19(6):e0304891. https://doi.org/10.1371/journal.pone.0304891.
36. Grogan M, Scott CG, Kyle RA, et al. Natural history of wild-type transthyretin cardiac amyloidosis and risk stratification using a novel staging system. J Am Coll Cardiol. 2016;68(10):1014–20. https://doi.org/10.1016/j.jacc.2016.06.033.
37. Finsterer J, Iglseder S, Wanschitz J, Topakian R, Löscher WN, Grisold W. Hereditary transthyretin-related amyloidosis. Acta Neurol Scand. 2019;139(2):92–105. https://doi.org/10.1111/ane.13035.
38. Schneider SM, Kochar K, Ruge M, et al. Cardiogenic shock due to atrial arrhythmia as the initial presentation of transthyretin cardiac amyloidosis. JACC Case Rep. 2022;4(22):1490–5. https://doi.org/10.1016/j.jaccas.2022.07.041.
39. Nativi-Nicolau J, Maurer MS. Amyloidosis cardiomyopathy: update in the diagnosis and treatment of the most common types. Curr Opin Cardiol. 2018;33(5):571–9. https://doi.org/10.1097/hco.0000000000000547.
40. González-López E, Gallego-Delgado M, Guzzo-Merello G, et al. Wild-type transthyretin amyloidosis as a cause of heart failure with preserved ejection fraction. Eur Heart J. 2015;36(38):2585–94. https://doi.org/10.1093/eurheartj/ehv338.
41. Ternacle J, Krapf L, Mohty D, et al. Aortic stenosis and cardiac amyloidosis: JACC review topic of

the week. J Am Coll Cardiol. 2019;74(21):2638–51. https://doi.org/10.1016/j.jacc.2019.09.056.
42. Westin O, Fosbøl EL, Maurer MS, et al. Screening for cardiac amyloidosis 5 to 15 years after surgery for bilateral carpal tunnel syndrome. J Am Coll Cardiol. 2022;80(10):967–77. https://doi.org/10.1016/j.jacc.2022.06.026.
43. Godara A, Riesenburger RI, Zhang DX, et al. Association between spinal stenosis and wild-type ATTR amyloidosis. Amyloid. 2021;28(4):226–33. https://doi.org/10.1080/13506129.2021.1950681.
44. Maurer MS, Smiley D, Simsolo E, et al. Analysis of lumbar spine stenosis specimens for identification of amyloid. J Am Geriatr Soc. 2022;70(12):3538–48. https://doi.org/10.1111/jgs.17976.
45. Geller HI, Singh A, Alexander KM, Mirto TM, Falk RH. Association between ruptured distal biceps tendon and wild-type transthyretin cardiac amyloidosis. JAMA. 2017;318(10):962–3. https://doi.org/10.1001/jama.2017.9236.
46. Cyrille NB, Goldsmith J, Alvarez J, Maurer MS. Prevalence and prognostic significance of low QRS voltage among the three main types of cardiac amyloidosis. Am J Cardiol. 2014;114(7):1089–93. https://doi.org/10.1016/j.amjcard.2014.07.026.
47. Cheng Z, Zhu K, Tian Z, Zhao D, Cui Q, Fang Q. The findings of electrocardiography in patients with cardiac amyloidosis. Ann Noninvasive Electrocardiol. 2013;18(2):157–62. https://doi.org/10.1111/anec.12018.
48. Boldrini M, Cappelli F, Chacko L, et al. Multiparametric echocardiography scores for the diagnosis of cardiac amyloidosis. JACC Cardiovasc Imaging. 2020;13(4):909–20. https://doi.org/10.1016/j.jcmg.2019.10.011.
49. Tipoo Sultan FA, Khan MT. Clinical presentation, diagnostic features on cardiac magnetic resonance imaging and outcome of patients with cardiac amyloidosis presenting to a tertiary care setting. J Pak Med Assoc. 2021;71(12):2802–5. https://doi.org/10.47391/jpma.385.
50. Clerc OF, Cuddy SAM, Robertson M, et al. Cardiac amyloid quantification using (124)I-Evuzamitide ((124)I-P5+14) versus (18)F-Florbetapir: a pilot PET/CT study. JACC Cardiovasc Imaging. 2023;16(11):1419–32. https://doi.org/10.1016/j.jcmg.2023.07.007.
51. Dorbala S, Cuddy S, Falk RH. How to image cardiac amyloidosis: a practical approach. JACC Cardiovasc Imaging. 2020;13(6):1368–83. https://doi.org/10.1016/j.jcmg.2019.07.015.
52. Muchtar E, Gertz MA, Kyle RA, et al. A modern primer on light chain amyloidosis in 592 patients with mass spectrometry-verified typing. Mayo Clin Proc. 2019;94(3):472–83. https://doi.org/10.1016/j.mayocp.2018.08.006.
53. Poterucha TJ, Elias P, Bokhari S, et al. Diagnosing transthyretin cardiac amyloidosis by technetium Tc 99m pyrophosphate: a test in evolution. JACC Cardiovasc Imaging. 2021;14(6):1221–31. https://doi.org/10.1016/j.jcmg.2020.08.027.
54. Bowen K, Shah N, Lewin M. AL-amyloidosis presenting with negative Congo Red staining in the setting of high clinical suspicion: a case report. Case Rep Nephrol. 2012;2012:593460. https://doi.org/10.1155/2012/593460.
55. Gonzalez-Lopez E, McPhail ED, Salas-Anton C, et al. Histological typing in patients with cardiac amyloidosis. J Am Coll Cardiol. 2024;83(11):1085–99. https://doi.org/10.1016/j.jacc.2024.01.010.
56. Nitsche C, Ioannou A, Patel RK, et al. Expansion of the National Amyloidosis Centre staging system to detect early mortality in transthyretin cardiac amyloidosis. Eur J Heart Fail. 2024; https://doi.org/10.1002/ejhf.3354.
57. Ioannou A, Cappelli F, Emdin M, et al. Stratifying disease progression in patients with cardiac ATTR amyloidosis. J Am Coll Cardiol. 2024;83(14):1276–91. https://doi.org/10.1016/j.jacc.2023.12.036.
58. Kristen AV, Scherer K, Buss S, et al. Noninvasive risk stratification of patients with transthyretin amyloidosis. JACC Cardiovasc Imaging. 2014;7(5):502–10. https://doi.org/10.1016/j.jcmg.2014.03.002.
59. Ozbay B, Satyavolu BS, Rearick C, et al. Right ventricular strain improves the echocardiographic diagnosis and risk stratification of transthyretin cardiac amyloidosis among other phenotypes of left ventricular hypertrophy. J Am Soc Echocardiogr. 2024; https://doi.org/10.1016/j.echo.2024.06.006.
60. Ney S, Gertz RJ, Pennig L, et al. Multiparametric monitoring of disease progression in contemporary patients with wild-type transthyretin amyloid cardiomyopathy initiating Tafamidis treatment. J Clin Med. 2024;13(1):284.
61. Ioannou A, Fumagalli C, Razvi Y, et al. Prognostic value of a 6-minute walk test in patients with transthyretin cardiac amyloidosis. J Am Coll Cardiol. 2024;84(1):43–58. https://doi.org/10.1016/j.jacc.2024.04.011.
62. Banydeen R, Eggleston R, Deney A, et al. Risk stratification in transthyretin cardiac amyloidosis: the added value of lung spirometry. J Clin Med. 2023;12(11) https://doi.org/10.3390/jcm12113684.
63. Kastritis E, Palladini G, Minnema MC, et al. Daratumumab-based treatment for immunoglobulin light-chain amyloidosis. N Engl J Med. 2021;385(1):46–58. https://doi.org/10.1056/NEJMoa2028631.
64. Kastritis E, Leleu X, Arnulf B, et al. Bortezomib, Melphalan, and Dexamethasone for light-chain amyloidosis. J Clin Oncol. 2020;38(28):3252–60. https://doi.org/10.1200/jco.20.01285.
65. Jaccard A, Moreau P, Leblond V, et al. High-dose Melphalan versus Melphalan plus Dexamethasone for AL amyloidosis. N Engl J Med. 2007;357(11):1083–93. https://doi.org/10.1056/NEJMoa070484.

66. D'Souza A, Dispenzieri A, Wirk B, et al. Improved outcomes after autologous hematopoietic cell transplantation for light chain amyloidosis: a Center for International Blood and Marrow Transplant Research Study. J Clin Oncol. 2015;33(32):3741–9. https://doi.org/10.1200/jco.2015.62.4015.
67. Dima D, Mazzoni S, Anwer F, et al. Diagnostic and treatment strategies for AL amyloidosis in an era of therapeutic innovation. JCO Oncol Pract. 2023;19(5):265–75. https://doi.org/10.1200/op.22.00396.
68. Comenzo RL, Reece D, Palladini G, et al. Consensus guidelines for the conduct and reporting of clinical trials in systemic light-chain amyloidosis. Leukemia. 2012;26(11):2317–25. https://doi.org/10.1038/leu.2012.100.
69. Gertz MA, Kyle RA, Greipp PR. Response rates and survival in primary systemic amyloidosis. Blood. 1991;77(2):257–62.
70. Griffin JM, Rosenthal JL, Grodin JL, Maurer MS, Grogan M, Cheng RK. ATTR amyloidosis: current and emerging management strategies: JACC: CardioOncology state-of-the-art review. JACC Cardio Oncol. 2021;3(4):488–505. https://doi.org/10.1016/j.jaccao.2021.06.006.
71. Alexander KM, Evangelisti A, Witteles RM. Emerging therapies for transthyretin cardiac amyloidosis. Curr Treat Options Cardiovasc Med. 2019;21(8):40. https://doi.org/10.1007/s11936-019-0743-2.
72. Maurer MS, Schwartz JH, Gundapaneni B, et al. Tafamidis treatment for patients with transthyretin amyloid cardiomyopathy. N Engl J Med. 2018;379(11):1007–16. https://doi.org/10.1056/NEJMoa1805689.
73. Miller M, Pal A, Albusairi W, et al. Enthalpy-driven stabilization of transthyretin by AG10 mimics a naturally occurring genetic variant that protects from transthyretin amyloidosis. J Med Chem. 2018;61(17):7862–76. https://doi.org/10.1021/acs.jmedchem.8b00817.
74. Gillmore JD, Judge DP, Cappelli F, et al. Efficacy and safety of Acoramidis in transthyretin amyloid cardiomyopathy. N Engl J Med. 2024;390(2):132–42. https://doi.org/10.1056/NEJMoa2305434.
75. Lohrmann G, Pipilas A, Mussinelli R, et al. Stabilization of cardiac function with Diflunisal in transthyretin (ATTR) cardiac amyloidosis. J Card Fail. 2020;26(9):753–9. https://doi.org/10.1016/j.cardfail.2019.11.024.
76. Crooke ST, Witztum JL, Bennett CF, Baker BF. RNA-targeted therapeutics. Cell Metab. 2018;27(4):714–39. https://doi.org/10.1016/j.cmet.2018.03.004.
77. Benson MD. Liver transplantation and transthyretin amyloidosis. Muscle Nerve. 2013;47(2):157–62. https://doi.org/10.1002/mus.23521.
78. Adams D, Tournev IL, Taylor MS, et al. Efficacy and safety of vutrisiran for patients with hereditary transthyretin-mediated amyloidosis with polyneuropathy: a randomized clinical trial. Amyloid. 2023;30(1):1–9. https://doi.org/10.1080/13506129.2022.2091985.
79. Solomon SD, Adams D, Kristen A, et al. Effects of Patisiran, an RNA interference therapeutic, on cardiac parameters in patients with hereditary transthyretin-mediated amyloidosis. Circulation. 2019;139(4):431–43. https://doi.org/10.1161/CIRCULATIONAHA.118.035831.
80. Maurer MS, Kale P, Fontana M, et al. Patisiran treatment in patients with transthyretin cardiac amyloidosis. N Engl J Med. 2023;389(17):1553–65. https://doi.org/10.1056/NEJMoa2300757.
81. Fontana M, Berk JL, Gillmore JD, et al. Vutrisiran in patients with transthyretin amyloidosis with cardiomyopathy. N Engl J Med. 2025; https://doi.org/10.1056/NEJMoa2409134.
82. Wang Y, Yu RZ, Henry S, Geary RS. Pharmacokinetics and clinical pharmacology considerations of GalNAc3-conjugated antisense oligonucleotides. Expert Opin Drug Metab Toxicol. 2019;15(6):475–85. https://doi.org/10.1080/17425255.2019.1621838.
83. Viney NJ, Guo S, Tai L-J, et al. Ligand conjugated antisense oligonucleotide for the treatment of transthyretin amyloidosis: preclinical and phase 1 data. ESC Heart Fail. 2021;8(1):652–61. https://doi.org/10.1002/ehf2.13154.
84. Falk R, Gertz M, Benson M, et al. Rationale and design of a phase 3 study to evaluate the efficacy and safety of ION-682884 in patients with transthyretin-mediated amyloid cardiomyopathy (ATTR-CM). Blood. 2019;134:5764. https://doi.org/10.1182/blood-2019-129269.
85. Kleinstiver BP, Pattanayak V, Prew MS, et al. High-fidelity CRISPR-Cas9 nucleases with no detectable genome-wide off-target effects. Nature. 2016;529(7587):490–5. https://doi.org/10.1038/nature16526.
86. Finn JD, Smith AR, Patel MC, et al. A single administration of CRISPR/Cas9 lipid nanoparticles achieves robust and persistent in vivo genome editing. Cell Rep. 2018;22(9):2227–35. https://doi.org/10.1016/j.celrep.2018.02.014.
87. Gillmore JD, Gane E, Taubel J, et al. CRISPR-Cas9 in vivo gene editing for transthyretin amyloidosis. N Engl J Med. 2021;385(6):493–502. https://doi.org/10.1056/NEJMoa2107454.
88. Ioannou A, Fontana M, Gillmore JD. RNA targeting and gene editing strategies for transthyretin amyloidosis. BioDrugs. 2023;37(2):127–42. https://doi.org/10.1007/s40259-023-00577-7.
89. Garcia-Pavia P, Siepen F, Donal E, et al. Phase 1 trial of antibody NI006 for depletion of cardiac transthyretin amyloid. N Engl J Med. 2023;389(3):239–50. https://doi.org/10.1056/NEJMoa2303765.
90. Griffin JM, Rosenblum H, Maurer MS. Pathophysiology and therapeutic approaches to cardiac amyloidosis. Circ Res.

2021;128(10):1554–75. https://doi.org/10.1161/circresaha.121.318187.
91. Michalon A, Hagenbuch A, Huy C, et al. A human antibody selective for transthyretin amyloid removes cardiac amyloid through phagocytic immune cells. Nat Commun. 2021;12(1):3142. https://doi.org/10.1038/s41467-021-23274-x.
92. Prothena. Prothena reports positive 9 month results from phase 1 long-term extension study of PRX004, the first investigational anti-amyloid immunotherapy for the treatment of ATTR amyloidosis. In. 2020.
93. Coelho T, Inês M, Conceição I, Soares M, de Carvalho M, Costa J. Natural history and survival in stage 1 Val30Met transthyretin familial amyloid polyneuropathy. Neurology. 2018;91(21):e1999–2009. https://doi.org/10.1212/wnl.0000000000006543.
94. Liepnieks JJ, Zhang LQ, Benson MD. Progression of transthyretin amyloid neuropathy after liver transplantation. Neurology. 2010;75(4):324–7. https://doi.org/10.1212/WNL.0b013e3181ea15d4.
95. Algalarrondo V, Antonini T, Théaudin M, et al. Prediction of long-term survival after liver transplantation for familial transthyretin amyloidosis. J Am Coll Cardiol. 2015;66(19):2154–6. https://doi.org/10.1016/j.jacc.2015.08.870.
96. Yamamoto S, Wilczek HE, Nowak G, et al. Liver transplantation for familial amyloidotic polyneuropathy (FAP): a single-center experience over 16 years. Am J Transplant. 2007;7(11):2597–604. https://doi.org/10.1111/j.1600-6143.2007.01969.x.
97. Dubrey SW, Burke MM, Hawkins PN, Banner NR. Cardiac transplantation for amyloid heart disease: the United Kingdom experience. J Heart Lung Transplant. 2004;23(10):1142–53. https://doi.org/10.1016/j.healun.2003.08.027.
98. Davis MK, Kale P, Liedtke M, et al. Outcomes after heart transplantation for amyloid cardiomyopathy in the modern era. Am J Transplant. 2015;15(3):650–8. https://doi.org/10.1111/ajt.13025.
99. Rosenbaum AN, AbouEzzeddine OF, Grogan M, et al. Outcomes after cardiac transplant for wild type transthyretin amyloidosis. Transplantation. 2018;102(11):1909–13. https://doi.org/10.1097/tp.0000000000002240.
100. Fine NM, Miller RJH. Heart transplantation for cardiac amyloidosis: the need for high-quality data to improve patient selection. Can J Cardiol. 2022;38(8):1144–6. https://doi.org/10.1016/j.cjca.2022.05.015.
101. Witteles RM. Cardiac transplantation and mechanical circulatory support in amyloidosis. JACC Cardio Oncol. 2021;3(4):516–21. https://doi.org/10.1016/j.jaccao.2021.05.007.
102. Bhimaraj A, Agrawal T, Duran A, et al. Percutaneous left axillary artery placement of intra-aortic balloon pump in advanced heart failure patients. JACC Heart Fail. 2020;8(4):313–23. https://doi.org/10.1016/j.jchf.2020.01.011.
103. Barrett CD, Alexander KM, Zhao H, et al. Outcomes in patients with cardiac amyloidosis undergoing heart transplantation. JACC Heart Fail. 2020;8(6):461–8. https://doi.org/10.1016/j.jchf.2019.12.013.
104. Kittleson MM, Ruberg FL, Ambardekar AV, et al. 2023 ACC expert consensus decision pathway on comprehensive multidisciplinary care for the patient with cardiac amyloidosis: a report of the American College of Cardiology Solution Set Oversight Committee. J Am Coll Cardiol. 2023;81(11):1076–126. https://doi.org/10.1016/j.jacc.2022.11.022.
105. Mehra MR, Canter CE, Hannan MM, et al. The 2016 International Society for Heart Lung Transplantation listing criteria for heart transplantation: a 10-year update. J Heart Lung Transplant. 2016;35(1):1–23. https://doi.org/10.1016/j.healun.2015.10.023.

Inherited Cardiac Conditions: Management of the Hypertrophic Cardiomyopathy Patient with Heart Failure

18

Sanjay Sivalokanathan, Alejandro De Feria Alsina, and Anjali Owens

Introduction

Hypertrophic cardiomyopathy (HCM) is the most common genetic cardiomyopathy globally, with a prevalence of 1:200–1:500, suggesting that as many as 750,000 Americans may be afflicted by this disorder [1]. It is a widely heterogeneous disorder with phenotypic variability, resulting in only a fraction (10–20%) of individuals being clinically diagnosed. However, highly effective diagnostic and treatment strategies have emerged, changing the paradigm of how HCM is identified and managed while substantially reducing disease-related morbidity and mortality rates. HCM can be classified as obstructive (oHCM), labile, or non-obstructive (nHCM). Obstructive HCM is diagnosed when the left ventricular outflow tract (LVOT) gradient is greater than 30 mmHg, which has a greater predilection of developing heart failure (HF) at a rate of 3% per year [1]. Symptoms of HCM can include fatigue, exercise intolerance, dyspnea, chest pain, palpitations, dizziness, and syncope, while some affected patients remain asymptomatic. Although HCM can be compatible with near-normal life expectancy, the risk of sudden cardiac death (0.32 per 1000 HCM person-years) and the prevalence (as high as 50%) of heart failure symptoms necessitates further development of non-invasive diagnostic tools and refinement of management strategies to accurately risk stratify patients and better evaluate disease progression [1]. This chapter focuses on the important distinctions in pathophysiology, clinical profile, and manifestation of HCM-related HF and the nuanced approach to diagnosis and management of this complex disorder.

Pathophysiology

A diverse array of mechanisms are implicated in the pathogenesis of HCM, with the clinical phenotype being a result of the complex interactions between genetic and environmental factors. In genotype-positive HCM, the initial defect is due to genetic variants resulting in changes in both the structure and function of cardiac sarcomere proteins, which subsequently instigates changes in gene expression and the activation of erroneous signaling pathways. Over time, these changes can result in molecular and histological alterations responsible for the clinical phenotypes of HCM [2]. However, it is important to acknowledge that approximately 50% of HCM patients

S. Sivalokanathan (✉)
Division of Internal Medicine, Pennsylvania Hospital of the University of Pennsylvania Health System, Philadelphia, PA, USA
e-mail: sanjay.sivalokanathan@pennmedicine.upenn.edu

A. D. F. Alsina · A. Owens (✉)
Division of Cardiovascular Medicine, Perelman School of Medicine, University of Pennsylvania, Philadelphia, PA, USA
e-mail: adeferia@pennmedicine.upenn.edu; anjali.owens@pennmedicine.upenn.edu

H. J. Eisen (ed.), *Heart Failure I*, https://doi.org/10.1007/978-3-032-12626-9_18

are genotype-negative and do not harbor an identifiable pathogenic variant. Within this cohort, development of left ventricular hypertrophy is likely the result of complex polygenic inheritance, which explains why approximately 0.5% of the population with the highest polygenic susceptibility are at a greater risk of developing HCM [3]. The pathological hallmarks of HCM include myocyte hypertrophy, myocyte disarray (affecting greater than 10% of the myocardium), interstitial fibrosis, and microvascular dysfunction. Several patterns of left ventricular hypertrophy (LVH) are described in HCM (Fig. 18.1), including either diffuse or segmental involvement, with the classic phenotype predominantly affecting the septum [4].

Furthermore, one-third of patients have obstruction at rest; the other third have labile obstruction, while the remaining third are non-obstructive. In oHCM, the subaortic (LVOT) obstruction is primarily attributed to the systolic anterior motion (SAM) of the mitral valve. Here, the anterior leaflet abuts the hypertrophied interventricular system during systole and is aided by the hydrodynamic force of the flow drag, causing obstruction to outflow. Further contributing factors include elongated mitral valve leaflets, abnormally positioned and hypertrophied papillary muscles, and accessory left ventricular (LV) muscle bundles. The subsequent subaortic obstruction can cause mechanical impedance, leading to LV systolic pressure overload and increased wall stress, associated with mild to severe mitral regurgitation and either a preserved or hyperdynamic LV function.

For the third of HCM patients, where the obstruction is dynamic and provokable, the diagnosis is typically made through stress (exercise) testing. However, Valsalva maneuver or amyl nitrate inhalation may be substituted in select patients who are unable to exercise with optimal effort [5]. More significantly, it may be influenced by factors such as ventricular volume, myocardial contractility, preload and afterload. Therefore, the obstruction arises when the ventricular volume is reduced during episodes of increased contractility and reductions in preload and afterload. Furthermore, in a subset of patients, the obstruction occurs in the mid-ventricle due to muscular apposition of the septum and anterolateral papillary muscle, which insert directly into the anterior leaflet or septal and LV free wall. Patients with the mid-cavitary variant of HCM are at risk of developing an apical aneurysm over time.

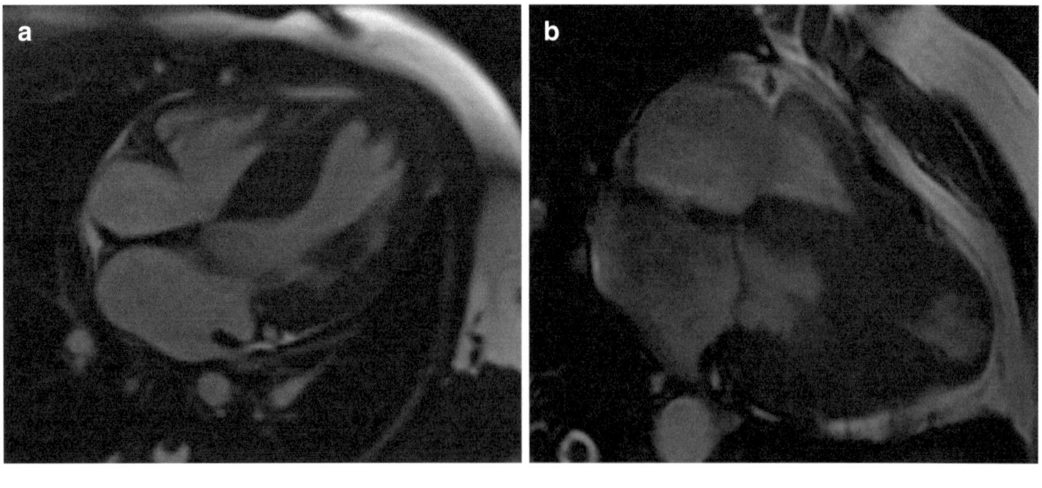

Fig. 18.1 Hypertrophic cardiomyopathy (HCM) may manifest in different phenotypes, with the most frequently observed being (**a**) asymmetric hypertrophy affecting the basal interventricular septum. The mid-ventricle may also be involved, with development of an apical aneurysm (**b**). Other types of HCM include symmetric/concentric, apical, masslike, and noncontiguous

Diagnosis

HCM is most often an autosomal dominant disorder caused by pathogenic variants affecting the sarcomere protein genes, resulting in metabolic inflexibility and inefficient muscular contraction that leads to the many sequelae of HCM, which include arrhythmias, heart failure, and sudden cardiac death. Both echocardiography and cardiovascular magnetic resonance (CMR) imaging are synergistic for diagnosis, describing a hypertrophied, non-dilated LV that is not associated with other cardiac, metabolic, or systemic diseases.

The clinical presentation of HCM is highly variable. While symptoms are often attributed to obstruction, it is important to remain vigilant for heart failure symptoms, even in the non-obstructive patients. Furthermore, although mortality associated with HCM-related HF is less common, up to 50% of patients experience a measure [New York Heart Association (NYHA) functional class II to IV] of HF disability, cementing the need for early and astute recognition [6]. Unlike the archetypal features of congestive heart failure (CHF), HCM-related HF is commonly due to dynamic mechanical impedance to flow in the LVOT, produced by the systolic anterior motion of the mitral valve, which results in high intracavitary pressures. Therefore, signs of extravascular volume overload, such as peripheral edema, are often absent in oHCM patients. In nHCM, exertional dyspnea and fatigue are becoming increasingly recognized symptoms of heart failure and are likely attributable to both diastolic dysfunction and microvascular ischemia [6]. On the opposite end of the spectrum, a small but growing subset (5–15%) of patients, labeled 'end-stage', are characterized by depressed LV systolic function which is defined by a LV ejection fraction (LVEF) < 50%, accompanied in some patients by left ventricular dilatation and wall thinning (Fig. 18.2) [7, 8]. Here, symptoms such as dyspnea, paroxysmal nocturnal dyspnea, orthopnea, and reduced exercise tolerance are more prevalent.

Differentiating between hypertensive cardiomyopathy and HCM may be challenging, particularly due to the age-dependent expression of cardiac hypertrophy and when the wall thickness ranges from 13–17 mm. However, markers that favor HCM include SAM and mitral valve-septal contact with a dynamic LV outflow tract gradient; septal thickness greater than 17 mm; LV hypertrophy that dominates the apex, anterolateral free wall or posterior septum; with diffuse or prominent late gadolinium enhancement (LGE) [9, 10].

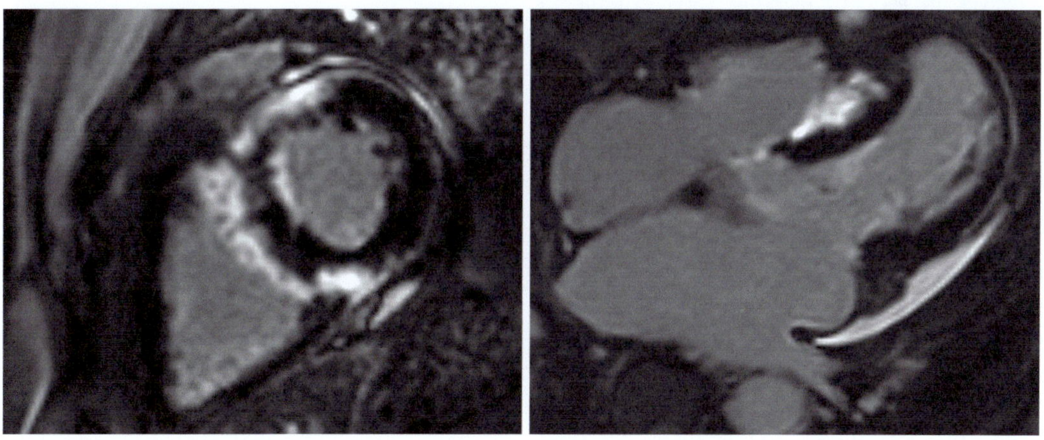

Fig. 18.2 Cardiac magnetic resonance imaging (MRI) demonstrating 'end-stage' hypertrophic cardiomyopathy with extensive late gadolinium enhancement (LGE)

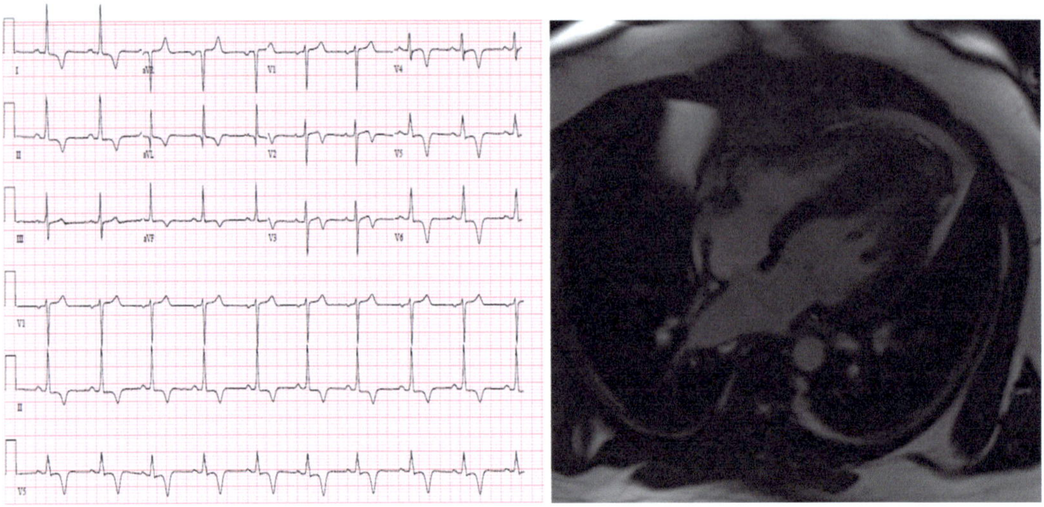

Fig. 18.3 Electrocardiogram (ECG) demonstrates deep T-wave inversions representative of apical HCM, confirmed by cardiovascular magnetic resonance (CMR) imaging

Electrocardiogram

The 12-lead electrocardiogram (ECG) is a vital tool for evaluating HCM. Nonetheless, it should be noted that the ECG may appear normal in 5–20% of adults with HCM [11, 12]. Abnormal ECG patterns seen in HCM include left atrial enlargement, ST-T wave abnormalities (prominent ST-segment elevation in anterior leads; biphasic, flat, or asymmetric T-wave inversion), increased voltages (deep S-waves in V1–V3, high R-waves in V4–V6) meeting LVH criteria, Q waves (detected in up to 53% of HCM patients) or pre-excitation. Notably, giant symmetric T-wave inversions are characteristic of apical HCM (Fig. 18.3). Additionally, ECG patterns that suggest fibrosis and an increased risk for arrhythmias include atrioventricular delay and QRS fragmentation [13]. Common patterns associated with HF include intraventricular delay and QT prolongation, also associated with LVOT obstruction [13].

The ECG can be utilized in sudden cardiac death (SCD) risk stratification. In particular, a wide QRS (>120 ms), ST-segment elevation ('pseudo-STEMI' pattern), and low QRS voltages are associated with an increased risk of SCD as well as an increase in appropriate implantable cardioverter defibrillator (ICD) discharges [14]. Moreover, ECG has a vital role in differential diagnosis. For instance, a discrepancy between the magnitude of LVH, as assessed by echocardiography, in comparison to the amplitude of the QRS voltage is typical of an infiltrative disorder [13].

Transthoracic Echocardiography

Transthoracic echocardiography (TTE) is the first imaging modality (Fig. 18.4) for diagnosing HCM. In adults, the criteria for identifying HCM include a ventricular wall thickness greater than or equal to 15 mm in the absence of abnormal loading conditions or greater than or equal to 13 mm in familial HCM. In adults with HCM, the average maximal LV thickness is reported to be around 21–22 mm [1]. TTE has several advantages, such as characterizing SAM, mechanical impedance, and mechanisms of LV outflow obstruction [1]. Moreover, it provides reliable and reproducible measurements of peak LV outflow gradient, the magnitude of mitral regurgitation, other concomitant valvular disorders, degree

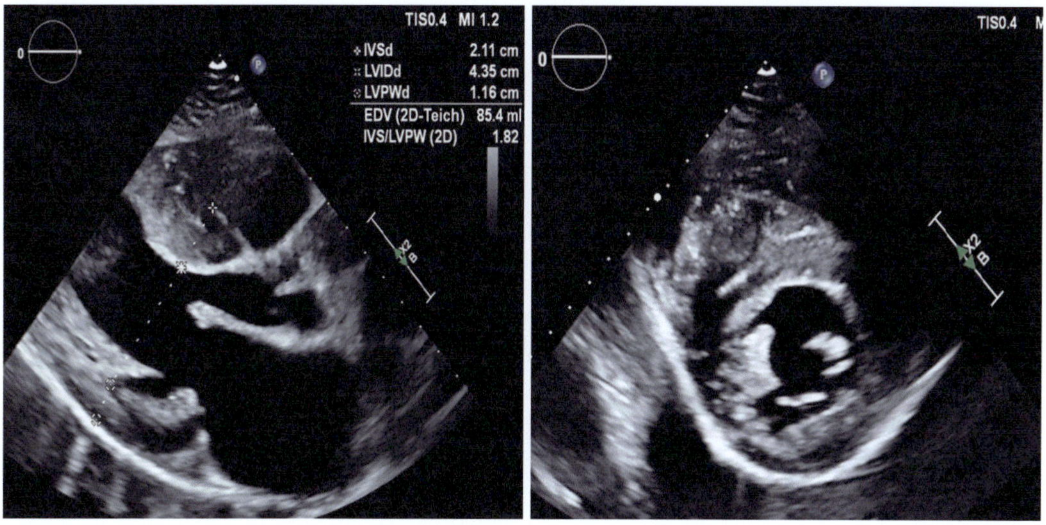

Fig. 18.4 Echocardiography demonstrating the archetypal features of hypertrophic cardiomyopathy (HCM)

of diastolic dysfunction, and estimation of the pulmonary arterial pressure. Features of HCM include a normal end-diastolic volume (EDV), reduced end-systolic volume, and a high (>70%) LVEF. Diastolic dysfunction is frequent in HCM and is a marker for both the diagnosis and progression of HF. This is characterized by increased LV end-diastolic pressure, impaired relaxation, filling and distensibility, and increased left atrial volume [6]. More importantly, subtle changes in diastology, such as mean early diastolic myocardial velocities (Ea ≤13.5 cm/s), are apparent in genotype-positive HCM individuals prior to the development of LVH [15].

In addition, HCM patients experience a reduction in global longitudinal strain, a measure of systolic function [16]. More significantly, continuous wave Doppler echocardiography at rest, with Valsalva, and with stress is essential in estimating subaortic gradients accurately. Exercise stress echocardiography may be necessary to provoke labile LV outflow gradients. This approach, combined with cardiopulmonary exercise testing (CPET), may identify candidates for septal reduction therapy (SRT) or for heart transplant in oHCM and nHCM patients, respectively. In addition, it may provide valuable insights into the clinical progression of the disorder. For instance, the risk of developing advanced HF symptoms is 1.6% per year in nHCM, in contrast to 3.2% per year in labile obstructive HCM [6]. However, limitations of echocardiography include poor acoustic windows in some patients and underestimation of the wall thickness.

Cardiovascular Magnetic Resonance Imaging

Cardiovascular magnetic resonance (CMR) imaging is complementary to echocardiogram for assessing HCM, providing high spatial and temporal resolution. More significantly, CMR can accurately identify focal hypertrophy and tissue characterization, which is important in differentiating between physiological remodeling (such as athlete's heart) and pathological disorders (such as hypertensive cardiomyopathy or infiltrative diseases). Table 18.1 outlines the advantages of CMR over TTE.

Furthermore, CMR offers a range of valuable applications for effectively characterizing and evaluating the risk associated with HCM. This includes the use of late gadolinium enhancement, parametric [T1-, T2- and extracellular volume (ECV)] mapping, and perfusion CMR [1]. LGE and parametric mapping can help identify the presence and extent of fibrosis (or scarring), which does not conform to a typical coronary vasculature distribution and is often found in patchy multiple foci (Fig. 18.5). The magnitude and distribution of LGE have been linked to adverse outcomes such as SCD, progression to HF, and ventricular arrhythmias. Stress perfusion MRI is another important tool for evaluating myocardial blood flow at rest and stress, often reduced in HCM patients and correlates with the degree of LV hypertrophy. In addition, when encountering mid-ventricular HCM, CMR is important in excluding apical aneurysm and thrombus formation.

Table 18.1 Advantages of Cardiac MRI in the assessment of HCM

Advantages
Optimal assessment of the left ventricle, providing accurate and reliable volumetric assessments
Better precision in assessing ventricular wall thickness
Identification of hypertrophy in areas of the left ventricle that are poorly visualized by echocardiography
Assessment for left ventricular apical aneurysm
Assessing microvascular dysfunction through stress perfusion MRI
Tissue characterization (late gadolinium enhancement, parametric mapping), which can help differentiate HCM from phenocopies
Pre-operative planning for septal reduction therapy
Sudden death risk stratification

Genetics and Screening

HCM is typically inherited in an autosomal dominant pattern, placing first-degree relatives with a 50% chance of carrying the disease. Pathogenic variants are most frequently observed in genes encoding sarcomere proteins, including MYBPC3, MYH7, MYL2, MYL3, ACTC1, TPM1, TNNI3, TNNT2 [2]. In addition, pathogenic variants in genes encoding Z disk proteins, sarcomere associated proteins, and calcium handling proteins have also been implicated in HCM. Identification of a genetic etiology in HCM patients can vary widely (30–60%) depending on the age of diagnosis, family history, and comorbid conditions. Heterogeneity in phenotypic expression and clinical course is typical and should be relayed to family members. Presently, specific variants are not utilized to predict prognosis, clinical course, or sudden death [1]. However, in aggregate, patients with pathogenic/likely pathogenic sarcomere variants have an increased risk for adverse outcomes [17]. One potential benefit of genetic testing is the ability to identify HCM phenocopies, including Fabry disease, cardiac amyloidosis, and other inherited conditions that cause the phenotype of left ventricular hypertrophy. In addition, genetic screen-

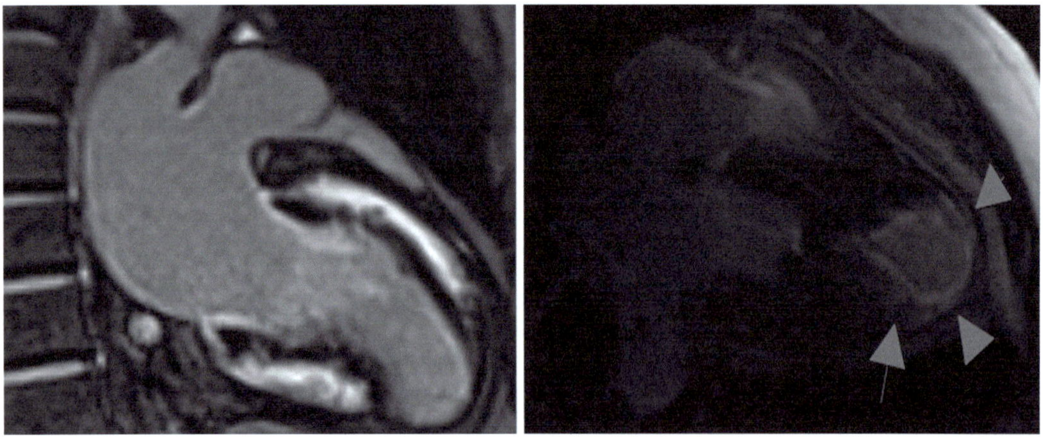

Fig. 18.5 Cardiovascular magnetic resonance (CMR) imaging demonstrating extensive late gadolinium enhancement in a patient with (**a**) end-stage and (**b**) mid-ventricular hypertrophic cardiomyopathy with apical aneurysm

ing offers a useful approach for discharging genotype-negative patients while maintaining longitudinal follow-up with genotype-positive but phenotype-negative individuals. In familial HCM, the preferred screening tool is echocardiography, which helps identify relatives with the HCM phenotype, potentially facilitating early intervention and management [1]. Subtle structural abnormalities include diastolic dysfunction, and with the use of speckle-tracking echocardiography, it may reveal increased LV rotation and twist, as well as increased apical rotation [18]. Furthermore, in certain cases, CMR may help identify pathological findings such as increased ECV as well as a reduction in myocardial blood flow (MBF), which underscores the significance of myocardial fibrosis and perfusion abnormalities, respectively, prior to the development of LVH [19]. Nevertheless, the natural history of this cohort remains unclear and unresolved, as phenotypic conversion is not universal and challenging to predict.

Cardiac Biomarkers

Cardiac biomarkers are useful additional tools in predicting outcomes and guiding treatment in patients with HCM and heart failure. N-terminal pro–B-type natriuretic peptide (NT-proBNP), can be useful in both risk stratifying HCM as well as playing a role in diagnosing and characterizing the severity of heart failure [1]. Additionally, in HCM, elevated levels of troponin reflect myocardial necrosis and interstitial fibrosis [1].

Management

Comprehensive evaluation of the HCM patient includes a detailed personal and family history, followed by a physical examination, 12-lead ECG and TTE. CMR, cardiac rhythm monitoring, stress echocardiography and cardiopulmonary exercise testing are essential but underutilized, often due to a lack of resources or expertise. The potential complications of HCM include LVOT obstruction with significant HF symptoms requiring SRT; sudden cardiac death; atrial and ventricular arrhythmias, including an increased burden of atrial fibrillation; and progression to end-stage, nonobstructive HCM [6]. It is customary for yearly or biennial follow-up, with the evaluation focusing on LV morphology, development of LVOT obstruction, complications such as HF or arrhythmias, and change in EF or SCD profile. Therefore, it is recommended that TTEs be performed annually, while CMRs be repeated every 3–5 years based on the clinical scenario. Accurate risk stratification of SCD plays a fundamental role in the assessment of HCM, with the American College of Cardiology (ACC)/American Heart Association (AHA) and the European Society of Cardiology (ESC) identifying several key risk factors such as a prior cardiac arrest, repeated runs of nonsustained ventricular tachycardia (NSVT), unexplained syncope, family history of SCD, and severe hypertrophy (greater than or equal to 30 mm) [1]. Moreover, additional risk factors that should be taken into account include the extent of LGE, the presence of an LV apical aneurysm, and the development of LVEF <50%. Of particular significance, LGE $\geq$15% is highly correlated with adverse cardiac events and may prompt consideration of prophylactic ICD. HCM patients with an LV apical aneurysm are not only at increased risk of SCD but also formation of intracavitary thrombus, thus necessitating consideration of primary prevention ICD and systemic anticoagulation, respectively [6]. CPET is an important measure of functional capacity and can provide valuable insights into the clinical profile of HCM patients. Here, it has been observed that HCM patients exhibit reduced peak myocardial oxygen consumption (VO_2) for age, at times even when they report no exercise limitation. CPET can be followed over time to assess for early changes in objective functional capacity and to assess response to treatment. In addition, pVO2 can be helpful in determining timing (<14 ml/kg/min or < 50% predicted for age) for heart transplantation in nHCM. Right heart catheterization can be utilized in conjunction with CPET for hemodynamic assessment of patients with advancing stage of nonobstructive HCM and can be critical in identifying the subset of patients who develop severe pulmonary hypertension and pulmonary vascular disease. Annual ambulatory ECG monitoring is an integral and necessary step in the continued evaluation of HCM patients. This, subsequently, allows detection of both ventricular and supraventricular arrhythmias. Extended ambulatory ECG monitoring should be considered in particular when screening for atrial fibrillation which occurs in up to 30% of patients with HCM and requires initiation of anticoagulation for prevention of stroke [20].

The current options for the treatment of HCM include addressing symptoms of obstruction, diastolic dysfunction, risk of SCD, arrhythmias, and heart failure (Fig. 18.6). In general, treatment may be directed by hemodynamic subtype; oHCM and nHCM. In symptomatic obstructive HCM, pharmacologic treatment options include beta-blockers, non-dihydropyridine calcium channel blockers, and disopyramide. Disopyramide, an antiarrhythmic, may be added onto beta blocker or calcium channel blocker as second line therapy due to its additional negative inotropic action. It is important to note that the outflow obstruction, and thus symptom burden, may vary greatly due to changes in physiological loading such as standing, hydration, meals or alcohol intake. Therefore, it is advisable to heed supportive measures such as adequate hydration and avoiding triggers such as prolonged standing or excessive alcohol consumption. If symptoms are not controlled adequately despite maximal medical therapy, invasive septal reduction therapy (SRT) may be necessary. There are two broad approaches to SRT, which include surgical septal myectomy or alcohol septal ablation (ASA). Surgical myectomy has low operative mortality (<1%, when performed in experienced centers) and produces reversal of HF and durable symptom relief in 90–95% of cases. Percutaneous ASA produces transmural basal septal infarction that relieves LV outflow gradient and, thus, HF symptoms in properly selected patients with

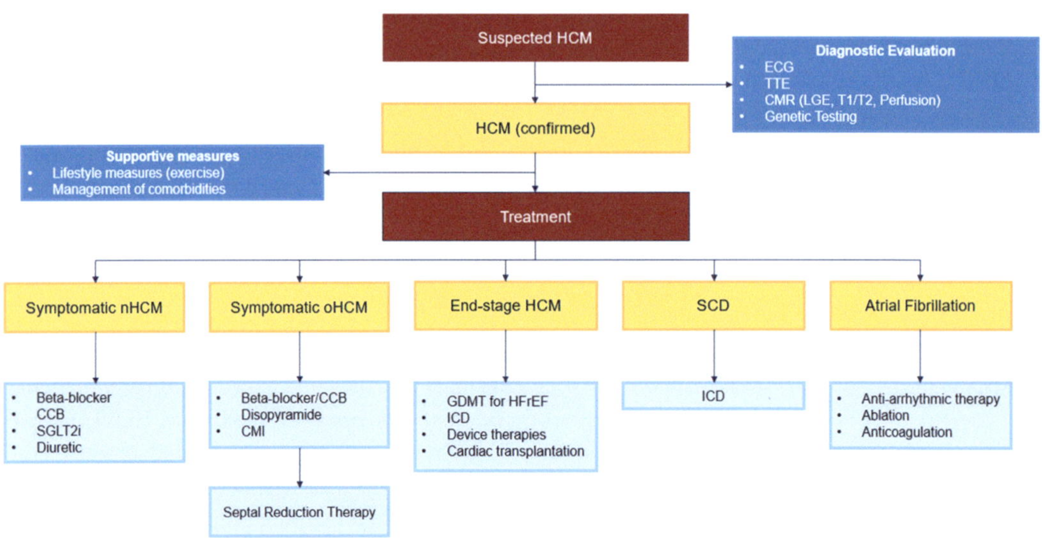

Fig. 18.6 Algorithm for the diagnosis and management of symptomatic hypertrophic cardiomyopathy. CCB calcium channel blocker; CMI cardiac myosin inhibitor, CMR cardiovascular magnetic resonance imaging; ECG electrocardiogram; GDMT guideline-directed medical therapy; HCM hypertrophic cardiomyopathy; HFrEF heart failure with reduced ejection fraction; ICD implantable cardioverter defibrillator; LA left atrium; LGE late gadolinium enhancement; LVH left ventricular hypertrophy; LVOTO LV outflow tract obstruction; nHCM nonobstructive HCM; NSVT non-sustained ventricular tachycardia; oHCM obstructive HCM; SCA sudden cardiac arrest; SCD sudden cardiac death; SGLT2i sodium-glucose transporter 2 inhibitor; TTE transthoracic echocardiogram

favorable coronary and septal anatomy and no significant intrinsic mitral valve disease.

Most recently, inhibition of myosin ATPase with the selective, reversible cardiac myosin inhibitors (CMIs) mavacamten and aficamten has been demonstrated to be effective in reducing LVOT gradients and improving symptoms and quality of life in oHCM patients. Clinical trials of mavacamten, including PIONEER-HCM, EXPLORER-HCM, VALOR-HCM, and MAVA-LTE, demonstrated significant improvements in peak oxygen consumption, cardiac biomarkers, patient-reported outcomes, and NYHA class, as well as the ability to delay or prevent the need for SRT in eligible patients. In addition to reduction in LVOT gradient, structural remodeling including reduction of LV mass and left atrial volume were observed over longer term follow up [21–23]. Mavacamten received US FDA approval as the first-in-class CMI in April 2022 for treatment of symptomatic patients with obstructive HCM. Dosing and titration require periodic surveillance with an echocardiogram to assess LVOT gradient and LVEF. If LVEF decreases to <50%, temporary drug discontinuation is required. The safety and efficacy of aficamten, a next-in-class CMI, were evaluated in both the Phase 2 and Phase 3 clinical trials REDWOOD-HCM and SEQUOIA-HCM, respectively [24, 25]. Reduction in LVOT gradient, improved cardiac biomarkers, and symptom improvement were seen within two weeks of starting aficamten and sustained throughout the treatment period. Aficamen has a relatively short half-life (3.4 days), which, in comparison to mavacamten (7–9 days), provides the option for more rapid up-titration and also faster washout in case LV dysfunction occurs [24, 25]. Ongoing longitudinal follow-up studies will determine if these agents have the potential to modify disease trajectory and assess long-term safety. It should be noted that the current European and US guidelines recommend the use of CMIs as an adjunct to AV nodal blockers to improve symptoms in patients with resting or labile obstruction [26, 27]. Alternatively, CMIs may be utilized as monotherapy in patients with resting or labile obstruction who are intolerant to or have contraindications for beta-blocker, calcium channel blocker, or disopyramide treatment [26].

In patients with symptomatic nonobstructive HCM, similar to oHCM, current guideline recommended treatment includes beta-blockers and non-dihydropyridine calcium channel blockers [27]. If congestive symptoms are present, diuretic therapy can be added. However, none of these therapies have undergone rigorous placebo-controlled trials. Given the efficacy of myosin inhibitors in oHCM, there are two phase 3 randomized controlled trials to assess the efficacy and safety of CMIs in patients with symptomatic nonobstructive HCM: ODYSSEY-HCM (NCT05582395) and ACACIA-HCM (NCT06081894).

Advanced or end-stage heart failure in HCM occurs as a result of progressive adverse remodeling and can result in regression of hypertrophy and subsequent LV dilation and dysfunction due to accumulation of replacement fibrosis. However, it is important to note that end-stage HCM can be present with normal *or* reduced LVEF, and cases with a restrictive end-stage phenotype can be particularly challenging to recognize. If LVEF <50%, pharmacologic treatment should transition to guideline-directed medical therapy (GDMT) for HF with reduced LVEF, as well as consideration for ICD placement. In this setting, calcium channel blockers and disopyramide should be discontinued [27]. The four pillars of heart failure with reduced ejection fraction (HFrEF) therapy [beta-blockers, renin-angiotensin-aldosterone system (RAAS) inhibitors or angiotensin receptor/neprilysin inhibitors (ARNIs), mineralocorticoid receptor antagonists (MRAs) and sodium-glucose cotransporter-2 (SGLT2) inhibitors] can be instituted with particular attention to LV cavitary size, systemic blood pressure, preload and renal function as determinants of extent to which systemic vasodilation will be tolerated. Diuretics may be useful for pulmonary congestion, but vigilance should remain to avoid hypovolemia and hypotension. Right heart catheterization can be helpful in guiding pharmacologic management of end-stage patients and determining if inotropes or pulmonary vasodilator therapy may be required as bridge to transplantation.

The introduction of ICDs has played an important role in the reduction of sudden deaths and includes both primary and secondary indications. The rate of appropriate discharges ranges from 3–15%, with its complication rate being less than 5% per year [6]. In end-stage HCM, heart transplantation is the only definitive treatment. Further supportive management of HCM-related HF patients includes cardiac rehabilitation, with recent evidence highlighting that exercise is not associated with adverse cardiac events, promoting a reduction in rates of obesity and coronary artery disease (CAD) [28].

Future Treatment Options

Increased understanding of the underlying pathophysiology of disease in HCM has led to the investigation and emergence of several new potential therapies. For instance, ninerafaxstat is a novel cardiac mitotrope that inhibits 3-ketoacyl CoA thiolase and shifts myocardial substrate utilization in favor of glucose, facilitating the restoration of myocardial energy hemostasis. As evidenced by the results of the Phase 2 IMPROVE-HCM study, ninerafaxstat has demonstrated a reduction in symptom burden and improved ventilatory efficiency in a subset of patients with nHCM [29]. Furthermore, SGLT2 inhibitors may have a role in HCM patients. Observational studies have demonstrated lower rates of mortality, hospitalization, and cardiovascular symptoms. A potential mechanism may be its beneficial effect on cardiac energetics, which may result in favorable LV remodeling [30]. Moreover, detailed genotyping is likely to play a critical role in guiding future therapeutic options in HCM. MicroRNAs may be a means of reversing myocyte hypertrophy and fibrosis, while in vivo CRISPR gene editing is emerging as a promising treatment choice that has demonstrated the reversion of genes to their wild-type function. However, phase 1 human clinical trials are needed to evaluate the safety and efficacy of this approach [31–33]. An important stride in gene therapy is TN-201, which utilizes an adeno-associated virus (AAV) serotype 9 vector, and is being investigated in a phase 1 study involving patients with MYBPC3 related nHCM [34].

References

1. Maron BJ, Desai MY, Nishimura RA, et al. Diagnosis and evaluation of hypertrophic cardiomyopathy: JACC state-of-the-art review. J Am Coll Cardiol. 2022;79(4):372–89.
2. Marian AJ, Braunwald E. Hypertrophic cardiomyopathy: genetics, pathogenesis, clinical manifestations, diagnosis, and therapy. Circ Res. 2017;121(7):749–70.
3. Harper AR, Goel A, Grace C, et al. Common genetic variants and modifiable risk factors underpin hypertrophic cardiomyopathy susceptibility and expressivity. Nat Genet. 2021;53(2):135–42.
4. Chun EJ, Choi SI, Jin KN, et al. Hypertrophic cardiomyopathy: assessment with MR imaging and multidetector CT. Radiographics. 2010;30(5):1309–28.
5. Maron MS, Olivotto I, Zenovich AG, et al. Hypertrophic cardiomyopathy is predominantly a disease of left ventricular outflow tract obstruction. Circulation. 2006;114(21):2232–9.
6. Maron BJ, Rowin EJ, Udelson JE, Maron MS. Clinical spectrum and management of heart failure in hypertrophic cardiomyopathy. JACC Heart Fail. 2018;6(5):353–63.
7. Melacini P, Basso C, Angelini A, et al. Clinicopathological profiles of progressive heart failure in hypertrophic cardiomyopathy. Eur Heart J. 2010;31(17):2111–23. https://doi.org/10.1093/eurheartj/ehq136. Epub 2010 May 31.
8. Maron BJ, Spirito P. Implications of left ventricular remodeling in hypertrophic cardiomyopathy. Am J Cardiol. 1998;81(11):1339–44.
9. Sipola P, Magga J, Husso M, et al. Cardiac MRI assessed left ventricular hypertrophy in differentiating hypertensive heart disease from hypertrophic cardiomyopathy attributable to a sarcomeric gene mutation. Eur Radiol. 2011;21(7):1383–9.
10. Burrage MK, Ferreira VM. Cardiovascular magnetic resonance for the differentiation of left ventricular hypertrophy. Curr Heart Fail Rep. 2020;17(5):192–204.
11. McLeod CJ, Ackerman MJ, Nishimura RA, et al. Outcome of patients with hypertrophic cardiomyopathy and a normal electrocardiogram. J Am Coll Cardiol. 2009;54(3):229–33.
12. Cronin H, Vaughan C, Gallagher M, et al. Promise or peril: the ECG in hypertrophic cardiomyopathy. Heart. 2022;108:A35.
13. Bernardini A, Crotti L, Olivotto I, Cecchi F. Diagnostic and prognostic electrocardiographic features in patients with hypertrophic cardiomyopathy. Eur Heart J Suppl. 2023;25(Suppl C):C173–8.
14. Biagini E, Pazzi C, Olivotto I, et al. Usefulness of electrocardiographic patterns at presentation to

predict long-term risk of cardiac death in patients with hypertrophic cardiomyopathy. Am J Cardiol. 2016;118(3):432–9.
15. Ho CY, Sweitzer NK, McDonough B, Maron BJ, Casey SA, Seidman JG, Seidman CE, Solomon SD. Assessment of diastolic function with Doppler tissue imaging to predict genotype in preclinical hypertrophic cardiomyopathy. Circulation. 2002;105(25):2992–7.
16. Tower-Radar A, Mohananey D, To A, et al. Prognostic value of global longitudinal strain in hypertrophic cardiomyopathy: a systematic review of existing literature. J Am Coll Cardiol Img. 2019;12:1930–42.
17. Ho CY, Day SM, Ashley EA, et al. Genotype and lifetime burden of disease in hypertrophic cardiomyopathy: insights from the sarcomeric human cardiomyopathy registry (SHaRe). Circulation. 2018;138(14):1387–98.
18. Forsey J, Benson L, Rozenblyum E, Friedberg MK, Mertens L. Early changes in apical rotation in genotype positive children with hypertrophic cardiomyopathy mutations without hypertrophic changes on two-dimensional imaging. J Am Soc Echocardiogr. 2014;27(2):215–21.
19. Ho CY, Abbasi SA, Neilan TG, et al. T1 measurements identify extracellular volume expansion in hypertrophic cardiomyopathy sarcomere mutation carriers with and without left ventricular hypertrophy. Circ Cardiovasc Imaging. 2013;6(3):415–22.
20. Rowin EJ, Hausvater A, Link MS, et al. Clinical profile and consequences of atrial fibrillation in hypertrophic cardiomyopathy. Circulation. 2017;136(25):2420–36.
21. Olivotto I, Oreziak A, Barriales-Villa R, et al. Mavacamten for treatment of symptomatic obstructive hypertrophic cardiomyopathy (EXPLORER-HCM): a randomised, double-blind, placebo-controlled, phase 3 trial [published correction appears in Lancet. 2020 Sep 12;396(10253):758]. Lancet. 2020;396(10253):759–69.
22. Milind DY, Owens A, Geske Jeffrey B, et al. Myosin inhibition in patients with obstructive hypertrophic cardiomyopathy referred for septal reduction therapy. J Am Coll Cardiol. 2022;80(2):95–108.
23. Rader F, Oręziak A, Choudhury L, et al. Mavacamten treatment for symptomatic obstructive hypertrophic cardiomyopathy: interim results from the MAVA-LTE study, EXPLORER-LTE Cohort. JACC Heart Fail. 2024;12(1):164–77.
24. Maron MS, Masri A, Choudhury L, et al. Phase 2 study of aficamten in patients with obstructive hypertrophic cardiomyopathy. J Am Coll Cardiol. 2023;81:34–45.
25. Maron MS, Masri A, Nassif ME et al. Aficamten for symptomatic obstructive hypertrophic cardiomyopathy. N Engl J Med. Published online May 13, 2024.
26. Arbelo E, Protonotarios A, Gimeno JR, et al. 2023 ESC guidelines for the management of cardiomyopathies. Eur Heart J. 2023;44(37):3503–626.
27. Ommen SR, Ho CY, Asif IM et al. 2024 AHA/ACC/AMSSM/HRS/PACES/SCMR guideline for the Management of Hypertrophic Cardiomyopathy: a report of the American Heart Association/American College of Cardiology Joint Committee on Clinical Practice Guidelines. Circulation. Published online May 8, 2024.
28. Lampert R, Ackerman MJ, Marino BS, et al. Vigorous exercise in patients with hypertrophic cardiomyopathy. JAMA Cardiol. 2023;8(6):595–605.
29. Maron M, Mahmod M, Abd Samat A, et al. Safety and efficacy of metabolic modulation with ninerafaxstat in patients with nonobstructive hypertrophic cardiomyopathy. J Am Coll Cardiol. 83:2037–48.
30. Aglan A, Fath A, Eldaly A et al. Impact of sodium-glucose cotransporter 2 inhibitors on mortality in hypertrophic cardiomyopathy. JACC Adv. 2024;3(3).
31. Chai AC, Cui M, Chemello F, et al. Base editing correction of hypertrophic cardiomyopathy in human cardiomyocytes and humanized mice. Nat Med. 2023;29(2):401–11.
32. Reichart D, Newby GA, Wakimoto H, et al. Efficient in vivo genome editing prevents hypertrophic cardiomyopathy in mice. Nat Med. 2023;29(2):412–21.
33. Strong A. CRISPR gene-editing therapies for hypertrophic cardiomyopathy. Nat Med. 2023;29(2):305–6.
34. Haroldson J, Harrison W, Lombardi L, et al. MyPeak-1: a phase 1b study to evaluate safety and efficacy of TN-201, an adeno-associated virus serotype 9 (AAV9) investigational gene therapy, in adults with MYBPC3-associated hypertrophic cardiomyopathy (HCM). J Card Fail. 2024;30(1):55.

Heart Failure in Adult Congenital Heart Disease

19

Amanda W. Cai and Elisa A. Bradley

Introduction

With advances in medical and surgical care, it is expected that children born with congenital heart disease (CHD) will survive to adulthood, compared just half a century ago when only 25% survival was reported [1]. Most interesting, is that definitive infant surgery for those with complex cardiac defects were not approached until the mid and late 1970s. This has led to an emerging ACHD population inclusive of those who are for the first time, are surviving beyond age 40 into mid and later adulthood, for example those with hypoplastic left heart syndrome (HLHS) and Dextro-Transposition of the great arteries (D-TGA). At present, approximately 84% of children with CHD are expected to survive to age 40 and beyond [2]. With changes in survival for complex groups, sudden cardiac death as the leading cause of death in the ACHD has been supplanted by chronic circulatory failure, which accounts for 21–40% of all deaths in this group [3–5]. Stratified data from the National Inpatient Sample additionally has demonstrated that heart failure (HF)-related hospitalizations in patients with underlying ACHD have increased 91% in the first decade since the turn of the twenty-first century (from 1998 to 2011), as compared to a 21% increase in those without underlying CHD [6]. The changing demographic of middle and older-aged adults with increasingly complex CHD requires healthcare teams to understand the unique characteristics of HF and management of late CHD. Comprehensive evaluation and treatment of lesion-specific heart failure is beyond the scope of this chapter; however, general concepts and emerging areas of focus regarding HF in the patient with ACHD are cursorily reviewed.

A. W. Cai
Pennsylvania State University Hershey S. Milton Medical Center, Heart and Vascular Institute, Division of Cardiovascular Medicine, Hershey, PA, USA
e-mail: acai1@pennstatehealth.psu.edu

E. A. Bradley (✉)
Pennsylvania State University Hershey S. Milton Medical Center, Heart and Vascular Institute, Division of Cardiovascular Medicine, Hershey, PA, USA

Pennsylvania State University College of Medicine, Hershey, PA, USA

Pennsylvania State University, College of Medicine, Department of Cellular and Molecular Physiology, Hershey, PA, USA
e-mail: ebradley3@pennstatehealth.psu

H. J. Eisen (ed.), *Heart Failure I*, https://doi.org/10.1007/978-3-032-12626-9_19

Classification of Heart Failure

There is no universally accepted definition for HF in the ACHD population due to the heterogeneity of underlying CHD. Further, the presentation of HF in ACHD is unique because abnormal myocardial architecture is often present from birth, and adaptation, perhaps through epigenetic changes among others, affect functional class and tolerability of the condition. In most cases, this is clinically characterized by a patient with severe anatomic and physiologic abnormalities, who appears to have reasonably good subjective functional class. In such cases, objective measures of function, such as VO2 are often abnormal, and small changes in these parameters suggest significant decline in function, albeit without apparent changes in New York Heart Association (NYHA) functional class [7]. Two iterations of the U.S. ACHD guidelines have been published to date: the first in 2008 and the more recent in 2018, with an anticipated update in 2025 [8, 9]. In the 2018 guidelines, a new classification system for evaluation of ACHD patients was created to more accurately capture the variable complexity of the CHD population (Tables 19.1 and 19.2). This system, the ACHD Anatomic Physiologic or AP Classification, subdivides CHD anatomy into 3 categories based on severity of the defect (simple, moderate complexity, and great complexity) and 4 subcategories of physiologic severity (A, B, C, and D) and are routinely used in clinical practice [9].

Table 19.1 Anatomic classification of adult congenital heart disease

Congenital heart disease anatomy
Simple
Isolated septal defects Mild isolated pulmonic stenosis Repaired PDA, ASD, or VSD without residual sequelae (shunt, chamber enlargement, valvular regurgitation)
Moderate Complexity
Anomalous pulmonary veins Anomalous coronaries Atrioventricular septal defect (AVSD) Coarctation of the aorta Congenital aortic or mitral valve disease Ebstein Anomaly Infundibular right ventricular outflow obstruction Moderate or large shunts, unrepaired or repaired with residual sequelae Pulmonary valve disease (moderate or greater) Subaortic stenosis or Shone Complex Tetralogy of Fallot
Great Complexity
Cyanotic congenital heart defects Double outlet ventricle Fontal procedure Interrupted aortic arch Mitral atresia Single ventricle Pulmonary atresia Transposition of the great arteries Truncus arteriosus Other abnormalities of atrioventricular or ventriculoarterial connection (e.g., heterotaxy syndromes)

Adapted from the 2018 AHA/ACC Guideline for the Management of Adults with Congenital Heart Disease [9]

Table 19.2 Physiologic classification of adult congenital heart disease

Physiologic Stage	NYHA FC symptoms	Hemodynamic or anatomic sequelae (e.g., aortic enlargement, ventricular enlargement, ventricular dysfunction, residual shunt, valve disease)	Arrhythmias	Exercise capacity	End-organ function	Hypoxemia, cyanosis, or pulmonary hypertension
A	I	None	None	Normal	Normal	None
B	II	Mild	Not requiring treatment	Abnormal objective cardiac limitation to exercise; may subjectively feel normal	Mild dysfunction, not requiring treatment	None
C	III	Moderate	Controlled with treatment	Moderately Reduced	End-organ dysfunction responsive to therapy	Mild or moderate
D	IV	Severe	Refractory to treatment	Severely Reduced	Refractory end-organ dysfunction	Severe including Eisenmenger Syndrome

Adapted from the 2018 AHA/ACC Guideline for the Management of Adults with Congenital Heart Disease [9]

Phenotypes in Adult Congenital Heart Disease Heart Failure (ACHD-HF)

2-Ventricle, Morphologic Systemic LV Failure

Patients with biventricular circulation and a systemic left ventricle (LV) most closely approximate acquired heart failure populations in terms of physiology and presentation. Most commonly this can be seen in those with repaired tetralogy of Fallot (TOF) and atrioventricular septal defects (AVSD), formerly known as atrioventricular canal defects. In patients with TOF, data has shown that it is the group over 40 years of age and beyond will develop heart failure [10]. Early in life, chronic cyanosis has been shown to deleteriously affect the myocardium, supported by prior research demonstrating that palliative shunt creation and the duration of shunting is an independent predictor of impaired LV function [11]. Later in life, valvular pathology, most notably severe pulmonary regurgitation in patients with a prior transannular patch, commonly contributes to severe right ventricular (RV) dilation and dysfunction, right-sided heart failure, and ventricular arrhythmias [12]. Coupled with ventriculo-ventricular dyssynchrony from abnormal electrical activation (right bundle branch block from transannular patch surgical repair), RV dilation and dysfunction with interventricular shift into the LV can lead to significant risk of LV dysfunction, which has been shown to portend worse prognoses in patients with TOF. [13–15]

Patients with AVSD, particularly those with complete defects involving both a large ASD and a large VSD, are at risk for pulmonary hypertension from overcirculation of the pulmonary bed as well as heart failure from left atrioventricular valve (LAVV) regurgitation and LV volume loading. Given the underlying structural abnormalities in the AVSD LAVV including significant clefts and dysplastic leaflets, abnormal chordal attachments to the septum are common and can also lead to LV outflow tract obstruction. While patients who had operations in a later surgical era, where earlier intervention reduced the amount of time for volume loading, demonstrate improved survival, significant LAVV regurgitation remains the most common reason for reoperation and is associated with increased mortality risk from heart failure [16, 17].

2-Ventricle, Morphologic Systemic RV Failure

In some forms of complex CHD, the morphologic right ventricle (RV) functions as the systemic ventricle, for example, in DTGA with (Mustard or Senning) atrial switch operation, and also in native levo-transposition of the great vessels (L-TGA). The morphologic characteristics of the RV make for a poor systemic pump, given its thin-walled, trabeculated structure and predominance of longitudinal contraction fibers, which result in lower overall reduced contractility compared to the more compacted LV [18, 19]. Adaptations in the systemic RV include hypertrophy and dilation to maintain stroke volume, but these lead to reduced compliance, elevated end-diastolic filling pressures, and progressive tricuspid annular dilation. The resultant systemic tricuspid regurgitation, made worse by abnormal, Ebsteinoid tricuspid leaflet morphology often seen in patients with L-TGA, poses a significant risk to the systemic RV and is often a target of early intervention [20]. The hypertrophied systemic RV is subject to coronary supply-demand mismatch given ventricular-coronary concordance, producing a degree of myocardial ischemia which has been postulated to contribute to sudden cardiac death in D-TGA [21]. Other mechanistic underpinnings of systemic RV failure include electrophysiologic issues such as atrioventricular node (AVN) dysfunction and chronotropic incompetence (particularly in the case of L-TGA, where ventricular inversion produces a more anterosuperior AVN with elongated His-Purkinje systems that are susceptible to both annular dilation and age-related fibrosis) as well as scar-mediated atrial arrhythmias as a result of atrial switch procedures in patients with D-TGA [1].

Fontan (Single Ventricle) Failure

Patients with single ventricle anatomy are palliated with a staged surgery culminating in a Fontan procedure, which is essentially a cavopulmonary anastomosis, resulting in dedication of the single pumping chamber to systemic circulation and a "bypass circuit" for systemic venous blood to circulate passively from the vena cava directly into the pulmonary arteries. Despite significant inter-stage mortality in the pediatric population, most patients with Fontan circulation survive to adulthood, and it is estimated that the probability of survival to 30 years after modern surgery is up to 85% [22]. Patients with Fontan physiology are one of the most complex cohorts of ACHD who develop HF. Fontan physiology is exceptionally unique, and circulatory failure may occur without gross signs of ventricular dysfunction. The so-called phenotypes of *Fontan failure* have been described to more precisely categorize the underlying physiology in this condition (Fig. 19.1) [23]. It is important to recognize that over time, the systemic ventricle can become progressively dilated due to significant volume overload, and may also demonstrate compensatory hypertrophy, leading to both systolic and diastolic ventricular dysfunction. Further insults including arrhythmia, increased neurohormonal activation, high systemic vascular resistance, and pulmonary venous congestion with relative increases in pulmonary vascular resistance can ultimately impair augmentation of cardiac output [23].

Fontan physiology is also associated with expectant extracardiac disease, more specifically, chronic high venous (Fontan) pressures lead to progressive congestion of the liver and result in the ubiquitous Fontan-associated liver disease (FALD) by adulthood. In FALD, congestive hepatopathy leads to fibrosis that in most cases, progresses to cirrhosis and predisposition to hepatocellular carcinoma [24]. The degree of FALD present contributes to the overall clinical HF presentation, and it is often difficult to determine which process is more significant.

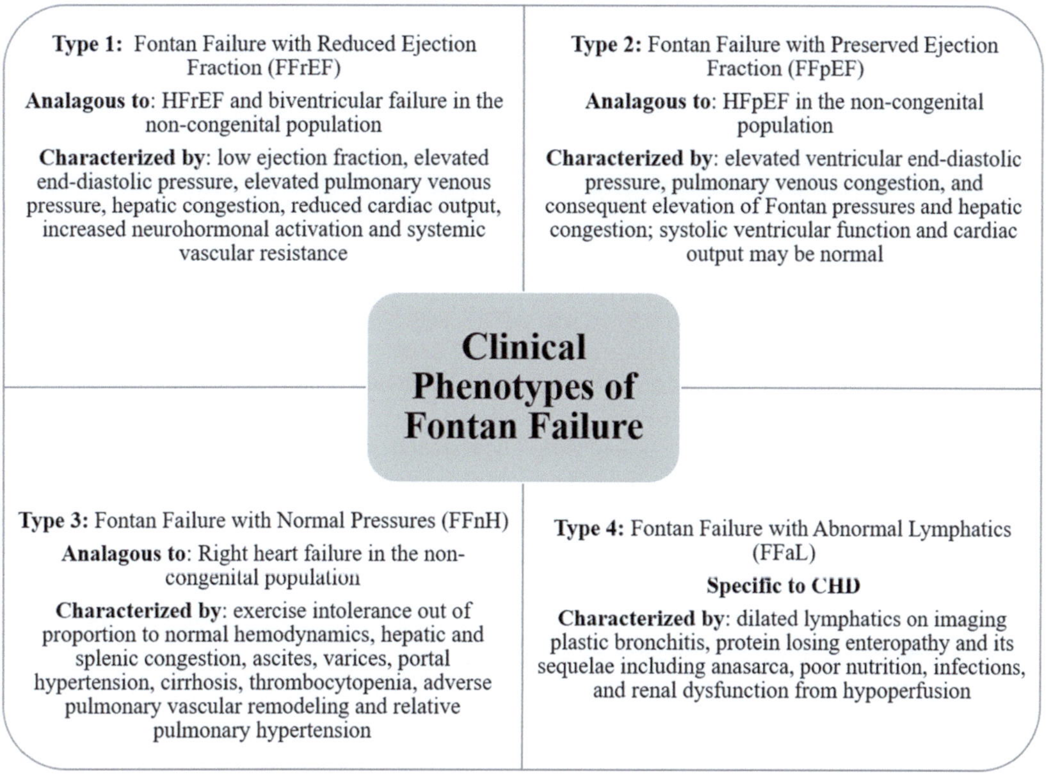

Fig. 19.1 Clinical Phenotypes of Fontan Failure. Types 1 and 4 are most prevalent in the pediatric population and less commonly seen in the ACHD population due to survival selection. HFrEF heart failure reduced ejection fraction, HFpEF heart failure preserved ejection fraction, CHD congenital heart disease. (Adapted from Book, et al. *Congenit Heart Dis*. 2016 [23])

Protein-losing enteropathy (PLE) is another condition for which Fontan patients are uniquely at risk for, and the presence of this condition often signifies a poor prognosis with 5-year mortality risk of up to 50% [25]. It is hypothesized that the lymphatic system plays an important role in the pathophysiology of PLE. Clinically, PLE is characterized by edema, hypoalbuminemia through gastrointestinal losses, congestion, coagulopathy, and increased risk for infections.

Pulmonary Hypertension

Pulmonary arterial hypertension (PAH) in patients with ACHD, denoted as CHD-PAH, is commonly caused by the presence of an unrepaired shunt, which results in over-circulation of the pulmonary vascular bed and the subsequent development of increasing pulmonary vascular resistance (PVR). The 2022 ESC Guidelines categorize CHD-PAH into 4 distinct phenotypes, of which 2 are cases of unrepaired shunts, including Eisenmenger syndrome (ES) and prevalent large systemic-to-pulmonary shunts [26]. These conditions are likely not unique, and represent a continuum whereby PVR rises over time in the setting of a large unrepaired shunt, and when it exceeds systemic vascular resistance (SVR), flow direction changes such that the shunt changes direction (right-to-left across the defect). Patients that develop ES demonstrate cyanosis at rest and often significant hypoxia with exercise. The clinical presentation of heart failure in this group often resembles the right heart failure phenotype, characterized by congestion, abdominal distention, and early satiety [27].

Treatment

Medical Therapy

Traditional goal-directed medical therapy (GDMT) studies often do not include sizable proportions of CHD patients, and limit the quality of data and confidence in application of such therapies to adults with CHD. While it would seem that it may be reasonable to offer GDMT based on use in 2 V anatomy with normally related vessels and a systemic morphologic LV, one needs to consider the risk of precipitating adverse events associated with the underlying congenital anatomy and physiology. For example, patients with L-TGA are at risk for atrioventricular node dysfunction and heart block which could affect the use of beta blockers, while those with Fontan physiology are at risk for sinus node dysfunction and hypotension due to preload dependency and reduced SVR, which may pose problems for the use of both beta blockers and afterload reducing agents [28–30]. While GDMT is still cautiously used in ACHD-HF, this practice is largely extrapolated from treatment of the failing systemic left ventricle in acquired heart failure groups and is not well studied in the ACHD-HF population. A 2018 systematic review on medical therapy for systemic right ventricles published by the AHA/ ACC Task Force on Clinical Practice Guidelines for Management of Adults with Congenital Heart Disease found no significant difference in mean ejection fraction, ventricular dimensions, or peak ventilatory equivalent of oxygen in patients with sRVs treated with at least 3 months of an ACE inhibitor, ARB, or aldosterone antagonist. The authors identified only 4 studies which included beta blockers as the treatment intervention for patients with sRVs and unfortunately could not provide data analysis due to the small number of patients and diversity of outcomes reported amongst the 4 studies [31]. Even less is known regarding the efficacy of traditional GDMT on heart failure in patients with Fontan circulation, though none of the available literature appears to show a significant benefit in the use of GDMT for this population [32–35].

Other therapeutic agents that have become a mainstay in the treatment of heart failure in the non-congenital patients including angiotensin receptor-neprolysin inhibitors (ARNIs) and sodium glucose cotransporter-2 inhibitors (SGLT2i). Existing single-center data support the use of ARNIs to improve sRV parameters, functional class, 6-minute walk distances in the sRV population [36], and prospective data from the currently enrolling ENTRUST ACHD HF study on the use of ARNIs in the ACHD population is anticipated in 2026 [37]. Currently, only case series exist to describe cardiovascular benefits of SGLT2i in the ACHD population [38–41].

Transcatheter and Device Therapies

Key developments in intervention have benefitted several growing groups of ACHD patients, and related to the focus of this chapter, are worth mentioning as interception for reversible causes of HF. For those with a history of pulmonary atresia and tetralogy of Fallot, the most common long-term complications include significant pulmonary valve disease (for both native and prosthetic homograft valves) and subsequent RV dysfunction and failure. Transcatheter pulmonary valve replacement (TPVR) developed in the early 2000s with the Medtronic Melody and Edwards SAPIEN stented balloon-expandable valves which were used for a valve-in-conduit TPVR approach. Following this, the need for larger valves to accommodate native RV outflow tracts in patients without conduits (e.g., patients with tetralogy of Fallot who underwent transannular patch repairs) led to the development of the Medtronic Harmony and Edwards SAPIEN 3 with the Alterra adaptive present docking system [42]. Several studies and meta analyses have demonstrated reduced in-hospital mortality, shorter hospital stays, comparable hemodynamic profiles and longevity associated with TPVR over surgical pulmonary valve replacement, though the risks of infective endocarditis are higher with TPVR [43, 44].

Use of cardiac resynchronization therapy (CRT) has suggested there is a mortality benefit to patients with CHD with symptomatic systolic heart failure and electrical dyssynchrony [45]. As such, the 2023 Heart Rhythm Society/ Asian Pacific Heart Rhythm Society/ Latin American

Heart Rhythm Society guidelines on cardiac physiologic pacing (CPP) for the avoidance and mitigation of heart failure included a IIa recommendation for CRT in CHD patients on GDMT with a *systemic LV*, symptomatic HF, EF <45%, and QRS duration z score of > + 3 or ventricular pacing >40%, and a IIb recommendation for CRT in CHD patients with a *systemic RV* and similar parameters [46]. The guidelines provide direction on optimal (apical) and alternative (non-apical or multisite) lead placements for patients with univentricular circulation, and for pacing strategies such as fusion-based pacing in patients with a right bundle branch block and subpulmonary RV dysfunction, as well as for and His bundle pacing or left bundle branch area pacing for patients with L-TGA and AV block [46, 47]. Nevertheless, defining responders to device therapy remains challenging due to the relatively small number of anatomically and physiologically unique ACHD patients meeting criteria for CPP in comparison to the non-congenital population, and further study is needed.

Transplant

Heart transplantation and multi-organ transplant for patients with ACHD account for only 3% of total heart transplantations performed annually, with this proportion increasing only 0.1% in the past 10 years [48]. Specific challenges facing the ACHD-HF population include: higher incidence of sensitization from prior surgery and transfusion, greater risk of bleeding due to prior sternotomies, collateral vessels with residual cyanosis, increased rates of post-transplant hepatic failure in specific cohorts such as those with FALD, and the need for additional surgery or intervention after transplantation (~30%) [49, 50]. Despite these challenges and higher 1-year perioperative mortality, a survival paradox exists, such that long-term survival in patients with ACHD who undergo heart transplant are better than that of patients transplanted for acquired heart disease indications, with median survival >20 years if survived to 1 year post-transplant [51]. The higher "up front" risks are often attributable to advanced disease at time of transplant, with increased risks of bleeding, stroke, primary graft dysfunction, and renal failure requiring dialysis [52, 53]. These risks, however, may be offset by younger average age and reduced number of comorbidities in patients who are transplanted for underlying CHD, which may be reflected in reduced long-term risks of developing coronary allograft vasculopathy, graft rejection, and malignancy [54, 55]. Short-term (30-day and 1-year) survival is increased when patients with ACHD are transplanted at high-volume centers, defined as centers with transplant volumes in the 75th percentile or greater nationally [56].

In October 2018, the United Network for Organ Sharing (UNOS) redesigned the donor heart allocation system with the intent to provide more equitable utilization of organs; this was done by incorporating frequently used status exceptions in the old, 3-tiered system into standard criteria in a new, 6-tiered system. As a result of this, patients with ACHD-HF, who previously spent longer times on the wait list in lower-urgency categories with risked increased mortality, could be listed under standard criteria rather than waiting to be listed under exception criteria. Data on ACHD transplant after implementation of the new allocation system show a reduction in wait list time, an increase in utilization of peripheral temporary MCS, an increase in transplantations, and no changes in 1-year post-transplant outcomes for patients with ACHD-HF [57–59]. In other efforts to address disparities in advanced therapies for ACHD patients, recent studies have identified late outcomes and produced risk scoring systems for specific groups of patients with CHD, such as those with D-TGA status post Mustard or Senning atrial switch, to identify optimal times for referral [60]. Further study is needed given that over the past two decades, evaluations for advanced therapies candidacy in patients with ACHD have increased five-fold and listings increased four-fold despite a smaller increase in actual transplantations [61].

Consideration for multiorgan transplant is often encountered in the ACHD population, given the effects of chronic circulatory failure on other organs such as the liver, lungs, and kidneys. Particularly in the Fontan-palliated single-ventricle patient population, FALD often necessitates consideration for combined heart-liver transplant (CHLT). In a recently published multicenter retrospective cohort study of 131 adult Fontan patients who underwent heart only versus CHLT, the FOSTER study found that compared with heart transplant alone, CHLT had similar overall survival and improved survival in patients with higher FALD scores [62]. Analysis of data from the Scientific Registry of Transplant Recipients over a 16-year period from 2000 to 2016 also showed no significant increased mortality with respect to combined heart-kidney transplant compared to heart transplant alone in patients with ACHD. The authors of this study did find that combined heart-lung transplant did show increased mortality compared to heart transplant alone in patients with ACHD, though this is similar to data available for the general population; notably, the study showed no significant differences in 30-day, 1-year, or 5-year survival for multiorgan transplant in the ACHD-HF group when compared to that in the non-congenital HF group [63].

Mechanical Circulatory Support

Mechanical circulatory support (MCS), including durable device therapy such as ventricular assist devices (VADs), also present challenges in patients with CHD, including anatomic complexity and variation, increased surgical risk, and limited experience and long-term data [64]. Anatomic barriers to temporary and durable MCS include single ventricles or systemic right ventricles, dextrocardia, and nonstandard anastomoses or vascular reconstruction of the great arteries, all of which may pose technical challenges to placing devices such as balloon pumps, Impellas, and LVADs [28, 57, 65]. In a specific example, implantation of VADs in patients with sRVs, which have a heavily trabeculated apex, require careful planning with selection of specific VADs with shorter cannulas, surgical resection of the trabeculations prior to implantation, and alternative placement of the inflow cannula (either in the right ventricular free wall or diaphragmatic surface), to prevent cannula obstruction [28, 29]. As such, MCS implantation for ACHD patients remains likely underutilized, and an option only at expert care centers where multidisciplinary teams including ACHD physicians and congenital surgeons are available to support the HF medical and transplant surgical teams.

Palliative Inotropes

Little is known about the outcomes of patients with ACHD who require long-term inotrope therapy to remain out of the hospital. Nearly a third of patients with ACHD-HF listed for heart transplant are inotrope dependent, which has been shown to be associated with an increased risk of death or delisting on the wait list [58]. The risks of ventricular arrhythmias, cardiac arrest, and sudden cardiac death with shortened survival are likely similar to that seen in patients with end-stage heart failure and no underlying congenital heart disease. In addition, patients with ACHD may be at increased risk for lesion-specific risks, such as paradoxical emboli and endocarditis due to unrepaired intracardiac shunts near the site of peripherally inserted central catheters. However, for many patients, chronic inotrope therapy may be the only option to improve quality of life irrespective of transplant candidacy, and therefore, should not be overlooked as part of the management toolkit for these patients.

Palliative and End-of-Life Care

Acute exacerbations of HF requiring hospitalization have increased disproportionately in the ACHD population compared to that in the general population; this discrepancy has been attributable to improvements in GDMT and earlier intervention for patients with acquired heart disease that have not been proven to have the same effect in the ACHD-HF population [66, 67]. Heart failure admissions in patients with underlying ACHD are associated with longer length of stay, increased procedural burden, and increased cost when compared to HF admissions in the general population [6]. In a multi-hospital healthcare system study, forty percent (40%) of all patients with ACHD-HF required inpatient and intensive care unit level of care in the terminal 30 days of life, and ultimately 64% of these patients died in the hospital [68].

Despite the lifelong medical challenges facing patients with ACHD, many are inadequately equipped to deal with declining health and end-of-life (EOL) care. The majority of patients with ACHD have a strong interest for participation in ACP discussions; yet, less than 30% of these patients reported actually having had these discussions with their providers [69]. Unfortunately, as a result, many patients will end up undergoing unsuccessful resuscitative measures, and a higher proportion of EOL care discussions, 41% in one study, occur with substitute decision makers at the time of terminal hospitalization, resulting in significant stress for surviving loved ones [70]. Recognizing these factors, it is strongly recommended that ACP should occur early in the treatment of heart failure [71, 72].

Conclusions

Patients with CHD demonstrate heterogenous anatomy and unique physiology, with many developing HF in the adult years. Understanding the common phenotypes of heart failure in ACHD can help clinicians recognize this disease and triage patients for appropriate expertise care. Optimal treatment strategies for the ACHD-HF population have yet to be defined but represent a new frontier in HF research that could benefit a largely underserved group of patients. With further advances in in medical, procedural, and advanced HF therapies, it is conceivable that in the future, patients born with complex CHD may achieve life expectancies that are similar to those of the general population, with parallel improvements in quality of life, yet more research in the application of traditional HF therapies to the ACHD group is needed.

References

1. Warnes CA. Transposition of the great arteries. Circulation. 2006;114(24):2699–709. https://doi.org/10.1161/CIRCULATIONAHA.105.592352.
2. Moons P, Bovijn L, Budts W, Belmans A, Gewillig M. Temporal trends in survival to adulthood among patients born with congenital heart disease from 1970 to 1992 in Belgium. Circulation. 2010;122(22):2264–72. https://doi.org/10.1161/circulationaha.110.946343.
3. Verheugt CL, Uiterwaal CS, van der Velde ET, et al. Mortality in adult congenital heart disease. Eur Heart J. 2010;31(10):1220–9. https://doi.org/10.1093/eurheartj/ehq032.
4. Oechslin EN, Harrison DA, Connelly MS, Webb GD, Siu SC. Mode of death in adults with congenital heart disease. Am J Cardiol. 2000;86(10):1111–6. https://doi.org/10.1016/s0002-9149(00)01169-3.
5. Nieminen HP, Jokinen EV, Sairanen HI. Causes of late deaths after pediatric cardiac surgery: a population-based study. J Am Coll Cardiol. 2007;50(13):1263–71. https://doi.org/10.1016/j.jacc.2007.05.040.
6. Burchill LJ, Gao L, Kovacs AH, et al. Hospitalization trends and health resource use for adult congenital heart disease-related heart failure. J Am Heart Assoc. 2018;7(15):e008775. https://doi.org/10.1161/JAHA.118.008775.
7. Stout KK, Broberg CS, Book WM, et al. Chronic heart failure in congenital heart disease: A scientific Sstatement from the American Heart Association. Circulation. 2016;133(8):770–801. https://doi.org/10.1161/CIR.0000000000000352.
8. Warnes CA, Williams RG, Bashore TM, et al. ACC/AHA 2008 guidelines for the management of adults with congenital heart disease: executive summary: a report of the American College of Cardiology/American Heart Association Task Force on Practice Guidelines (writing committee to develop guidelines for the management of adults with congenital heart disease). Circulation. 2008;118(23):2395–451. https://doi.org/10.1161/CIRCULATIONAHA.108.190811.
9. Stout KK, Daniels CJ, Aboulhosn JA, et al. 2018 AHA/ACC guideline for the management of adults with congenital heart disease: a report of the American College of Cardiology/American Heart Association Task Force on Clinical Practice Guidelines. J Am Coll Cardiol. 2019;73(12):e81–192. https://doi.org/10.1016/j.jacc.2018.08.1029.
10. Kalogeropoulos AP, Savvoulidis P, Saraf A, et al. Prevalence and incidence of heart failure in adolescents and adults with repaired tetralogy of FALLOT. J Am Coll Cardiol. 2017;69(11, Supplement):563. https://doi.org/10.1016/S0735-1097(17)33952-9.
11. Broberg CS, Aboulhosn J, Mongeon F-P, et al. Prevalence of left ventricular systolic dysfunction in adults with repaired tetralogy of Fallot. Am J Cardiol. 2011;107(8):1215–20. https://doi.org/10.1016/j.amjcard.2010.12.026.
12. Mueller AS, McDonald DM, Singh HS, Ginns JN. Heart failure in adult congenital heart disease: tetralogy of Fallot. Heart Fail Rev. 2020;25(4):583–98. https://doi.org/10.1007/s10741-019-09903-0.
13. Andrade AC, Jerosch-Herold M, Wegner P, et al. Determinants of left ventricular dysfunction and remodeling in patients with corrected tetralogy of Fallot. J Am Heart Assoc. 2019;8(17):e009618. https://doi.org/10.1161/jaha.118.009618.

14. Jiang L, Li Y, Huang S, et al. Right-left ventricular interdependence in repaired tetralogy of Fallot patients with right ventricular heart failure. J Magn Reson Imaging. 2024;60(2):628–39. https://doi.org/10.1002/jmri.29080.
15. Ghai A, Silversides C, Harris L, Webb GD, Siu SC, Therrien J. Left ventricular dysfunction is a risk factor for sudden cardiac death in adults late after repair of tetralogy of Fallot. J Am Coll Cardiol. 2002;40(9):1675–80. https://doi.org/10.1016/S0735-1097(02)02344-6.
16. Fong LS, Betts K, Ayer J, et al. Predictors of reoperation and mortality after complete atrioventricular septal defect repair. Eur J Cardiothorac Surg. 2021;61(1):45–53. https://doi.org/10.1093/ejcts/ezab221.
17. Ginde S, Lam J, Hill GD, et al. Long-term outcomes after surgical repair of complete atrioventricular septal defect. J Thorac Cardiovasc Surg. 2015;150(2):369–74. https://doi.org/10.1016/j.jtcvs.2015.05.011.
18. Rüssel IK, Tecelão SR, Kuijer JP, Heethaar RM, Marcus JT. Comparison of 2D and 3D calculation of left ventricular torsion as circumferential-longitudinal shear angle using cardiovascular magnetic resonance tagging. J Cardiovasc Magn Reson. 2009;11(1):8. https://doi.org/10.1186/1532-429x-11-8.
19. Vitarelli A, Terzano C. Do we have two hearts? New insights in right ventricular function supported by myocardial imaging echocardiography. Heart Fail Rev. 2010;15(1):39–61. https://doi.org/10.1007/s10741-009-9154-x.
20. Mongeon FP, Connolly HM, Dearani JA, Li Z, Warnes CA. Congenitally corrected transposition of the great arteries ventricular function at the time of systemic atrioventricular valve replacement predicts long-term ventricular function. J Am Coll Cardiol. 2011;57(20):2008–17. https://doi.org/10.1016/j.jacc.2010.11.021.
21. Khairy P. Sudden cardiac death in transposition of the great arteries with a Mustard or Senning Baffle: the myocardial ischemia hypothesis. Curr Opin Cardiol. 2017;32(1):101–7. https://doi.org/10.1097/HCO.0000000000000353.
22. Schilling C, Dalziel K, Nunn R, et al. The Fontan epidemic: population projections from the Australia and New Zealand Fontan Registry. Int J Cardiol. 2016;219:14–9. https://doi.org/10.1016/j.ijcard.2016.05.035.
23. Book WM, Gerardin J, Saraf A, Marie Valente A, Rodriguez F 3rd. Clinical phenotypes of Fontan failure: implications for management. Congenit Heart Dis. 2016;11(4):296–308. https://doi.org/10.1111/chd.12368.
24. Rychik J, Atz AM, Celermajer DS, et al. Evaluation and management of the child and adult with Fontan circulation: a scientific statement from the American Heart Association. Circulation. 2019;140(6):e234–84. https://doi.org/10.1161/CIR.0000000000000696.
25. Mertens L, Hagler DJ, Sauer U, Somerville J, Gewillig M. Protein-losing enteropathy after the Fontan operation: an international multicenter study. PLE study group. J Thorac Cardiovasc Surg. 1998;115(5):1063–73. https://doi.org/10.1016/s0022-5223(98)70406-4.
26. Humbert M, Kovacs G, Hoeper MM, et al. 2022 ESC/ERS Guidelines for the diagnosis and treatment of pulmonary hypertension. Eur Respir J. 2023;61(1). https://doi.org/10.1183/13993003.00879-2022.
27. Arvanitaki A, Giannakoulas G, Baumgartner H, Lammers AE. Eisenmenger syndrome: diagnosis, prognosis and clinical management. Heart. 2020;106(21):1638. https://doi.org/10.1136/heartjnl-2020-316665.
28. Vaikunth S, Sundaravel S, Saef J, Ortega-Legaspi J. Novel therapeutic strategies in heart failure in adult congenital heart disease: of medicines and devices. Curr Heart Fail Rep. 2023;20(5):401–16. https://doi.org/10.1007/s11897-023-00621-1.
29. Chaudhry A, Selwyn J, Adams E, Bradley EA. Heart failure in complex congenital heart disease of the adult. Curr Cardiol Rep. 2022;24(11):1727–35. https://doi.org/10.1007/s11886-022-01788-0.
30. Tompkins R, Romfh A. General principles of heart failure management in adult congenital heart disease. Heart Fail Rev. 2020;25(4):555–67. https://doi.org/10.1007/s10741-019-09895-x.
31. Zaragoza-Macias E, Zaidi AN, Dendukuri N, Marelli A. Medical therapy for systemic right ventricles: a systematic review (part 1) for the 2018 AHA/ACC guideline for the management of adults with congenital heart disease: a report of the American College of Cardiology/American Heart Association Task Force on Clinical Practice Guidelines. Circulation. 2019;139(14):e801–13. https://doi.org/10.1161/CIR.0000000000000604.
32. Butts R, Atz AM, BaezHernandez N, Sutcliffe D, Reisch J, Mahony L. Carvedilol does not improve exercise performance in Fontan patients: results of a crossover trial. Pediatr Cardiol. 2021;42(4):934–41. https://doi.org/10.1007/s00246-021-02565-6.
33. Kouatli AA, Garcia JA, Zellers TM, Weinstein EM, Mahony L. Enalapril does not enhance exercise capacity in patients after Fontan procedure. Circulation. 1997;96(5):1507–12. https://doi.org/10.1161/01.cir.96.5.1507.
34. Wilson TG, Iyengar AJ, d'Udekem Y. The use and misuse of ACE inhibitors in patients with single ventricle physiology. Heart Lung Circ. 2016;25(3):229–36. https://doi.org/10.1016/j.hlc.2015.10.005.
35. Mahle WT, Wang A, Quyyumi AA, McConnell ME, Book WM. Impact of spironolactone on endothelial function in patients with single ventricle heart. Congenit Heart Dis. 2009;4(1):12–6. https://doi.org/10.1111/j.1747-0803.2008.00240.x.
36. Fusco F, Scognamiglio G, Merola A, et al. Safety and efficacy of sacubitril/valsartan in patients with a failing systemic right ventricle: a prospective single-

center study. Circ Heart Fail. 2023;16(2):e009848. https://doi.org/10.1161/circheartfailure.122.009848.
37. Appadurai V, Nicolae M, Aboulhosn J, Lluri G. The protocol and rationale for the efficacy and Tolerability of sacubitril-valsartan in adult congenital heart disease patients with heart failure (ENTRUST ACHD HF) registry. Int J Cardiol Congenit Heart Dis. 2021;3:100096. https://doi.org/10.1016/j.ijcchd.2021.100096.
38. Egorova AD, Nederend M, Tops LF, Vliegen HW, Jongbloed MRM, Kiès P. The first experience with sodium-glucose cotransporter 2 inhibitor for the treatment of systemic right ventricular failure. ESC Heart Fail. 2022;9(3):2007–12. https://doi.org/10.1002/ehf2.13871.
39. Newland DM, Law YM, Albers EL, et al. Early clinical experience with dapagliflozin in children with heart failure. Pediatr Cardiol. 2023;44(1):146–52. https://doi.org/10.1007/s00246-022-02983-0.
40. Muneuchi J, Sugitani Y, Kobayashi M, Ezaki H, Yamada H, Watanabe M. Feasibility and safety of sodium glucose Cotransporter-2 inhibitors in adults with heart failure after the Fontan procedure. Case Rep Cardiol. 2022;2022:5243594. https://doi.org/10.1155/2022/5243594.
41. Saef J, Sundaravel S, Ortega-Legaspi J, Vaikunth S. Safety and treatment experience with sodium/glucose Cotransporter-2 inhibitors in adult patients with congenital heart disease. J Card Fail. 2023;29(6):974–5. https://doi.org/10.1016/j.cardfail.2023.03.011.
42. Patel ND, Levi DS, Cheatham JP, Qureshi SA, Shahanavaz S, Zahn EM. Transcatheter pulmonary valve replacement: a review of current valve technologies. J Soc Cardiovasc Angiogr Intervent. 2022;1(6) https://doi.org/10.1016/j.jscai.2022.100452.
43. Zhou Y, Xiong T, Bai P, Chu C, Dong N. Clinical outcomes of transcatheter versus surgical pulmonary valve replacement: a meta-analysis. J Thorac Dis. 2019;11(12):5343–51. https://doi.org/10.21037/jtd.2019.11.64.
44. Ribeiro JM, Teixeira R, Lopes J, Costa M, Pires A, Gonçalves L. Transcatheter versus surgical pulmonary valve replacement: a systemic review and meta-analysis. Ann Thorac Surg. 2020;110(5):1751–61. https://doi.org/10.1016/j.athoracsur.2020.03.007.
45. Chubb H, Rosenthal DN, Almond CS, et al. Impact of cardiac resynchronization therapy on heart transplant-free survival in pediatric and congenital heart disease patients. Circ Arrhythm Electrophysiol. 2020;13(4):e007925. https://doi.org/10.1161/CIRCEP.119.007925.
46. Chung MK, Patton KK, Lau CP, et al. 2023 HRS/APHRS/LAHRS guideline on cardiac physiologic pacing for the avoidance and mitigation of heart failure. Heart Rhythm. 2023;20(9):e17–91. https://doi.org/10.1016/j.hrthm.2023.03.1538.
47. Karpawich PP, Chubb H. Indications for cardiac resynchronization therapy in patients with congenital heart disease. Card Electrophysiol Clin. 2023;15(4):433–45. https://doi.org/10.1016/j.ccep.2023.07.005.
48. https://unos.org/
49. Schweiger M, Lorts A, Conway J. Mechanical circulatory support challenges in pediatric and (adult) congenital heart disease. Curr Opin Organ Transplant. 2018;23(3):301–7. https://doi.org/10.1097/MOT.0000000000000522.
50. Stiller B, Fleck T. Transplant challenges in adults with congenital heart disease. Int J Cardiol. 2020;300:145–6. https://doi.org/10.1016/j.ijcard.2019.10.038.
51. Burchill LJ, Edwards LB, Dipchand AI, Stehlik J, Ross HJ. Impact of adult congenital heart disease on survival and mortality after heart transplantation. J Heart Lung Transplant. 2014;33(11):1157–63. https://doi.org/10.1016/j.healun.2014.05.007.
52. Shah DK, Deo SV, Althouse AD, et al. Perioperative mortality is the Achilles heel for cardiac transplantation in adults with congenital heart disease: evidence from analysis of the UNOS registry. J Card Surg. 2016;31(12):755–64. https://doi.org/10.1111/jocs.12857.
53. Menachem JN, Schlendorf KH, Mazurek JA, et al. Advanced heart failure in adults with congenital heart disease. JACC Heart Fail. 2020;8(2):87–99. https://doi.org/10.1016/j.jchf.2019.08.012.
54. Monaco J, Khanna A, Khazanie P. Transplant and mechanical circulatory support in patients with adult congenital heart disease. Heart Fail Rev. 2020;25(4):671–83. https://doi.org/10.1007/s10741-020-09976-2.
55. Doumouras BS, Alba AC, Foroutan F, Burchill LJ, Dipchand AI, Ross HJ. Outcomes in adult congenital heart disease patients undergoing heart transplantation: a systematic review and meta-analysis. J Heart Lung Transplant. 2016;35(11):1337–47. https://doi.org/10.1016/j.healun.2016.06.003.
56. Menachem JN, Lindenfeld J, Schlendorf K, et al. Center volume and post-transplant survival among adults with congenital heart disease. J Heart Lung Transplant. 2018;37(11):1351–60. https://doi.org/10.1016/j.healun.2018.07.007.
57. Bravo-Jaimes K, Axsom K, Menachem J, Danford D, Kutty S, Cedars A. Impact of the new UNOS donor heart allocation system on waitlist outcomes and early posttransplant mortality among adults with congenital heart disease. Am J Transplant. 2022;22(4):1123–32. https://doi.org/10.1111/ajt.16900.
58. Kainuma A, Ning Y, Kurlansky PA, et al. Changes in waitlist and posttransplant outcomes in patients with adult congenital heart disease after the new heart transplant allocation system. Clin Transpl. 2021;35(11):e14458. https://doi.org/10.1111/ctr.14458.
59. Zhou AL, Menachem JN, Danford DA, Kutty S, Cedars AM. UNOS listing status-related changes in mechanical circulatory support utilization and outcomes in adult congenital heart disease patients. J

Heart Lung Transplant. 2022;41(7):889–95. https://doi.org/10.1016/j.healun.2022.03.001.
60. Broberg CS, van Dissel A, Minnier J, et al. Long-term outcomes after atrial switch operation for transposition of the great arteries. J Am Coll Cardiol. 2022;80(10):951–63. https://doi.org/10.1016/j.jacc.2022.06.020.
61. Crossland DS, Van De Bruaene A, Silversides CK, Hickey EJ, Roche SL. Heart failure in adult congenital heart disease: from advanced therapies to end-of-life care. Can J Cardiol. 2019;35(12):1723–39. https://doi.org/10.1016/j.cjca.2019.07.626.
62. Lewis MJ, Reardon LC, Aboulhosn J, et al. Clinical outcomes of adult Fontan-associated liver disease and combined heart-liver transplantation. J Am Coll Cardiol. 2023;81(22):2149–60. doi:10.1016/j.jacc.2023.03.421.
63. Wong K, Tecson K, Cedars A. Outcomes of multi-organ transplant in adult patients with congenital heart disease. J Am Heart Assoc. 2019;8(22):e014088. https://doi.org/10.1161/jaha.119.014088.
64. Saef J, Montgomery R, Cedars A, et al. Durable mechanical circulatory support in adult congenital heart disease: reviewing clinical considerations and experience. J Clin Med. 2022;11(11). https://doi.org/10.3390/jcm11113200.
65. Gurvitz M, Burns KM, Brindis R, et al. Emerging research firections in adult congenital heart disease: A report from an NHLBI/ACHA Working Group. J Am Coll Cardiol. 2016;67(16):1956–64. https://doi.org/10.1016/j.jacc.2016.01.062.
66. Hellermann JP, Goraya TY, Jacobsen SJ, et al. Incidence of heart failure after myocardial infarction: is it changing over time? Am J Epidemiol. 2003;157(12):1101–7. https://doi.org/10.1093/aje/kwg078.
67. Shafazand M, Rosengren A, Lappas G, Swedberg K, Schaufelberger M. Decreasing trends in the incidence of heart failure after acute myocardial infarction from 1993-2004: a study of 175,216 patients with a first acute myocardial infarction in Sweden. Eur J Heart Fail. 2011;13(2):135–41. https://doi.org/10.1093/eurjhf/hfq205.
68. Steiner JM, Kirkpatrick JN, Heckbert SR, et al. Hospital resource utilization and presence of advance directives at the end of life for adults with congenital heart disease. Congenit Heart Dis. 2018;13(5):721–7. https://doi.org/10.1111/chd.12638.
69. Ludmir J, Steiner JM, Wong HN, et al. Palliative care opportunities among adults with congenital heart disease-a systematic review. J Pain Symptom Manag. 2019;58(5):891–8. https://doi.org/10.1016/j.jpainsymman.2019.07.025.
70. Tobler D, Greutmann M, Colman JM, Greutmann-Yantiri M, Librach LS, Kovacs AH. End-of-life care in hospitalized adults with complex congenital heart disease: care delayed, care denied. Palliat Med. 2012;26(1):72–9. https://doi.org/10.1177/0269216311407694.
71. Deng LX, Gleason LP, Khan AM, et al. Advance care planning in adults with congenital heart disease: a patient priority. Int J Cardiol. 2017;231:105–9. https://doi.org/10.1016/j.ijcard.2016.12.185.
72. Troost E, Roggen L, Goossens E, et al. Advanced care planning in adult congenital heart disease: transitioning from repair to palliation and end-of-life care. Int J Cardiol. 2019;279:57–61. https://doi.org/10.1016/j.ijcard.2018.10.078.

20 Atrial Arrhythmias and Heart Failure

S. Luke Kusmirek and Howard J. Eisen

Introduction

Congestive heart failure and atrial arrhythmias, in particular atrial fibrillation are the two major cardiovascular epidemics of the current era with a major impact on the healthcare economics [1]. Incidence of both atrial fibrillation (AF) and congestive heart failure (CHF) is rapidly increasing [2]. These two conditions frequently coexist; onset of one often predates and predicts the occurrence of the other [3, 4]. In a prospective study that examined the temporal relations of AF and CHF, the incidence of CHF among AF patients was 33 per 1000 person-years, and the incidence of AF among CHF subjects was 64 per 1000 person-years. In patients with AF or CHF, subsequent development of the other is associated with increased mortality [2]. Patients with CHF are at excess risk of developing AF and the more advanced CHF is the more often AF occurs [4–8]. In the CONSENSUS trial, AF prevalence as high as 50% was observed in NYHA class IV CHF population [8]. Conversely, presence of AF with uncontrolled ventricular response may lead to tachycardia-induced cardiomyopathy and precipitate CHF symptoms.

S. L. Kusmirek (✉)
Drexel University College of Medicine, Tower Health Medical Group-Cardiology, Phoenixville, Phoenixville, PA, USA
e-mail: skusmire@drexelmed.edu

H. J. Eisen
Division of Cardiology, Thomas Jefferson University, Philadelphia, PA, USA
e-mail: howard.eisen@jefferson.edu

Pathophysiology

Failing heart undergoes mechanical and electrical remodeling that promotes proarrhythmic changes at the cellular and organ level. All major arrhythmia mechanisms are promoted and facilitated by the typical progression of the myocardial injury from the time of the acute insult, through the compensated phase of recovery to the long-term myocardial dysfunction and progressive loss of the cellular integrity and organ function. The increased levels of the serum and tissue norepinephrine, beta-receptor down regulation and unopposed activation of the sympathetic autonomic nervous system with the associated loss of the vagal input promote enhanced normal and pathological automaticity of the atrial pacemaker cells. Similarly, intracellular calcium perturbations, increased catecholamines levels, ischemia and proarrhythmic effects of the medications and electrolyte disorders facilitate triggered activity. Reentry, both functional as well as based on the presence of a fixed anatomical obstacle is also more likely to occur in CHF. The substrate necessary for reentry is created by the diffuse or focal cardiac tissue fibrosis leading to the loss of the gap junction function and enhancement in the anisotropic conduction properties. While the cellular changes are potentially reversible if

H. J. Eisen (ed.), *Heart Failure I*, https://doi.org/10.1007/978-3-032-12626-9_20

addressed early, the loss of electrical and mechanical function of the atrium is generally irreversible once extensive tissue necrosis and fibrosis has occurred [9, 10].

Classification

Atrial arrhythmias are usually classified on the basis of the anatomical structures involved in their initiation and propagation. Supraventricular tachycardias including atrioventricular node re-entrant tachycardia, atrioventricular re-entrant tachycardia and focal automatic atrial tachycardia are typically seen in younger patients without structural heart disease. Their prevalence is approximately 0.22% in general population [11]. Diagnosis is usually established when a 12 lead electrocardiogram or a rhythm strip is recorded during the symptomatic episode of arrhythmia. There are only sporadically associated with the development of structural heart disease and carry overall benign prognosis. In rare cases of the rapid incessant arrhythmia, tachycardia-induced cardiomyopathy may develop. Cardiomyopathy is usually reversible once the tachycardia is controlled. Options of the therapy include rate control with atrioventricular node blocking agents (β-blockers, calcium channel blockers, digoxin), antiarrhythmic drugs (sotalol, amiodarone) or catheter ablation. Catheter ablation of all types of supraventricular tachycardia is very effective and carries a very low risk of the periprocedural complications. Thus, it is the therapy of choice for the majority of patients regardless of the status of the underlying cardiac disease. Moreover, in the cases of supraventricular tachycardia occurring in patients with the preexisting structural heart disease, CHF and tachycardia-induced cardiomyopathy catheter ablation should be used preferentially to maximize the likelihood of the arrhythmia cure and avoid the long-term risks and complications of drug therapy.

Conversely, micro and macro reentrant atrial tachycardias, atrial flutters and atrial fibrillation are the typical atrial arrhythmias associated with structural heart disease and CHF. Despite the occasional differences in the underlying basic arrhythmia mechanism, atrial rates and the anatomical substrates involved, they are all producing similar clinical symptoms and share the same long term impact on the atrial transport mechanics and overall cardiac performance. They also create similar increased risk of thromboembolic complications and respond to similar therapies. They will collectively be addressed as atrial fibrillation (AF) and as such will be the focus of this chapter. AF is often classified as first detected or recurrent as well as paroxysmal (when it terminates spontaneously), persistent (when it lasts more than 7 days or requires some form of cardioversion for termination) or permanent (when it no longer responds to any therapeutic intervention). These categories are not mutually exclusive as the dominant pattern of AF may change over time depending on the patient's clinical status and the therapies used for arrhythmia control.

Epidemiology

AF is the most common heart rhythm abnormality. It is uncommon in young healthy individuals but rapidly increases in prevalence after the age of 50 up to approximately 10% of patients over the age of 80 years old. Men are affected earlier in life but women catch up rapidly when in their 70s and 80s with the slight overall higher prevalence in women. Lifetime risk of AF development in the Western countries is about 1 in 4. The AF association with structural heart disease is well established. The most common associated conditions are hypertensive heart disease, coronary artery disease, and congestive heart failure [2]. The AF epidemiology in the non-Caucasian populations is not well studied but the available data reveals risk factors pattern similar to Caucasian patients but overall lower AF age-adjusted incidence and prevalence.

Diagnosis

Atrial fibrillation is diagnosed with a combination of clinical history, physical examination findings and electrocardiographic recordings.

Patient's usually report palpitations, sensation of irregular pulse, dizziness, fatigue, shortness of breath and decreased exercise capacity. On physical examination pulse and heart rate are irregularly irregular and excessive resting or exercional tachycardia or bradycardia may be present. Findings of associated decompensated heart failure including low peripheral pulses, cool extremities, peripheral or pulmonary congestion and S3 gallop often coexist. Recording of at least single lead electrocardiographic rhythm strip is necessary to confirm the diagnosis. AF may also be asymptomatic and the diagnosis is made solely on the basis of abnormal physical examination and/or electrocardiographic recordings. There is a wide spectrum of the ECG recording methods useful in AF diagnosis including "spot check" 12-lead ECG, ambulatory 24 h Holter monitors, extended use ECG loop recorders as well as implantable loop recorders. The accuracy of AF detection varies substantially between the methods but generally improves with the length of the monitoring and the patient compliance. The implantable loop recorders provide the best compliance and their overall accuracy for AF detection was reported at 98.5% in the XPECT trial [12]. The ECG monitoring is also useful in the long term rate control assessment, monitoring the symptoms and evaluation of the efficacy of the therapy.

Once the diagnosis of AF is established, basic ancillary testing is recommended including blood tests (CBC, serum electrolytes, hepatic, renal and thyroid function tests) transthoracic echocardiography and in selected patients chest x-ray, transesophageal echocardiography, 6-min walk test, stress testing and electrophysiological study.

Many of these tests are also routinely used for evaluation of congestive heart failure status and if available may not need to be repeated [13].

Therapy

Therapy of atrial arrhythmias in CHF is focused on preventing thromboembolic complications and controlling the arrhythmia associated symptoms. Successful restoration and maintenance of normal sinus rhythm should bring about the theoretical benefits of restoring the atriventricular synchrony, improvement in the atrial transport, reduction in the long-term thromboembolic risk and return of the normal chronotropic competency. However these potential advantages were thus far not demonstrated to provide survival benefit in the clinical trials comparing diverse rhythm controlling strategies to rate control only.

Prevention of the Thromboembolic Complications

CHF is a prothrombotic state. The neurohormonal changes triggered by CHF lead to increased risk of intracardiac thrombus formation leading to systemic thromboembolism. In the WARCEF study, patients with CHF in normal sinus rhythm were treated with either oral aspirin or warfarin. The risk of the ischemic stroke in the anticoagulated patient was 2.5% in warfarin group and 4.7% in aspirin group, significantly exceeding the stroke risk in general population [14]. However, the association of CHF and stroke in patients with preexisting AF is not as robust although the data is largely from older trials with variable CHF definitions [15]. AF is known to substantially increase the risk of stroke and systemic embolization in all patients with the possible exception of young patients with no structural heart disease and no associated risk factors who have paroxysmal AF only. No single risk assessment scale is proven to predict the individual occurrence of stroke with a high accuracy. In clinical practice CHADS2 and CHA2DS2-VASc scores serve as a convenient while imperfect tool for a rapid stroke risk assessment. Other scales like HAS-BLED are helpful in assessing the risk of anticoagulation related complications [16]. Coincidentally, CHF patients often have additional stroke risk factors and generally should be considered for chronic anticoagulation with warfarin with the international normalized ratio (INR) target of 2.0–3.0. Currently approved and available oral anticoagulant alternatives to warfarin include direct thrombin inhibitor dabigatran and oral factor Xa inhibitors rivaroxiban and apixaban. The pivotal trials of the newer anticoagulants included a significant number of patients with clinical CHF and systolic LV dysfunction. In all these trials, the outcomes in the CHF subgroup were similar to the overall positive results of the general study population without excess risk of complications thus, the newer anticoagulants are considered safe and effective in CHF patients [17–19]. Given their decreased level of bleeding complications and excellent efficacy, novel oral anticoagulants are a valuable option for most of the patients with existing stroke risk factors including CHF population. Individuals who are intolerant to oral anticoagulants may be treated with aspirin or aspirin and clopidogrel combination. However, the antiplatelet therapy is less effective than warfarin while the risk of bleeding complications is as high as with the oral anticoagulants [20, 21]. The alternative strategies of the thromboembolic risk reduction in AF in a form of a percutaneous left atrial appendage occlusion device, percutaneous left atrial appendage ligation or surgical ligation may be considered in selected patient even if no outcomes data for their use in CHF patients is yet available.

Rate Control Versus Rhythm Control in CHF

Rate control and rhythm control strategies result in similar outcomes in both mildly symptomatic patients as well as patients with more advanced CHF. AFFIRM trial of rate versus rhythm control in mildly symptomatic AF patients included over 4000 patients. 23% of patients had a history of mild CHF. No advantage of restoration of normal sinus rhythm over rate control was seen [22]. AF-CHF trial studied 1376 AF patients with more advanced CHF. Sinus rhythm restoration and maintenance primarily with amiodarone resulted in the same outcomes for mortality, stroke and CHF hospitalization as rate control only [23]. Interestingly, the ability to maintain normal sinus rhythm with the antiarrhythmic drug therapy is associated with improved prognosis both in patients with mild and advanced CHF. It is not clear whether this phenomenon represents a true causative effect or is simply a marker of a lower risk patient.

Rate Control

Rate control of AF is an accepted goal of therapy and an alternative to the restoration and maintenance of normal sinus rhythm. Effective rate control of AF can be accomplished with medications as well as atrioventricular node ablation and permanent pacemaker implantation. Pharmacological approach is usually the initial strategy given its less invasive nature and reasonable efficacy. Pace and ablate strategy is reserved for situations where medications are ineffective or are not tolerated. β-blockers are the drugs of choice in AF rate control and are particularly valuable in CHF patients. In general, β-blockers that have proven outcomes benefit in CHF including carvedilol, metoprolol succinate and bisoprolol should be use preferentially. However, unstable patient may not be able to tolerate the higher doses needed for effective rate control. In addition, CHF patients with AF naive to β-blocker therapy are more likely to be β-blocker intolerant and have a lesser chance to respond to the therapy including less reduction in mortality as compared to their non-AF counterparts. Digoxin maybe added to β-blocker for an improved rate control efficacy and to allow for a lower dose of either drug to be used. Digoxin alone or in combination is less effective rate controlling agent during acute CHF decompensation. In refractory cases, intravenous or oral amiodarone may also be utilized but this strategy increases bradycardic complications and the need for a pacemaker implantation. Calcium channel antagonist especially nondihydropyridines should be avoided in patients with depressed left ventricular function. Dronaderone was evaluated as a rate control strategy in patients with persistent AF. In PALLAS trial, active therapy with dronaderone resulted in increased cardiovascular events including mortality. Moreover, the use of dronaderone in patients with moderate to severe heart failure resulted in significant increase in mortality and worsening of heart failure status. Thus, dronaderone should not be used in patients with active CHF symptoms and AF [24, 25]. The targets of strict rate control (<80/min at rest, <110/min with moderate exercise) were historically based on the values adopted from the AFFIRM trial [22]. The same targets were used in AF-CHF trial [23]. More recently, the strategy of strict versus lenient rate control (<110/min at rest) was evaluated in RACE II study. Both approaches were found to have equivalent results however; patients with CHF and left ventricular dysfunction were underrepresented [26]. Periodic monitoring of left ventricular function is recommended for patients who are treated with lenient rate control to avoid the insidious onset of tachycardia-induced cardiomyopathy.

Pace and ablate approach to permanent AF rate control in CHF has significant benefits but also carries a risk of short and long term complications. The benefits are related to the immediate complete rate control, rhythm regularization and reversal of the tachycardia mediated left ventricular dysfunction. Poorly tolerated rate controlling drugs can be discontinued. On the other hand, patient is rendered pacemaker dependent and faces the inherent risk of a random device failure or infection as well as hemodynamic consequences of the permanent pacing including progressive left ventricular failure and mitral regurgitation. Studies of pace and ablate strategy in unselected general population conducted prior to the era of cardiac resynchronization suggested net positive effect on symptoms control, improvement in left ventricular systolic performance and decreased rate of hospitalizations. However the same strategy studied in patients with low ejection fraction (EF) and CHF revealed more diverse outcomes with significant improvement in some patients but progressive deterioration associated with a very high early mortality rates in majority of patients. The PAVE study examined the effect of right ventricular versus biventricular pacing after AV node ablation in patients with permanent AF. Biventricular pacing protected from LV systolic function deterioration and improved quality of life and functional measures. The effect was particularly apparent in the population of patients with preexisting CHF and reduced EF [27]. Similar improved outcomes were subsequently reported in pace and ablate patients with initial RV pacing only after the upgrade to biventricular system was performed and patients with de novo biventricular pacing [28, 29]. Recent systematic review of the AV node ablation in the cardiac resynchronization therapy recipients with CHF and AF suggested not only improvement in symptoms but also mortality benefit [30]. Therefore, pace and ablate strategy utilizing isolated RV pacing should not be used in heart failure patients while cardiac resynchronization therapy should be strongly considered in all patients with LV dysfunction and anticipated high rate of ventricular pacing or pacemaker dependency.

Rhythm Control

Dofetilide and amiodarone are the only two antiarrhythmic drugs recommended for the pharmacological rhythm control of AF in CHF patients [31, 32]. The recommendation is based on their lack of negative inotropic effect on myocardial contractility and neutral effect on survival in patients with CHF. Dofetilide is usually well tolerated and moderately effective for the sinus rhythm maintenance in patients with CHF or ischemic heart disease as reported in the DIAMOND study. The risk of drug-induced proarrhythmia, most commonly in a form of torsades de pointes is acceptably low as long as the renal function and serum electrolytes are stable and excessive QTc interval prolongation is avoided. Dofetilide should only be initiated in the hospital settings. Amiodarone is also safe and more effective than placebo for normal sinus rhythm maintenance in variety of clinical setting including CHF patients. Frequent occurrence of intolerance and potential for serious organ toxicity limits the utility of amiodarone in long-term AF therapy. In DIONYSOS trial, amiodarone had to be stopped prematurely in 13.3% of patients while 44.5% of patients reported drug side effects at 12 months of its use [33]. It should be noted that the use of all other antiarrhythmic drugs including class I drugs, D-sotalol and dronaderone is associated with increased mortality in CHF patients and should be avoided.

Pacing Therapy

Cardiac pacing therapy outside of the pace and ablate situation is often necessary in CHF population with and without AF. The need for pacing is triggered by the increased frequency of sinus and atrioventricular node dysfunction as well as degenerative His-Purkinje conduction system disease driven by the cardiomyopathic process and frequent iatrogenic bradyarrhythmic complications of medical therapy with βblockers, digoxin and amiodarone. In addition, biventricular pacing is indicated in patients with decreased left ventricular systolic function, widened QRS and at least mild heart failure. Atrial pacing in patients with sinus node dysfunction may reduce occurrences of AF precipitated by severe bradycardia. Overdrive atrial pacing, multisite pacing and unconventional site pacing for AF prevention or AF burden reduction is controversial and the benefit is not clearly documented. High frequency conventional right ventricular pacing is known to increase incidence of both AF and CHF regardless of the baseline LV systolic function [34]. Optimal pacemaker programming set to minimize right ventricular pacing should be utilized in all pacemaker recipients when appropriate. Cardiac resynchronization therapy is reasonable in the setting of the coexisting AF. Despite the improvements in the left ventricular systolic performance and CHF functional status associated with biventricular pacing the effect on AF is not as favorable. In CARE-HF study, biventricular pacing was not protective against the future development of AF. In the MADIT-CRT the subgroup of clinical responders to resynchronization therapy defined as reduction in left atrial volume had lower incidence of new onset atrial fibrillation [35]. Presence of AF at the time of the biventricular pacemaker implantation is associated with decreases likelihood of clinical response and predicts increased risk of cardiac mortality particularly if the pacing therapy is not delivered at all times. Atrioventricular node ablation assures complete rate control and near 100% delivery of cardiac resynchronization therapy and should be considered under these circumstances [36].

Atrial Fibrillation Ablation

Catheter ablation of AF is an accepted therapy for symptomatic patients intolerant or unresponsive to medical management. It is postulated that ablation therapy in CHF patients would offer superior arrhythmia control translating into improvement in symptoms, myocardial systolic function parameters and potential mortality benefit. Some observational or non-randomized studies in AF ablation suggest that CHF patients may be effectively treated by ablation and often have significant improvement in left ventricular function when arrhythmia is controlled [37–40]. These observations from non-randomized trials were corroborated by meta-analysis that reviewed outcomes of 1851 patients undergoing catheter ablation of AF. Subgroup of CHF patients required more redo procedures but experienced an average EF improvement of 11% [41]. Randomized catheter ablation trial data in patients with LV dysfunction remains sparse. PABA-CHF randomized trial compared AF ablation to AV node ablation and biventricular pacing in patients with LV dysfunction and found the AF ablation to be more effective resulting in improvement in left ventricular EF, 6-min walk test and quality of life [42]. Another randomized trial compared ablation to medical management in patients with symptomatic CHF and EF <35% and found that the improvements in EF were restricted to the ablation patients who were able to maintain sinus rhythm [43]. ARC HF trial randomized persistent AF patients with stable moderate to severe CHF and EF <35% to extensive biatrial AF ablation versus rate control. Sinus rhythm was restored in 92% of patients. At 12 months of follow up the ablation group had significant improvement in peak oxygen consumption as well as significant improvement in quality of life, decreased B-type naturetic peptide levels and regression of left atrial dilatation. A trend towards improved left ventricular EF was observed as well [44]. Large scale randomized trials enrolling CHF patients with EF 35% or less and assigning them to either AF ablation or conventional medical therapy are ongoing and should provide more definitive data for the role of AF ablation in CHF population [45–47]. Accordingly, 2011 ACCF/AHA/HRS Focused Update on the Management of Patients With Atrial Fibrillation positions AF catheter ablation in patients with CHF in a " may be considered" category where more studies are needed before a definitive assessment and recommendation for the therapy can be made [13].

Atrial Fibrillation Ablation: The Fifth Pillar of Goal Directed Medical Therapy for Heart Failure?

Atrial fibrillation is frequently associated with heart failure with the incidence increasing as heart failure becomes more advanced (incidence ranging from 5% for patients with NYHA Class I heart failure to 50% for patients with Class IV heart failure) [48, 49]. The presence of atrial fibrillation in patients with heart failure increases the likelihood of heart failure related hospitalizations and mortality [48, 49]. Atrial fibrillation has a potentiating effect on the progression of heart failure through neurohormonal activation, increased inflammation, adverse cardiac remodeling and tachycardia-induced hemodynamic derangement and decompensation [49]. In turn, worsening heart failure can increase the burden of atrial fibrillation, further exacerbating heart failure progression. In essence these are reinforcing and reciprocal syndromes. Interrupting this cycle can potentially mitigate the progression of heart failure, improve hemodynamics and tamp down neurohormonal activation and inflammation as well as improving outcomes. Given the toxicity of many anti-arrhythmic agents in heart failure patients and the limited pharmacologic options available, more effective therapies for managing and treating atrial fibrillation are highly desirable. Catheter ablation of atrial fibrillation is an invasive, often successful approach for reducing atrial fibrillation burden and occasionally curing atrial fibrillation [50, 51]. It may be more challenging technically and in terms of achieving successful outcomes in patients with heart failure, specifically advanced heart failure [51, 52]. Until recently, information regarding the efficacy of catheter ablation for atrial fibrillation and its effect on outcomes in patients with advanced heart failure were not known. The recent CASTLE-HTx trial provided insight into these issues in patients with advanced heart failure and atrial fibrillation [53].

CASTLE-HTx was a single center European study of 194 patients with NYHA Class II-IV heart failure, an LV ejection fraction <35% and symptomatic atrial fibrillation who, because of their heart failure, were being evaluated for cardiac transplantation [53]. Patients were randomized to undergo catheter ablation for atrial fibrillation plus continue GDMT for heart failure versus GDMT without ablation. There was a median follow-up of 18 months.The likelihood of a composite of death from any cause, implantation of a left ventricular assist device, or urgent heart transplantation (primary end point) was lower in the ablation group than in the medical-therapy group, with a hazard ratio of 0.24. The composite endpoint results were driven by reductions in cardiovascular death and all cause mortality [53]. Death from any cause occurred in 6% of the patients in the ablation group and 20% of those in the medical-therapy group. Many of the deaths in the medical-therapy group resulted from advanced therapies such as implantation of a left ventricular assist device or after heart transplantation and which were more common in the medical therapy group likely because of progression of heart failure [53]. At 12 month follow up, LVEF improved by an absolute percentage of 6.4% in the ablation group. Atrial fibrillation burden declined by 22.7% [53].

In summary, catheter ablation of atrial fibrillation in addition to GDMT, improves outcomes in patients with advanced heart failure being evaluated for advanced therapies such as cardiac transplantation and LVADs. While this single center provides evidence of the utility of atrial fibrillation ablation in these sick patients with heart failure, stronger evidence could be obtained from a larger, multi-center study focused on the sickest patients, i.e., those with NYHA Class III and IV heart failure.

Summary

Atrial arrhythmias and CHF are common and often coexisting cardiac conditions. When present in the same patient, they tend to signify more advanced stage of cardiac disease and lower probability of the successful control of either problem. All patients with AF and CHF should receive β-blockers and angiotensin receptor inhibitors in addition to arrhythmia directed therapy. Therapeutic options for arrhythmia control are sparser when CHF is present. Traditional pharmacological therapies offer modest success while more contemporary therapies are more promising but not extensively studied yet. The current approach to the therapy of AF is based on stroke prevention with systemic anticoagulation and adequate heart rate control. Atrioventricular node ablation and biventricular pacing is appropriate for patient who fail to achieve rate control targets with medications or are unable to tolerate medical therapy. Aggressive rhythm control with increasingly important role of the catheter ablation is reserved for patients who remain symptomatic despite successful rate control.

References

1. Braunwald E. Shattuck Lecture—cardiovascular medicine at the turn of the millennium: triumphs, concerns, and opportunities. N Engl J Med. 1997;337:1360–9. CrossRef PubMed.
2. Wang TJ, Larson MG, Levy D, et al. Temporal relations of atrial fibrillation and congestive heart failure and their joint influence on mortality: the Framingham Heart Study. Circulation. 2003;107:2920–5. CrossRef PubMed.
3. Stevenson WG, Stevenson LW. Atrial fibrillation in heart failure. N Engl J Med. 1999;341:910–1. CrossRef PubMed.
4. Ehrlich JR, Nattel S, Hohnloser SH. Atrial fibrillation and congestive heart failure: specific considerations at the intersection of two common and important cardiac disease sets. J Cardiovasc Electrophysiol. 2002;13:399–405. CrossRef PubMed.
5. Carson PE, Johnson GR, Dunkman WB for the V-HeFT VA Cooperative Studies Group. The influence of atrial fibrillation on prognosis in mild to moderate heart failure. The V-HeFT studies. Circulation 1993;87:VI-102–VI-110.
6. Deedwania PC, Singh BN, Ellenbogen KA, et al. Spontaneous conversion and maintenance of sinus rhythm by amiodarone in patients with heart failure and atrial fibrillation. Observation from the Veterans Affairs Congestive Heart Failure Trial on Antiarrhythmic Therapy (CHF-STAT). Circulation. 1998;98:2574–9. CrossRef PubMed.
7. Middlekauff HR, Stevenson WG, Stevenson LW. Prognostic significance of atrial fibrillation in advanced heart failure. A study of 390 patients. Circulation. 1991;84:40–8. CrossRef PubMed.
8. The CONSENSUS Trial Study Group: effects of enalapril on mortality in severe congestive heart failure. Results of the Cooperative North Scandinavian Enalapril Survival Study (CONSENSUS). N Engl J Med 1987;316:1429–1435.
9. Allessie MA, Boyden PA, Camm AJ, et al. Pathophysiology and prevention of atrial fibrillation. Circulation. 2001;103:769–77. s
10. Wakili R, Voigt N, Kääb S, et al. Recent advances in the molecular pathophysiology of atrial fibrillation. J Clin Invest. 2011;121(8):2955–68. CrossRef PubMed PubMedCentral.
11. Orejarena L, Vidaillet H, DeStefano F, et al. Paroxysmal supraventricular tachycardia in the general population. J Am Coll Cardiol. 1998;31(1):150–7. CrossRef PubMed.
12. Hindricks G, Pokushalov E, Urban L, et al. Performance of a new leadless implantable cardiac monitor in detecting and quantifying atrial fibrillation: results of the XPECT trial. Circ Arrhythm Electrophysiol. 2010;3(2):141–7. CrossRef PubMed.
13. 2011 ACCF/AHA/HRS focused update on the management of patients with atrial fibrillation (Updating the 2006 Guideline): a report of the American College of Cardiology Foundation/American Heart Association Task Force on Practice Guidelines. J Am Coll Cardiol 2011;57(2):223–242.
14. Homma S, Thompson JL, Pullicino PM, WARCEF Investigators Warfarin and aspirin in patients with heart failure and sinus rhythm. N Engl J Med. 2012;366(20):1859–69. CrossRef PubMed PubMedCentral.
15. Stroke Prevention in Atrial Fibrillation Investigators. Stroke prevention in atrial fibrillation study: final results. Circulation. 1991;84:527–39. CrossRef.
16. Lane DA, Lip GYH. Use of the CHA2DS2-VASc and HAS-BLED scores to aid decision making for thromboprophylaxis in non-valvular atrial fibrillation. Circulation. 2012;126:860–5. CrossRef PubMed.
17. Connolly SJ, Ezekowitz MD, Yusuf S, et al. Dabigatran versus warfarin in patients with atrial fibrillation. N Engl J Med. 2009;361:1139–51. CrossRef PubMed.

18. Patel MR, Mahaffey KW, Garg J, et al. Rivaroxaban vs. warfarin in nonvalvular atrial fibrillation. N Engl J Med. 2011;365:883–91. CrossRef PubMed.
19. Granger CB, Alexander JH, McMurray JJ, et al. Apixaban vs. warfarin in patients with atrial fibrillation. N Engl J Med. 2011;365:981–92. CrossRef PubMed.
20. Connolly SJ, Pogue J, Hart RG, et al. Effect of clopidogrel added to aspirin in patients with atrial fibrillation. N Engl J Med. 2009;360:2066–78. CrossRef PubMed.
21. Connolly SJ, Pogue J, Hart R, et al. Clopidogrel plus aspirin versus oral anticoagulation for atrial fibrillation in the Atrial fibrillation Clopidogrel Trial with Irbesartan for prevention of Vascular Events (ACTIVE W): a randomised controlled trial. Lancet. 2006;367:1903–12. CrossRef PubMed.
22. Olshansky B, Rosenfeld LE, Warner AL, et al. The Atrial Fibrillation Follow-up Investigation of Rhythm Management (AFFIRM) study: approaches to control rate in atrial fibrillation. J Am Coll Cardiol. 2004;43:1201–8. CrossRef PubMed.
23. Roy D, Talajic M, Nattel S, et al. Rhythm control versus rate control for atrial fibrillation and heart failure. N Engl J Med. 2008;358:2667–77. CrossRef PubMed.
24. Kober L, Torp-Pedersen C, McMurray JJ, et al. Increased mortality after dronedarone therapy for severe heart failure. N Engl J Med. 2008;358:2678–87. CrossRef PubMed.
25. Connolly SJ, Camm AJ, Halperin JL, et al. Dronedarone in high-risk permanent atrial fibrillation. N Engl J Med. 2011;365:2268–76. CrossRef PubMed.
26. Van Gelder IC, Groenveld HF, Crijns HJ, et al. Lenient versus strict rate control in patients with atrial fibrillation. N Engl J Med. 2010;362:1363–73. CrossRef PubMed.
27. Doshi RN, Daoud EG, Fellows C, et al. Left ventricular-based cardiac stimulation post AV nodal ablation evaluation (the PAVE study). J Cardiovasc Electrophysiol. 2005;16:1160–5. CrossRef PubMed.
28. Leon AR, Greenberg JM, Kanuru N, et al. Cardiac resynchronization in patients with congestive heart failure and chronic atrial fibrillation: effect of upgrading to biventricular pacing after chronic right ventricular pacing. J Am Coll Cardiol. 2002;39:1258–63. CrossRef PubMed.
29. Valls-Bertault V, Fatemi M, Gilard M, et al. Assessment of upgrading to biventricular pacing in patients with right ventricular pacing and congestive heart failure after atrioventricular junctional ablation for chronic atrial fibrillation. Europace. 2004;6:438–43. CrossRef PubMed.
30. Ganesan AN, Brooks AG, Roberts-Thomson KC, et al. Role of AV nodal ablation in cardiac resynchronization in patients with coexistent atrial fibrillation and heart failure a systematic review. J Am Coll Cardiol. 2012;59:719–26. CrossRef PubMed.
31. Torp-Pedersen C, Moller M, Bloch-Thomsen PE, et al. Dofetilide in patients with congestive heart failure and left ventricular dysfunction. Danish Investigations of Arrhythmia and Mortality on Dofetilide Study Group. N Engl J Med. 1999;341:857–65. CrossRef PubMed.
32. Singh SN, Fletcher RD, Fisher SG, et al. Amiodarone in patients with congestive heart failure and asymptomatic ventricular arrhythmia. Survival trial of antiarrhythmic therapy in congestive heart failure. N Engl J Med. 1995;333:77–82. CrossRef PubMed.
33. Le Heuzey JY, De Ferrari GM, Radzik D, et al. A short-term, randomized, double-blind, Parallel-Group Study to evaluate the efficacy and safety of dronedarone versus amiodarone in patients with persistent atrial fibrillation: the DIONYSOS Study. J Cardiovasc Electrophysiol. 2010;21(6):597–605. CrossRef PubMed.
34. Sweeney MO, Bank AJ, Nsah E, et al. Minimizing ventricular pacing to reduce atrial fibrillation in sinus-node disease. N Engl J Med. 2007;357(10):1000–8. CrossRef PubMed.
35. Brenyo A, Link MS, Barsheshet A, et al. Cardiac resynchronization therapy reduces left atrial volume and the risk of atrial tachyarrhythmias in MADIT-CRT. J Am Coll Cardiol. 2011;58:1682–9. CrossRef PubMed.
36. Gasparini M, Auricchio A, Regoli F, et al. Four-year efficacy of cardiac resynchronization therapy on exercise tolerance and disease progression: the importance of performing atrioventricular junction ablation in patients with atrial fibrillation. J Am Coll Cardiol. 2006;48:734–43. CrossRef PubMed.
37. Haissaguerre M, Jais P, Shah DC, et al. Electrophysiological end point for catheter ablation of atrial fibrillation initiated from multiple pulmonary venous foci. Circulation. 2000;101:1409–17. CrossRef PubMed.
38. Pappone C, Oreto G, Rosanio S, et al. Atrial electroanatomic remodeling after circumferential radiofrequency pulmonary vein ablation: efficacy of an anatomic approach in a large cohort of patients with atrial fibrillation. Circulation. 2001;104:2539–44. CrossRef PubMed.
39. Oral H, Knight BP, Tada H, et al. Pulmonary vein isolation for paroxysmal and persistent atrial fibrillation. Circulation. 2002;105:1077–81. CrossRef PubMed.
40. Hsu L-F, Jaïs P, Sanders P, et al. Catheter ablation for atrial fibrillation in congestive heart failure. N Engl J Med. 2004;351:2373–83. CrossRef PubMed.
41. Wilton SB, Fundytus A, WA G, et al. Meta-analysis of the effectiveness and safety of catheter ablation of atrial fibrillation in patients with versus without left ventricular systolic dysfunction. Am J Cardiol. 2010;106(9):1284–91. CrossRef PubMed.
42. Khan MN, Jaïs P, Cummings J, et al. Pulmonary-vein isolation for atrial fibrillation in patients with heart failure. N Engl J Med. 2008;359(17):1778–85. CrossRef PubMed.
43. MacDonald MR, Connelly DT, Hawkins NM, et al. Radiofrequency ablation for persistent atrial fibrillation in patients with advanced heart failure and severe left ventricular systolic dysfunction: a randomised

controlled trial. Heart. 2011;97(9):740–7. CrossRef PubMed.
44. Jones DG, Haldar SK, Hussain W, et al. A randomized trial to assess catheter ablation versus rate control in the management of persistent atrial fibrillation in heart failure. J Am Coll Cardiol. 2013;61:1894–903.
45. Marrouche NF, Brachmann J. Catheter ablation versus standard conventional treatment in patients with left ventricular dysfunction and atrial fibrillation (CASTLE-AF)—study design. PACE. 2009;32:987–94. CrossRef PubMed.
46. Rate versus catheter ablation rhythm control in patients with heart failure and high burden atrial fibrillation (RAFT-AF). US National Library of Medicine. NCT01420393. ClinicalTrials.gov; 2016.
47. Atrial fibrillation management in congestive heart failure with ablation (AMICA). US National Library of Medicine. NCT00652522. ClinicalTrials.gov; 2016.
48. Carlisle MA, Fudim M, DeVore AD, Piccini JP. Heart failure and atrial fibrillation, like fire and fury. JACC Heart Fail. 2019;7:44756.
49. Lewis EF. Catheter ablation for atrial fibrillation in heart failure—an option to defer transplantation? New Engl J Med. 2023;389:1429–30.
50. Verma A, Kalman JM, Callans DJ. Treatment of patients with atrial fibrillation and heart failure with reduced ejection fraction. Circulation. 2017;135:154763.
51. Marrouche NF, Brachmann J, Andresen D, et al. Catheter ablation for atrial fibrillation with heart failure. N Engl J Med. 2018;378:417–27.
52. Prabhu S, Taylor AJ, Costello BT, et al. Catheter ablation versus medical rate control in atrial fibrillation and systolic dysfunction: the CAMERA-MRI study. J Am Coll Cardiol. 2017;70:1949–61.
53. Sohns C, Fox H, Marrouche NF, et al. Catheter ablation in end-stage heart failure with atrial fibrillation. New Eng J Med. 2023;389:1380–9.

Ventricular Arrhythmias and Heart Failure

21

Stephen C. Keane, Ethan R. Ellis, Mark E. Josephson, and David J. Callans

Introduction

Sudden death is a common cause of mortality in heart failure patients, mainly due to ventricular tachyarrhythmias [1]. Ventricular tachycardia (VT) is frequently observed in heart failure, and its evaluation and treatment necessitate special attention. Pathophysiologic changes in heart failure make patients susceptible to the development of ventricular arrhythmias. In this chapter, we will discuss the mechanisms of arrhythmogenesis associated with the heart failure syndrome, the clinical manifestations of ventricular arrhythmias in heart failure and appropriate treatment strategies to prevent recurrent arrhythmias and sudden cardiac death (SCD).

Mark E. Josephson died before publication of this work was completed.

S. C. Keane · D. J. Callans (✉)
Department of Cardiac Electrophysiology, Hospital of the University of Pennsylvania, Philadelphia, PA, USA
e-mail: stephen.keane@pennmedicine.upenn.edu; david.callans@pennmedicine.upenn.edu

E. R. Ellis
Cardiac Electrophysiologist, University of Colorado Health, Fort Collins, CO, USA
e-mail: ethan.ellis@uchealth.org

M. E. Josephson (Deceased)
Harvard Medical School, Cardiovascular Division, Beth Israel Deaconess Medical Center Harvard-Thorndike Electrophysiology Institute and Arrhythmia Service, Boston, MA, USA

Mechanisms of Arrhythmogenesis

There are three fundamental mechanisms of VT which include reentry, automaticity, and triggered activity due to early or delayed afterdepolarizations. Each heart failure etiology has a propensity for a specific mechanism of arrhythmogenesis.

Automaticity

Automaticity in cardiac myocytes may be normal or abnormal. Normal automaticity occurs in cells with intrinsic pacemaker properties and occurs in cells with normal resting potential, while abnormal automaticity happens in partially depolarized cells. Pathological environments lead to a reduction in resting membrane potential and when reduced sufficiently, spontaneous diastolic depolarization may occur and lead to impulse initiation. Some cells, such as Purkinje system myocytes, can display normal and abnormal automaticity, expressing normal automaticity at high levels of membrane potential and abnormal automaticity when the membrane potential is reduced [2]. Ventricular myocytes, on the other hand, only develop automaticity when they are partially depolarized due to underlying pathology and automaticity in ventricular myocytes is always abnormal. Under normal conditions, there is a hierarchy of intrinsic pacemaker rates with the sinus node being the most rapid, followed by

H. J. Eisen (ed.), *Heart Failure I*, https://doi.org/10.1007/978-3-032-12626-9_21

the atria, the AV node, the His bundle, and the Purkinje fibers respectively. In this hierarchy, latent pacemaker cells are depolarized by propagating wave fronts, which prevent them from reaching their own spontaneous depolarization threshold potential and are inhibited by repeated depolarization, known as overdrive suppression [2, 3]. For automatic VT to occur, the pacemaker rate in the Purkinje cells or ventricular myocytes must increase above that of the sinus node and higher pacemaker cells. The most important cause of this is sympathetic activation, which enhances the rate of spontaneous diastolic depolarization in latent ventricular pacemakers more than the sinus node. Catecholamine stimulation is generally required for the development of automatic ventricular arrhythmias.

Triggered Activity

Triggered activity initiates impulses that depend on after-depolarizations, which are oscillations in membrane potential that follow the upstroke of an action potential. Two types of after-depolarizations are observed: early after-depolarizations (EADs) occurring during repolarization and delayed after-depolarizations (DADs) occurring after repolarization is complete or nearly complete [2]. When an after-depolarization depolarizes a cell to its threshold potential, a triggered impulse is initiated, which leads to the initiation of an action potential. A series of additional triggered action potentials can occur, each arising from the after-potential caused by the previous action potential when an after-depolarization reaches the threshold potential.

DADs occur due to calcium overload, which is an increase in Ca^{2+} in the myoplasm and sarcoplasmic reticulum (SR) above normal levels. Abnormalities in the sequestration and release of Ca^{2+} by the SR may also contribute to their occurrence. When intracellular Ca^{2+} is elevated, a critical level may be reached during repolarization causing a secondary, spontaneous release of Ca^{2+} after the action potential which generates a transient inward current (the DAD) [2]. The increase in intracellular Ca^{2+} may result from an increase in heart rate or premature stimulation, digitalis inhibition of Na^+/K^+ pump, catecholamine-enhanced L-type Ca^{2+} current, or other pathological effects that increase Ca^{2+} loading such as heart failure or hypertrophy [2].

EADs occur when repolarization of an action potential suddenly shifts in a depolarizing direction, which happens when the outward current slows or the inward current increases, causing depolarization to reach the threshold potential, leading to reactivation of inward current and an action potential upstroke [2, 4, 5]. EADs prolong action potential duration and occur more easily in Purkinje fibers than in ventricular or atrial muscle. Class III antiarrhythmic drugs like sotalol and dofetilide or class IA AADs such as quinidine can cause EADs by inhibiting the IKr repolarizing current [6]. Other causes of EADs include hypoxia, hypoxia with acidosis and catecholamines, and stretch [2]. All EAD causes can be observed as QT prolongation on the surface ECG. EADs are responsible for functional reentrant excitation leading to polymorphic VT.

Slow Conduction and Reentry

Reentrant excitation requires a region of unidirectional block, at least transiently, allowing for impulse propagation in one direction while preventing excitation in the other direction. Block can occur after rapid repetitive activation or premature excitation, or even when there is permanent unidirectional block. For reentry to recur, the impulse must find excitable tissue, which requires longer conduction time around the circuit than the effective refractory period of the myocardium from which it originated. Slow conduction and short refractory periods allow reentry which is often the result of the underlying pathology. The reentrant circuit can have an anatomical component with a central obstacle, or it may be functional with its size and shape determined by the electrophysiological properties of the involved tissue.

Myocardial fibrosis and scarring in a diseased heart affect conduction by several mechanisms.

It increases the extracellular resistivity of myocyte bundles leading to slow conduction and block (Fig. 21.1). Fibrosis can also distort the size and shape of myocardial bundles trapped in scar tissue leading to changes in their conductive properties. Gap junctions are specialized regions of close interaction between neighboring myocytes in which clusters of transmembrane channels bridge the paired plasma membranes. Gap junctions allow the direct exchange of ions and small molecules between adjacent cardiac cells during the normal conduction of an impulse [7]. Connexins are proteins that form gap junctions in the heart, which are specialized intercellular channels that allow the direct exchange of ions and small molecules between adjacent cardiac cells. Connexin 43 is the primary connexin found in the ventricles [8, 9] whereas connexin 40 is primarily found in the His-Purkinje system (HPS) as well as the AV node [10, 11]. The most important causes of slow conduction and reentry are connexin dysfunction and fibrosis, which often coexist. Abnormal tissue architecture such as fibrosis may lead to reduced connexin 43 expression which may eventually result in arrhythmias [12].

Heart Failure and Arrhythmogenesis

All the previous mechanisms of arrhythmogenesis can contribute to the development of ventricular arrhythmias in heart failure. Fibrosis and scarring of the ventricles due to myocardial infarction (MI), pathologic hypertrophy, non-infarct related fibrosis, or myocardial dysplasia predispose patients with cardiomyopathy to reentrant ventricular arrhythmias. Additionally, heart failure can cause alterations in cardiac ion channel currents, leading to abnormal depolarization and repolarization, which increase the likelihood of automatic and triggered activity. These changes are thought to be due to neurohormonal activation and biomechanical abnormalities asso-

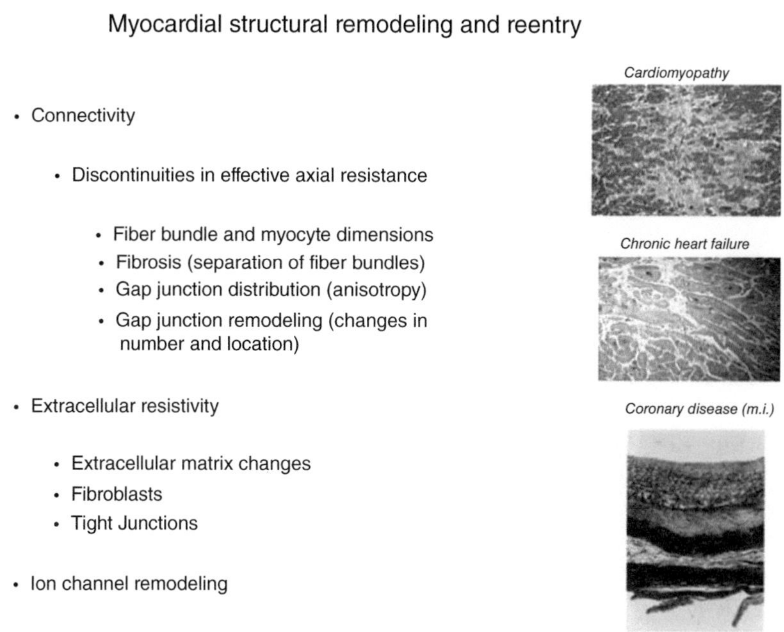

Fig. 21.1 Myocardial structural remodeling promotes conditions for reentry**.** Structural heart disease in heart failure and cardiomyopathy leads to pathophysiologic changes which result in abnormal impulse formation and propagation setting the stage for reentrant excitation. Abnormalities in cell-to-cell connectivity, extracellular resistance, and ion channel remodeling all contribute to the increased likelihood of reentrant arrhythmias in heart failure and cardiomyopathy. See text for discussion

ciated with heart failure. Thus, structural heart disease and the heart failure syndrome are often interdependent for the production of ventricular arrhythmias.

Fibrosis

Fibrosis is the most common cause of functional and anatomic block leading to slow conduction and reentry and occurs in both infarct-related and non-ischemic cardiomyopathies. The pattern and extent of fibrosis may range from patchy areas in some forms of heart failure to extensive fibrotic scars in MI. In infarct-related cardiomyopathies, fibrosis replaces necrotic regions and may extend into non-infarcted bordering regions. The number of cell-to-cell contacts is reduced with side-to-side connections selectively affected [13, 14]. In healing infarct border zones, increased interstitial collagen disrupts the long transversely oriented gap junctions enhancing anisotropy by increasing the axial resistivity transverse to the long fiber axis [14]. Gap junctions at the ends of myocytes undergo fewer changes. Thus the normal property of uniform anisotropy is converted to non-uniform anisotropy [13, 14].

When there is a large scar such as in hearts with myocardial infarcts, bridges of intact myocytes can project into or completely across areas of fibrosis termed "channels". Myocytes in these bridges sometimes link with normal myocytes on the outer borders of the infarct [15]. Slow conduction can result from circuitous, non-uniform propagation through these myocardial bundles trapped in scar tissue [16]. The effects of fibrosis on conduction is often detectable by low amplitude, long duration, fractionated electrograms with delayed activation, the basis for substrate mapping for ablation of VT [17]. The number of fractionated electrograms seen during endocardial substrate mapping has been shown to correlate with the likelihood of inducible monomorphic VT at the time of electrophysiology study [18]. Fractionated electrograms are also more likely to be seen during endocardial mapping in patients with infarct-related and non-ischemic cardiomyopathy (NICM) who present with VT when compared to patients with no VT, non-sustained ventricular tachycardia (NSVT), or cardiac arrest [19].

Ischemia

Acute ischemia may result in abnormal automaticity or focal discharges from calcium overload and triggered activity in the form of delayed or early after-depolarizations [20, 21]. Acute ischemia activates the ATP-sensitive potassium (K_{ATP}) channels, causing an increase in extracellular potassium in the cardiac muscle. Minor increases in extracellular potassium depolarize the myocyte's resting membrane potential, which can increase tissue excitability in the early phase of ischemia [22]. Further hyperkalemia causes greater resting membrane depolarization, decreased conduction velocity and tissue excitability, and shortening of the action potential duration, but prolongs the effective refractory period due to post-repolarization refractoriness [22]. These changes provide a substrate for injury current to flow between ischemic and non-ischemic cells located in border zones, which can promote focal abnormal automaticity and initiate VT [23, 24]. In addition to acute ischemia, chronic ischemia and infarction can also lead to abnormal automaticity and triggered activity. Changes in neurohormonal signaling and mechanical stress on the heart may also contribute to arrhythmogenesis in the setting of chronic ischemia and infarction [25].

Action Potential Prolongation and Abnormal Calcium Handling

Prolongation of the action potential duration is a common feature of heart failure and can contribute to the development of arrhythmias. This prolongation is caused by alterations in the activity of several ionic currents in the heart. Downregulation of the transient outward current (I_{to}) is the most consistent ionic current change observed in heart failure [26–28] but downregulation of other potassium channel currents including I_{K1}, I_{Kr}, and I_{Ks} have also been observed in animal models [26, 29–33]. In addition to the downregulation of repolarizing potassium currents and alterations in calcium handling, a late sodium current is another mechanism for altered repolarization in animals with chronic heart failure [34].

The dysregulation of calcium handling is another mechanism that can contribute to action potential prolongation and arrhythmia development in heart failure [35]. This dysregulation can lead to abnormal intracellular calcium handling, which is a common feature of myocytes from failing hearts. An increase in the function of the Na^+/Ca^{2+} exchanger has been observed in many studies, while downregulation of the sarcoplasmic reticulum calcium ATPase (SERCA) is also consistently found across studies [36–41]. These changes can result in an increased open probability of the ryanodine receptor, which is the calcium release channel of the sarcoplasmic reticulum [42, 43]. Spontaneous calcium release from the sarcoplasmic reticulum, facilitated by the presence of beta-adrenergic stimulation and the increased open probability of the ryanodine receptor, can give rise to delayed afterdepolarizations. Adrenergic stimulation is necessary for this effect, and the electrogenic Na^+/Ca^{2+} exchanger removes the released calcium from the cell, causing a transient inward Na^+ current that can cause a delayed afterdepolarization [44]. This is facilitated by the higher resting membrane potential created by a decrease in outward potassium current.

Purkinje myocytes, which are often the sources of afterdepolarizations associated with triggered arrhythmias, undergo substantial remodeling of both potassium and calcium currents. This remodeling can result in prolonged action potential duration and labile repolarization, predisposing these cells to afterdepolarization-mediated triggered activity and functional reentry [45]. The prolonged action potential duration is caused by a decrease in the repolarizing currents and an increase in depolarizing currents, which in turn leads to an unstable and labile repolarization pattern that occurs both spatially and temporally. This instability can predispose the heart to after-depolarization-mediated triggered activity, as well as functional reentry, where electrical impulses are able to travel repeatedly in a circular path, maintaining an arrhythmia. Although afterdepolarizations and reentry are not mutually exclusive, afterdepolarizations that are of sufficient amplitude to elicit an action potential may initiate an arrhythmia, while reentry may sustain it [46].

Mechanical Factors

Mechanical abnormalities in patients with heart failure, such as increased wall stress and cavitary dilatation, can cause changes in the electrophysiologic properties of the myocardium through a phenomenon known as mechanoelectric feedback [47, 48]. In the normal heart, acute myocardial stretch exaggerates the normal rate-dependent shortening of refractoriness but does not influence transverse or longitudinal conduction velocity [49]. However, in animal models with dilated cardiomyopathy, the refractoriness and repolarization can be significantly prolonged and this effect cannot be reversed by reducing the load with drugs [49]. Stretch has also been shown to cause a reduction of connexin 43 as well as its redistribution to the lateral sarcolemmal membranes resulting in slowing of conduction in the transverse direction, predisposing these cells to reentry [50]. In human studies, direct correlations have been found between left ventricular end-diastolic volume and the prevalence of ventricular arrhythmias, and the QT prolongation seen in patients with advanced heart failure can be significantly reversed by mechanically unloading the left ventricle with a left ventricular assist device [51, 52].

Altered Neurohormonal Signaling

The adrenergic and renin-angiotensin-aldosterone systems (RAAS) are known to play a significant role in the progression of heart failure. Inhibiting these pathways through pharmacological intervention has been shown to be associated with a reduction in overall mortality as well as SCD mortality, as demonstrated in randomized clinical trials [53–58]. In patients with heart failure, there is an enhancement in sympathetic activity and a reduction in parasympathetic activity [59]. This neurohormonal activation is thought to influence the substrate and triggers for ventricular arrhythmias in heart failure. Studies of ventricular biopsies and autopsy specimens have shown an increased density and exaggerated spatial heterogeneity of sympathetic nerves in patients with a prior history of ventricular arrhythmias in cardiomyopathies [60]. In the normal ventricle, sympathetic stimulation shortens the action potential duration and reduces the dispersion of repolarization, both associated with a decrease in arrhythmia potential [61]. However, in heart failure, sympathetic stimulation is a potent stimulus for the generation of arrhythmias perhaps by enhancing the dispersion of repolarization. Beta-adrenergic stimulation has significant effects on calcium handling in cardiac myocytes, which can alter the electrophysiological properties of myocardial tissue, as discussed earlier [46]. Elevated levels of sympathetic stimulation enhance the rate of spontaneous diastolic depolarization in latent ventricular pacemakers more than the sinus node, which can lead to the development of automatic arrhythmias. Increases in intrinsic heart rate in the setting of sympathetic stimulation can also increase the likelihood of the occurrence of triggered arrhythmias [2]. Furthermore, catecholamines can alter conduction and refractoriness, which may promote functional block and facilitate reentry.

RAAS signaling has numerous effects on the cardiovascular system that increase heart failure patients' propensity to develop ventricular arrhythmias. The two major effectors of the RAAS axis, angiotensin II and aldosterone, are upregulated in heart failure and have prominent effects on the properties of myocardial cells [46]. Angiotensin II can indirectly promote arrhythmia formation via potassium and magnesium loss in the urine resulting in prolongation of repolarization. It can also potentiate the effects of the sympathetic nervous system. Vasoconstriction caused by RAAS activation alters loading conditions, affecting wall stress and mechanical factors. Angiotensin II and aldosterone also promote generation of fibrosis in the myocardium by myofibroblasts [62]. Angiotensin II has also been shown to influence gap junction coupling in cardiac cells [63]. Abnormal phosphorylation of connexin 43, a protein important in cell-to-cell communication, may occur as a result of angiotensin II activation, leading to non-uniform anisotropy and promoting reentry. Angiotensin II can also inhibit a number of K^+ currents including the transient outward K^+ current (I_{to}) and delayed rectifier K^+ currents (I_{Kr}) in the myocardium [64–67]. By inhibiting these K+ currents, angiotensin II can prolong the duration of the action potential, which can increase the risk of arrhythmias.

Conduction System Disease and Bundle Branch Reentry

Bundle branch reentrant ventricular tachycardia (BBRVT) is a unique form of VT that can occur in patients with QRS prolongation due to underlying myocardial disease [68, 69]. BBRVT occurs when there is sustained reentry within the His-Purkinje system (HPS), which is normally protected from reentry by its rapid conduction and long refractory periods. In BBRVT, the conduction delay within one or both of the bundle branches can facilitate the development of reentry circuits [70]. Three circuits have been described in BBRVT. The first circuit involves anterograde conduction over the right bundle branch and retrograde conduction over the left bundle branch, with the His bundle located adjacent to but separate from the circuit. The second circuit utilizes the left bundle branch as the anterograde limb and the right bundle branch for retrograde conduction. In rare cases, intrafascicular reentry can also occur with the separate fascicles of the left bundle branch being used for the reentrant circuit [71]. Most patients that develop BBRVT tend to have advanced structural heart disease and QRS prolongation in the form of bundle branch block or non-specific conduction delay. Although most have a baseline bundle branch block, the QRS prolongation in these patients is generally due to delayed conduction in one or both of the bundle branches rather than true block as complete block would not allow propagation of wavefronts retrogradely, which is required to facilitate reentry. This delay tends to be a result of the severity of the underlying heart disease with cardiac enlargement and heart failure being common.

Ventricular Arrhythmias and Heart Failure Etiology

Ventricular arrhythmias have varying prognoses and are managed based on the underlying cardiomyopathy and clinical arrhythmia characteristics. Although certain types of cardiomyopathy may predispose patients to the development of certain types of arrhythmias, all mechanisms of arrhythmogenesis can exist in all forms of heart failure. For example, infarct-related cardiomyopathy often involves sustained monomorphic VT due to reentry, but patients may also have tachycardias from triggered activity from other sites. Arrhythmias may also arise from areas outside of classic sites in patients with certain cardiomyopathies. Similarly, certain cardiomyopathies may have a predisposition towards the development of arrhythmias originating in certain anatomic areas, such as the right ventricular inflow and outflow tracts in arrhythmogenic right ventricular cardiomyopathy. However, arrhythmias may originate from areas outside of these more classic sites in the same patients.

Infarct-Related Cardiomyopathy

Sustained monomorphic VT most frequently occurs after a healed myocardial infarction (MI), either in the subacute phase or long after the acute ischemic injury. The extent of myocardial necrosis, fibrosis, and left ventricular dysfunction are important factors influencing the risk of arrhythmias post-MI. The incidence of sustained VT after MI has declined from 3–5% to about 1% due to advances in revascularization strategies resulting in smaller infarct size as well as improved utilization of guideline-directed pharmacologic therapy. Although most VTs in infarct-related cardiomyopathy are caused by a reentrant mechanism, focal activation by abnormal automaticity or triggered activity from the ischemic border zone may serve to initiate the tachycardia, especially in the setting of ischemia. Reentry is the mechanism underlying VT associated with healed or healing MIs in more than 95% of cases [72].

The 12-lead ECG during VT can provide valuable information for localization of VT origin. In patients with prior MI, VT typically originates subendocardially in the region of myocardial scarring, resulting in qR or QR patterns in the QRS complexes overlying areas of infarction, reflecting terminal activation of the subepicardium. However, a QS pattern may occur in full-thickness MI, representing a cavity potential and not useful in localizing VT origin. In NICM, the absence of prior MI, and a QS pattern in the QRS complex may suggest an epicardial origin of VT [73] (Fig. 21.2).

Reentry, which is the most common mechanism of VT in the setting of prior MI, is believed to occur through surviving bundles of myocardium within the scarred tissue, which are separated by connective tissue, fibrosis, and disrupted intercellular coupling (Fig. 21.3) [74]. This hypothesis is supported by the observation that fixed areas of slow conduction can be mapped during sinus rhythm in patients with VT, and ablation at these sites has been shown to effectively eliminate VT. Furthermore, the triggers for initiating VT in the presence of MI are known to increase in certain situations, such as during acute heart failure decompensation, which can lead to surges in autonomic tone, electrolyte imbalances, and acute ischemia [72]. These factors may further promote the occurrence of reentry and contribute to the development of VT in patients with MI. Understanding the underlying mechanisms of VT in the presence of MI is crucial for effective management and treatment strategies for these patients.

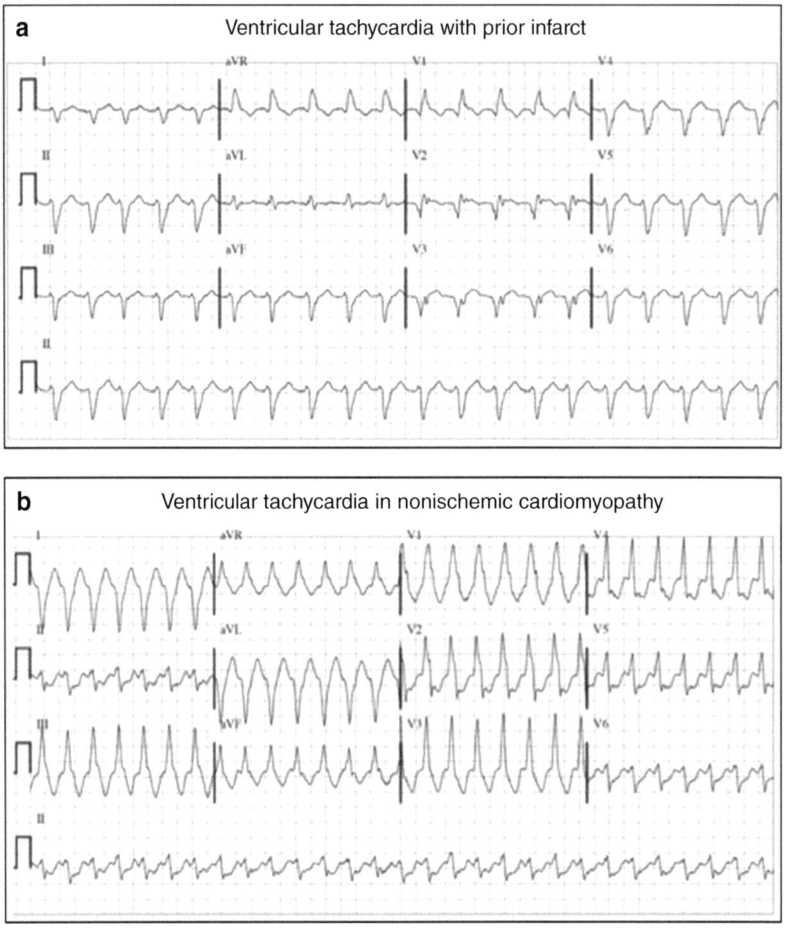

Fig. 21.2 The 12-lead ECG of VT in the presence and absence of prior myocardial infarction. Panel (**a**) is the ECG of a monomorphic VT in a patient with a prior anteroseptal MI. The QRS complexes in the anterior precordial leads demonstrate a qR pattern in a distribution consistent with the previous anteroseptal MI representing terminal activation of the subepicardium in this region. Panel (**b**) is the ECG of a monomorphic ventricular tachycardia in a patient with non-ischemic cardiomyopathy and no history of prior MI. None of the QRS complexes demonstrate a qR pattern consistent with the non-ischemic substrate. The QS pattern seen in the lateral leads suggests an epicardial origin of the VT given the absence of prior infarction

Dilated Cardiomyopathy

Dilated cardiomyopathy, a condition marked by ventricular dilation and reduced contraction in one or both ventricles, is associated with impaired systolic function and may or may not lead to overt heart failure. The presenting manifestations include ventricular arrhythmias, and sudden death can occur at any stage of the disease. The pathophysiologic basis for ventricular arrhythmias in dilated cardiomyopathies is not fully understood, although several possible mechanisms have been proposed [72]. Extensive myocardial abnormalities, fibrosis, and loss of cell-to-cell coupling in patients with dilated cardiomyopathy may create a substrate for reentry, whereby surviving bundles of myocardium within the scarred tissue may facilitate the occurrence of reentry due to the development of conduction block in lines parallel to the epicardial fiber orientation between the epicardium and endocardium [75]. In addition, increased levels of fibrosis in the endocardium and epicardium can lead to increased tissue anisotropy,

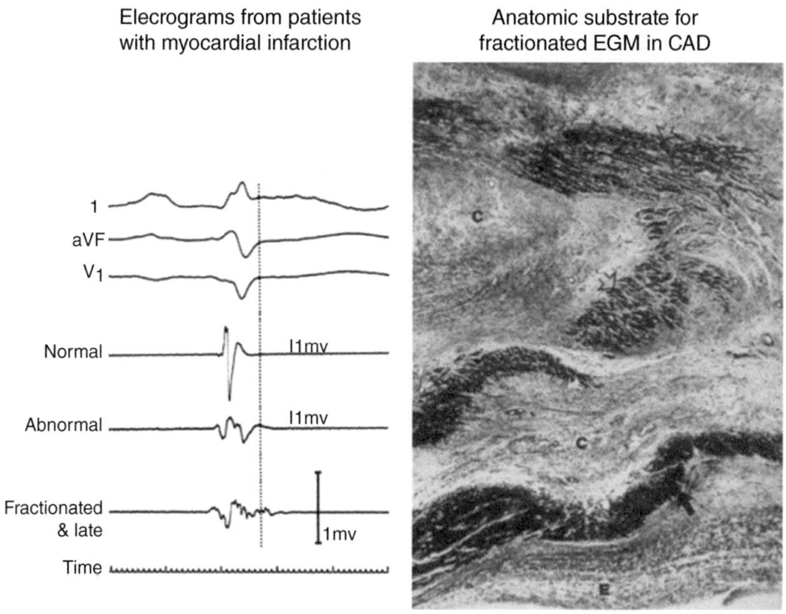

Fig. 21.3 The Anatomic substrate for fractionated electrograms in coronary artery disease (CAD). Most VT in the setting of prior myocardial infarction are sustained through a reentrant mechanism. Reentry is facilitated by slow conduction through surviving myocardial bundles trapped inside fibrotic myocardium. This slow conduction is detectable by low amplitude fractionated and late potentials with delayed activation represented above, *left*. Above *right*, fibrosis and scar from a prior myocardial infarction is pictured at the microscopic level. See text for discussion

particularly from epicardium to endocardium, which may further contribute to the development of ventricular arrhythmias [75]. Although the pathophysiology that causes this substrate is not well understood, it is especially prominent in sarcoidosis and some genetic cardiomyopathies (Lamin and Titin gene defects), in which ventricular arrhythmias are often prominent well before the onset of clinical heart failure.

Focal mechanisms may also play a role in the genesis of ventricular arrhythmias in dilated cardiomyopathy. Spontaneous and induced VT in patients with dilated cardiomyopathy have been found to arise in the subendocardium through triggered activity from early or delayed afterdepolarizations, without evidence of reentry [76].

Moreover, patients with dilated cardiomyopathy have been shown to have a non-homogeneous distribution of sympathetic fibers. Regions with dense fibrosis may show myocardial denervation, similar to what is seen in a scar due to myocardial infarction, while other regions may exhibit an increase in sympathetic innervation. It is postulated that denervation hypersensitivity could lead to a regional increase in sensitivity to catecholamines, which may contribute to the development of ventricular arrhythmias in dilated cardiomyopathy [77].

Furthermore, autoantibodies against beta-1 adrenergic receptors have been detected in up to 50% of patients with dilated cardiomyopathy, and some subgroups of these autoantibodies can exert sympathomimetic activity [78]. These autoantibodies have been associated with increased rates of ventricular arrhythmias in heart failure patients [78, 79].

Hypertrophic Cardiomyopathy

Hypertrophic cardiomyopathy (HCM) is a type of genetic cardiomyopathy characterized by abnormal hypertrophy, of the left ventricular muscle. It is estimated that HCM affects at least

1 in every 500 individuals [80]. There are multiple variations of HCM, which can manifest differently depending on the location and extent of hypertrophy. These patients have an increased likelihood of developing ventricular arrhythmias [80]. The annual incidence of SCD in adult patients with HCM is approximately 1%, but it is notably higher in pediatric patients with HCM. In patients with HCM, the hemodynamic consequences of myocardial hypertrophy can result in various complications, such as left ventricular outflow tract obstruction, mitral regurgitation, diastolic dysfunction, and myocardial ischemia. Similar to all other etiologies of heart failure, it is thought that myocardial fibrosis, potentially related to micro-ischemic changes, plays an important role in the arrhythmogenic substrate of HCM [81]. Late gadolinium enhancement (LGE) on cardiovascular magnetic resonance (CMR) imaging is a common finding in HCM patients, likely reflecting collagen deposition and fibrosis [82–84]. The extent of LGE in HCM patients has been correlated with SCD risk factors [85] as well as the frequency of ventricular premature depolarizations (VPDs) and NSVT on ambulatory monitoring [85]. Although sustained monomorphic VT may occur in the presence of HCM, similar to dilated cardiomyopathies, these patients more commonly have cardiac arrest due to polymorphic VT or VF [72]. The most recent guidelines have advised that if a patient with HCM does not have evidence of increased SCD risk after assessment with family/personal history, echocardiography, and ambulatory monitoring, cardiac MRI with extensive LGE, which is defined as ≥15% of LV mass, can aid decision making regarding potential ICD implantation [86].

Arrhythmogenic Cardiomyopathy

Arrhythmogenic cardiomyopathy is characterized by fibrous or fibro-fatty replacement of either the right or left ventricular myocardium or a combination of both. Arrhythmogenic Right Ventricular Cardiomyopathy (ARVC) is the most common form of this disease. The right ventricular myocardial scarring initially produces regional wall motion abnormalities but as the disease progresses, it may involve the free wall and become global with right ventricular dilatation [87, 88]. These areas of scarring tend to be the focus of ventricular arrhythmias in patients with ARVC who often present with sustained or non-sustained monomorphic VT originating in the right ventricle. VTs originate from areas where scarring develops, most commonly the inflow tract, apex, or outflow tract of the right ventricle. As in the case of dilated cardiomyopathy, the fibrosis and scarring in this setting tend to be more pronounced in the epicardium than the endocardium. For individuals with advanced fibrosis, VT tends to be due to macroreentry in areas of epicardial scar. However, in patients with earlier stages of disease, VT may be due to triggered or automatic activity in the diseased myocardium, often related to adrenergic stimulation. In such instances, VT and SCD are often exercise-induced [89]. Exercise is thought to increase the risk of sudden death in ARVC patients, potentially due to catecholamine effects on triggered or automatic activity or due to the increased stress placed on the right ventricle during exercise [90, 91]. Animal models of ARVC have suggested that exercise increases right ventricular dilatation and worsens manifestations of the disease [90]. In regard to the relationship of catecholamines and VT in patients with ARVC, a higher frequency of induced ventricular arrhythmias in patients with ARVC on isoproterenol infusion has been reported when compared to control patients [92]. The onset of VT has also been shown to be associated with gradual rises in sinus rates and shortening of coupling intervals prior to initiation suggesting an increase in sympathetic tone may play a role in initiation [93].

Ventricular Arrhythmias and Risk of Sudden Death

Ventricular arrhythmias in heart failure patients may range from VPDs to VF leading to SCD. VPDs occur in 70–95% of patients with heart failure [94–96]. The significance of these beats varies according to the etiology of the cardiomyopathy. VPDs in a patient with prior MI are associated with an increased risk of death. However, in patients with non-infarct-related cardiomyopathy, VPDs have not been uniformly shown to be associated with a worse prognosis [97]. The use of AADs to suppress VPDs has been shown to be harmful regardless of the etiology of heart failure due to their proarrhythmic effects [98, 99]. On the other hand, beta-blockers can often suppress VPDs and are indicated for most forms of heart failure regardless of the presence or absence of arrhythmias. In rare cases, very frequent VPDs may cause or worsen left ventricular dysfunction or patients may be highly symptomatic despite beta blockade. In such circumstances, treatment with AADs and catheter ablation is often necessary and can improve left ventricular function [100, 101]. When AADs are necessary, amiodarone has been shown to be safe in heart failure patients but it is not used for the routine suppression of ventricular arrhythmias as it has not been shown to provide any survival benefit [102, 103].

NSVT has been reported in 50–80% of heart failure patients on ambulatory monitoring [95, 104, 105]. The significance of NSVT in heart failure is similar to that of VPDs. In patients with infarct-related cardiomyopathy [106] and hypertrophic cardiomyopathy [107–109], NSVT has been associated with increased mortality. However, this has not been reliably shown in other forms of heart failure such as dilated cardiomyopathy [95, 105, 110] and heart failure related to valvular disease [111]. As is the case with VPDs, there is no clear role for pharmacologic suppression of NSVT to reduce the risk of SCD, but NSVT can be an indication for electrophysiology study in order to better risk stratify heart failure patients with the hopes of determining who may benefit from implantable cardioverter-defibrillator (ICD) therapy [112, 113] . Like VPDs, in rare cases, very frequent NSVT can contribute to or exacerbate left ventricular dysfunction and may require more aggressive therapies such as AADs or catheter ablation.

Sustained VT is far less frequent than VPDs and NSVT in heart failure patients. Several studies have reported an incidence of sustained VT in patients with heart failure or cardiomyopathy of 5% or less [95, 104, 105]. However, VT and VF cause the majority of sudden deaths in heart failure patients. It is notable that all types of ventricular arrhythmias, including VPDs, NSVT, and sustained VT have been associated with increased mortality for most groups of heart failure patients. Despite the increased mortality associated with ventricular arrhythmias in heart failure, the rates of sudden cardiac death are not increased. Even as total mortality rises, the percentage of patients dying suddenly remains the same across groups. Approximately half of all deaths in heart failure patients are sudden, regardless of the amount of ventricular ectopy. For any given patient, the greater the severity of the heart failure, the more likely they are to die suddenly, irrespective to their history of ventricular arrhythmias [1].

Effect of Heart Failure Medications

Multiple classes of medications have been shown to improve mortality in heart failure patients due to systolic dysfunction. Standard therapy includes beta-blockers, ACE inhibitors, angiotensin receptor blockers (ARBs), aldosterone antagonists, Angiotensin Receptor-Neprilysin Inhibitor (ARNi) and most recently Sodium-Glucose Transport Protein 2 (SGLT-2) inhibitors. Beta-blockers have been shown in multiple trials to impart a survival benefit to heart failure patients, mainly due to a significant reduction in SCD [56, 57, 114]. As previously discussed, heart failure is associated with enhancement of sympathetic activity and a reduction in parasympathetic activity [59, 115]. An increase in sinus rates in heart failure patients may be associated with an increased risk of sudden death, most likely due to an excess of sympathetic activity [25]. This may be because rapid rates increase the likelihood of triggered arrhythmias [2]. Although heart rate reduction has been associated with a survival benefit in heart failure patients, for any given reduction in heart rate and any baseline heart rate, beta blockade has been shown to further improve survival compared to placebo. This suggests that heart rate reduction is not the only mechanism responsible for the beneficial effects of beta blocker therapy [56].

Ace inhibitors and ARBs have been shown to improve all-cause mortality in heart failure. However, their effects on SCD are less clear. Several major trials found that the survival benefit was primarily due to slowed progression of heart failure with little or no reduction in sudden death [55, 116, 117]. However, other large trials have found ACE inhibitors and ARBs to be associated with significant reductions in sudden death [118–120]. Less controversial is the effect of aldosterone antagonists on sudden death. Both spironolactone and eplerenone have been shown to significantly reduce overall mortality and sudden death in patients with advanced heart failure [54, 121]. Spironolactone has also been shown to reduce the frequency of VPDs and NSVT [122]. The mechanisms by which modulation of the RAAS axis might decrease the risk of sudden death is not well understood. However, possible effects may include reverse remodeling of the arrhythmogenic substrate, decreased proliferation of fibrosis, and fewer effects of angiotensin II and aldosterone on active membrane properties [25]. ACE inhibitors and ARBs have been shown to prevent myocyte uncoupling and improve gap junction conductance through modulation of connexin 43 which may decrease the likelihood of sustained reentrant arrhythmias [50, 123] . Ace inhibitors, ARBs, and aldosterone antagonists may also decrease the risk of ventricular arrhythmias through maintenance of a higher serum potassium concentration and decreased prolongation of action potential duration.

ARNi have been shown to improve outcomes in heart failure. Sacubatril/valsartan has been shown in meta-analyses to lower the frequency of VT compared to those treated with ACEi alone [124, 125]. Although the precise mechanism by which sacubatril/valsartan decreases the rate of VT is not completely understood, it is believed to be related to the drug's ability to alleviate the pressure on the heart and enhance its overall function.

SGLT2 inhibitors are the newest heart failure therapy and have been shown to improve heart failure outcomes. Dapagliflozin has been shown to reduce the risk of ventricular arrhythmia, or sudden death when added to conventional therapy in patients with HFrEF [126].

Therapies for Ventricular Arrhythmias

Patients with heart failure are at increased risk of developing ventricular arrhythmias that can lead to sudden cardiac death (SCD). Although antiarrhythmic medications and implantable cardioverter-defibrillators (ICD) can prevent or abort SCD in some patients, these interventions carry risks that need to be carefully considered. Antiarrhythmic drugs have been shown to have significant and often fatal proarrhythmic effects in multiple randomized controlled trials [98, 99]. Similarly, ICDs have potential complications such as infections, inappropriate discharges, and device malfunction. Furthermore, while heart failure patients represent a high-risk group for SCD, only a minority of patients actually develop fatal ventricular arrhythmias. Therefore, it is crucial to improve our ability to identify high-risk patients who would benefit from these interventions. Developing better risk stratification tools and biomarkers for SCD is an important area of ongoing research.

Catheter ablation is increasingly used to treat patients with VT that is refractory to medical therapy. Although catheter ablation techniques have advanced, the procedure still poses a significant risk of complications. It is essential to balance the benefits and risks of these interventions and make informed decisions about their use.

Antiarrhythmic Drug Therapy

The role of AADs for ventricular arrhythmias in patients with heart failure is limited. The use of AADs for suppression of ventricular arrhythmias fell out of favor after the CAST trial demonstrated that AADs had significant, often proarrhythmic effects [99]. This was later confirmed in large randomized trials, suggesting AADs might harm more patients than they benefit. Beyond their proarrhythmic effects, most antiarrhythmic drugs also have some negative inotropic activity, which can produce heart failure in patients with ventricular dysfunction [127].

Low cardiac output and the associated renal dysfunction that is common in heart failure can impair the elimination of these drugs, increasing the risk of drug toxicity. Some of the AADs, particularly the class I and class III agents exert a strong proarrhythmic effect. Heart failure is a risk factor for the development of torsades de pointes in patients receiving the class III agents ibutilide, sotalol, and dofetilide. Amiodarone is considered less proarrhythmic than other AADs and is often the preferred drug for the treatment of ventricular arrhythmias in heart failure. Some studies suggest that amiodarone may reduce SCD in patients with left ventricular dysfunction caused by previous MI or NICM. However, SCD-HeFT study did not show any survival benefit of amiodarone compared to placebo. A secondary analysis of SCD-HeFT revealed increased mortality risk with amiodarone in patients with NYHA class III symptoms [113, 128–130]. Long-term use of amiodarone can lead to complex drug interactions and a range of adverse effects involving the lungs, liver, thyroid, skin, and nervous system. Generally, higher doses and longer durations of amiodarone therapy increase the risk of adverse effects, often necessitating the discontinuation of the medication. Therefore, in younger patients, chronic amiodarone treatment should be reserved as a temporary measure until more definitive treatment options such as catheter ablation can be pursued.

Catheter Ablation

Radiofrequency ablation (RFA) has emerged as an effective treatment for VT. For patients with ischemic cardiomyopathy catheter ablation has been demonstrated to be highly effective in reducing the incidence of ICD shocks and VT. For patients with NICM, catheter ablation can be more challenging due to the diffuse nature of myocardial disease and the presence of multiple reentrant circuits on both the endocardium and epicardium [131]. However, recent studies have demonstrated the safety and efficacy of catheter ablation in these patients. RFA can be used in conjunction with an ICD to reduce the frequency of subsequent ICD therapies in patients with frequent arrhythmias and shocks. Additionally, catheter ablation can be used as an alternative treatment strategy in patients who do not want an ICD or who are not considered candidates for ICD implantation.

The choice of treatment approach depends on the specific patient and the underlying cardiac condition. Catheter ablation has also been shown to be effective at reducing the incidence of ICD shocks prophylactically in patients with a history of MI who received ICDs for secondary prevention of sudden death [132]. The VANISH and SURVIVE-VT trials both examined ICD patients with ischemic cardiomyopathy and VT. When compared to escalating antiarrhythmic therapy, catheter ablation demonstrated a significantly lower rate of the composite primary outcome of death, VT storm, or appropriate ICD shocks [133, 134].

The timing of VT ablation, again, depends on the specific patient and the etiology of the VT. Two recent studies that investigated the safety and efficacy of first-line catheter ablation of VT in ICD patients with cardiomyopathy, and both found that early catheter ablation significantly reduced the incidence of the composite outcome of appropriate ICD therapy, death, and hospitalization for heart failure compared to conventional medical therapy [132, 135].

The role of catheter ablation in non-ischemic cardiomyopathies has not been as well informed by prospective clinical trials. Contemporary observational trials suggest the following: 1. The effectiveness of VT ablation varies considerably by disease entity [136], 2. Patients with inferobasal substrate, which is typically more epicardial and endocardial respond to ablation better than patients with mid-septal substrate [137] and 3. Patients with advanced NICM have a poor prognosis despite VT ablation [138].

For patients with bundle branch reentrant VT (BBRVT), RFA is front line therapy where catheter ablation of the right bundle branch can eliminate the arrhythmia. The 2017 ACC/AHA/ESC guidelines recommend patients with BBRVT undergo electrophysiology study and ablation [138].

Cardiac Stereotactic Body Radiotherapy

Since its first use in 2015, stereotactic body radiotherapy (SBRT) has grown in popularity as a strategy for patients with VT refractory to medical therapy and catheter ablation or patients who would not tolerate an invasive procedure [139]. In particular cases, the arrhythmogenic substrate may not be amenable to catheter ablation due to inaccessibility or an inability to deliver transmural RF lesions. SBRT involves delivering a radiation dose to a specific area of myocardium leading to tissue destruction. The steps involved in SBRT include identifying the arrhythmogenic scar using cardiac MRI, CT, PET or echocardiography. Electroanatomic maps or electrocardiographic imaging are then fused with this imaging and the scar is delineated. The treatment is done in a single or a few sessions and can be completed on an outpatient basis.

The ENCORE-VT trial examined 19 patients with treatment resistant VT and PVC induced cardiomyopathy. SBRT lead to a significant reduction in ICD shocks and VT episodes along with an improvement in quality of life [140]. Despite this and numerous other studies that have demonstrated SBRTs effectiveness in the short term, longer-term data is still lacking [139–141]. Protocols for planning and radiation delivery differ from center to center, thus, significant collaboration between EP centers is required in order to form standardized protocols. More research is needed to fully understand the long-term effectiveness and safety of SBRT but it has shown promise as a non-invasive alternative to traditional treatments.

Surgical Treatment

Surgical ablative therapy guided by mapping is an effective treatment for VT in patients with prior MI and scar-related reentrant VT, although it is not as useful for patients with diffuse NICM [142, 143]. Although it was more common before the introduction of catheter ablation and ICD therapy, VT surgery is now relatively uncommon. However, appropriately selected patients in experienced centers achieved over 90% freedom from recurrent clinical VT with more than half not requiring adjuvant antiarrhythmic therapy [144].

Implantable Cardioverter Defibrillators

Implantable cardioverter-defibrillator (ICD) therapy has proven effective in preventing sudden arrhythmic death for patients with cardiomyopathy and heart failure. Implanting an ICD is crucial for stopping life-threatening VT and VF from recurring. Current guidelines recommend considering a secondary prevention ICD implantation when there is no reversible cause identified and when it aligns with the patient's preferences.

Regarding primary prevention ICDs, various trials focused on preventing sudden death have demonstrated that ICDs can effectively reduce the risk in patients with a reduced left ventricular ejection fraction. Notably, the MADIT II and SCD-HeFT trials established ICD implantation as the standard of care by showing a 5–7% decrease in mortality compared to the control group [145, 146].

Recent evidence from two large prospective registries, involving over 5000 patients, further supports the reported mortality reduction. Specifically, the EU-CERT-ICD trial found a significant 27% decrease in mortality associated with primary prevention ICD implantation [147]. These results were consistent for patients with both coronary artery disease and NICM. However, the DANISH trial provided insights suggesting that the mortality benefit of ICD implantation may be less apparent in patients with NICM who are already receiving contemporary medical therapies [148].

Risk stratification of NICM patients for ICD placement remains challenging, as those with NICM and reduced left ventricular ejection fraction have varying risks for sudden cardiac death (SCD). However, relying solely on left ventricular ejection fraction as a predictor of clinical events has limitations in terms of sensitivity and specificity. Despite these limitations, the current guidelines still primarily rely on left ventricular ejection fraction to determine eligibility for an ICD [149]. The NICM-SCAR study demonstrated that both myocardial scar on cardiac MRI and left ventricular ejection fraction are risk markers for all-cause death, but only myocardial scar had additional prognostic value in assessing the risk of sudden cardiac death [150].

Although left ventricular ejection fraction is a better predictor of SCD in patients with ischemic cardiomyopathy than non-ischemic, more than 70% of sudden deaths in coronary artery disease occur in individuals with left ventricular ejection fraction greater than 35%, who do not qualify for an ICD according to the most recent guidelines [151, 152].

When evaluating a patient for ICD therapy, it is crucial to consider their life expectancy, quality of life, and comorbidities. Patients with end-stage renal disease, diabetes, and elderly individuals may derive less benefit or no benefit at all from primary prevention ICDs. Balancing the risk of sudden cardiac death with non-arrhythmic death is important. Shared decision-making plays a vital role, involving patients in discussions about ICD implantation, generator replacement, and end-of-life care. Effective communication and understanding of the benefits, risks, and consequences are essential. While clinical prediction scores provide additional information, they should not be the sole basis for decision-making.

It is important to note that ICD implantation is not without risks. Potential complications include infection, inappropriate shocks, the potential for proarrhythmia, device malfunctions, and procedural complications [152]. While there are certain patients who may potentially benefit from ICD implantation to prevent ventricular arrhythmias and sudden death, applying simplified guidelines to a complex patient population poses risks to patients without guaranteed benefits. An individualized approach to these patients is crucial.

Left Ventricular Assist Devices and Cardiac Transplantation

Sustained VT in patients with advanced heart failure can be a potentially life-threatening arrhythmia, especially when associated with hemodynamic embarrassment. This becomes of particular concern when such patients are refractory to antiarrhythmic drugs and hemodynamic stability limits the safety of catheter or surgical ablation strategies. Percutaneous circulatory assist devices are now being used to provide hemodynamic support during VT ablation allowing for entrainment mapping of sustained VT as well as prolonged substrate mapping and ablation [153, 154]. Unfortunately, durable cure of sustained recurrent VT with catheter ablation in the setting of advanced heart failure can be difficult to achieve. For patients with a high burden of ventricular arrhythmias, ventricular assist devices (VADs) can provide circulatory support to the failing ventricle even if a patient is in VT for a substantial amount of time. Surgical implantation of a VAD has been used to hemodynamically stabilize patients with VT storm and advanced cardiomyopathy [155]. Such an intervention may prevent further episodes of VT by unloading the left ventricle and can also provide a bridge to cardiac transplantation [156]. Empiric or electrophysiologically-guided surgical ablation can be performed during LVAD implantation [157]. If VT does recur after VAD implant, the device will provide hemodynamic support for potential mapping and successful ablation has been reported in VAD patients [158, 159].

Autonomic Nervous System Modulation

Heart failure is characterized by sympathetic hyperactivity, which increases the risk for ventricular arrhythmias. This makes autonomic modulation a promising treatment option. Autonomic modulation utilizes the ability of neural tissue to remodel itself for therapeutic benefits. Examples of autonomic modulation methods include vagus nerve stimulation, tragus stimulation, renal denervation, baroreceptor activation therapy, and cardiac sympathetic denervation.

Left cardiac sympathetic denervation (LCSD) is a well-established treatment for patients with refractory ventricular arrhythmias in long QT syndrome and arrhythmogenic channelopathies and has recently been shown to be effective in patients with cardiomyopathy [160–162]. The procedure involves resection of the lower half of the left stellate ganglion and thoracic ganglia 2–4, which diminishes noradrenergic input to the left ventricular myocardium. The result is an adequate denervation without a significant Horner's syndrome since most sympathetic innervation to the eye arises from the upper ganglion. Early studies have also shown that LCSD may have beneficial effects in heart failure patients irrespective of its effects on ventricular arrhythmias [163]. Percutaneous stellate ganglia and thoracic sympathetic blocks or ablation have also been utilized for refractory VT and have the benefit of being less invasive [164–166].

Transcutaneous magnetic stimulation of the left stellate ganglia has been shown in a small study to reduce the burden of VT in patients with VT storm but larger trials are required to confirm its effectiveness [167, 168].

Vagal nerve stimulation has also been shown to provide a protective effect against ventricular arrhythmias and preclinical studies have suggested that VNS will be effective at improving heart failure as well [169, 170]. Multiple studies have demonstrated a reduced incidence of ventricular arrhythmias with VNS in animals with cardiomyopathy and heart failure [171]. While early human trials suggested that VNS might improve quality of life and left ventricular function, two larger randomized trials, NECTAR-HF and INOVATE-HF failed to show a significant benefit in heart failure hospitalizations or mortality [172–174].

Conclusion

Understanding the mechanisms of arrhythmogenesis and the pathophysiologic changes in heart failure that predispose patients to ventricular tachycardia is important in the overall management of these complex cardiovascular patients. Through advances in medical knowledge and technologies, treatment strategies continue to target the underlying arrhythmia substrate and the pathologic changes of the heart failure syndrome, which will remain the cornerstone of VT treatment in cardiomyopathy.

References

1. Janse MJ. Electrophysiological changes in heart failure and their relationship to arrhythmogenesis. Cardiovasc Res. 2004;61(2):208–17.
2. Wit AL. Cellular electrophysiologic mechanisms of cardiac arrhythmias. Cardiol Clin. 1990;8(3):393–409.
3. Mangoni ME, Nargeot J. Genesis and regulation of the heart automaticity. Physiol Rev. 2008;88(3):919–82.
4. Luo CH, Rudy Y. A dynamic model of the cardiac ventricular action potential. II. Afterdepolarizations, triggered activity, and potentiation. Circ Res. 1994;74(6):1097–113.
5. Szabo B, Sweidan R, Rajagopalan CV, Lazzara R. Role of Na+:Ca2+ exchange current in Cs(+)-induced early afterdepolarizations in Purkinje fibers. J Cardiovasc Electrophysiol. 1994;5(11):933–44.
6. Kannankeril PJ, Roden DM. Drug-induced long QT and torsade de pointes: recent advances. Curr Opin Cardiol. 2007;22(1):39–43.
7. Kléber AG, Rudy Y. Basic mechanisms of cardiac impulse propagation and associated arrhythmias. Physiol Rev. 2004;84(2):431–88.
8. Severs NJ, Bruce AF, Dupont E, Rothery S. Remodelling of gap junctions and connexin expression in diseased myocardium. Cardiovasc Res. 2008;80(1):9–19.
9. Söhl G, Willecke K. Gap junctions and the connexin protein family. Cardiovasc Res. 2004;62(2):228–32.
10. Roberts DE, Hersh LT, Scher AM. Influence of cardiac fiber orientation on wavefront voltage,

conduction velocity, and tissue resistivity in the dog. Circ Res. 1979;44(5):701–12.
11. Saffitz JE, Davis LM, Darrow BJ, Kanter HL, Laing JG, Beyer EC. The molecular basis of anisotropy: role of gap junctions. J Cardiovasc Electrophysiol. 1995;6(6):498–510.
12. Fontes MS, van Veen TA, de Bakker JM, van Rijen HV. Functional consequences of abnormal Cx43 expression in the heart. Biochim Biophys Acta. 2012;1818(8):2020–9.
13. Spach MS, Dolber PC. Relating extracellular potentials and their derivatives to anisotropic propagation at a microscopic level in human cardiac muscle. Evidence for electrical uncoupling of side-to-side fiber connections with increasing age. Circ Res. 1986;58(3):356–71.
14. Luke RA, Saffitz JE. Remodeling of ventricular conduction pathways in healed canine infarct border zones. J Clin Invest. 1991;87(5):1594–602.
15. Smith JH, Green CR, Peters NS, Rothery S, Severs NJ. Altered patterns of gap junction distribution in ischemic heart disease. An immunohistochemical study of human myocardium using laser scanning confocal microscopy. Am J Pathol. 1991;139(4):801–21.
16. de Bakker JM, Wittkampf FH. The pathophysiologic basis of fractionated and complex electrograms and the impact of recording techniques on their detection and interpretation. Circ Arrhythm Electrophysiol. 2010;3(2):204–13.
17. Gardner PI, Ursell PC, Fenoglio JJ Jr, Wit AL. Electrophysiologic and anatomic basis for fractionated electrograms recorded from healed myocardial infarcts. Circulation. 1985;72(3):596–611.
18. Miller JM, Vassallo JA, Kussmaul WG 3rd, Cassidy DM, Hargrove WC 3rd, Josephson ME. Anterior left ventricular aneurysm: factors associated with the development of sustained ventricular tachycardia. J Am Coll Cardiol. 1988;12(2):375–82.
19. Cassidy DM, Vassallo JA, Buxton AE, Doherty JU, Marchlinski FE, Josephson ME. The value of catheter mapping during sinus rhythm to localize site of origin of ventricular tachycardia. Circulation. 1984;69(6):1103–10.
20. Rubart M, Zipes DP. Mechanisms of sudden cardiac death. J Clin Invest. 2005;115(9):2305–15.
21. Benito B, Josephson ME. Ventricular tachycardia in coronary artery disease. Rev Esp Cardiol (Engl Ed). 2012;65(10):939–55.
22. Carmeliet E. Cardiac ionic currents and acute ischemia: from channels to arrhythmias. Physiol Rev. 1999;79(3):917–1017.
23. Coronel R, Wilms-Schopman FJ, Dekker LR, Janse MJ. Heterogeneities in [K+]o and TQ potential and the inducibility of ventricular fibrillation during acute regional ischemia in the isolated perfused porcine heart. Circulation. 1995;92(1):120–9.
24. Arnar DO, Bullinga JR, Martins JB. Role of the Purkinje system in spontaneous ventricular tachycardia during acute ischemia in a canine model. Circulation. 1997;96(7):2421–9.
25. Tomaselli GF, Marbán E. Electrophysiological remodeling in hypertrophy and heart failure. Cardiovasc Res. 1999;42(2):270–83.
26. Beuckelmann DJ, Näbauer M, Erdmann E. Alterations of K+ currents in isolated human ventricular myocytes from patients with terminal heart failure. Circ Res. 1993;73(2):379–85.
27. Näbauer M, Beuckelmann DJ, Erdmann E. Characteristics of transient outward current in human ventricular myocytes from patients with terminal heart failure. Circ Res. 1993;73(2):386–94.
28. Wettwer E, Amos GJ, Posival H, Ravens U. Transient outward current in human ventricular myocytes of subepicardial and subendocardial origin. Circ Res. 1994;75(3):473–82.
29. Kääb S, Nuss HB, Chiamvimonvat N, O'Rourke B, Pak PH, Kass DA, et al. Ionic mechanism of action potential prolongation in ventricular myocytes from dogs with pacing-induced heart failure. Circ Res. 1996;78(2):262–73.
30. Tsuji Y, Opthof T, Kamiya K, Yasui K, Liu W, Lu Z, et al. Pacing-induced heart failure causes a reduction of delayed rectifier potassium currents along with decreases in calcium and transient outward currents in rabbit ventricle. Cardiovasc Res. 2000;48(2):300–9.
31. Li GR, Lau CP, Ducharme A, Tardif JC, Nattel S. Transmural action potential and ionic current remodeling in ventricles of failing canine hearts. Am J Physiol Heart Circ Physiol. 2002;283(3):H1031–41.
32. Koumi S, Backer CL, Arentzen CE. Characterization of inwardly rectifying K+ channel in human cardiac myocytes. Alterations in channel behavior in myocytes isolated from patients with idiopathic dilated cardiomyopathy. Circulation. 1995;92(2):164–74.
33. Furukawa T, Bassett AL, Furukawa N, Kimura S, Myerburg RJ. The ionic mechanism of reperfusion-induced early afterdepolarizations in feline left ventricular hypertrophy. J Clin Invest. 1993;91(4):1521–31.
34. Maltsev VA, Sabbah HN, Higgins RS, Silverman N, Lesch M, Undrovinas AI. Novel, ultraslow inactivating sodium current in human ventricular cardiomyocytes. Circulation. 1998;98(23):2545–52.
35. Beuckelmann DJ, Näbauer M, Erdmann E. Intracellular calcium handling in isolated ventricular myocytes from patients with terminal heart failure. Circulation. 1992;85(3):1046–55.
36. Sipido KR, Volders PG, Vos MA, Verdonck F. Altered Na/ca exchange activity in cardiac hypertrophy and heart failure: a new target for therapy? Cardiovasc Res. 2002;53(4):782–805.
37. Mercadier JJ, Lompré AM, Duc P, Boheler KR, Fraysse JB, Wisnewsky C, et al. Altered sarcoplasmic reticulum Ca2(+)-ATPase gene expression in the human ventricle during end-stage heart failure. J Clin Invest. 1990;85(1):305–9.

38. Arai M, Alpert NR, MacLennan DH, Barton P, Periasamy M. Alterations in sarcoplasmic reticulum gene expression in human heart failure. A possible mechanism for alterations in systolic and diastolic properties of the failing myocardium. Circ Res. 1993;72(2):463–9.
39. O'Rourke B, Kass DA, Tomaselli GF, Kääb S, Tunin R, Marbán E. Mechanisms of altered excitation-contraction coupling in canine tachycardia-induced heart failure, I: experimental studies. Circ Res. 1999;84(5):562–70.
40. Marx SO, Reiken S, Hisamatsu Y, Jayaraman T, Burkhoff D, Rosemblit N, et al. PKA phosphorylation dissociates FKBP12.6 from the calcium release channel (ryanodine receptor): defective regulation in failing hearts. Cell. 2000;101(4):365–76.
41. Yano M, Ono K, Ohkusa T, Suetsugu M, Kohno M, Hisaoka T, et al. Altered stoichiometry of FKBP12.6 versus ryanodine receptor as a cause of abnormal ca(2+) leak through ryanodine receptor in heart failure. Circulation. 2000;102(17):2131–6.
42. Baartscheer A, Schumacher CA, Belterman CN, Coronel R, Fiolet JW. SR calcium handling and calcium after-transients in a rabbit model of heart failure. Cardiovasc Res. 2003;58(1):99–108.
43. Vermeulen JT, MA MG, Opthof T, Coronel R, de Bakker JM, Klöpping C, et al. Triggered activity and automaticity in ventricular trabeculae of failing human and rabbit hearts. Cardiovasc Res. 1994;28(10):1547–54.
44. Pogwizd SM, Sipido KR, Verdonck F, Bers DM. Intracellular Na in animal models of hypertrophy and heart failure: contractile function and arrhythmogenesis. Cardiovasc Res. 2003;57(4):887–96.
45. Han W, Chartier D, Li D, Nattel S. Ionic remodeling of cardiac Purkinje cells by congestive heart failure. Circulation. 2001;104(17):2095–100.
46. Tomaselli GF, Zipes DP. What causes sudden death in heart failure? Circ Res. 2004;95(8):754–63.
47. Dean JW, Lab MJ. Arrhythmia in heart failure: role of mechanically induced changes in electrophysiology. Lancet. 1989;1(8650):1309–12.
48. White CW, Mirro MJ, Lund DD, Skorton DJ, Pandian NG, Kerber RE. Alterations in ventricular excitability in conscious dogs during development of chronic heart failure. Am J Phys. 1986;250(6 Pt 2):H1022–9.
49. Reiter MJ, Landers M, Zetelaki Z, Kirchhof CJ, Allessie MA. Electrophysiological effects of acute dilatation in the isolated rabbit heart: cycle length-dependent effects on ventricular refractoriness and conduction velocity. Circulation. 1997;96(11):4050–6.
50. Hussain W, Patel PM, Chowdhury RA, Cabo C, Ciaccio EJ, Lab MJ, et al. The renin-angiotensin system mediates the effects of stretch on conduction velocity, connexin43 expression, and redistribution in intact ventricle. J Cardiovasc Electrophysiol. 2010;21(11):1276–83.
51. Xydas S, Rosen RS, Ng C, Mercando M, Cohen J, DiTullio M, et al. Mechanical unloading leads to echocardiographic, electrocardiographic, neurohormonal, and histologic recovery. J Heart Lung Transplant. 2006;25(1):7–15.
52. Koilpillai C, Quiñones MA, Greenberg B, Limacher MC, Shindler D, Pratt CM, et al. Relation of ventricular size and function to heart failure status and ventricular dysrhythmia in patients with severe left ventricular dysfunction. Am J Cardiol. 1996;77(8):606–11.
53. Yusuf S, Sleight P, Pogue J, Bosch J, Davies R, Dagenais G. Effects of an angiotensin-converting-enzyme inhibitor, ramipril, on cardiovascular events in high-risk patients. N Engl J Med. 2000;342(3):145–53.
54. Pitt B, Zannad F, Remme WJ, Cody R, Castaigne A, Perez A, et al. The effect of spironolactone on morbidity and mortality in patients with severe heart failure. Randomized Aldactone evaluation study investigators. N Engl J Med. 1999;341(10):709–17.
55. Yusuf S, Pitt B, Davis CE, Hood WB, Cohn JN. Effect of enalapril on survival in patients with reduced left ventricular ejection fractions and congestive heart failure. N Engl J Med. 1991;325(5):293–302.
56. The Cardiac Insufficiency Bisoprolol Study II (CIBIS-II): a randomised trial. Lancet. 1999;353(9146):9–13.
57. Effect of metoprolol CR/XL in chronic heart failure: Metoprolol CR/XL Randomised Intervention Trial in Congestive Heart Failure (MERIT-HF). Lancet. 1999;353(9169):2001–7.
58. Køber L, Torp-Pedersen C, Carlsen JE, Bagger H, Eliasen P, Lyngborg K, et al. A clinical trial of the angiotensin-converting-enzyme inhibitor trandolapril in patients with left ventricular dysfunction after myocardial infarction. Trandolapril Cardiac Evaluation (TRACE) Study Group. N Engl J Med. 1995;333(25):1670–6.
59. Binkley PF, Nunziata E, Haas GJ, Nelson SD, Cody RJ. Parasympathetic withdrawal is an integral component of autonomic imbalance in congestive heart failure: demonstration in human subjects and verification in a paced canine model of ventricular failure. J Am Coll Cardiol. 1991;18(2):464–72.
60. Cao JM, Fishbein MC, Han JB, Lai WW, Lai AC, Wu TJ, et al. Relationship between regional cardiac hyperinnervation and ventricular arrhythmia. Circulation. 2000;101(16):1960–9.
61. Takei M, Sasaki Y, Yonezawa T, Lakhe M, Aruga M, Kiyosawa K. The autonomic control of the transmural dispersion of ventricular repolarization in anesthetized dogs. J Cardiovasc Electrophysiol. 1999;10(7):981–9.
62. Kim S, Iwao H. Molecular and cellular mechanisms of angiotensin II-mediated cardiovascular and renal diseases. Pharmacol Rev. 2000;52(1):11–34.

63. Dhein S. Pharmacology of gap junctions in the cardiovascular system. Cardiovasc Res. 2004;62(2):287–98.
64. Yu H, Gao J, Wang H, Wymore R, Steinberg S, McKinnon D, et al. Effects of the renin-angiotensin system on the current I(to) in epicardial and endocardial ventricular myocytes from the canine heart. Circ Res. 2000;86(10):1062–8.
65. Daleau P, Turgeon J. Angiotensin II modulates the delayed rectifier potassium current of Guinea pig ventricular myocytes. Pflugers Arch. 1994;427(5):553–5.
66. Clément-Chomienne O, Walsh MP, Cole WC. Angiotensin II activation of protein kinase C decreases delayed rectifier K+ current in rabbit vascular myocytes. J Physiol. 1996;495(Pt 3):689–700.
67. Caballero R, Delpón E, Valenzuela C, Longobardo M, Tamargo J. Losartan and its metabolite E3174 modify cardiac delayed rectifier K(+) currents. Circulation. 2000;101(10):1199–205.
68. Caceres J, Jazayeri M, McKinnie J, Avitall B, Denker ST, Tchou P, et al. Sustained bundle branch reentry as a mechanism of clinical tachycardia. Circulation. 1989;79(2):256–70.
69. Lloyd EA, Zipes DP, Heger JJ, Prystowsky EN. Sustained ventricular tachycardia due to bundle branch reentry. Am Heart J. 1982;104(5 Pt 1):1095–7.
70. Balasundaram R, Rao HB, Kalavakolanu S, Narasimhan C. Catheter ablation of bundle branch reentrant ventricular tachycardia. Heart Rhythm. 2008;5(6 Suppl):S68–72.
71. Tchou P, Mehdirad AA. Bundle branch reentry ventricular tachycardia. Pacing Clin Electrophysiol. 1995;18(7):1427–37.
72. Josephson ME. Recurrent ventricular tachycardia. In: Clinical cardiac electrophysiology. 4th ed. Philadelphia: Lippincott Williams & Wilkins; 2008.
73. Vallès E, Bazan V, Marchlinski FE. ECG criteria to identify epicardial ventricular tachycardia in nonischemic cardiomyopathy. Circ Arrhythm Electrophysiol. 2010;3(1):63–71.
74. Lazzara R, Scherlag BJ. Mechanisms of monomorphic ventricular tachycardia in coronary artery disease. J Interv Card Electrophysiol. 2003;8(2):87–92.
75. Wu TJ, Ong JJ, Hwang C, Lee JJ, Fishbein MC, Czer L, et al. Characteristics of wave fronts during ventricular fibrillation in human hearts with dilated cardiomyopathy: role of increased fibrosis in the generation of reentry. J Am Coll Cardiol. 1998;32(1):187–96.
76. Pogwizd SM, McKenzie JP, Cain ME. Mechanisms underlying spontaneous and induced ventricular arrhythmias in patients with idiopathic dilated cardiomyopathy. Circulation. 1998;98(22):2404–14.
77. Schofer J, Spielmann R, Schuchert A, Weber K, Schlüter M. Iodine-123 meta-iodobenzylguanidine scintigraphy: a noninvasive method to demonstrate myocardial adrenergic nervous system disintegrity in patients with idiopathic dilated cardiomyopathy. J Am Coll Cardiol. 1988;12(5):1252–8.
78. Chiale PA, Ferrari I, Mahler E, Vallazza MA, Elizari MV, Rosenbaum MB, et al. Differential profile and biochemical effects of antiautonomic membrane receptor antibodies in ventricular arrhythmias and sinus node dysfunction. Circulation. 2001;103(13):1765–71.
79. Iwata M, Yoshikawa T, Baba A, Anzai T, Mitamura H, Ogawa S. Autoantibodies against the second extracellular loop of beta1-adrenergic receptors predict ventricular tachycardia and sudden death in patients with idiopathic dilated cardiomyopathy. J Am Coll Cardiol. 2001;37(2):418–24.
80. Maron BJ. Clinical course and management of hypertrophic cardiomyopathy. N Engl J Med. 2018;379(7):655–68.
81. Basso C, Thiene G, Corrado D, Buja G, Melacini P, Nava A. Hypertrophic cardiomyopathy and sudden death in the young: pathologic evidence of myocardial ischemia. Hum Pathol. 2000;31(8):988–98.
82. Choudhury L, Mahrholdt H, Wagner A, Choi KM, Elliott MD, Klocke FJ, et al. Myocardial scarring in asymptomatic or mildly symptomatic patients with hypertrophic cardiomyopathy. J Am Coll Cardiol. 2002;40(12):2156–64.
83. Moon JC, Reed E, Sheppard MN, Elkington AG, Ho SY, Burke M, et al. The histologic basis of late gadolinium enhancement cardiovascular magnetic resonance in hypertrophic cardiomyopathy. J Am Coll Cardiol. 2004;43(12):2260–4.
84. Moon JC, McKenna WJ, McCrohon JA, Elliott PM, Smith GC, Pennell DJ. Toward clinical risk assessment in hypertrophic cardiomyopathy with gadolinium cardiovascular magnetic resonance. J Am Coll Cardiol. 2003;41(9):1561–7.
85. Adabag AS, Maron BJ, Appelbaum E, Harrigan CJ, Buros JL, Gibson CM, et al. Occurrence and frequency of arrhythmias in hypertrophic cardiomyopathy in relation to delayed enhancement on cardiovascular magnetic resonance. J Am Coll Cardiol. 2008;51(14):1369–74.
86. Ommen SR, Mital S, Burke MA, Day SM, Deswal A, Elliott P, et al. AHA/ACC guideline for the diagnosis and treatment of patients with hypertrophic cardiomyopathy. Circulation. 2020;142(25):e558–631.
87. Towbin JA, McKenna WJ, Abrams DJ, Ackerman MJ, Calkins H, Darrieux FCC, et al. HRS expert consensus statement on evaluation, risk stratification, and management of arrhythmogenic cardiomyopathy. Heart Rhythm. 2019;16(11):e301–e72.
88. Pinamonti B, Sinagra G, Salvi A, Di Lenarda A, Morgera T, Silvestri F, et al. Left ventricular involvement in right ventricular dysplasia. Am Heart J. 1992;123(3):711–24.
89. Corrado D, Basso C, Schiavon M, Thiene G. Screening for hypertrophic cardiomyopathy in young athletes. N Engl J Med. 1998;339(6):364–9.

90. Kirchhof P, Fabritz L, Zwiener M, Witt H, Schäfers M, Zellerhoff S, et al. Age- and training-dependent development of arrhythmogenic right ventricular cardiomyopathy in heterozygous plakoglobin-deficient mice. Circulation. 2006;114(17):1799–806.
91. Douglas PS, O'Toole ML, Hiller WD, Reichek N. Different effects of prolonged exercise on the right and left ventricles. J Am Coll Cardiol. 1990;15(1):64–9.
92. Haissaguerre M, Le Métayer P, D'Ivernois C, Barat JL, Montserrat P, Warin JF. Distinctive response of arrhythmogenic right ventricular disease to high dose isoproterenol. Pacing Clin Electrophysiol. 1990;13(12 Pt 2):2119–26.
93. Leclercq JF, Potenza S, Maison-Blanche P, Chastang C, Coumel P. Determinants of spontaneous occurrence of sustained monomorphic ventricular tachycardia in right ventricular dysplasia. J Am Coll Cardiol. 1996;28(3):720–4.
94. Francis GS. Development of arrhythmias in the patient with congestive heart failure: pathophysiology, prevalence and prognosis. Am J Cardiol. 1986;57(3):3b–7b.
95. Teerlink JR, Jalaluddin M, Anderson S, Kukin ML, Eichhorn EJ, Francis G, et al. Ambulatory ventricular arrhythmias in patients with heart failure do not specifically predict an increased risk of sudden death. PROMISE (prospective randomized Milrinone survival evaluation) investigators. Circulation. 2000;101(1):40–6.
96. Podrid PJ, Fogel RI, Fuchs TT. Ventricular arrhythmia in congestive heart failure. Am J Cardiol. 1992;69(18):82G–95G; discussion G-6G.
97. Packer M. Lack of relation between ventricular arrhythmias and sudden death in patients with chronic heart failure. Circulation. 1992;85(1 Suppl):I50–6.
98. Echt DS, Liebson PR, Mitchell LB, Peters RW, Obias-Manno D, Barker AH, et al. Mortality and morbidity in patients receiving encainide, flecainide, or placebo. The cardiac arrhythmia suppression trial. N Engl J Med. 1991;324(12):781–8.
99. Teo KK, Yusuf S, Furberg CD. Effects of prophylactic antiarrhythmic drug therapy in acute myocardial infarction. An overview of results from randomized controlled trials. JAMA. 1993;270(13):1589–95.
100. Duffee DF, Shen WK, Smith HC. Suppression of frequent premature ventricular contractions and improvement of left ventricular function in patients with presumed idiopathic dilated cardiomyopathy. Mayo Clin Proc. 1998;73(5):430–3.
101. Bogun F, Crawford T, Reich S, Koelling TM, Armstrong W, Good E, et al. Radiofrequency ablation of frequent, idiopathic premature ventricular complexes: comparison with a control group without intervention. Heart Rhythm. 2007;4(7):863–7.
102. Cairns JA, Connolly SJ, Roberts R, Gent M. Randomised trial of outcome after myocardial infarction in patients with frequent or repetitive ventricular premature depolarisations: CAMIAT. Canadian Amiodarone Myocardial Infarction Arrhythmia Trial Investigators. Lancet. 1997;349(9053):675–82.
103. Julian DG, Camm AJ, Frangin G, Janse MJ, Munoz A, Schwartz PJ, et al. Randomised trial of effect of amiodarone on mortality in patients with left-ventricular dysfunction after recent myocardial infarction: EMIAT. European Myocardial Infarct Amiodarone Trial Investigators. Lancet. 1997;349(9053):667–74.
104. Meinertz T, Hofmann T, Kasper W, Treese N, Bechtold H, Stienen U, et al. Significance of ventricular arrhythmias in idiopathic dilated cardiomyopathy. Am J Cardiol. 1984;53(7):902–7.
105. Singh SN, Fisher SG, Carson PE, Fletcher RD. Prevalence and significance of nonsustained ventricular tachycardia in patients with premature ventricular contractions and heart failure treated with vasodilator therapy. Department of Veterans Affairs CHF STAT Investigators. J Am Coll Cardiol. 1998;32(4):942–7.
106. Bigger JT Jr, Fleiss JL, Rolnitzky LM. Prevalence, characteristics and significance of ventricular tachycardia detected by 24-hour continuous electrocardiographic recordings in the late hospital phase of acute myocardial infarction. Am J Cardiol. 1986;58(13):1151–60.
107. McKenna WJ, England D, Doi YL, Deanfield JE, Oakley C, Goodwin JF. Arrhythmia in hypertrophic cardiomyopathy. I: influence on prognosis. Br Heart J. 1981;46(2):168–72.
108. Elliott PM, Poloniecki J, Dickie S, Sharma S, Monserrat L, Varnava A, et al. Sudden death in hypertrophic cardiomyopathy: identification of high risk patients. J Am Coll Cardiol. 2000;36(7):2212–8.
109. Monserrat L, Elliott PM, Gimeno JR, Sharma S, Penas-Lado M, McKenna WJ. Non-sustained ventricular tachycardia in hypertrophic cardiomyopathy: an independent marker of sudden death risk in young patients. J Am Coll Cardiol. 2003;42(5):873–9.
110. Larsen L, Markham J, Haffajee CI. Sudden death in idiopathic dilated cardiomyopathy: role of ventricular arrhythmias. Pacing Clin Electrophysiol. 1993;16(5 Pt 1):1051–9.
111. Kligfield P, Hochreiter C, Niles N, Devereux RB, Borer JS. Relation of sudden death in pure mitral regurgitation, with and without mitral valve prolapse, to repetitive ventricular arrhythmias and right and left ventricular ejection fractions. Am J Cardiol. 1987;60(4):397–9.
112. Buxton AE, Lee KL, Fisher JD, Josephson ME, Prystowsky EN, Hafley G. A randomized study of the prevention of sudden death in patients with coronary artery disease. Multicenter Unsustained Tachycardia Trial Investigators. N Engl J Med. 1999;341(25):1882–90.
113. Moss AJ, Hall WJ, Cannom DS, Daubert JP, Higgins SL, Klein H, et al. Improved survival with an implanted defibrillator in patients with coronary disease at high risk for ventricular

arrhythmia. Multicenter Automatic Defibrillator Implantation Trial Investigators. N Engl J Med. 1996;335(26):1933–40.

114. Packer M, Bristow MR, Cohn JN, Colucci WS, Fowler MB, Gilbert EM, et al. The effect of carvedilol on morbidity and mortality in patients with chronic heart failure. U.S. Carvedilol Heart Failure Study Group. N Engl J Med. 1996;334(21):1349–55.
115. Porter TR, Eckberg DL, Fritsch JM, Rea RF, Beightol LA, JF S Jr, et al. Autonomic pathophysiology in heart failure patients. Sympathetic-cholinergic interrelations. J Clin Invest. 1990;85(5):1362–71.
116. Swedberg K, Kjekshus J. Effects of enalapril on mortality in severe congestive heart failure: results of the Cooperative North Scandinavian Enalapril Survival Study (CONSENSUS). Am J Cardiol. 1988;62(2):60a–6a.
117. Pratt CM, Gardner M, Pepine C, Kohn R, Young JB, Greenberg B, et al. Lack of long-term ventricular arrhythmia reduction by enalapril in heart failure. SOLVD Investigators. Am J Cardiol. 1995;75(17):1244–9.
118. Cleland JG, Erhardt L, Murray G, Hall AS, Ball SG. Effect of ramipril on morbidity and mode of death among survivors of acute myocardial infarction with clinical evidence of heart failure. A report from the AIRE Study Investigators. Eur Heart J. 1997;18(1):41–51.
119. Fletcher RD, Cintron GB, Johnson G, Orndorff J, Carson P, Cohn JN. Enalapril decreases prevalence of ventricular tachycardia in patients with chronic congestive heart failure. The V-HeFT II VA Cooperative Studies Group. Circulation. 1993;87(6 Suppl):Vi49–55.
120. Cohn JN, Johnson G, Ziesche S, Cobb F, Francis G, Tristani F, et al. A comparison of enalapril with hydralazine-isosorbide dinitrate in the treatment of chronic congestive heart failure. N Engl J Med. 1991;325(5):303–10.
121. Pitt B, Remme W, Zannad F, Neaton J, Martinez F, Roniker B, et al. Eplerenone, a selective aldosterone blocker, in patients with left ventricular dysfunction after myocardial infarction. N Engl J Med. 2003;348(14):1309–21.
122. Ramires FJ, Mansur A, Coelho O, Maranhão M, Gruppi CJ, Mady C, et al. Effect of spironolactone on ventricular arrhythmias in congestive heart failure secondary to idiopathic dilated or to ischemic cardiomyopathy. Am J Cardiol. 2000;85(10):1207–11.
123. Iravanian S, Sovari AA, Lardin HA, Liu H, Xiao HD, Dolmatova E, et al. Inhibition of renin-angiotensin system (RAS) reduces ventricular tachycardia risk by altering connexin43. J Mol Med (Berl). 2011;89(7):677–87.
124. Fernandes ADF, Fernandes GC, Ternes CMP, Cardoso R, Chaparro SV, Goldberger JJ. Sacubitril/valsartan versus angiotensin inhibitors and arrhythmia endpoints in heart failure with reduced ejection fraction. Heart Rhythm O2. 2021;2(6Part B):724–32.
125. Mujadzic H, Prousi GS, Napier R, Siddique S, Zaman N. The impact of angiotensin receptor-neprilysin inhibitors on arrhythmias in patients with heart failure: a systematic review and meta-analysis. J Innov Card Rhythm Manag. 2022;13(9):5164–75.
126. Curtain JP, Docherty KF, Jhund PS, Petrie MC, Inzucchi SE, Køber L, et al. Effect of dapagliflozin on ventricular arrhythmias, resuscitated cardiac arrest, or sudden death in DAPA-HF. Eur Heart J. 2021;42(36):3727–38.
127. Amabile CM, Spencer AP. Keeping your patient with heart failure safe: a review of potentially dangerous medications. Arch Intern Med. 2004;164(7):709–20.
128. Doval HC, Nul DR, Grancelli HO, Perrone SV, Bortman GR, Curiel R. Randomised trial of low-dose amiodarone in severe congestive heart failure. Grupo de Estudio de la Sobrevida en la Insuficiencia Cardiaca en Argentina (GESICA). Lancet. 1994;344(8921):493–8.
129. Effect of prophylactic amiodarone on mortality after acute myocardial infarction and in congestive heart failure: meta-analysis of individual data from 6500 patients in randomised trials. Amiodarone Trials Meta-Analysis Investigators. Lancet. 1997;350(9089):1417–1424.
130. Singh SN, Fletcher RD, Fisher SG, Singh BN, Lewis HD, Deedwania PC, et al. Amiodarone in patients with congestive heart failure and asymptomatic ventricular arrhythmia. Survival Trial of Antiarrhythmic Therapy in Congestive Heart Failure. N Engl J Med. 1995;333(2):77–82.
131. Soejima K, Stevenson WG, Sapp JL, Selwyn AP, Couper G, Epstein LM. Endocardial and epicardial radiofrequency ablation of ventricular tachycardia associated with dilated cardiomyopathy: the importance of low-voltage scars. J Am Coll Cardiol. 2004;43(10):1834–42.
132. Reddy VY, Reynolds MR, Neuzil P, Richardson AW, Taborsky M, Jongnarangsin K, et al. Prophylactic catheter ablation for the prevention of defibrillator therapy. N Engl J Med. 2007;357(26):2657–65.
133. Sapp JL, Wells GA, Parkash R, Stevenson WG, Blier L, Sarrazin J-F, et al. Ventricular Tachycardia Ablation versus Escalation of Antiarrhythmic Drugs. N Engl J Med. 2016;375(2):111–21.
134. Arenal Á, Ávila P, Jiménez-Candil J, Tercedor L, Calvo D, Arribas F, et al. Substrate Ablation vs Antiarrhythmic Drug Therapy for Symptomatic Ventricular Tachycardia. J Am Coll Cardiol. 2022;79(15):1441–53.
135. Della Bella P, Baratto F, Vergara P, Bertocchi P, Santamaria M, Notarstefano P, et al. Does timing of ventricular tachycardia ablation affect prognosis in patients with an implantable cardioverter defibrillator? Results from the Multicenter Randomized PARTITA Trial. Circulation. 2022;145(25):1829–38.
136. Vaseghi M, Hu TY, Tung R, Vergara P, Frankel DS, Di Biase L, et al. Outcomes of catheter ablation of ventricular tachycardia based on etiology in non-

ischemic heart disease: an international ventricular tachycardia ablation center collaborative study. JACC Clin Electrophysiol. 2018;4(9):1141–50.
137. Oloriz T, Silberbauer J, Maccabelli G, Mizuno H, Baratto F, Kirubakaran S, et al. Catheter ablation of ventricular arrhythmia in nonischemic cardiomyopathy: anteroseptal versus inferolateral scar sub-types. Circ Arrhythm Electrophysiol. 2014;7(3):414–23.
138. Zeppenfeld K, Wijnmaalen AP, Ebert M, Baldinger SH, Berruezo A, Catto V, et al. Clinical outcomes in patients with dilated cardiomyopathy and ventricular tachycardia. J Am Coll Cardiol. 2022;80(11):1045–56.
139. Cuculich PS, Schill MR, Kashani R, Mutic S, Lang A, Cooper D, et al. Noninvasive cardiac radiation for ablation of ventricular tachycardia. N Engl J Med. 2017;377(24):2325–36.
140. Robinson CG, Samson PP, Moore KMS, Hugo GD, Knutson N, Mutic S, et al. Phase I/II trial of electrophysiology-guided noninvasive cardiac radioablation for ventricular tachycardia. Circulation. 2019;139(3):313–21.
141. Ninni S, Gallot-Lavallée T, Klein C, Longère B, Brigadeau F, Potelle C, et al. Stereotactic radioablation for ventricular tachycardia in the setting of electrical storm. Circ Arrhythm Electrophysiol. 2022;15(9):e010955.
142. Josephson ME, Harken AH, Horowitz LN. Endocardial excision: a new surgical technique for the treatment of recurrent ventricular tachycardia. Circulation. 1979;60(7):1430–9.
143. Swerdlow CD, Mason JW, Stinson EB, Oyer PE, Winkle RA, Derby GC. Results of operations for ventricular tachycardia in 105 patients. J Thorac Cardiovasc Surg. 1986;92(1):105–13.
144. Krishnan SC, Josephson ME. Surgery for postinfarction ventricular tachycardia: is it obsolete? Pacing Clin Electrophysiol. 2000;23(8):1295–301.
145. Bardy GH, Lee KL, Mark DB, Poole JE, Packer DL, Boineau R, et al. Amiodarone or an implantable cardioverter–defibrillator for congestive heart failure. N Engl J Med. 2005;352(3):225–37.
146. Moss AJ, Zareba W, Hall WJ, Klein H, Wilber DJ, Cannom DS, et al. Prophylactic implantation of a defibrillator in patients with myocardial infarction and reduced ejection fraction. N Engl J Med. 2002;346(12):877–83.
147. Zabel M, Willems R, Lubinski A, Bauer A, Brugada J, Conen D, et al. Clinical effectiveness of primary prevention implantable cardioverter-defibrillators: results of the EU-CERT-ICD controlled multicentre cohort study. Eur Heart J. 2020;41(36):3437–47.
148. Køber L, Thune JJ, Nielsen JC, Haarbo J, Videbæk L, Korup E, et al. Defibrillator implantation in patients with nonischemic systolic heart failure. N Engl J Med. 2016;375(13):1221–30.
149. Khatib S, Stevenson W, Ackerman M. 2017 AHA/ACC/HRS guideline for management of patients with ventricular arrhythmias and the prevention of sudden cardiac death: a report of the American College of Cardiology/American Heart Association Task Force on Clinical Practice Guidelines and the Heart Rhythm Society (vol 72, e91, 2018). J Am Coll Cardiol. 2018;72(14).
150. Klem I, Klein M, Khan M, Yang EY, Nabi F, Ivanov A, et al. Relationship of LVEF and myocardial scar to long-term mortality risk and mode of death in patients with nonischemic cardiomyopathy. Circulation. 2021;143(14):1343–58.
151. Chatterjee NA, Moorthy MV, Pester J, Schaecter A, Panicker GK, Narula D, et al. Sudden death in patients with coronary heart disease without severe systolic dysfunction. JAMA Cardiol. 2018;3(7):591–600.
152. Al-Khatib SM, Stevenson WG, Ackerman MJ, Bryant WJ, Callans DJ, Curtis AB, et al. 2017 AHA/ACC/HRS guideline for management of patients with ventricular arrhythmias and the prevention of sudden cardiac death: a report of the American College of Cardiology/American Heart Association Task Force on Clinical Practice Guidelines and the Heart Rhythm Society. J Am Coll Cardiol. 2018;72(14):e91–e220.
153. Abuissa H, Roshan J, Lim B, Asirvatham SJ. Use of the Impella microaxial blood pump for ablation of hemodynamically unstable ventricular tachycardia. J Cardiovasc Electrophysiol. 2010;21(4):458–61.
154. Friedman PA, Munger TM, Torres N, Rihal C. Percutaneous endocardial and epicardial ablation of hypotensive ventricular tachycardia with percutaneous left ventricular assist in the electrophysiology laboratory. J Cardiovasc Electrophysiol. 2007;18(1):106–9.
155. Maile S, Kunz M, Oechslin E, Zund G, Rahn M, Lachat ML, et al. Intractable ventricular tachycardia and bridging to heart transplantation with a non-pulsatile flow assist device in a patient with isolated left-ventricular non-compaction. J Heart Lung Transplant. 2004;23(1):147–9.
156. Cesario DA, Saxon LA, Cao MK, Bowdish M, Cunningham M. Ventricular tachycardia in the era of ventricular assist devices. J Cardiovasc Electrophysiol. 2011;22(3):359–63.
157. Moss JD, Flatley EE, Beaser AD, Shin JH, Nayak HM, Upadhyay GA, et al. Characterization of ventricular tachycardia after left ventricular assist device implantation as destination therapy: a single-center ablation experience. JACC Clin Electrophysiol. 2017;3(12):1412–24.
158. Osaki S, Alberte C, Murray MA, Brahmbhatt RD, Johnson MR, Edwards NM, et al. Successful radiofrequency ablation therapy for intractable ventricular tachycardia with a ventricular assist device. J Heart Lung Transplant. 2008;27(3):353–6.
159. Dandamudi G, Ghumman WS, Das MK, Miller JM. Endocardial catheter ablation of ventricular tachycardia in patients with ventricular assist devices. Heart Rhythm. 2007;4(9):1165–9.

160. Coleman MA, Bos JM, Johnson JN, Owen HJ, Deschamps C, Moir C, et al. Videoscopic left cardiac sympathetic denervation for patients with recurrent ventricular fibrillation/malignant ventricular arrhythmia syndromes besides congenital long-QT syndrome. Circ Arrhythm Electrophysiol. 2012;5(4):782–8.
161. Zipes DP, Festoff B, Schaal SF, Cox C, Sealy WC, Wallace AG. Treatment of ventricular arrhythmia by permanent atrial pacemaker and cardiac sympathectomy. Ann Intern Med. 1968;68(3):591–7.
162. Collura CA, Johnson JN, Moir C, Ackerman MJ. Left cardiac sympathetic denervation for the treatment of long QT syndrome and catecholaminergic polymorphic ventricular tachycardia using video-assisted thoracic surgery. Heart Rhythm. 2009;6(6):752–9.
163. Conceição-Souza GE, Pêgo-Fernandes PM, Cruz F, Guimarães GV, Bacal F, Vieira ML, et al. Left cardiac sympathetic denervation for treatment of symptomatic systolic heart failure patients: a pilot study. Eur J Heart Fail. 2012;14(12):1366–73.
164. Tan AY, Abdi S, Buxton AE, Anter E. Percutaneous stellate ganglia block for acute control of refractory ventricular tachycardia. Heart Rhythm. 2012;9(12):2063–7.
165. Allen F, Weaver B, Burkey A. Bilateral thoracic sympathetic block for refractory polymorphic tachycardia. Can J Anaesth. 2011;58(12):1110–4.
166. Patel RA, Priore DL, Szeto WY, Slevin KA. Left stellate ganglion blockade for the management of drug-resistant electrical storm. Pain Med. 2011;12(8):1196–8.
167. Markman TM, NVK P, Zghaib T, Smietana J, McBride D, Amankwah NA, et al. Effect of transcutaneous magnetic stimulation in patients with ventricular tachycardia storm: a randomized clinical trial. JAMA Cardiol. 2022;7(4):445–9.
168. Markman TM, Hamilton RH, Marchlinski FE, Nazarian S. Case series of transcutaneous magnetic stimulation for ventricular tachycardia storm. JAMA. 2020;323(21):2200–2.
169. Zhang Y, Mazgalev TN. Arrhythmias and vagus nerve stimulation. Heart Fail Rev. 2011;16(2):147–61.
170. Lopshire JC, Zipes DP. Device therapy to modulate the autonomic nervous system to treat heart failure. Curr Cardiol Rep. 2012;14(5):593–600.
171. Vanoli E, De Ferrari GM, Stramba-Badiale M, Hull SS Jr, Foreman RD, Schwartz PJ. Vagal stimulation and prevention of sudden death in conscious dogs with a healed myocardial infarction. Circ Res. 1991;68(5):1471–81.
172. De Ferrari GM, Crijns HJ, Borggrefe M, Milasinovic G, Smid J, Zabel M, et al. Chronic vagus nerve stimulation: a new and promising therapeutic approach for chronic heart failure. Eur Heart J. 2011;32(7):847–55.
173. De Ferrari GM, Stolen C, Tuinenburg AE, Wright DJ, Brugada J, Butter C, et al. Long-term vagal stimulation for heart failure: Eighteen month results from the NEural Cardiac TherApy foR Heart Failure (NECTAR-HF) trial. Int J Cardiol. 2017;244:229–34.
174. Gold MR, Van Veldhuisen DJ, Hauptman PJ, Borggrefe M, Kubo SH, Lieberman RA, et al. Vagus nerve stimulation for the treatment of heart failure: the INOVATE-HF Trial. J Am Coll Cardiol. 2016;68(2):149–58.

22 Cardiac Defibrillators and Heart Failure

Fergie J. Losiniecki, George S. Waits, and Michael R. Gold

Introduction

Sudden Cardiac Death (SCD) is the leading cause of mortality in the United States and annually claims over 500,000 lives [1]. Initial efforts to prevent SCD focused on patients who had survived SCD or who had sustained ventricular arrhythmias. However, given the low rate of survival of an out-of-hospital arrest (improved from <5% to 9.1% in the 2021 CARES registry), a substantial portion of the population remained at high risk for an initial SCD event [2, 3]. Several landmark trials assessing the impact of implantable cardioverter defibrillators (ICDs), in addition to conventional medical therapy, demonstrated significant reduction in mortality for patients in whom ICDs were implanted. Currently, over 250,000 ICDs are implanted annually in the US with primary prevention serving as the most common indication [4]. Presently, most patients undergoing ICD implantation suffer from congestive heart failure (CHF). A summary of indications for ICD implantation in heart failure patients is included in Table 22.1 [4, 5].The standard of care for patients with persistent moderate to severe systolic dysfunction despite procedural and pharmacologic therapy includes implantation of ICDs in addition to conventional optimal medical therapy. It is important to note that medical therapy for heart failure has evolved since trials first validated the use of ICDs; however, even in contemporary randomized trials of drug therapy for heart failure (largely with reduced ejection fraction) the rate of ICD use was low, but still associated with a decreased risk in both all-cause mortality and sudden cardiac death. [6].

This review will address the role of ICDs in the heart failure population with the most updated guidelines of treatment in the current era.

F. J. Losiniecki · G. S. Waits · M. R. Gold (✉)
Division of Cardiology, Medical University of South Carolina, Charleston, SC, USA
e-mail: fjr@musc.edu; waitsg@musc.edu; goldmr@musc.edu

H. J. Eisen (ed.), *Heart Failure I*, https://doi.org/10.1007/978-3-032-12626-9_22

Table 22.1 AHA/ACC/HRS ICD guidelines for heart failure patients

Secondary prevention
Class I
ICD therapy is indicated in patients who are survivors of cardiac arrest due to VF or hemodynamically unstable sustained VT after evaluation to define the cause of the event and to exclude any completely reversible causes
ICD therapy is indicated in patients with structural heart disease and spontaneous sustained VT, whether hemodynamically stable or unstable
ICD therapy is indicated in patients with syncope of undetermined origin with clinically relevant, hemodynamically significant sustained VT or VF induced at electrophysiological study
ICD therapy is indicated in patients with non-sustained VT due to prior MI, LVEF less than or equal to 40%, and inducible VF or sustained VT at electrophysiological study
Class IIa
ICD implantation is reasonable for patients with unexplained syncope, significant LV dysfunction, and nonischemic DCM
ICD implantation is reasonable for patients with sustained VT and normal or near-normal ventricular function
Primary prevention
Class I
ICD therapy is indicated in patients with LVEF less than or equal to 35% due to prior MI who are at least 40 days post-MI and are in NYHA functional class II or III
ICD therapy is indicated in patients with nonischemic DCM who have an LVEF less than or equal to 35% and who are in NYHA functional class II or III
ICD therapy is indicated in patients with LV dysfunction due to prior MI who are at least 40 days post
ICD in combination with biventricular pacing is indicated for patients who have LVEF less than or equal to 35%, sinus rhythm, LBBB with a QRS duration greater than or equal to 150 ms, and NYHA class II, III, or ambulatory IV symptoms
Class IIa
ICD implantation is reasonable for non-hospitalized patients awaiting transplantation
ICD in combination with biventricular pacing in patients with NYHA functional class II, III or IV, receiving optimal medical therapy, in sinus rhythm with a LBBB QRS 120–149 ms, and a reasonable survival expectation of >1 year
Patients who are at high risk of SCA due to genetic disorders, such as long QT syndrome, Brugada syndrome, hypertrophic cardiomyopathy and arrhythmogenic right ventricular cardiomyopathy (ARVC), and have reasonable expectation of survival with a good functional status at >1 year
ICD implantation is reasonable for patients with cardiac sarcoidosis, giant cell myocarditis, or Chagas disease
Class IIb
ICD therapy may be considered in patients with nonischemic heart disease who have an LVEF of less than or equal to 30% and who are in NYHA functional class I
ICD therapy may be considered in patients with syncope and advanced structural heart disease in whom thorough invasive and noninvasive investigations have failed to define a cause
ICD therapy may be considered in patients with a familial cardiomyopathy associated with sudden death
ICD therapy may be considered in patients with LV noncompaction

DMC dilated cardiomyopathy, *LBBB* left bundle branch block, *LV* left ventricular, *LVEF* left ventricular ejection fraction, *MI* myocardial infarction, *NYHA* New York Heart Association, *VF* ventricular fibrillation, *VT* ventricular tachycardia

Secondary Prevention Trials

ICDs were initially studied in patients who survived SCD or in those patients with sustained ventricular arrhythmias. From such secondary prevention trials, several findings suggested that patients with reduced systolic function had the greatest benefit from ICD implantation. In the AVID study, patients who survived SCD or had sustained ventricular arrhythmias were randomized to ICD or Class III anti-arrhythmic drug therapy [7]. Left Ventricular Ejection Fraction (LVEF) was 0.31 and 0.32 in the ICD and medical treatment arms, respectively. Fifty-five percent of the ICD group and 60% of the medical therapy group had clinical heart failure symptoms. The primary outcome was a significant reduction in mortality for patients in the ICD arm. The benefit of ICD therapy was more pronounced among patients with LVEF <0.35. CIDS (Canadian Implantable Defibrillator Study) randomized patients with ventricular arrhythmias to ICD implantation versus amiodarone therapy [8]. The mean LVEF was 0.33 and 0.34 in the ICD and amiodarone groups, respectively, with half of both groups diagnosed with clinical heart failure. Sub-analysis of the CIDS population revealed that depressed LVEF (<0.35) and advanced NYHA (New York Heart Association) heart failure class were independent predictors of benefit from ICD therapy [9]. CASH evaluated the effect of metoprolol, propafenone, amiodarone or ICD therapy in survivors of SCD [10]. All patients had clinical heart failure with mean LVEF ranging from 0.44 to 0.47 in the treatment arms. Again, ICD implantation provided a significant reduction in mortality compared with AADs. Furthermore, the class Ic antiarrhythmic drug propafenone increased mortality leading to early cessation of this treatment arm. A meta-analysis of the AVID, CIDS and CASH trials showed a 28% relative risk reduction in mortality with ICD therapy compared with amiodarone therapy [11]. Moreover, the difference in mortality was attributed to a 50% reduction to arrhythmic deaths in the ICD group. There was no statistical difference between mortality for patients with LVEF >0.35; however, among patient(s) with LVEF <0.35, there was a 34% reduction in mortality with ICD therapy. For patients with VT/VF arrest and an ejection fraction >24%, ICDs are used in the absence of STEMI within 48 h of the arrhythmic event or other clear reversible cause. The AVID registry data showed a 19.4% 2-year mortality in patients with transient/correctable VT/VF [12]. Secondary prevention of SCD trials provided the basis for future studies investigating ICD implantation as a primary prevention therapy. Patients with reduced LVEF were identified from these studies as a sub-population with the potential for significant benefit from ICD implantation. Additionally, ICD therapy reduced mortality compared with AAD therapy supporting ICD implantation as first-line therapy for patients with history of SCD or ventricular arrhythmia.

Groups of patients with specific etiologies of nonischemic cardiomyopathy have demonstrated benefit of ICDs. For example, in patients with cardiac sarcoidosis receiving ICDs for secondary prevention, 58.4% of these patients received appropriate shocks or SCD events [13]. An observational series of patients with Chagas disease showed mortality rates as high as 16.6% (compared with 7.7%, 8.3%, and 10.0% for CASH, CIDS and AVID respectively), underscoring strength of indication in this population [14]. Patients with congenital heart disease—especially Tetralogy of Fallot and Transposition of the Great Arteries—showed appropriate ICD interventions in 35% of patients who had undergone ICD implant for secondary prevention during a mean follow-up of 4.3 years [15]. Conversely, data supporting ICD implantation in patients with cardiac amyloidosis has not been robust [16, 17].

Notably, within the ischemic cardiomyopathy cohort, appropriate ICD therapies occurred with greater left ventricular end-diastolic diameter (62.3 ± 1.3 vs. 54.6 ± 1.1 mm, $P < 0.001$), lower left ventricular ejection fraction (LVEF; $36.3 \pm 2.0\%$ vs. $45.7 \pm 1.8\%$, $P < 0.001$), less complete revascularization (ICR; 70.7% vs. 45.5%, $P = 0.014$) than those without appropriate guideline direceted medical therapy [18].

Primary Prevention Trials

Due to the results of secondary prevention trials, the focus of ICD investigation became primary prevention of SCD. Summaries of primary prevention ICD trials are included in Table 22.2. The MADIT and MUSTT trials were the first large primary prevention trials evaluating the impact ICD therapy on mortality. In both studies, the population included those with coronary artery disease, LV systolic dysfunction, non-sustained ventricular tachycardia, and inducible sustained ventricular tachycardia with programmed stimulation.

Table 22.2 Primary prevention ICD trials

Trial	No. of patients	Etiology	Major inclusion criteria	Hazard ratio for overall mortality (ICD)	P value
MADIT	196	ICM	EF ≤35%, NSVT, inducible VT	0.46	0.009
MUSTT	704	ICM	EF ≤40%, NSVT, inducible VT	0.45[a]	<0.001
MADIT II	1232	ICM	EF ≤30%, prior MI	0.69	0.016
SCD-HeFT	2521	ICM & NICM	EF ≤35%, CHF NYHA class II or III	0.77	0.007
DEFINITE	458	NICM	EF ≤35%, PVCs or NSVT	0.65	0.08
COMPANION	1520	ICM & NICM	EF ≤35%, CHF NYHA class II or III, QRS >120	0.64[b]	0.003
DINAMIT	676	ICM	EF ≤35%, ¯HRV, recent MI (<40 days)	1.08	0.66
CABG-PATCH	900	ICM	EF ≤35%, CABG, abnormal SAECG	1.07	0.64

MADIT Multicenter Automatic Defibrillator Implantation Trial, *MUSTT* Multicenter Unsustained Tachycardia Trial, *SCD-HeFT* Sudden Cardiac Death in Heart Failure Trial, *DEFINITE* Defibrillators in Non-Ischemic Cardiomyopathy Treatment Evaluation; *COMPANION* Comparison of Medical Therapy, Pacing, and Defibrillation in Heart Failure Trial; *DINAMIT* Defibrillator in Acute Myocardial Infarction Trial, *CABG-PATCH* Coronary Artery Bypass Graft Patch, *ICM* ischemic cardiomyopathy, *EF* ejection fraction, *NSVT* nonsustained VT, *VT* ventricular tachycardia, *MI* myocardial infarction, *NICM* nonischemic cardiomyopathy, *CHF* congestive heart failure, *NYHA* New York Heart Association, *PVC* premature ventricular contraction, *HRV* heart rate variability, *SAECG* signal-averaged ECG

[a]COMPANION results listed are for CRT + ICD vs. medical therapy alone. The hazard ratio for overall mortality for CRT alone vs. medical therapy was 0.76 (P = 0.059)

[b]MUSTT results listed are the adjusted relative risk for overall mortality for patients receiving electrophysiologically guided therapy with an ICD compared with no antiarrhythmic therapy

In the MADIT trial, ICD therapy resulted in a 54% reduction in mortality compared with antiarrhythmic drug (AAD) therapy. The mean LVEF was ~0.25 in the study population and two-thirds of the patients had clinical heart failure. Amiodarone consisted of 74% of the AAD group and was associated with increased mortality compared with beta blocker therapy. Guideline directed medical therapy was suboptimal in this study.

In the MUSTT trial patients with coronary artery disease, LVEF <0.40, and non-sustained ventricular tachycardia underwent an electrophysiology study. Patients with inducible sustained ventricular tachycardia were randomized to conservative medical therapy with beta blockade and/or ACE inhibitors or a strategy of AAD therapy. In the latter arm, they received antiarrhythmic drugs and if unsuccessful for rendering VT/VF non-inducible with programmed ventricular stimulation then an ICD was implanted.

Although ICD was not a treatment arm of the MUSTT trial, the results in those who did receive an ICD suggested that patients with inducible ventricular tachycardia at the time of electrophysiology study were at high risk for SCD and had major benefit from ICD therapy.

Patients who were non-inducible at baseline were not randomized in MUSTT, but were included in a registry. Fourteen percent (49/353) of patients randomized to conservative therapy after inducible ventricular tachycardia had syncope, sustained ventricular tachycardia or SCD leading to ICD implantation. It should be noted that this was similar to the 14% of patients in the registry who were non-inducible and had similar events leading to ICD implantation suggesting that electrophysiology study alone may not be a reliable tool. Nevertheless, the results from the MUSTT trial suggested that depressed LVEF and inducible ventricular tachycardia were associated with a high risk of SCD. Specifically, in a subgroup analysis, the patients who received an ICD clearly performed better than any other group, with 92% being alive at 60 months. Furthermore, if the ICD patients were removed from the antiarrhythmic therapy group, there was no significant difference between the conservative group and the antiarrhythmic drug group. Total mortality was less strongly affected by inducibility of VT [19].

Several trials explored the effect of primary prevention ICD implantation at the time of coronary artery revascularization or shortly after myocardial infarction. CABG-PATCH assessed the impact of ICD implantation with epicardial patches at the time of coronary artery bypass graft (CABG) surgery for patients at high risk for SCD [20]. There were 900 patients with reduced LVEF and abnormal signal averaged ECG randomized to CABG with or without ICD implantation. The mean age was 62 years old, LVEF was 0.27, and greater than 70% had NYHA Class II/III heart failure. At the end of 4 years there was no statistical difference in mortality among the two groups. Subsequent analysis demonstrated that ICD implantation significantly reduced arrhythmic deaths between groups by 45% [21]. However, due to high percentages of non-arrhythmic death in the population the protective effect of ICD therapy was not effective in reducing all-cause mortality. Furthermore, revascularization may have led to improvements in LVEF that was protective from arrhythmic deaths.

The DINAMIT trial evaluated ICD implantation in a high-risk population at the time of acute myocardial infarction [22]. Patients with recent (6–40 days) myocardial infarction who had reduced LVEF and autonomic dysfunction (reduced heart rate variability or elevated 24 h average heart rate) were randomized to optimal medical therapy with and without ICD implantation. In 676 patients, the mean LVEF was 0.28, >85% had NYHA Class II/III heart failure and >70% of patients suffered a new ST elevation myocardial infarction. All-cause mortality was not statistically different between the two groups; however, there was a statistically significant reduction in arrhythmic mortality in the ICD group (HR 0.42). This was offset by an increase in non-arrhythmic deaths in the ICD group compared with control. These findings did not support implantation of primary prevention ICDs at the time of myocardial infarction. Accordingly, this trial was the basis for the 40-day post-MI requirement for ICD implantation in the current guidelines. In a secondary analysis of DINAMIT, mortality in patients with ICD implantation differed by whether they had received appropriate ICD shocks [23]. Patients in the ICD arm with inappropriate ICD shocks had 15% annual mortality compared with 6% annual mortality in ICD patients with appropriate shocks. Effectively, the reduction in arrhythmic mortality observed in the ICD arm was negated by non-arrhythmic death in the other patients. The DINAMIT results were supported by the IRIS trial in which 898 patients with recent (5–31 days) myocardial infarction were randomized to conventional medical therapy with or without ICD implantation [24]. In the IRIS trial many more patients underwent PCI (72%) compared with the DINAMIT trial (27%). There were similar rates of beta blocker and ACE/ARB use in both studies. All-cause mortality at an average of 37 months (about 3 years) was not different in the ICD arm (HR 1.04) compared with control. Subgroup analysis demonstrated that patients with left main disease benefitted from ICD therapy whereas those with thrombolytic therapy fared better in the control group. There was a non-significant trend toward NYHA Class III/IV and smoking as predictors of ICD benefit. Like the DINAMIT trial, reduction in arrhythmic death in the ICD arm (HR 0.55) was offset by increase in non-arrhythmic death (HR 1.92). In a secondary analysis of DINAMIT, assessing the risk factors for arrhythmic and non-arrhythmic death in an attempt to explain the lack of an effect of ICD therapy on all-cause mortality, it was observed that arrhythmic events treated by an ICD in patients with recent MI are associated with intercurrent cardiac events such as heart failure or ischemic events, resulting in overall poor prognosis after ICD therapy [23].

In summary, the results of the CABG-Patch, DINAMIT and IRIS trials found no mortality benefit of primary prevention ICD implantation in patients with reduced LVEF at the time of CABG or acute myocardial infarction.

MADIT II randomized 1232 patients with prior myocardial infarction and LVEF <0.30 to conventional medical therapy with and without ICD implantation [25]. Compared with MADIT, sustained VT or electrophysiology studies were not required for enrollment. The population was 85% male with mean LVEF 0.23 in each group. Approximately two-thirds of the patients had NYHA Class II or greater heart failure symptoms and 15% were on AADs. There were 105/742 (14.2%) and 97/490 (17.9%) deaths in the ICD and conventional groups, respectively ($p = 0.016$), with a hazard ratio for ICD implantation of 0.69. The trial was stopped prematurely once superiority of ICD therapy was detected. The effect of ICD on survival was not influenced by age, sex, LVEF or NYHA Class. These results supported ICD implantation for primary prevention of SCD in patients with reduced LVEF and ischemic cardiomyopathy, a majority of whom have symptomatic heart failure.

The next generation of primary prevention trials included patients with non-ischemic cardiomyopathy as well as ischemic cardiomyopathy. The CAT trial randomized 104 patients with reduced LVEF <0.30 and recent onset (<9 months) of dilated cardiomyopathy to conventional medical therapy with or without ICD implantation [26]. At a mean follow up of 5.5 years there was no statistical difference in mortality with ICD implantation. Of note, the trial was stopped prematurely due to lower-than-expected SCD event rates in the control arm at 1 year. AMIOVERT randomized 103 patients with non-ischemic cardiomyopathy, LVEF >0.35 and asymptomatic non-sustained ventricular tachycardia to amiodarone versus ICD implantation [27]. There was no statistical difference in mortality at 1 and 3 years with a non-statistical trend toward reduced arrhythmic burden in the amiodarone arm. The DEFINITE trial [28] enrolled 458 patients with non-ischemic cardiomyopathy and ventricular ectopy to optimal medical therapy versus optimal medical therapy plus ICD. The mean LVEF was 0.21, roughly 80% had NYHA Class II/III symptoms and clinical heart failure duration was 2.8 years. Beta blocker and ACE/ARB use was ~85% in the population. ICD therapy reduced all-cause mortality by 35%, although this was not statistically significant (HR 0.65, CI 0.4–1.06). In the ICD arm, there was a significant reduction of arrhythmic deaths (HR 0.2) without changing deaths related to heart failure. Subgroup analysis demonstrated that men and patients with NYHA Class III symptoms benefitted the most from ICD implantation. Age, LVEF and QRS duration had no significant impact on the outcome. All these studies were underpowered, so it is difficult to draw conclusions regarding the role of ICD therapy in this population based on these trials.

SCD-HeFT (Sudden Cardiac Death Heart Failure Trial) was the first large, randomized trial appropriately powered to evaluate the efficacy of ICD therapy in systolic HF patients with reduced LVEF, regardless of etiology [29]. In contrast to the MADIT trials, patients with non-ischemic cardiomyopathy, in addition to those with ischemic cardiomyopathy, were included in the study. Over 2500 patients with NYHA Class II or III heart failure, LVEF <0.35 were randomized to placebo, amiodarone, or ICD implantation. The mean ejection fraction of the population was 0.25 and there were roughly equal non-ischemic and ischemic cardiomyopathy patients. The use of evidence-based medical therapy and other appropriate medications were strongly encouraged. ACE/ARBs and beta blockers were being used by 95 and 70% of patients, respectively, at the time of last follow up. The primary finding was that single chamber ICD implantation imparted a 23% relative risk reduction (HR 0.77) of all-cause mortality that was statistically significant compared with placebo (Fig. 22.1).

The effect was similar in patients with either ischemic cardiomyopathy (HR 0.79) or non-ischemic cardiomyopathy (HR 0.73), although absolute mortality was higher in the ischemic population as expected. The mortality benefit was markedly pronounced in patients with NYHA Class II heart failure (HR 0.54) compared with those with NYHA Class III (HR 1.16). Amiodarone did not significantly reduce mortality (HR 1.06) compared with placebo. There was a statistical trend toward worsened outcomes in NYHA Class III patients on amiodarone therapy (HR 1.44). SCD-HeFT demonstrated that regardless of etiology, patients with reduced LVEF benefited from ICD implantation.

A meta-analysis of primary prevention ICD therapy versus conventional medical therapy in non-ischemic patients from SCD-HeFT,

Study	Years of enrollment	No. of patients	Risk ratio (95% CI)
CAT [17]	1991–1997	104	0.83 (0.45–1.82)
AMIOVIRT [18]	1996–2000	103	0.87 (0.31–2.42)
DEFINITE [20]	1998–2002	458	0.65 (0.40–1.06)
SCD-HeFT [19]	1997–2001	792	0.73 (0.50–1.04)
COMPANION [21]	2000–2002	397	0.50 (0.29–0.88)
Combined		**1854**	**0.69 (0.55–0.87)**

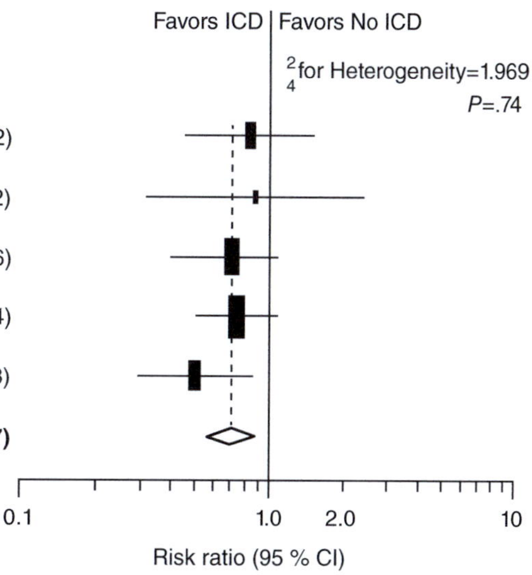

Fig. 22.1 All-cause mortality among patients with NICM randomized to ICD or CRT-D vs. medical therapy in primary prevention. The number of patients with nonischemic cardiomyopathy (NICM) enrolled is reported. Size of the data marker corresponds to the relative weight assigned in the pooled analysis using fixed-effects models. *ICD* indicates implantable cardioverter defibrillator, *CRT-D* cardiac resynchronization plus defibrillator, *CI* confidence interval. (Reprinted with permission *JAMA/American Medical Association*, from Desai et al. [30], ©2004 American Medical Association. All rights reserved)

DEFINITE, CAT, AMIOVERT and COMPANION [31] trials included over 1800 patients. The mean ejection fraction of the population was 0.28 with advanced heart failure (NYHA Class III/IV) present in roughly one third of the population. The analysis demonstrated a 31% relative risk reduction in mortality in ICD recipients [30].

The results of the primary prevention trials strongly supported ICD implantation in addition to optimal medical therapy for patients with reduced LVEF regardless of type of cardiomyopathy. Additionally, these trials placed less emphasis on the requirement of inducible ventricular arrhythmias for high-risk patients prior to ICD implantation.

In 2016, the DANISH trial added to the available body of data to formulate the indications for ICD implantation among patients with nonischemic systolic heart failure. The DANISH trial was a randomized, controlled trial of 556 patients with symptomatic systolic heart failure and left ventricular ejection fraction <0.35 with nonischemic cardiomyopathy. Subjects were assigned to receive an ICD vs. usual clinical care (control group). In both groups, 58% of the patients received cardiac resynchronization therapy (CRT) with CRT pacemakers in the control arm. The primary outcome of the trial was death from any cause. The secondary outcomes were sudden cardiac death and cardiovascular death.

This study showed that implantation of an ICD in patients who had heart failure that was not caused by ischemic heart disease did not provide an overall survival benefit, although the risk of sudden cardiac death was halved with an ICD (4.3 vs. 8.2% HR 0.50; 95% CI, 0.31–0.82; P = 0.005). These results were independent of whether a patient received a CRT device.

In this study, almost every patient received beta-blockers and inhibitors of the renin–angiotensin system and 60% of the patients received mineralocorticoid-receptor antagonists, which is improved medical therapy when compared to prior primary prevention studies.

The DANISH results suggest an attenuation of ICD advantage when compared to contemporary medical and cardiac resynchronization therapy. However, until large trials confirm this finding, ICD therapy should remain the recommendation for primary prevention of SCD in systolic heart failure in non-ischemic cardiomyopathy patients [32]. Of note, on long-term follow up of DANISH, younger patients (<70 years) had reduced mortality in the ICD arm with lower incidence of all-cause mortality, cardiovascular death and sudden cardiac death [33].

An important issue that has arisen from the DANISH trial is whether all patients who are eligible for CRT should routinely receive an ICD. Previous studies of implantable cardiac resynchronization therapy plus defibrillator (CRT-D) therapy used for primary prevention of sudden cardiac death have suggested that CRT-D therapy is less effective in patients with mild heart failure and a wide QRS complex. A meta-analysis of randomized trials analyzed three studies (3858 patients) with a mean follow-up of 66 months. Overall, CRT-D therapy was associated with significantly lower all-cause mortality than implantable cardioverter defibrillator (ICD) therapy (OR, 0.78; 95% CI, 0.63–0.96; $P = 0.02$; I (2) = 19%). However, the risk of cardiac mortality was comparable between two groups (OR, 0.74; 95% CI, 0.53–1.01; $P = 0.06$). CRT-D treatment was associated with a significantly lower risk of hospitalization for heart failure (OR, 0.67; 95% CI, 0.50–0.89; $P = 0.005$; I (2) = 55%). The composite outcome of all-cause mortality and hospitalization for heart failure was also markedly lower with CRT-D therapy than with ICD treatment alone (OR, 0.67; 95% CI, 0.57–0.77; $P < 0.0001$; I (2) = 0%). CRT-D therapy decreased the long-term risk of mortality and heart failure events in patients with mild heart failure with QRS prolongation. However, long-term risk of cardiac mortality was similar between the two groups. A study in which patients are randomly assigned to receive a CRT pacemaker or a CRT defibrillator would be of potential clinical importance [34].

In the current American Heart Association guidelines, ICD implantation for primary prevention of sudden cardiac death in patients with symptomatic systolic heart failure is a class 1A recommendation, with no differentiation between patients with ischemic and nonischemic causes [32].In the European guidelines, ICD implantation is a class 1B recommendation for patients with nonischemic heart failure, as opposed to a class 1A recommendation for patients with ischemic heart failure [32].The American Heart Association guidelines refer solely to the SCD-HeFT trial for their recommendations regarding ICD implantation in patients with nonischemic causes of heart failure. However, SCD-HeFT enrolled patients between 1997 and 2001, and only 69% of enrolled patients received beta-blockers at baseline, 20% of patients received a mineralocorticoid-receptor antagonist, and no patients received concomitant CRT. In addition, the designation of ischemic or nonischemic causes in the SCD-HeFT trial was based primarily on patient history, with results from coronary angiography used to designate the cause only if such results were available. The DEFINITE trial, which enrolled patients between 1998 and 2002, included a larger proportion of patients who received beta-blockers (85%) but, again, no patients who received CRT.

In the present era, new therapies in addition to the continuing aging of the population, the impact of patient age on the risks of death or rehospitalization after primary prevention implantable cardioverter-defibrillator (ICD) demands special attention. In a study by Hess et al., data from 5 major ICD trials were merged: the Multicenter Automatic Defibrillator Implantation Trial I (MADIT-I), the Multicenter UnSustained Tachycardia Trial (MUSTT), the Multicenter Automatic Defibrillator Implantation Trial II (MADIT-II), the Defibrillators in Nonischemic Cardiomyopathy Treatment Evaluation Trial (DEFINITE), and the Sudden Cardiac Death in Heart Failure Trial (SCD-HeFT). The median age at enrollment was 62 (interquartile range 53–70) years. Compared with their younger counterparts, older patients had a greater burden of comorbid illness. In unadjusted exploratory analyses, ICD recipients were less likely to die than nonrecipients in all age groups. Sample sizes were limited among patients aged ≥75 years in this analysis. Point estimates indicate ICD efficacy persists but is attenuated with increasing age. There was no evidence that age modifies the association between ICD treatment and rehospitalization. The impact of patient age on the risks of death or rehospitalization after primary prevention implantable cardioverter-defibrillator (ICD) placement is uncertain [33, 35]. A number of models have been developed to help stratify those patients more likely to benefit from ICD therapy based on competing co-morbidities for mortality [36–38].

Similarly in the DANISH study, 31% of deaths were attributed to non-cardiovascular causes. This is not surprising in an elderly population, but it highlights the importance of selecting patients for ICD implantation carefully. Importantly, ICD therapy for primary prevention of SCD in the non-ischemic heart disease population in most trials included patients with systolic heart failure classified as "idiopathic, valvular, hypertensive, or other" and thus special groups such as cardiac amyloid, cardiac sarcoid, Brugada syndrome, hypertrophic cardiomyopathy, and arrhythmogenic right ventricular dysplasia which carry indications for primary prevention ICD therapy were not distinctly investigated.

Cardiac Resynchronization Therapy (CRT)

Cardiac resynchronization therapy was developed based on observations that interventricular conduction disturbances, commonly observed in heart failure patients, were markers for poor ventricular function and increased mortality [39]. One of the most observed conduction disturbances, LBBB, was associated with delayed activation of the left ventricular free wall. When early CRT investigators evaluated left ventricular pacing in conjunction with conventional right ventricular pacing, there were immediate improvements in hemodynamic performance as well as long term improvement in clinical symptoms [40, 41]. Based on these observations, larger clinical trials exploring CRT were performed demonstrating the benefit of CRT on mortality, left ventricular function, heart failure class and quality of life in symptomatic heart failure patients with depressed systolic function and prolonged (>130 ms) QRS duration [31, 42–48]. A full discussion of the effect of CRT on heart failure patients will be presented in a subsequent chapter; however, the decision to implant an ICD should include consideration of a left ventricular lead where indicated. While the incremental benefit of CRT when added to ICD therapy has been reported [31, 43, 44], the benefit of a defibrillator lead with CRT (CRT-D) versus CRT without an ICD lead (CRT-P) is less well studied. The COMPANION trial randomized 1520 advanced heart failure (NYHA Class III/IV) patients with wide QRS morphologies to optimal medical therapy, CRT-P and CRT-D in a 1:2:2 ratio. Compared with optimal medical therapy, death and hospitalization were reduced by 36 and 40% in the CRT-P and CRT-D groups, respectively, and all-cause mortality was reduced by 24 and 36% in the CRT-P and CRT-D arms, respectively. A secondary analysis of mode of death in the COMPANION trial showed that CRT-D significantly reduced the number of cardiac deaths and, in particular, SCD compared with CRT-P [49]. Cardiac causes comprised 78% of deaths in the COMPANION trial. CRT-D reduced all cardiac deaths by 38% compared with optimal medical therapy whereas CRT-P reduced all cardiac deaths by 14.5%, which was not statistically different than optimal medical therapy (Fig. 22.2). The difference was due primarily to a significant reduction in SCD in the CRT-D arm of 56%. Of note, both groups statistically reduced the rate of heart failure deaths by almost 30% suggesting that CRT-D did not diminish the favorable hemodynamic effects of CRT-P. In fact, a meta-analysis of both COMPANION and Cardiac Resynchronization-Heart Failure (CARE-HF) trials showed CRT-P reduced morbidity and mortality in appropriately selected patients when compared to optimal medical therapy alone [50]. In an analysis of NYHA Class IV patients from COMPANION, CRT-D but not CRT-P significantly reduced sudden cardiac death compared with optimal medical therapy [51]. Since most patients with an indication for CRT also have an indication for an ICD and vise-versa, CRT-D is the usual choice for a biventricular implantable device for patients with heart failure.

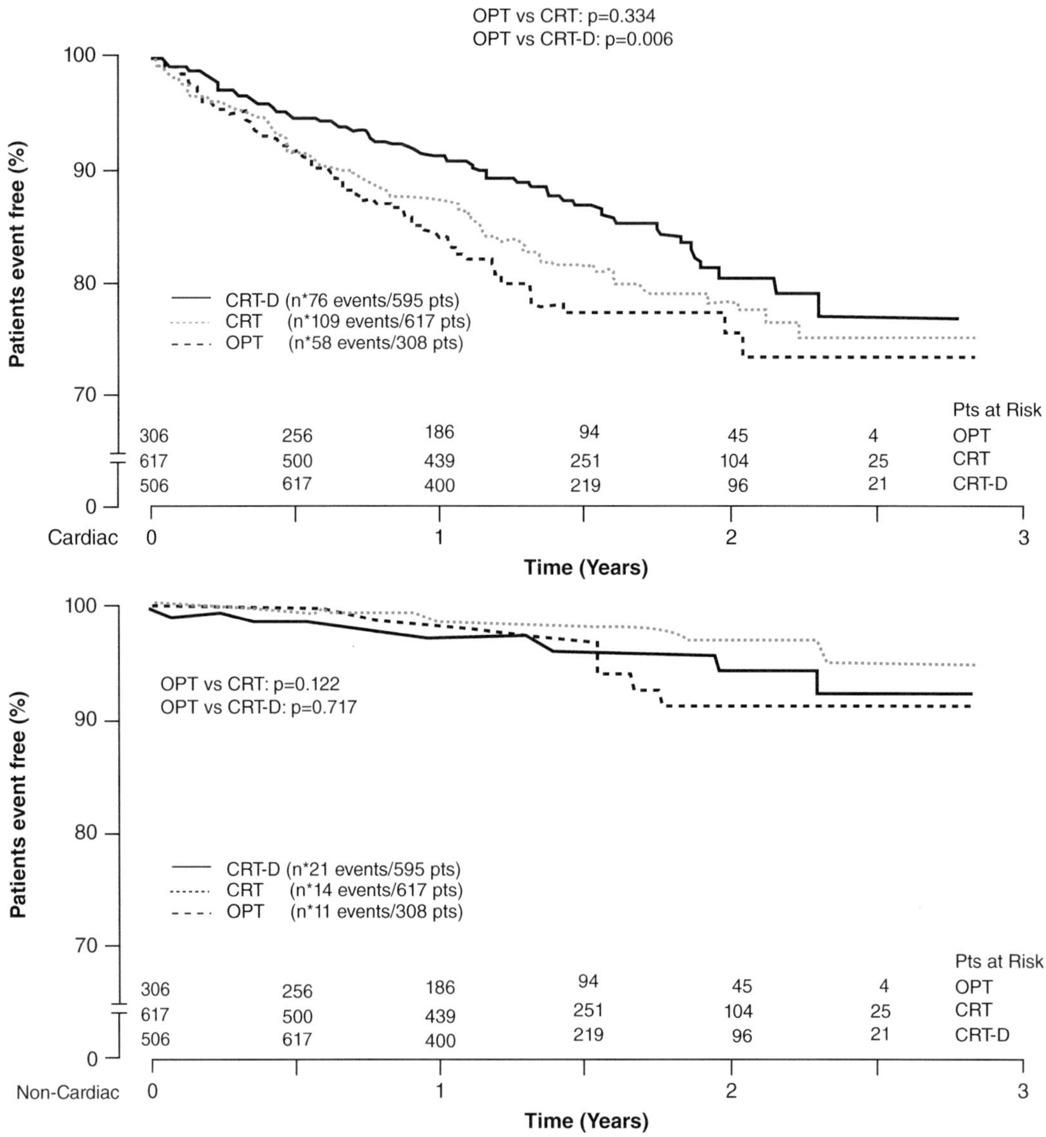

Fig. 22.2 Kaplan-Meier estimates of the time to first cardiac death. (**b**) Kaplan-Meier estimates of the time to first non-cardiac death. *CRT* cardiac resynchronization therapy, *CRT-D* cardiac resynchronization therapy with defibrillation, *OPT* optimal pharmacologic therapy (Reprinted with permission from *Journal of the American College of Cardiology* [49], © 2005 with permission from Elsevier)

As noted previously, the role of ICDs for patients with nonischemic cardiomyopathy was questioned when the DANISH study showed no difference in all-cause mortality in patients with defibrillators compared with those receiving usual clinical care. However, the event rates were low (4.3% and 8.2% in ICD and control groups, respectively) and 58% of the participants in both groups had undergone CRT therapy. It is reasonable to conclude that the low event rates and high prevalence of CRT may have contributed to a statistical type II error. It is also worth noting recent studies have evaluated the incremental benefit of CRT-D over CRT-P including a systematic review and meta-analysis showing no difference in all-cause mortality between CRT-D and CRT-P [52].

However, a large meta-analysis from China analyzing more than 69,000 patients showed a mortality benefit in CRT-D over CRT-P, particularly in patients with ischemic cardiomyopathy and those under age 75 [53].

Certain ECG features of delayed conduction can yield prognostic information that may inform ICD decision-making. For example, T-waves discordant with the polarity of the left bundle branch block QRS pattern may portend a worse prognosis, even in patients receiving CRT-D compared with those with concordant T-waves [54].

Subcutaneous/Extravascular ICDS

Subcutaneous leads have been used in conjunction with transvenous defibrillator systems for patients with abnormal defibrillation thresholds. A subcutaneous ICD system, avoiding transvenous leads, was subsequently developed [55]. Initial studies showed that subcutaneous ICDs (S-ICDs) appropriately recognized and treated ventricular arrhythmias in 12 patients [56]. The S-ICD also performed as well or better than transvenous systems for SVT discrimination [57]. For patients requiring ICD implantation without a pacing indication, the subcutaneous ICD remains an attractive option as it was shown in the PRAETORIAN trial to be noninferior to transvenous systems with respect to device-related complications and inappropriate shocks [58] and lead-related complications were more prevalent and more severe in transvenous systems as compared with subcutaneous ICDs [59]. These results were similar to the ATLAS trial in which 503 patients were randomized to S-ICD or TV-ICD. Major lead complications occurred more often in TV-ICD and no statistical difference in inappropriate shocks or failed appropriate shocks was detected, but the study is ongoing to detect potential differences [60]. Large observational data show overall similar complication rates between TV-ICD and S-ICD systems but more lead-related complications in the former and non-lead related complications in the latter [61]. The post-approval study is the largest prospective study of the S-ICD to date and had 5-year follow-up. All prespecified endpoints were met demonstrating excellent safety and efficacy [62]. A secondary analysis demonstrated infection rates similar to transvenous systems with no associated blood-borne infections [63], the EFFORTLESS registry also showed enduring safety and efficacy data for the subcutaneous system [64] in an early cohort with fewer co-morbidities compared with contemporary trials of this device. A secondary analysis of the UNTOUCHED study demonstrated an inappropriate annual shock rate of 3.1%, among device with contemporary electrogram filtering, which was lower than many transvenous ICD studies [65]. The generator is placed in the left lateral costal margin and the lead courses subcutaneously to the xiphoid process and then along the left parasternal region. Avoiding the transvenous and intracardiac areas eliminates risk of intravascular infections, valvular damage, cardiac perforation, and pneumothorax. The S-ICD is also an alternative to traditional transvenous ICDs for patient with obstructive vascular access, prosthetic tricuspid valves and high risk of systemic infection such as dialysis or immunocompromised subjects. It is commonly used in young patients given high long-term risk of lead failures with transvenous systems.

Ongoing studies are investigating the potential role for subcutaneous ICDs in patients with diabetes and a recent myocardial infarction with only mild-to-moderate LV dysfunction [66]. Whether these findings result in an expanded indication for extravascular ICDs remains to be determined. In addition, the combination of leadless pacing and an S-ICD is being studied.

A notable limitation of the S-ICD is the lack of antitachycardial or pause prevention pacing, except for a brief post-shock period. A novel extravascular ICD implanted substernally is designed to offer the same benefits as traditional subcutaneous systems, with the added functions of antitachycardia—and pause prevention pacing. A multicenter trial showed efficacy and safety of this system [67] but FDA approval remains pending at the time of this publication.

Left Ventricular Assist Devices and ICDS

Left ventricular assist device (LVAD) implantation has become an increasingly used method for both short and long-term stabilization of end-stage heart failure. Technological improvements and advancements in operative experience have propelled LVAD numbers over the last decade. Since almost every patient with an LVAD meets criteria for an ICD, there are issues unique to concomitant LVAD and ICD recipients that need to be considered. Interference between LVAD and older ICD electromagnetic properties have been reported which impaired ICD function, often due to inability to communicate with the device [68–70]. In some cases, the pulse generator was exchanged for an LVAD-compatible device. Current ICD systems have adapted to account for interference by LVAD implantation. The effect of LVADs on VT/VF burden has yet to be comprehensively evaluated. In a retrospective analysis, LVAD implantation reduced the number of ventricular arrhythmias but 21% of patients had appropriate therapy for ventricular arrhythmias despite the beneficial effects of continuous mechanical support [71]. Little is also known regarding the impact of ICDs on LVAD patients' overall mortality [72–74].

Ventricular arrhythmia (VA) is a common complication after LVAD implantation, including ventricular tachycardia and ventricular fibrillation, both of which may cause abnormal circulation. In a review of 12 original research articles 0.83 [95% CI: 0.77, 0.89] were studied. More than half (53%) of VA patients had a history of atrial fibrillation and 61% had a history of VA. Importantly, 39% of the participants had no prior history of VA and experienced new VA following LVAD implantation. Following CF-LVAD implantation, 59% of patients developed early VA (VA $\leq$30 days). The reported incidence of VA after LVAD implantation is not identical in different medical centers and ranges from 20% to 60%. The mechanism of VA after LVAD implantation is summarized as primary cardiomyopathy-related, device mechanical stimulation, myocardial scarring, ventricular displacement, electrolyte regulation, and other processes [73].

A metanalysis of studies comparing the use of ICD in patients with LVADs looked at two primary outcomes: all-cause mortality, and a successful bridge to heart transplantation. In this review, the use of an ICD was not associated with all-cause mortality in patients with LVADs (OR: 0.85, 95% CIs: 0.64–1.12, p = 0.24). The presence of an ICD, however, was associated with a trend towards increased likelihood of successful bridge to heart transplantation (OR: 1.12, 95% CI: 1.0–1.3, p = 0.06). Furthermore, a subgroup analysis of studies published by European centers revealed a significant decrease in pooled mortality (OR: 0.58, 95% CI: 0.4–0.83, p = 0.003) with the use of ICD, contrary to an increase in pooled mortality among studies published by US centers (OR: 1.2, 95% CI 1.02–1.33, p = 0.025). These observations shed light to potential significant differences in the derived benefit, in distinct patient populations. This might reflect differences in baseline patient characteristics and warrant further investigation [73].

There remains controversy whether patients without ICDs prior to LVAD implantation should receive an ICD for primary prevention [75]. Further studies are needed to definitively address this matter.

ICD Programming Optimization of Shock Zones in Patients with LVADs

Multiple studies have investigated the delivery of shocks following LVAD implantation. In a small single-center study including pulsatile and continuous flow LVADs placed as bridge to transplant and destination therapy, 42% of patients received either an appropriate or inappropriate shock from their ICD following LVAD implantation over an average follow-up of 238 days, with similar numbers of patients receiving appropriate and inappropriate ICD shocks. ICD shocks were associated with worse outcomes compared to those who did not receive ICD shocks [76]. In this study, there were no data provided on the

ICD zone programming, use of ATP, differentiation of pulsatile versus continuous flow LVADs, or differentiation in outcomes in patients receiving destination therapy LVADs.

Many patients with LVADs will tolerate sustained VT, VF, or even asystole, with published reports demonstrating clinically stable presentation with continuous VT/VF for >24 h. However, there are concerns about a reduction in pump flow and cardiac output during sustained ventricular arrhythmias (VAs), as well as potential adverse effects on RV function or thrombosis in a fibrillating RV. On the other hand, tachycardia monitor zone–only programming could lead to failure to treat sustained slow VT. In patients with severe RV dysfunction or pulmonary hypertension, this could worsen HF and systemic perfusion. In patients who have hemodynamically significant slow VT or in whom there are concerns about hemodynamic or thrombotic complications, ablation may be the most advantageous strategy.

Richardson et al. in a single-center prospective randomized trial of 83 patients, compared an ultraconservative ICD programming strategy (maximal allowable intervals to detection in the VF and VT zone with use of ATP) with standard ICD programming [77].

The primary outcome was time to first ICD shock. There was no significant difference between groups in time to first ICD shock or total ICD shocks. No harmful effects on mortality or hospitalization were seen with extending VT/VF zones to the maximum allowable detection times. Thus, an ultraconservative programming strategy appears to be reasonable utilizing a combination of high rate cut off limits for tachycardia therapies, prolonged tachycardia detection programming, and aggressive use of ATP algorithms. The AHA Scientific Statement recommends guidance regarding ICD programming [78]. The consensus of the panel is to provide a high-rate cutoff VF zone (240–250 bpm) with the longest programmable detection time available on the device. For patients with a known history of VT, a second zone (VT zone) can be added with the highest detection cutoff allowed by the device unless the tachycardia is known to result in hemodynamic instability. The VT zone (unlike the VF zone) can be programmed as an ATP only for patients with recurrent VAs that are amenable to ATP. If ATP is unsuccessful at terminating a VT episode, elective cardioversion or defibrillation under sedation is advised. Alternatively, on an individualized basis, shocks can be programmed to be delivered in the VT zone after extensive sequences of ATP.

The goal of this protocol is to standardize peri-operative (pre and post) ICD interrogation around the time of LVAD placement and to provide standardized ICD programming to reduce the incidence of unnecessary and inappropriate ICD shocks.

Quality of Life and Other Considerations

The impact of implantable defibrillators on quality of life is important to recognize and should be incorporated into patient education and shared decision-making. Quality of life was comparable between S-ICD over transvenous systems in a survey-based case-controlled study with an advantage to S-ICDs with respect to physical well-being [79]. A systematic review and meta-analysis of 37 trials found a moderate-to-large pre-post effect on quality of life in patients undergoing ICD implant [80]. As technology advances to improve the safety and efficacy of implantable defibrillators, one anticipates the psychological benefit would track favorably as well but future studies are needed.

Failed Shocks and Inappropriate Shocks

Inappropriate device-delivered therapy, defined as therapy delivered for non-ventricular tachyarrhythmias, affects 8–40% of patients with ICDs [81]. The best method for programming ICD devices to reduce inappropriate therapy is unknown. The investigators of MADIT RIT (Multicenter Automatic Defibrillator Implantation Trial–Reduce Inappropriate Therapy) conducted a large-scale, randomized study designed to evaluate specific programming features for reducing inappropriate therapy in patients with ICDs [82]. The primary objective was to determine whether programmed high-rate therapy (with a 2.5-second delay before the initiation of therapy at a heart rate of ≥200 beats per minute) or delayed therapy (with a 60-second delay at 170–199 beats per minute, a 12-second delay at 200–249 beats per minute, and a 2.5-second delay at ≥250 beats per minute) was associated with a decrease in the number of patients with a first occurrence of inappropriate anti-tachycardia pacing or shocks, as compared with conventional programming (with a 2.5-second delay at 170–199 beats per minute and a 1.0-second delay at ≥200 beats per minute). The investigators found that programming of ICD therapies for tachyarrhythmias of 200 beats per minute or higher or with a prolonged delay in therapy at 170 beats per minute or higher, as compared with conventional programming, was associated with reductions in inappropriate therapy and all-cause mortality during long-term follow-up in 1500 patients with a primary-prevention indication to receive an ICD. Similarly, The ADVANCE III trial randomized patients receiving a VVI ICD to programming either a long- (30 of 40 intervals) or standard short- (18 of 24 intervals) detection length and found the long detection length arm significantly reduced appropriate therapies by 48%, overall shocks by 40%, and also a survival benefit [83].

In a similar fashion, The UNTOUCHED trial (Understanding Outcomes With the S-ICD in Primary Prevention Patients with Low Ejection Fraction) was designed to evaluate the inappropriate shock (IAS) rate in a more typical, contemporary ICD patient population implanted with the S-ICD using standardized programming and enhanced discrimination algorithms. Primary prevention patients with left ventricular ejection fraction ≤35% and no pacing indications were included. Generation 2 or 3 S-ICD devices were implanted and programmed with rate-based therapy delivery for rates ≥250 beats per minute and morphology discrimination for rates ≥200 and <250 beats per minute.

Patients were followed for 18 months. A total of 1111 patients were included in postimplant follow-up analysis. The mean left ventricular ejection fraction was 26.4 ± 5.8%. Eighteen-month freedom from IAS was 95.9% (lower confidence limit, 94.8%). Predictors of reduced incidence of IAS were implanting the most recent generation of device, using the 3-incision technique, no history of atrial fibrillation, and ischemic cause. All primary endpoints were met. The 18-month all-cause shock-free rate was 90.6% (lower confidence limit, 89.0%). Conversion success rate for appropriate, discrete episodes was 98.4%. Complication-free rate at 18 months was 92.7%. The inappropriate shock rate of 3.1% at 1 year was the lowest reported for the S-ICD and lower than many transvenous ICD studies using contemporary programming to reduce IAS [65].

Conclusion

In addition to survivors of sudden cardiac death, heart failure patients have an elevated risk of fatal ventricular arrhythmias. ICD implantation for secondary prevention of SCD is established. For either ischemic or non-ischemic heart failure patients with reduced LVEF <0.35 and NYHA Class II–III symptoms, primary prevention ICD implantation in addition to optimal medical therapy has become the standard of care. When combined with medical therapy, ICDs offer an additional 20–30% mortality benefit that is most pronounced in those with the lowest LVEF. Mortality reduction is primarily driven by preventing sudden cardiac death rather than preventing heath failure deaths. CRT when combined with a defibrillator lead offers the greatest magnitude of mortality advantage as well as improving heart failure symptoms in the appropriate patient. Although LVAD interference has been reported, current ICDs are designed to accommodate LVAD implantation. Modern technologies such as subcutaneous ICDs offer an alternative to traditional transvenous systems. Finally, despite advancements in identifying high risk patients for SCD, over half of SCD victims do not meet current indications for ICD therapy [84, 85]. In addition to optimizing device-based therapy, efforts to identify factors associated with SCD should be explored such as those with less severe LV dysfunction, as well as those with genetic abnormalities or other unusual etiologies of increased SCD risk.

References

1. Heron M. Deaths: leading causes for 2008. Natl Vital Stat Rep. 2012;60(6):1–94. PubMed PMID: 22827019
2. Goldberger JJ, Cain ME, Hohnloser SH, Kadish AH, Knight BP, Lauer MS, Maron BJ, Page RL, Passman RS, Siscovick D, Siscovick D, Stevenson WG, Zipes DP, American Heart A, American College of Cardiology F, Heart Rhythm S. American Heart Association/American College of Cardiology Foundation/Heart Rhythm Society scientific statement on noninvasive risk stratification techniques for identifying patients at risk for sudden cardiac death: a scientific statement from the American Heart Association Council on Clinical Cardiology Committee on Electrocardiography and Arrhythmias and Council on Epidemiology and Prevention. Circulation. 2008;118(14):1497–1518. PubMed PMID: 18833586.
3. Correction to: heart disease and stroke Statistics-2023 update: a report from the American Heart Association. Circulation 2023;147(8):e622. https://doi.org/10.1161/CIR.0000000000001137. PubMed PMID: 36802886.
4. Epstein AE, Dimarco JP, Ellenbogen KA, Estes NA, 3rd, Freedman RA, Gettes LS, Gillinov AM, Gregoratos G, Hammill SC, Hayes DL, Hlatky MA, Newby LK, Page RL, Schoenfeld MH, Silka MJ, Stevenson LW, Sweeney MO, American College of C, American Heart Association Task Force on Practice G, American Association for Thoracic S, Society of Thoracic S. ACC/AHA/HRS 2008 Guidelines for device-based therapy of cardiac rhythm abnormalities. Heart Rhythm. 2008;5(6):e1–62. https://doi.org/10.1016/j.hrthm.2008.04.014. PubMed PMID: 18534360.
5. Writing Group M, Tracy CM, Epstein AE, Darbar D, DiMarco JP, Dunbar SB, Estes NA, 3rd, Ferguson TB, Jr., Hammill SC, Karasik PE, Link MS, Marine JE, Schoenfeld MH, Shanker AJ, Silka MJ, Stevenson LW, Stevenson WG, Varosy PD, Writing Committee M, Epstein AE, DiMarco JP, Ellenbogen KA, Estes NA, 3rd, Freedman RA, Gettes LS, Gillinov AM, Gregoratos G, Hammill SC, Hayes DL, Hlatky MA, Newby LK, Page RL, Schoenfeld MH, Silka MJ, Stevenson LW, Sweeney MO, Members AATF, Anderson JL, Jacobs AK, Halperin JL, Albert NM, Creager MA, DeMets D, Ettinger SM, Guyton RA, Hochman JS, Kushner FG, Ohman EM, Stevenson W, Yancy CW, American College of Cardiology F, American Heart Association Task Force on Practice G, American Association for Thoracic S, Heart Failure Society of A, Society of Thoracic S. 2012 ACCF/AHA/HRS focused update of the 2008 guidelines for device-based therapy of cardiac rhythm abnormalities: a report of the American College of Cardiology Foundation/American Heart Association Task Force on Practice Guidelines. J Thorac Cardiovasc Surg. 2012;144(6):e127–e145. https://doi.org/10.1016/j.jtcvs.2012.08.032. PubMed PMID: 23140976.
6. Gama F, Ferreira J, Carmo J, Costa FM, Carvalho S, Carmo P, Cavaco D, Morgado FB, Adragao P, Mendes M. Implantable cardioverter-defibrillators in trials of drug therapy for heart failure: a systematic review and meta-analysis. J Am Heart Assoc. 2020;9(8):e015177. https://doi.org/10.1161/JAHA.119.015177. PubMed PMID: 32290732; PMCID: PMC7428541.
7. Antiarrhythmics versus implantable defibrillators I. A comparison of antiarrhythmic-drug therapy with implantable defibrillators in patients resuscitated from near-fatal ventricular arrhythmias. N Engl J Med 1997;337(22):1576–1583. https://doi.org/10.1056/NEJM199711273372202. PubMed PMID: 9411221.
8. Connolly SJ, Gent M, Roberts RS, Dorian P, Roy D, Sheldon RS, Mitchell LB, Green MS, Klein GJ, O'Brien B. Canadian implantable defibrillator study (CIDS) : a randomized trial of the implantable cardioverter defibrillator against amiodarone. Circulation. 2000;101(11):1297–302. https://doi.org/10.1161/01.cir.101.11.1297. PubMed PMID: 10725290.
9. Sheldon R, Connolly S, Krahn A, Roberts R, Gent M, Gardner M. Identification of patients most likely to benefit from implantable cardioverter-defibrillator therapy: the Canadian Implantable Defibrillator Study. Circulation. 2000;101(14):1660–4. https://doi.org/10.1161/01.cir.101.14.1660. PubMed PMID: 10758047.
10. Kuck KH, Cappato R, Siebels J, Ruppel R. Randomized comparison of antiarrhythmic drug therapy with implantable defibrillators in patients resuscitated from cardiac arrest : the Cardiac Arrest Study Hamburg (CASH). Circulation. 2000;102(7):748–54. https://doi.org/10.1161/01.cir.102.7.748. PubMed PMID: 10942742.
11. Connolly SJ, Hallstrom AP, Cappato R, Schron EB, Kuck KH, Zipes DP, Greene HL, Boczor S, Domanski M, Follmann D, Gent M, Roberts RS. Meta-analysis of the implantable cardioverter defibrillator secondary prevention trials. AVID, CASH and CIDS studies. Antiarrhythmics vs Implantable Defibrillator study. Cardiac Arrest Study Hamburg. Canadian Implantable Defibrillator Study. Eur Heart J. 2000;21(24):2071–8. https://doi.org/10.1053/euhj.2000.2476. PubMed PMID: 11102258.
12. Anderson JL, Hallstrom AP, Epstein AE, Pinski SL, Rosenberg Y, Nora MO, Chilson D, Cannom DS, Moore R. Design and results of the antiarrhythmics vs

implantable defibrillators (AVID) registry. The AVID Investigators. Circulation. 1999;99(13):1692–9. https://doi.org/10.1161/01.cir.99.13.1692. PubMed PMID: 10190878.
13. Franke KB, Marshall H, Kennewell P, Pham HD, Tully PJ, Rattanakosit T, Mahadevan G, Mahajan R. Risk and predictors of sudden death in cardiac sarcoidosis: a systematic review and meta-analysis. Int J Cardiol. 2021;328:130–40. https://doi.org/10.1016/j.ijcard.2020.11.044. PubMed PMID: 33242509
14. Rassi FM, Minohara L, Rassi A Jr, Correia LCL, Marin-Neto JA, Rassi A, da Silva Menezes A Jr. Systematic review and meta-analysis of clinical outcome after implantable cardioverter-defibrillator therapy in patients with Chagas heart disease. JACC Clin Electrophysiol. 2019;5(10):1213–23. https://doi.org/10.1016/j.jacep.2019.07.003. PubMed PMID: 31648747.
15. Vehmeijer JT, Brouwer TF, Limpens J, Knops RE, Bouma BJ, Mulder BJ, de Groot JR. Implantable cardioverter-defibrillators in adults with congenital heart disease: a systematic review and meta-analysis. Eur Heart J. 2016;37(18):1439–48. https://doi.org/10.1093/eurheartj/ehv735. PubMed PMID: 26873095; PMCID: PMC4914887.
16. Halawa A, Woldu HG, Kacey KG, Alpert MA. Effect of ICD implantation on cardiovascular outcomes in patients with cardiac amyloidosis: a systematic review and meta-anaylsis. J Cardiovasc Electrophysiol. 2020;31(7):1749–58. https://doi.org/10.1111/jce.14541. PubMed PMID: 32391952.
17. Kim EJ, Holmes BB, Huang S, Lugo R, Al Aboud A, Goodman S, Hung RR, Slosky D, Stevenson WG, Michaud GF, John RM. Outcomes in patients with cardiac amyloidosis and implantable cardioverter-defibrillator. Europace. 2020;22(8):1216–23. https://doi.org/10.1093/europace/euaa094. PubMed PMID: 32514579.
18. Takano T, Tanaka K, Ozaki K, Sato A, Iijima K, Yanagawa T, Izumi D, Ozawa T, Fuse K, Sato M, Tanabe N, Minamino T. Clinical predictors of recurrent ventricular arrhythmias in secondary prevention implantable cardioverter defibrillator recipients with coronary artery disease – lower left ventricular ejection fraction and incomplete revascularization. Circ J. 2018;82(12):3037–43. https://doi.org/10.1253/circj.CJ-18-0646. PubMed PMID: 30305485.
19. Buxton AE, Lee KL, DiCarlo L, Gold MR, Greer GS, Prystowsky EN, O'Toole MF, Tang A, Fisher JD, Coromilas J, Talajic M, Hafley G. Electrophysiologic testing to identify patients with coronary artery disease who are at risk for sudden death. Multicenter Unsustained Tachycardia Trial Investigators. N Engl J Med. 2000;342(26):1937–45. https://doi.org/10.1056/NEJM200006293422602. PubMed PMID: 10874061.
20. Bigger JT Jr. Prophylactic use of implanted cardiac defibrillators in patients at high risk for ventricular arrhythmias after coronary-artery bypass graft surgery. Coronary Artery Bypass Graft (CABG) Patch Trial Investigators. N Engl J Med. 1997;337(22):1569–75. https://doi.org/10.1056/NEJM199711273372201. PubMed PMID: 9371853
21. Bigger JT Jr, Whang W, Rottman JN, Kleiger RE, Gottlieb CD, Namerow PB, Steinman RC, Estes NA 3rd. Mechanisms of death in the CABG Patch trial: a randomized trial of implantable cardiac defibrillator prophylaxis in patients at high risk of death after coronary artery bypass graft surgery. Circulation. 1999;99(11):1416–21. https://doi.org/10.1161/01.cir.99.11.1416. PubMed PMID: 10086963.
22. Hohnloser SH, Kuck KH, Dorian P, Roberts RS, Hampton JR, Hatala R, Fain E, Gent M, Connolly SJ, Investigators D. Prophylactic use of an implantable cardioverter-defibrillator after acute myocardial infarction. N Engl J Med. 2004;351(24):2481–8. https://doi.org/10.1056/NEJMoa041489. PubMed PMID: 15590950.
23. Dorian P, Hohnloser SH, Thorpe KE, Roberts RS, Kuck KH, Gent M, Connolly SJ. Mechanisms underlying the lack of effect of implantable cardioverter-defibrillator therapy on mortality in high-risk patients with recent myocardial infarction: insights from the defibrillation in acute myocardial infarction Trial (DINAMIT). Circulation. 2010;122(25):2645–52. https://doi.org/10.1161/CIRCULATIONAHA.109.924225. PubMed PMID: 21135366.
24. Steinbeck G, Andresen D, Seidl K, Brachmann J, Hoffmann E, Wojciechowski D, Kornacewicz-Jach Z, Sredniawa B, Lupkovics G, Hofgartner F, Lubinski A, Rosenqvist M, Habets A, Wegscheider K, Senges J, Investigators I. Defibrillator implantation early after myocardial infarction. N Engl J Med. 2009;361(15):1427–36. https://doi.org/10.1056/NEJMoa0901889. PubMed PMID: 19812399.
25. Moss AJ, Zareba W, Hall WJ, Klein H, Wilber DJ, Cannom DS, Daubert JP, Higgins SL, Brown MW, Andrews ML, Multicenter Automatic Defibrillator Implantation Trial III. Prophylactic implantation of a defibrillator in patients with myocardial infarction and reduced ejection fraction. N Engl J Med. 2002;346(12):877–83. https://doi.org/10.1056/NEJMoa013474. PubMed PMID: 11907286.
26. Bansch D, Antz M, Boczor S, Volkmer M, Tebbenjohanns J, Seidl K, Block M, Gietzen F, Berger J, Kuck KH. Primary prevention of sudden cardiac death in idiopathic dilated cardiomyopathy: the Cardiomyopathy Trial (CAT). Circulation. 2002;105(12):1453–8. https://doi.org/10.1161/01.cir.0000012350.99718.ad. PubMed PMID: 11914254.
27. Strickberger SA, Hummel JD, Bartlett TG, Frumin HI, Schuger CD, Beau SL, Bitar C, Morady F, Investigators A. Amiodarone versus implantable cardioverter-defibrillator:randomized trial in patients with non-ischemic dilated cardiomyopathy and asymptomatic nonsustained ventricular tachycardia—AMIOVIRT. J Am Coll Cardiol. 2003;41(10):1707–12. https://doi.org/10.1016/s0735-1097(03)00297-3. PubMed PMID: 12767651.

28. Kadish A, Dyer A, Daubert JP, Quigg R, Estes NA, Anderson KP, Calkins H, Hoch D, Goldberger J, Shalaby A, Sanders WE, Schaechter A, Levine JH. Defibrillators in non-ischemic cardiomyopathy treatment evaluation I. Prophylactic defibrillator implantation in patients with nonischemic dilated cardiomyopathy. N Engl J Med. 2004;350(21):2151–8. https://doi.org/10.1056/NEJMoa033088. PubMed PMID: 15152060.
29. Bardy GH, Lee KL, Mark DB, Poole JE, Packer DL, Boineau R, Domanski M, Troutman C, Anderson J, Johnson G, McNulty SE, Clapp-Channing N, Davidson-Ray LD, Fraulo ES, Fishbein DP, Luceri RM, Ip JH, Sudden Cardiac Death in Heart Failure Trial I. Amiodarone or an implantable cardioverter-defibrillator for congestive heart failure. N Engl J Med. 2005;352(3):225–37. https://doi.org/10.1056/NEJMoa043399. PubMed PMID: 15659722.
30. Desai AS, Fang JC, Maisel WH, Baughman KL. Implantable defibrillators for the prevention of mortality in patients with nonischemic cardiomyopathy: a meta analysis of randomized controlled trials. JAMA. 2004;292(23):2874–9. https://doi.org/10.1001/jama.292.23.2874. PubMed PMID: 15598919.
31. Bristow MR, Saxon LA, Boehmer J, Krueger S, Kass DA, De Marco T, Carson P, DiCarlo L, DeMets D, White BG, DW DV, Feldman AM, Comparison of Medical Therapy P, Defibrillation in Heart Failure I. Cardiac-resynchronization therapy with or without an implantable defibrillator in advanced chronic heart failure. N Engl J Med. 2004;350(21):2140–50. https://doi.org/10.1056/NEJMoa032423. PubMed PMID: 15152059.
32. Kober L, Thune JJ, Nielsen JC, Haarbo J, Videbaek L, Korup E, Jensen G, Hildebrandt P, Steffensen FH, Bruun NE, Eiskjaer H, Brandes A, Thogersen AM, Gustafsson F, Egstrup K, Videbaek R, Hassager C, Svendsen JH, Hofsten DE, Torp-Pedersen C, Pehrson S, Investigators D. Defibrillator implantation in patients with nonischemic systolic heart failure. N Engl J Med. 2016;375(13):1221–30. https://doi.org/10.1056/NEJMoa1608029. PubMed PMID: 27571011.
33. Yafasova A, Butt JH, Elming MB, Nielsen JC, Haarbo J, Videbaek L, Olesen LL, Steffensen FH, Bruun NE, Eiskjaer H, Brandes A, Thogersen AM, Egstrup K, Gustafsson F, Hassager C, Svendsen JH, Hofsten DE, Torp-Pedersen C, Pehrson S, Thune JJ, Kober L. Long-term follow-up of DANISH (the Danish study to assess the efficacy of ICDs in patients with nonischemic systolic heart failure on mortality). Circulation. 2022;145(6):427–36. https://doi.org/10.1161/CIRCULATIONAHA.121.056072. PubMed PMID: 34882430.
34. Sun WP, Li CL, Guo JC, Zhang LX, Liu R, Zhang HB, Zhang L. Long-term efficacy of implantable cardiac resynchronization therapy plus defibrillator for primary prevention of sudden cardiac death in patients with mild heart failure: an updated meta-analysis. Heart Fail Rev. 2016;21(4):447–53. https://doi.org/10.1007/s10741-016-9550-y. PubMed PMID: 27043219.
35. Hess PL, Al-Khatib SM, Han JY, Edwards R, Bardy GH, Bigger JT, Buxton A, Cappato R, Dorian P, Hallstrom A, Kadish AH, Kudenchuk PJ, Lee KL, Mark DB, Moss AJ, Steinman R, Inoue LY, Sanders G. Survival benefit of the primary prevention implantable cardioverter-defibrillator among older patients: does age matter? An analysis of pooled data from 5 clinical trials. Circ Cardiovasc Qual Outcomes. 2015;8(2):179–86. https://doi.org/10.1161/CIRCOUTCOMES.114.001306. PubMed PMID: 25669833; PMCID: PMC4408540.
36. Levy WC, Lee KL, Hellkamp AS, Poole JE, Mozaffarian D, Linker DT, Maggioni AP, Anand I, Poole-Wilson PA, Fishbein DP, Johnson G, Anderson J, Mark DB, Bardy GH. Maximizing survival benefit with primary prevention implantable cardioverter-defibrillator therapy in a heart failure population. Circulation. 2009;120(10):835–42. https://doi.org/10.1161/CIRCULATIONAHA.108.816884. PubMed PMID: 19704100; PMCID: PMC3774781.
37. Barsheshet A, Moss AJ, Huang DT, McNitt S, Zareba W, Goldenberg I. Applicability of a risk score for prediction of the long-term (8-year) benefit of the implantable cardioverter-defibrillator. J Am Coll Cardiol. 2012;59(23):2075–9. https://doi.org/10.1016/j.jacc.2012.02.036. PubMed PMID: 22651863.
38. Kramer DB, Mitchell SL, Monteiro J, Jones PW, Normand SL, Hayes DL, Reynolds MR. Patient activity and survival following implantable cardioverter-defibrillator implantation: the ALTITUDE activity study. J Am Heart Assoc. 2015;4(5). https://doi.org/10.1161/JAHA.115.001775. PubMed PMID: 25979902; PMCID: PMC4599410.
39. Abraham WT. Cardiac resynchronization therapy for heart failure: biventricular pacing and beyond. Curr Opin Cardiol. 2002;17(4):346–52. https://doi.org/10.1097/00001573-200207000-00004. PubMed PMID: 12151867.
40. Cazeau S, Ritter P, Lazarus A, Gras D, Backdach H, Mundler O, Mugica J. Multisite pacing for end-stage heart failure: early experience. Pacing Clin Electrophysiol. 1996;19(11 Pt 2):1748–57. https://doi.org/10.1111/j.1540-8159.1996.tb03218.x. PubMed PMID: 8945034.
41. Cazeau S, Ritter P, Bakdach S, Lazarus A, Limousin M, Henao L, Mundler O, Daubert JC, Mugica J. Four chamber pacing in dilated cardiomyopathy. Pacing Clin Electrophysiol. 1994;17(11 Pt 2):1974–9. https://doi.org/10.1111/j.1540-8159.1994.tb03783.x. PubMed PMID: 7845801.
42. Linde C, Abraham WT, Gold MR, St John Sutton M, Ghio S, Daubert C, Group RS. Randomized trial of cardiac resynchronization in mildly symptomatic heart failure patients and in asymptomatic patients with left ventricular dysfunction and previous heart failure symptoms. J Am Coll Cardiol. 2008;52(23):1834–43.

https://doi.org/10.1016/j.jacc.2008.08.027. PubMed PMID: 19038680.

43. Moss AJ, Hall WJ, Cannom DS, Klein H, Brown MW, Daubert JP, Estes NA 3rd, Foster E, Greenberg H, Higgins SL, Pfeffer MA, Solomon SD, Wilber D, Zareba W, Investigators M-CT. Cardiac-resynchronization therapy for the prevention of heart-failure events. N Engl J Med. 2009;361(14):1329–38. https://doi.org/10.1056/NEJMoa0906431. PubMed PMID: 19723701.
44. Young JB, Abraham WT, Smith AL, Leon AR, Lieberman R, Wilkoff B, Canby RC, Schroeder JS, Liem LB, Hall S, Wheelan K, Multicenter InSync ICDRCETI. Combined cardiac resynchronization and implantable cardioversion defibrillation in advanced chronic heart failure: the MIRACLE ICD Trial. JAMA. 2003;289(20):2685–94. https://doi.org/10.1001/jama.289.20.2685. PubMed PMID: 12771115.
45. Cleland JG, Daubert JC, Erdmann E, Freemantle N, Gras D, Kappenberger L, Tavazzi L, Cardiac Resynchronization-Heart Failure Study I. The effect of cardiac resynchronization on morbidity and mortality in heart failure. N Engl J Med. 2005;352(15):1539–49. https://doi.org/10.1056/NEJMoa050496. PubMed PMID: 15753115.
46. Higgins SL, Hummel JD, Niazi IK, Giudici MC, Worley SJ, Saxon LA, Boehmer JP, Higginbotham MB, De Marco T, Foster E, Yong PG. Cardiac resynchronization therapy for the treatment of heart failure in patients with intraventricular conduction delay and malignant ventricular tachyarrhythmias. J Am Coll Cardiol. 2003;42(8):1454–9. https://doi.org/10.1016/s0735-1097(03)01042-8. PubMed PMID: 14563591.
47. Abraham WT, Fisher WG, Smith AL, Delurgio DB, Leon AR, Loh E, Kocovic DZ, Packer M, Clavell AL, Hayes DL, Ellestad M, Trupp RJ, Underwood J, Pickering F, Truex C, McAtee P, Messenger J, Evaluation MSGMIRC. Cardiac resynchronization in chronic heart failure. N Engl J Med. 2002;346(24):1845–53. https://doi.org/10.1056/NEJMoa013168. PubMed PMID: 12063368.
48. Gras D, Leclercq C, Tang AS, Bucknall C, Luttikhuis HO, Kirstein-Pedersen A. Cardiac resynchronization therapy in advanced heart failure the multicenter InSync clinical study. Eur J Heart Fail. 2002;4(3):311–20. https://doi.org/10.1016/s1388--9842(02)00018-1. PubMed PMID: 12034157.
49. Carson P, Anand I, O'Connor C, Jaski B, Steinberg J, Lwin A, Lindenfeld J, Ghali J, Barnet JH, Feldman AM, Bristow MR. Mode of death in advanced heart failure: the Comparison of Medical, Pacing, and Defibrillation Therapies in Heart Failure (COMPANION) trial. J Am Coll Cardiol. 2005;46(12):2329–34. https://doi.org/10.1016/j.jacc.2005.09.016. PubMed PMID: 16360067.
50. Cleland JGF, Bristow MR, Freemantle N, Olshansky B, Gras D, Saxon L, Tavazzi L, Boehmer J, Ghio S, Feldman AM, Daubert JC, de Mets D. The effect of cardiac resynchronization without a defibrillator on morbidity and mortality: an individual patient data meta-analysis of COMPANION and CARE-HF. Eur J Heart Fail. 2022;24(6):1080–90. https://doi.org/10.1002/ejhf.2524. PubMed PMID: 35490339; PMCID: PMC9543287.
51. Lindenfeld J, Feldman AM, Saxon L, Boehmer J, Carson P, Ghali JK, Anand I, Singh S, Steinberg JS, Jaski B, DeMarco T, Mann D, Yong P, Galle E, Ecklund F, Bristow M. Effects of cardiac resynchronization therapy with or without a defibrillator on survival and hospitalizations in patients with New York Heart Association class IV heart failure. Circulation. 2007;115(2):204–12. https://doi.org/10.1161/CIRCULATIONAHA.106.629261. PubMed PMID: 17190867.
52. Patel D, Kumar A, Black-Maier E, Morgan RL, Trulock K, Wilner B, Nemer D, Donnellan E, Tarakji KG, Cantillon DJ, Varma N, Saba SF, Al-Khatib SM, Wilkoff BL, Rickard JW. Cardiac resynchronization therapy with or without defibrillation in patients with nonischemic cardiomyopathy: a systematic review and meta-analysis. Circ Arrhythm Electrophysiol. 2021;14(6):e008991. https://doi.org/10.1161/CIRCEP.120.008991. PubMed PMID: 33999647.
53. Long YX, Hu Y, Cui DY, Hu S, Liu ZZ. The benefits of defibrillator in heart failure patients with cardiac resynchronization therapy: a meta-analysis. Pacing Clin Electrophysiol. 2021;44(2):225–34. https://doi.org/10.1111/pace.14150. PubMed PMID: 33372697.
54. Padeletti L, Aimo A, Vishenvsky B, Schwartz A, McNitt S, Wang PJ, Moss AJ, Emdin M, Zareba W. The prognostic benefit of cardiac resynchronization therapy is greater in concordant vs. discordant left bundle branch block in the Multicenter Automatic Defibrillator Implantation Trial-Cardiac Resynchronization Therapy (MADIT-CRT). Europace. 2018;20(5):794–800. https://doi.org/10.1093/europace/euw446. PubMed PMID: 28398490.
55. Rowley CP, Lobodzinski SS, Gold MR. The subcutaneous defibrillator. Curr Treat Options Cardiovasc Med. 2012;14(5):550–7. https://doi.org/10.1007/s11936-012-0196-3. PubMed PMID: 22836713
56. Bardy GH, Smith WM, Hood MA, Crozier IG, Melton IC, Jordaens L, Theuns D, Park RE, Wright DJ, Connelly DT, Fynn SP, Murgatroyd FD, Sperzel J, Neuzner J, Spitzer SG, Ardashev AV, Oduro A, Boersma L, Maass AH, Van Gelder IC, Wilde AA, van Dessel PF, Knops RE, Barr CS, Lupo P, Cappato R, Grace AA. An entirely subcutaneous implantable cardioverter-defibrillator. N Engl J Med. 2010;363(1):36–44. https://doi.org/10.1056/NEJMoa0909545. PubMed PMID: 20463331.
57. Gold MR, Theuns DA, Knight BP, Sturdivant JL, Sanghera R, Ellenbogen KA, Wood MA, Burke MC. Head-to-head comparison of arrhythmia discrimination performance of subcutaneous and transvenous ICD arrhythmia detection algorithms: the START study. J Cardiovasc Electrophysiol.

2012;23(4):359–66. https://doi.org/10.1111/j.1540--8167.2011.02199.x. PubMed PMID: 22035049.
58. Knops RE, Olde Nordkamp LRA, Delnoy PHM, Boersma LVA, Kuschyk J, El-Chami MF, Bonnemeier H, Behr ER, Brouwer TF, Kaab S, Mittal S, Quast ABE, Smeding L, van der Stuijt W, de Weger A, de Wilde KC, Bijsterveld NR, Richter S, Brouwer MA, de Groot JR, Kooiman KM, Lambiase PD, Neuzil P, Vernooy K, Alings M, Betts TR, Bracke F, Burke MC, de Jong J, Wright DJ, Tijssen JGP, Wilde AAM, Investigators P. Subcutaneous or transvenous defibrillator therapy. N Engl J Med. 2020;383(6):526–36. https://doi.org/10.1056/NEJMoa1915932. PubMed PMID: 32757521.
59. Knops RE, Pepplinkhuizen S, Delnoy P, Boersma LVA, Kuschyk J, El-Chami MF, Bonnemeier H, Behr ER, Brouwer TF, Kaab S, Mittal S, Quast ABE, van der Stuijt W, Smeding L, de Veld JA, Tijssen JGP, Bijsterveld NR, Richter S, Brouwer MA, de Groot JR, Kooiman KM, Lambiase PD, Neuzil P, Vernooy K, Alings M, Betts TR, Bracke F, Burke MC, de Jong J, Wright DJ, Jansen WPJ, Whinnett ZI, Nordbeck P, Knaut M, Philbert BT, van Opstal JM, Chicos AB, Allaart CP, Borger van der Burg AE, Dizon JM, Miller MA, Nemirovsky D, Surber R, Upadhyay GA, Weiss R, de Weger A, Wilde AAM, Olde Nordkamp LRA. Device-related complications in subcutaneous versus transvenous ICD: a secondary analysis of the PRAETORIAN trial. Eur Heart J. 2022;43(47):4872–83. https://doi.org/10.1093/eurheartj/ehac496. PubMed PMID: 36030464; PMCID: PMC9748587.
60. Rordorf R. The ATLAS randomised clinical Trial: what do the superiority results mean for subcutaneous ICD therapy and sudden cardiac death prevention as a whole? Arrhythm Electrophysiol Rev. 2022;11. https://doi.org/10.15420/aer.2022.11.S1. PubMed PMID: 36313240; PMCID: PMC9611761.
61. Brouwer TF, Yilmaz D, Lindeboom R, Buiten MS, Olde Nordkamp LR, Schalij MJ, Wilde AA, van Erven L, Knops RE. Long-term clinical outcomes of subcutaneous versus transvenous implantable defibrillator therapy. J Am Coll Cardiol. 2016;68(19):2047–55. https://doi.org/10.1016/j.jacc.2016.08.044. PubMed PMID: 27810043.
62. Gold MR, El-Chami MF, Burke MC, et al. Postapproval study of a subcutaneous implantable cardioverter-defibrillator system. J Am Coll Cardiol. 2023;82:383–97.
63. Gold MR, Aasbo JD, Weiss R, Burke MC, Gleva MJ, Knight BP, Miller MA, Schuger CD, Carter N, Leigh J, Brisben AJ, El-Chami MF. Infection in patients with subcutaneous implantable cardioverter-defibrillator: results of the S-ICD Post Approval Study. Heart Rhythm. 2022;19(12):1993–2001. https://doi.org/10.1016/j.hrthm.2022.07.031. PubMed PMID: 35944889.
64. Boersma L, Barr C, Knops R, Theuns D, Eckardt L, Neuzil P, Scholten M, Hood M, Kuschyk J, Jones P, Duffy E, Husby M, Stein K, Lambiase PD, Group EI. Implant and midterm outcomes of the subcutaneous implantable cardioverter-defibrillator registry: the EFFORTLESS study. J Am Coll Cardiol. 2017;70(7):830–41. https://doi.org/10.1016/j.jacc.2017.06.040. PubMed PMID: 28797351.
65. Gold MR, Lambiase PD, El-Chami MF, Knops RE, Aasbo JD, Bongiorni MG, Russo AM, Deharo JC, Burke MC, Dinerman J, Barr CS, Shaik N, Carter N, Stoltz T, Stein KM, Brisben AJ, Boersma LVA, Investigators* U. Primary results from the understanding outcomes with the S-ICD in primary prevention patients with low ejection fraction (UNTOUCHED) Trial. Circulation. 2021;143(1):7–17. https://doi.org/10.1161/CIRCULATIONAHA.120.048728. PubMed PMID: 33073614; PMCID: PMC7752215.
66. Kutyifa V, Beck C, Brown MW, Cannom D, Daubert J, Estes M, Greenberg H, Goldenberg I, Hammes S, Huang D, Klein H, Knops R, Kosiborod M, Poole J, Schuger C, Singh JP, Solomon S, Wilber D, Zareba W, Moss AJ, Committee MSIE. Multicenter automatic defibrillator implantation Trial-subcutaneous implantable cardioverter defibrillator (MADIT S-ICD): design and clinical protocol. Am Heart J. 2017;189:158–66. https://doi.org/10.1016/j.ahj.2017.04.014. PubMed PMID: 28625372.
67. Friedman P, Murgatroyd F, Boersma LVA, Manlucu J, O'Donnell D, Knight BP, Clementy N, Leclercq C, Amin A, Merkely BP, Birgersdotter-Green UM, Chan JYS, Biffi M, Knops RE, Engel G, Munoz Carvajal I, Epstein LM, Sagi V, Johansen JB, Sterlinski M, Steinwender C, Hounshell T, Abben R, Thompson AE, Wiggenhorn C, Willey S, Crozier I, Extravascular ICDPSI. Efficacy and safety of an extravascular implantable cardioverter-defibrillator. N Engl J Med. 2022;387(14):1292–302. https://doi.org/10.1056/NEJMoa2206485. PubMed PMID: 36036522.
68. Oswald H, Klein G, Struber M, Gardiwal A. Implantable defibrillator with left ventricular assist device compatibility. Interact Cardiovasc Thorac Surg. 2009;8(5):579–80. https://doi.org/10.1510/icvts.2009.202077. PubMed PMID: 19223309.
69. Matthews JC, Betley D, Morady F, Pelosi F Jr. Adverse interaction between a left ventricular assist device and an implantable cardioverter defibrillator. J Cardiovasc Electrophysiol. 2007;18(10):1107–8. https://doi.org/10.1111/j.1540-8167.2007.00805.x. PubMed PMID: 17403078.
70. Netzler PC, Vasuki N, Peura JL, Gold MR. Interactions between a left ventricular assist device and implantable cardioverter-defibrillator. Pacing Clin Electrophysiol. 2012;35(9):e272–3. https://doi.org/10.1111/j.1540--8159.2012.03370.x. PubMed PMID: 22452670.
71. Refaat MM, Tanaka T, Kormos RL, McNamara D, Teuteberg J, Winowich S, London B, Simon MA. Survival benefit of implantable cardioverter-defibrillators in left ventricular assist device-supported heart failure patients. J Card Fail. 2012;18(2):140–5. https://doi.org/10.1016/j.cardfail.2011.10.020. PubMed PMID: 22300782; PMCID: PMC3272629.

72. Vakil K, Kazmirczak F, Sathnur N, Adabag S, Cantillon DJ, Kiehl EL, Koene R, Cogswell R, Anand I, Roukoz H. Implantable cardioverter-defibrillator use in patients with left ventricular assist devices: a systematic review and meta-analysis. JACC Heart Fail. 2016;4(10):772–9. https://doi.org/10.1016/j.jchf.2016.05.003. PubMed PMID: 27395347.
73. Rorris FP, Antonopoulos CN, Kyriakopoulos CP, Drakos SG, Charitos C. Implantable cardioverter defibrillators in left ventricular assist device patients: alpha systematic review and meta-analysis. J Heart Lung Transplant. 2021;40(10):1098–106. https://doi.org/10.1016/j.healun.2021.05.014. PubMed PMID: 34176727.
74. Elkaryoni A, Badarin FA, Khan MS, Ellakany K, Potturi N, Poonia J, Kennedy KF, Magalski A, Sperry BW, Wimmer AP. Implantable cardioverter-defibrillators and survival in advanced heart failure patients with continuous-flow left ventricular assist devices: a systematic review and meta-analysis. Europace. 2019;21(9):1353–9. https://doi.org/10.1093/europace/euz125. PubMed PMID: 31086951.
75. Pettit SJ, Petrie MC, Connelly DT, Japp AG, Payne JR, Haj-Yahia S, Gardner RS. Use of implantable cardioverter defibrillators in patients with left ventricular assist devices. Eur J Heart Fail. 2012;14(7):696–702. https://doi.org/10.1093/eurjhf/hfs062. PubMed PMID: 22547745.
76. Ambardekar AV, Allen LA, Lindenfeld J, Lowery CM, Cannon AP, Cleveland JC Jr, Brieke A, Sauer WH. Implantable cardioverter-defibrillator shocks in patients with a left ventricular assist device. J Heart Lung Transplant. 2010;29(7):771–6. https://doi.org/10.1016/j.healun.2010.02.001. PubMed PMID: 20347337.
77. Richardson TD, Hale L, Arteaga C, Xu M, Keebler M, Schlendorf K, Danter M, Shah A, Lindenfeld J, Ellis CR. Prospective randomized Evaluation of implantable cardioverter-defibrillator programming in patients with a left ventricular assist device. J Am Heart Assoc. 2018;7(5). https://doi.org/10.1161/JAHA.117.007748. PubMed PMID: 29475875; PMCID: PMC5866326.
78. Kusumoto FM, Calkins H, Boehmer J, Buxton AE, Chung MK, Gold MR, Hohnloser SH, Indik J, Lee R, Mehra MR, Menon V, Page RL, Shen WK, Slotwiner DJ, Warner Stevenson L, Varosy PD, Welikovitch L. HRS/ACC/AHA expert consensus statement on the use of implantable cardioverter-defibrillator therapy in patients who are not included or not well represented in clinical trials. Heart Rhythm. 2014;11(7):1271–303. https://doi.org/10.1016/j.hrthm.2014.03.041. PubMed PMID: 24819194.
79. Kobe J, Hucklenbroich K, Geisendorfer N, Bettin M, Frommeyer G, Reinke F, Dechering D, Burgmer M, Eckardt L. Posttraumatic stress and quality of life with the totally subcutaneous compared to conventional cardioverter-defibrillator systems. Clin Res Cardiol. 2017;106(5):317–21. https://doi.org/10.1007/s00392-016-1055-0. PubMed PMID: 27878381.
80. Willy K, Ellermann C, Reinke F, Rath B, Wolfes J, Eckardt L, Doldi F, Wegner FK, Kobe J, Morina N. The impact of cardiac devices on patients' quality of life-a systematic review and meta-analysis. J Cardiovasc Dev Dis. 2022;9(8). https://doi.org/10.3390/jcdd9080257. PubMed PMID: 36005421; PMCID: PMC9409697.
81. Moss AJ, Schuger C, Beck CA, Brown MW, Cannom DS, Daubert JP, Estes NA 3rd, Greenberg H, Hall WJ, Huang DT, Kautzner J, Klein H, McNitt S, Olshansky B, Shoda M, Wilber D, Zareba W, Investigators M-RT. Reduction in inappropriate therapy and mortality through ICD programming. N Engl J Med. 2012;367(24):2275–83. https://doi.org/10.1056/NEJMoa1211107. PubMed PMID: 23131066.
82. Schuger C, Daubert JP, Brown MW, Cannom D, Estes NA 3rd, Hall WJ, Kayser T, Klein H, Olshansky B, Power KA, Wilber D, Zareba W, Moss AJ. Multicenter automatic defibrillator implantation trial: reduce inappropriate therapy (MADIT-RIT): background, rationale, and clinical protocol. Ann Noninvasive Electrocardiol. 2012;17(3):176–85. https://doi.org/10.1111/j.1542-474X.2012.00531.x. PubMed PMID: 22816536; PMCID: PMC6932441.
83. Gasparini M, Lunati MG, Proclemer A, Arenal A, Kloppe A, Martinez Ferrer JB, Hersi AS, Gulaj M, Wijffels MCE, Santi E, Manotta L, Varma N. Long detection programming in single-chamber Defibrillators reduces unnecessary therapies and mortality: the ADVANCE III Trial. JACC Clin Electrophysiol. 2017;3(11):1275–82. https://doi.org/10.1016/j.jacep.2017.05.001. PubMed PMID: 29759624.
84. de Vreede-Swagemakers JJ, Gorgels AP, Dubois-Arbouw WI, van Ree JW, Daemen MJ, Houben LG, Wellens HJ. Out-of-hospital cardiac arrest in the 1990's: a population-based study in the Maastricht area on incidence, characteristics and survival. J Am Coll Cardiol. 1997;30(6):1500–5. https://doi.org/10.1016/s0735-1097(97)00355-0. PubMed PMID: 9362408.
85. Stecker EC, Vickers C, Waltz J, Socoteanu C, John BT, Mariani R, JH MA, Gunson K, Jui J, Chugh SS. Population-based analysis of sudden cardiac death with and without left ventricular systolic dysfunction: two-year findings from the Oregon Sudden Unexpected Death Study. J Am Coll Cardiol. 2006;47(6):1161–6. https://doi.org/10.1016/j.jacc.2005.11.045. PubMed PMID: 16545646.

23 Cardiac Resynchronization Therapy in Heart Failure

Kiran Sidhu, Joyce Wald, and David Feldman

Introduction

Heart failure pharmacotherapy including beta-blockers (BB), angiotensin converting enzyme inhibitors/Angiotensin II Receptor Blockers/Angiotensin Receptor -Neprilysin Inhibitor (ACEi/ARB/ARNI), SGLT2 inhibitors and aldosterone antagonists have resulted in dramatic improvements in the morbidity and mortality of patients with heart failure (HF) with a reduced ejection fraction. However, in many patients, medical management alone is insufficient to achieve adequate symptom control and HF associated morbidity and mortality remains high. In a subgroup of these patients with prolonged QRS duration, particularly with left bundle branch block (LBBB) morphology, cardiac resynchronization therapy (CRT) has demonstrated additional benefit. Currently CRT is indicated for patients with NYHA functional class II-IV heart failure, severe systolic dysfunction (left ventricular ejection fraction (LVEF) $\leq 35\%$) and interventricular conduction delay. Over the last two decades it has become a key component of the staged treatment of HF [1].

K. Sidhu (✉) · J. Wald
Penn Heart and Vascular Center, Philadelphia, PA, USA
e-mail: kiran.sidhu@pennmedicine.upenn.edu

D. Feldman
Trinity Cardiology, Buffalo, NY, USA

Background and Rationale for Use

The deleterious effects of dyssynchronous activation of the ventricular myocardium were first noted almost 90 years ago when Wiggers demonstrated a reduction in the rate of LV pressure rise (dP/dt) and peak power production with right ventricular (RV) pacing [2]. More recently Askenazi et al. demonstrated the incremental reduction in dp/dT and LV peak pressure incurred when moving from right atrial pacing with normal ventricular conduction, to RV (AV sequential) pacing, to direct RV pacing with loss of AV synchrony. They further demonstrated that RV pacing not only had acute hemodynamic effects, but also led to a significant reductions in the LVEF over time [3]. Burkhoff and colleagues demonstrated that an inverse linear relationship existed between the QRS duration and LV pressure production [4]. In addition to detrimental effects on systolic function, Zile et al. demonstrated that diastolic properties and LV filling were also degraded with RV pacing with reductions in the isovolumic pressure decline and myocardial emptying rate [5]. In addition to the acute effects on hemodynamics and medium term effects on LV remodeling, increasing degrees of QRS prolongation are at least a marker for worse prognosis in advanced systolic HF. This was demonstrated in post-hoc analysis of the VEST (Vesnarinone) trial demonstrating a fivefold reduction in cumulative survival for patients with

H. J. Eisen (ed.), *Heart Failure I*, https://doi.org/10.1007/978-3-032-12626-9_23

a QRS duration >220 ms versus those with normal QRS duration [6].

The prevalence of interventricular conduction delays in patients with advanced systolic HF (perhaps up to 1/3 of all HF patients) and the aforementioned observations led several groups to question whether resynchronization of myocardial activation could result in improved hemodynamics and long-term outcomes. Mower and colleagues were the first to formally theorize that simultaneous pacing of both ventricles would reduce both electrical and mechanical dyssynchrony [7]. Cazeau et al., were the first to experiment with this approach in humans at Paris' Hôpital Lariboisière. A standard dual chamber AV pacemaker was modified to pace both atria and both ventricles simultaneously—the LV lead having been implanted via thoracotomy. The group demonstrated that in eight subjects with QRS prolongation and end-stage HF despite maximal medical therapy, biventricular (BiV) pacing increased the mean cardiac index by 25% and decreased the pulmonary capillary wedge pressure by 17% [8]. Following their initial success, a number of small observational studies were performed demonstrating a variety of clinical benefits ultimately confirmed in large randomized studies.

Nelson and colleagues went on to demonstrate that in patients with LBBB (mean QRS duration 179 ± 3 ms) and severe systolic dysfunction, LV or BiV pacing resulted in a nearly instantaneous improvement in dP/dt and pulse pressure with a reduction in the arterial-coronary sinus oxygen difference and thus the myocardial oxygen consumption [9]. This critical observation underscores the key difference between CRT and inotropic agents which achieve their augmentation of contractility via an increase in myocardial oxygen consumption likely accounting for the adverse long-term effects that have been observed in clinical trials of these agents [10].

Not surprisingly, electrical and mechanical dyssynchrony are associated with cellular pathophysiology with important regional changes in myocardial gene expression for stress remodeling proteins such as mitogen-activated protein kinases, altered cell survival signaling, reduced L-type calcium currents, and decreased adrenergic responsiveness with varying degrees of reversibility following resynchronization therapy [11].

Types of Dyssynchrony and Physiologic Consequences

The normal electrical activation of the ventricular myocardium results in simultaneous activation of the right and left bundles of the Purkinje system culminating in the generation of symmetric counterforces during cardiac ejection. The normal Purkinje system is electrically isolated from the myocardium except at the apically located terminal Purkinje-myocardial junctions facilitating the normal apical to basal mechanical activation and contraction. When this is interrupted due to conduction block, dyssynchronous activation of the myocardium results. Also common in the setting of advanced systolic heart failure is first degree AV delay with associated alterations in atrioventricular synchrony. Cumulatively these conduction disturbances (particularly in the context of LBBB) result in three types of dyssynchrony with important implications for cardiac performance.

Intraventricular Dyssynchrony

Dyssynchronous activation of the LV myocardium with LBBB results in early, unloaded contraction of the interventricular septum. Rather than contributing to a rise in LV pressure, this contraction is primarily converted to prestretch of the lateral wall. This results in reductions in stroke volume, dP/dt, and pulse pressure and ultimately worsening LV systolic function and mitral regurgitation due to uncoordinated contraction of the papillary muscles. These derangements in turn contribute to progressive adverse remodeling and the "vicious cycle" of HF pathophysiology.

Interventricular Dyssynchrony

With LBBB and RV pacing there is early RV activation resulting in a disadvantageous pressure gradient between the RV and LV. This gradient precipitates a reduction in the RV stroke volume and concordant reduction in LV preload. While CRT is conventionally thought of as a therapy for LV failure there is emerging evidence that correcting interventricular dyssynchrony may have benefits for RV performance. Haddad et al. recently presented data suggesting that patients undergoing CRT-D implantation had significant improvements in their RV ejection fraction, end-systolic volume, and RV peak filling rate [12].

AV Dyssynchrony

While not the primary target of CRT, correction of AV dyssynchrony has increasingly been regarded as a critical function of CRT. Advanced first degree AV block is common in systolic heart failure and results in increased left atrial pressures, decreased LV diastolic filling times and diastolic mitral regurgitation due to the superimposition of atrial contraction (which occurs too early) and early diastolic LV filling. The echocardiographic hallmark of this phenomenon is fusion of the A and E waves. In contrast, short AV delays also reduce LV preload by causing interruption of active atrial transport via premature closure of the mitral valve.

Clinical Trial Data

Investigators have taken a stepwise approach to the evaluation of CRT beginning with small studies investigating the acute hemodynamic effects of CRT in patients with severe HF and culminating in large studies assessing mortality and long-term clinical outcomes in thousands of patients with milder degrees of HF. The seminal studies from this clinical trial program are summarized below:

NYHA FC III-IV

Early clinical trials on CRT focused on patients with NYHA class III or IV HF despite optimal medical therapy (OMT), and severe LV systolic dysfunction (LVEF < 35%) with evidence of electrical dyssynchrony defined as QRS prolongation of at least 120–150 (ms).

PATH-CHF

Encouraged by the short-term results of hemodynamic studies involving CRT, Auricchio et al. set out to define the longer term effects of biventricular or univentricular (LV) stimulation on functional capacity in 41 patients [13]. They demonstrated a net increase in peak oxygen consumption (peak VO_2) from 12.5 to 15.2 ml/kg/m/in ($p = 0.002$) and an improvement in 6-min walk from 342 to 416 m. PATH-CHF was the first study to establish the durability of CRTs effects with these clinical benefits persisting after 12 months of therapy [13].

MUSTIC

Cazeau et al. performed a single-blind, randomized, controlled crossover study assessing the clinical effects of CRT in patients with NYHA class III–IV symptoms and QRS durations >150 ms. Their unique crossover design overcame some of the methodological barriers of PATH-CHF which as a non-blinded study relying on effort dependent clinical endpoints like peak VO_2 and 6-min walk was susceptible to obvious biases. The study consisted of two phases including a 3-month period of active therapy (AV sequential pacing with CRT) and a 3-month period of inactive (ventricular inhibited pacing) allowing each patient to function as his/her own control. The group found that patients receiving CRT had improved 6-min walk distances, an 8% increase in peak VO_2, improved quality-of-life scores as assessed by the Minnesota Living With Heart Failure Questionnaire (MLWHFQ), and a 2/3 reduction in HF hospitalizations [14].

MIRACLE

Abraham et al., performed the first large-scale, double-blind, randomized clinical trial assessing the efficacy of CRT in patients with QRS durations >130 ms. All enrolled patients (n = 453) were implanted with CRT capable devices and then randomized to atrial-biventricular pacing vs. no pacing [15]. At 6 months of follow-up the CRT group experienced improvements in 6-min walk (+39 vs. +10 m, $p = 0.005$), functional class, quality of life, and EF (+4.6% vs. −0.2%, $p < 0.001$). Also observed was a reduction in HF hospitalizations (8 vs. 15%). While generally safe, this large scale study highlighted some of the potential complications of CRT implantation including failure to place a coronary sinus lead in 8% of patients, coronary sinus perforation, and death [15]. The MIRACLE trial led to approval of CRT by the Food and Drug Administration (FDA).

MIRACLE-ICD

CRTs rise was contemporaneous with a period of rapidly evolving guidelines for implantable cardioverter defibrillator (ICD) therapy. Young et al. went on to perform an analogous study in and identical patient population receiving devices with combined CRT and ICD functionality [16]. Three hundred sixty-nine patients were randomized to a control (ICD on/CRT off) or CRT group (ICD on/CRT on). At 6 months the CRT group had greater improvements in quality of life, functional class, and peak VO_2, but no difference in 6-min walk, EF, HF hospitalizations, or survival. Of critical importance, MIRACLE ICD highlighted the fact that the benefits of CRT could be achieved without evidence of proarrhythmia or compromise in ICD function.

Meta-Analysis of Studies with NYHA Class III-IV HF

A 2007 Meta-analysis published in the *Journal of the American Medical Association* summarized the results of the 14 randomized trials performed up to that point including 4420 patients [17]. This demonstrated improvements in NYHA functional class, 6-min walk, and quality of life metrics. There was an overall reduction in the rate of HF associated hospitalizations (RR 0.63, 95% CI 0.43–0.93) as well as a reduction in all-cause mortality (RR 0.78, 95% CI 0.67–0.91) driven by a reduction in deaths from "pump-failure" (RR 0.64; 95% CI 0.49–0.84) [17]. These benefits were achieved with a high rate of procedural success (93%) and low risk of complications.

COMPANION

While early studies hinted towards a potential improvement in hard clinical outcomes such as HF hospitalizations and HF and all-cause mortality, this question was first directly addressed in an appropriately powered study by Bristow et al. who randomized 1520 patients with QRS duration >120 ms in a 1:2:2 ratio to OMT, CRT-pacemaker (CRT-P), or CRT-defibrillator (CRT-D) [18]. In addition to conventional criteria for CRT enrolled patients had to have at least one HF hospitalization in the year prior to randomization. Compared to OMT, CRT-P and CRT-D both demonstrated reductions in the primary composite endpoint of time to death from or hospitalization for any cause (Hazard ratio 0.81 and 0.80 respectively). The combined end point of death from or hospitalization for HF was reduced by 34% in the CRT-P group and 40% in the CRT-D group. CRT-P patients had a non-significant reduction in all cause mortality whereas patients with CRT-D had a significant 36% reduction in the risk of all cause mortality ($p = 0.003$) [18]. The COMPANION trial led to FDA approval of combined CRT-D devices.

CARE-HF

Cleland et al. further examined the effects of CRT-P versus OMT on morbidity and mortality in 813 patients followed for 29 months and established for the first time that CRT-P alone provided a mortality benefit in patients with QRS duration >120 ms. Patients with CRT-P had a 37% reduction in the primary endpoint a composite of death from any cause or unplanned hospitalization for a major cardiovascular event. Similarly there was a 36% reduction in the secondary endpoint of all cause mortality [19]. The study also demonstrated a reduction in end-systolic volume index, mitral regurgitant jet volume, and improvement in LVEF and QoL. Subsequent longer-term follow-up from the CARE-HF investigators demonstrated that these reductions in mortality are durable and that they were due to a reduction in both sudden cardiac death and pump failure [20]. It is interesting to note that unlike prior studies (including COMPANION) the inclusion criteria for patients with intermediate QRS durations (i.e., between 120 and 149 ms) required two of three additional echocardiographic features of dyssynchrony including: aortic preejection delay of more than 140 ms, an interventricular mechanical delay of more than 40 ms, or delayed activation of the posterolateral LV wall [19].

NYHA FC I-II

The clinical trial program outlined above provided conclusive evidence that CRT reduced HF associated morbidity and mortality in patients with severe systolic heart failure. However, as the majority of HF patients are NYHA FC I and II, investigators began to ask whether earlier application of CRT could result in an inflexion point in the natural history of the disease.

MIRACLE-ICD II

Abraham et al. first assessed the efficacy of CRT-D in patients with NYHA class II symptoms and a QRS duration >130 ms [21]. CRT-D treated patients had no significant improvement in peak VO_2 but did see improvement in ventricular remodeling (LV systolic and diastolic volumes and LVEF). CRT-D patients demonstrated significant improvements in NYHA class and ventilator efficiency (VE/VCO_2) a well validated and effort-independent predictor of survival in patients with advanced HF [21].

REVERSE

Linde and Packer et al., examined the effects of CRT-D in patients with NYHA I and II HF with QRS durations >120 ms and with LVEF $\leq 40\%$ [22]. The large, randomized, double-blind trial enrolled 610 patients randomized 2:1 to CRT-D versus ICD alone. The primary endpoint was the novel clinical composite score which classified patients as "improved," "unchanged," or "worsened" based on a combination of mortality, HF hospitalizations, withdrawal from the study, or worsening NYHA class. The study included an American arm that proceeded for 12 months and a European arm that extended follow-up to 24 months. While there was no difference In the clinical composite score, CRT-D patients demonstrated significant reductions in the LV end-systolic volume index, improvements in LVEF, and a delay in the time-to-first HF hospitalization (hazard ratio: 0.47, $p = 0.03$).

RAFT

Tang et al., assessed the efficacy of CRT added to ICD therapy to reduce HF morbidity and hospitalizations in patients with NYHA FC II and III HF, QRS duration >120 ms, and LVEF < 30% [23]. In pre-specified subgroup analysis both patients with NYHA FC II and III symptoms had significant reductions in the composite endpoint of death or hospitalization for HF. Somewhat surprisingly, only the patients with NYHA II symptoms had a statistically significant reduction in all cause mortality (Hazard ratio 0.71; 95% CI 0.56–0.91).

MADIT-CRT

Moss et al. performed the largest and longest follow-up study to date of CRT in patients with mild HF (NYHA class I–II) in 1820 patients with LVEF of 30% or less and QRS duration >120 ms [24]. Importantly only NYHA class I patients with ischemic cardiomyopathy were included in the study. They demonstrated that during an average follow-up of 2.4 years CRT lead to a 34% reduction in the primary endpoint of death from any cause or nonfatal HF event. This was driven largely by a 41% reduction in HF events in the CRT group. Pre-specified subgroup analysis demonstrated that the majority of the clinical benefit was seen in patients with LBBB and QRS duration of ≥150 ms. In contrast to RAFT there was no demonstrable reduction in the risk of mortality in the CRT group.

Meta-Analysis of Studies with NYHA Class I-II HF

A meta-analysis and systematic review of CRT in patients with mild HF (NYHA FC I–II) was performed by Santangeli et al. [25]. These authors reviewed results from CONTAK-CD, MIRACLE-ICD-II, REVERSE, MADIT-CRT, and RAFT with 4213 patients (91% of whom were NYHA II functional class). They demonstrated a reduction in mortality (OR 0.78, 95% CI 0.63–0.97) and HF events (OR 0.63; 95% CI 0.52–0.76) [25]. In addition, they demonstrated beneficial reverse remodeling with an improvement in LVEF of 4.8% (95% CI 0.9–8.7%) and reduction in LV end-systolic volume index of -19.4 ml/m^2 (95% CI -18.2 to -20.7 ml/m^2).

While it is tempting to lump NYHA I and II patients together in this analysis, it is essential to note that only 372 patients (<20% of patients enrolled in REVERSE and MADIT-CRT and no patients in RAFT or MIRACLE-ICD II) were NYHA FC I. In fact in REVERSE, patients were required to have previously had NYHA II symptoms before enrollment. In the European REVERSE study, results trended toward favoring CRT-OFF in the NYHA I cohort. Subgroup analysis from MADIT-CRT demonstrated inconclusive results in NYHA I patients with ischemic cardiomyopathy. With uncertainty about benefit and increased early risk of adverse events (13% in CRT-D patients vs. 6.7% in ICD only patients in RAFT) guideline societies have generally tempered or removed recommendations for implantation in patients with NYHA I symptoms [23, 26].

Poor Uptake

Despite strong evidence for the use of CRT in certain populations, the uptake remains poor. A study of over 72,000 patients with data extracted from the GWTG-HF database and CMS showed that only 26.3% of eligible patients underwent CRT implant. While CRT utilization improved early in the study period from 2005–2007, it subsequently plateaued. As well, despite evidence showing women derive more benefit from CRT, white women were less likely to get CRT compared to white men. Black patients were also less likely to receive CRT compared to their white counterparts [27].

Observational data out of Europe suggests that 20–30% of patients have HFrEF with a prolonged QRS in a LBBB pattern. After implementation of GDMT—5–10% of patients remain CRT eligible which is ~400 patients/million inhabitants in Europe. Unfortunately, the actual CRT implant rates are 106–123 patients/million inhabitants suggesting that up to 2/3rds of eligible patients are going without CRT. Factors cited as reasons for non-referral include older age, lack of CRT implant centers, shorter duration of HF, absence of a HF nurses or non-cardiology follow-up [28].

Current Guidelines

In 2023, the Heart Rhythm Society, the Asia-Pacific HRS and the Latin America HRS released a joint guideline reviewing the evidence for cardiac physiologic pacing in the prevention and improvement of heart failure.

Pacing Strategies in Patients with Heart Failure

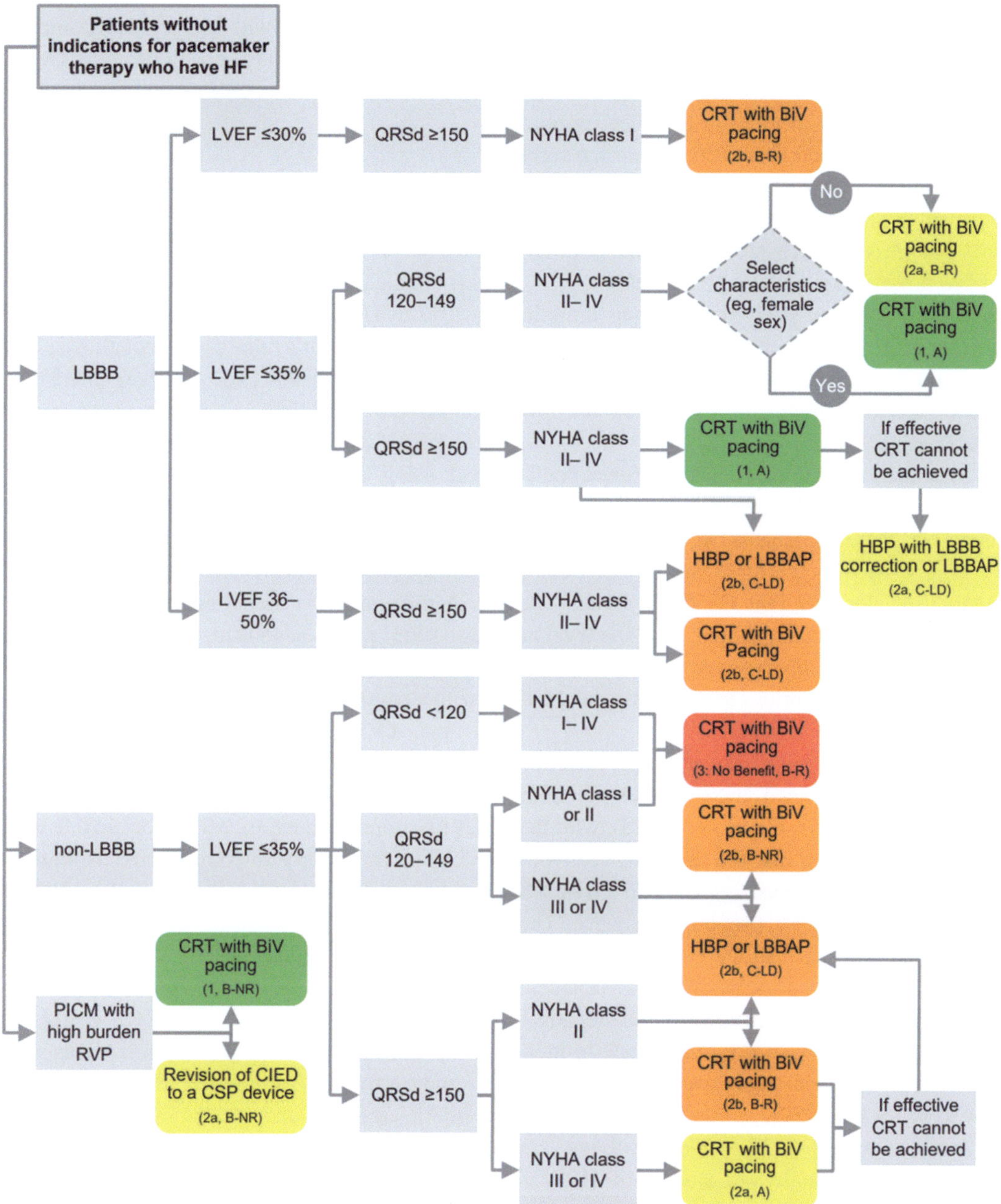

Reprinted from the 2023 HRS/APHRS/LAHRS guideline on cardiac physiologic pacing for the avoidance and mitigation of heart failure, Heart Rhythm 2023; 20(9), page e32, with permission from Elsevier.

Conduction System Pacing (CSP)

His Bundle Pacing

His bundle pacing (HBP) paces using the His-Purkinje system with the aim to reflect normal physiology. The lead is entirely within the right atrium and as such, AV and VV synchrony can be achieved simultaneously. As well, since the lead does not cross the tricuspid valve, HBP does not lead to downstream tricuspid regurgitation.

The first clinical study of HBP was done in the late 90's and in it, 12/14 patients were successfully paced but it was noted that procedure times were long, with high thresholds and low sensing [29].

Over time, more implanters have gained confidence with HBP leading to improved procedural times but there remains a significant learning curve. The Medtronic 3830 lead has been commonly used along with the C315 His sheath. The sheath allows the lead to be placed at the level of the His bundle, though implants may still be challenging if the right atrium is enlarged or the tricuspid annulus is displaced.

Early studies focused on attaining selective HBP which is defined by: stimulus to QRS (S-QRS) = native His to QRS (H-QRS), with the paced QRS looking like the native QRS. Non-selective HBP is defined as: S-QRS < H-QRS with the presence of a pseudo-delta wave. The paced QRS is wider than the native QRS by the H-QRS interval in non-selective HBP. In recent years, registry data from the Rush and Geisinger HBP registries has shown no difference in mortality/HF hospitalizations between selective and non-selective HBP [30].

A meta-analysis of 13 studies involving 503 patients, mostly single-arm studies of HBP as CRT, with 2 studies comparing HBP to conventional BiVP. Implant success rates were roughly 80%. An impressive reduction was seen in QRS duration from 165 to 123 ms and mean increases in LVEF of 14.7%. NYHA class by >1 class. With respect to safety, there was an increase in HB capture threshold in 6% of patients with repeat procedures needed in only 4 patients. Early battery depletion was seen in 5 patients [31].

The HIS SYNC II is underway currently which will enroll 987 patients and compare HBP to conventional CRT with the primary compsite outcome being time to HF hospitalization, LVAD or death.

Left Bundle Branch Area Pacing (LBBAP)

Left bundle area pacing was first done clinically in 2017 by Huang et al. and since then has gained popularity due to it's relative procedural ease and ability to capture the LBB at lower thresholds compared to HBP [32].

LBBAP is also done using the Medtronic 3830 lead using a fixed curve sheath. The lead is advanced across the septum until the LBBB changes to RBB delay or the QRS near normalizes suggesting that the LBB has been captured.

A meta-analysis including 10 studies enrolling 1063 patients looked at outcomes with LBBAP vs. conventional BiVP for CRT. LBBAP led to a significant reduction in QRS duration of 30 ms. LVEF improved by ~6% and more patients were classified as responders (LVEF improvement of >5%) and super responders (LVEF improvement of >20% or final LVEF > 50%). The primary outcome of HF hospitalizations was significantly reduced in the LBBAP arm by 40% [33].

The only RCT of LBBAP vs. BiVP for CRT called the LBBP RESYNC trial enrolled 40 patients. The LBBAP arm had a 5.6% change of LVEF in addition to that seen with BiVP as well as more patients were super responders. The LBBAP arm also had greater improvements in NT-proBNP as well as LVESV. QRS duration decreased similarly between the arms and was reduced by ~45 ms [34].

CSP was featured prominently in the 2023 HRS pacing guidelines. HBP with LBBB correction or LBBAP has a 2a recommendation for those where effective CRT cannot be achieved. In addition, in those with a wide QRS > 150 ms and a LVEF 36–50%, NYHA II-IV, both conventional CRT as well as CSP had a 2b recommendation. CSP also has a 2b recommendation in those with a non-LBBB, LVEF< 35% and an intermediate QRS duration (120–149 ms) with NYHA III/IV symptoms [35].

CSP can also be considered in lieu of conventional CRT in those who there is concern for high burden ventricular pacing with an LVEF of 36–50% with a class 2a recommendation. In addition, those who have AF and are undergoing an AVJ ablation with a LVEF < 50%, conventional CRT has a 2a recommendation, with a 2b recommendation for either a HBP lead or a LBBAP lead [35].

Implantation and Follow-Up

While initial studies in CRT necessitated epicardial LV lead placement via thoracotomy, currently the vast majority of patients can be successfully provided LV pacing via transvenous coronary sinus lead placement. The procedure is performed in an electrophysiology laboratory. Following creation of a subcutaneous pocket, RA and RV leads are placed with a standard approach via the axillary or cephalic vein (Fig. 23.1). A coronary sinus occlusion venogram is performed to identify a target vein and then using various guidewires and catheters the coronary sinus lead is positioned. This lead should ideally be positioned in the mid posterolateral aspect of the LV, thereby maximizing spatial separation from the RV lead. This degree of separation when assessed by a standard lateral chest roentogram has been shown to be predictive of acute hemodynamic response to CRT [36]. Pacing thresholds are assessed and because of the proximity of the posterolateral LV to both the left phrenic nerve and the diaphragm itself, diaphragmatic capture is assessed for.

Maximizing the likelihood of CRT response requires maintenance of continuous or near-continuous BiV pacing. While the precise threshold for optimal effect is unknown, prior retrospective analysis of large CRT trials demonstrated that the maximum benefit in reduction of HF hospitalizations and mortality was seen in patients receiving ≥92% BiV pacing [37] (See Fig. 23.2). Maximizing BiV pacing requires programming algorithms allowing for AV intervals short enough to minimize native conduction but long enough to facilitate optimal ventricular loading. Individual optimization of the AV delay was incorporated into most of the landmark CRT trials listed above.

Many methods for echo guided AV optimization exist. These rely on achieving optimal separation of the A and E waves on pulsed-wave Doppler of the mitral inflow, optimizing the Doppler-derived rate of pressure rise (derived from analysis of the mitral regurgitant jet), optimizing the myocardial performance index (Tei Index), or maximizing the LV outflow tract or

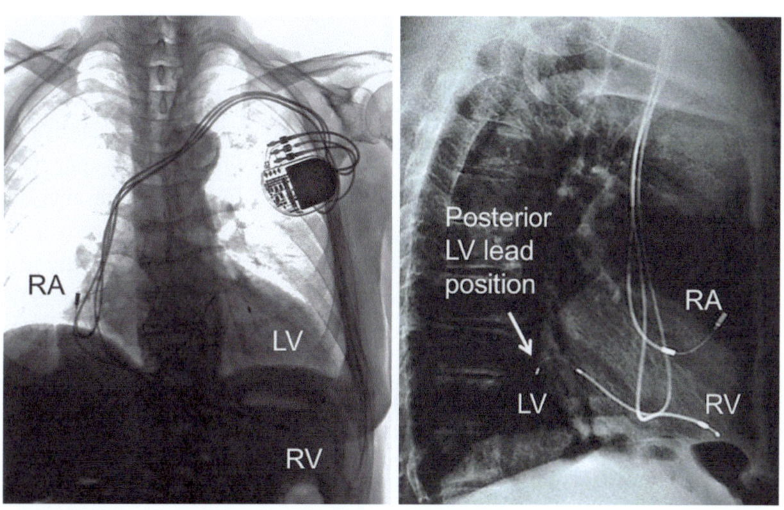

Fig. 23.1 Ideal lead position by AP and lateral CXR. Note the position of the LV lead in the mid to basal aspect of the posterolateral wall. Also note the degree of spatial separation between the RV and LV lead tips in the lateral projection

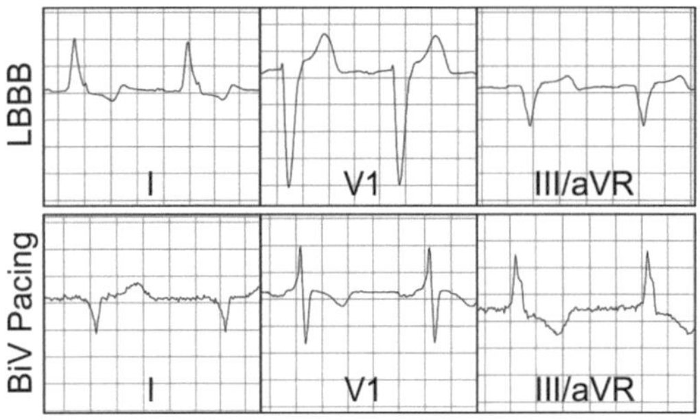

Fig. 23.2 ECG changes associated with biventricular stimulation. Top row demonstrates typical ECG findings of complete left bundle branch block (*LBBB*). The bottom row demonstrates desired changes in the ECG accompanying biventricular (*BiV*) pacing. Stimulation from the posterolateral aspect of the LV generates anterior forces represented as a positive deflection in the anteroseptal pre-precordial leads (V1–V3). The left-to-right and basal-to-apical progression of electrical activation from an optimally positioned lead should also result in the reversal of polarity in leads I, III, and aVR demonstrated above

aortic flow velocity profile (VTI) [38]. Prospective studies assessing the effect of automated or echo-guided AV optimization have demonstrated no benefit in functional status, quality-of-life, or ventricular remodeling versus a fixed AV delay of 120 milliseconds [39]. Similarly, while current devices allow for multiple configurations of biventricular or LV pacing, recent studies have failed to demonstrate a clear benefit of biventricular pacing over LV only pacing [40]. While failing to consistently demonstrate efficacy in clinical trials, in individual patients, AV optimization can be critical to maximizing the frequency of ventricular pacing.

Safety and Complications

Between 2 and 6% of LV leads cannot be placed via the transvenous approach and require epicardial lead placement via thoracotomy [41] Between 4 and 10% of patients experience a clinically significant lead dislodgement necessitating repositioning [17]. The incidence of other complications has been assessed and reported in a recent review in the *Journal of the American Medical Association* [17]. In 54 reviewed studies including over 6000 patients the implant success rate was 93% with peri-procedural complications occurring in 4% of cases and peri-procedural death occurring in 0.3% of patients [17]. Coronary sinus dissection or perforation can occur, but is rarely a fatal complication owing to the relatively low pressure of the cardiac venous system with pericardial effusion/tamponade complicating only 0.6–1.2% of cases. Just over 1% of patients developed device site infections consistent with the reported risk of infectious complications of 1–2% for all implanted electrophysiologic devices.

Clinical Response and Non-responders

One of the challenges in assessing CRT efficacy in clinical trials has been disagreement regarding what outcomes should be used to assess response. Fornwalt et al. recently assessed the agreement among the 15 most common response-criteria used in 26 published CRT studies (Table 23.1). They found that 99% of patients in these studies were CRT "responders" on the basis of at least 1 criteria, but that 75% of comparisons between response-criteria demonstrated poor agreement [42]. The selection of response-criteria also has important implications on trial design as end-points such as quality of life, 6-min walk, and peak VO_2 are either subjective or effort dependent measures that are susceptible to bias. Substudy analysis from MADIT-CRT began to identify characteristics associated with patients who are "super-responders" to CRT [43] Table 23.2 presents other clinical features demonstrating efficacy in predicting response to CRT along with supporting references [43–51]. Importantly, to date, no features have demonstrated more reliability in predicting response to CRT than QRS duration and the presence of LBBB [52].

Table 23.1 Definition of CRT response [35]

Response	Criteria
Clinical response	1. Reduction in mortality
	2. Reduction in HF hospitalization
	3. Improvement in NYHA class
	4. Improvement in quality of life, symptoms, or clinical composite scores
	5. Increase in peak VO_2 (eg, >10%)
	6. Improvement in 6-minute walk distance
	7. Reduction in HF medications, such as diuretic therapy (note: continuation of GDMT is advised)
Echocardiographic response	1. Improvement or stability in LVEF (eg, ≥5% absolute increase or absence of worsening)
	2. Reduction in LV size (eg, reduction in LV systolic or diastolic dimensions or volume indices)
	3. Increase in LV stroke volume
	4. Reduction in mitral regurgitation

Reprinted from the 2023 HRS/APHRS/LAHRS guideline on cardiac physiologic pacing for the avoidance and mitigation of heart failure, Heart Rhythm 2023; 20(9), page e25, with permission from Elsevier

While the majority of appropriately selected patients derive clinical benefit from CRT, approximately 30% of patients with appropriate QRS criteria are nonresponders without improvement in symptoms, ventricular remodeling, or HF hospitalizations. Mullens et al. demonstrated that a multi-disciplinary CRT nonresponder clinic could successfully identify and intervene on omissions or insufficiencies in the care of CRT nonresponders in a positive way. Interventions addressed suboptimal AV delay, loss of BiV pacing due to arrhythmia, suboptimal LV lead position, and suboptimal HF pharmacotherapy [28, 53, 54].

Table 23.2 Conventional predictors of CRT response [43–51]

	Response more likely	Response less likely
Qrs duration [43]	≥150 ms	<150 ms
BBB pattern [43]	LBBB	RBBB or IVCD
Cardiomyopathy [43]	Nonischemic	Ischemic
Gender [43]	Female	Male
Dyssynchrony [44, 48]	Present	Absent
BMI < 30 kg/m^2 [43]	Present	Absent
Left atrial size [43]	Smaller	Larger
Scar burden [49, 50]	Low burden	High Burden
	Non-transmural	Transmural
	Posterolateral viable	Posterolateral scar
Mitral regurgitation [45, 46]	Mild-moderate	Severe
RV dysfunction [47]	None-mild	Severe
Lead position [51]	Posterior or lateral	Anterior or apical

Strategies in Non-responders

Studies have shown that more biventricular pacing (BiVP) is associated with improved outcomes namely HF and mortality [55–57] and as such, efforts should be made to attain near 100% biventricular pacing.

PVC Ablation

In those with reduced biventricular pacing secondary to frequent PVCs, studies have shown that PVC suppression is beneficial in improving BiVP percentage. One study of 64 patients who either underwent PVC/VT ablation compared to medical therapy, found that the former group had a higher increase in BiVP and more patients also showed improvements in NYHA class [58].

Another study of CRT non-responders who underwent PVC ablation for a significant PVC burden (>10,000 PVCs/day) showed improvements in BiVP from 76% to 98% and associated improvements in LV function, decreased LV size as well as improvements in NYHA functional class [59].

AV and VV Optimization

While physiologically, AV optimization makes sense, it has not been shown to improve outcomes in randomized trials, but a subset may benefit. While ECHO guided optimization of the AV interval is the gold standard, it is laborious and requires multiple providers at the bedside. Several device-based AV optimization algorithms now exist that allow for repeated AV delay adjustments.

AdaptivCRT (Medtronic) was compared to echo optimization in the Adaptive CRT trial. This device-based algorithm works to assess intrinsic conduction every minute. In the setting of normal AV conduction, adaptive LV pacing occurs. In the setting of prolonged AV conduction, the algorithm switches to adaptive BiVP. Studies have shown AdaptivCRT to be non-inferior to echo based optimization when looking at a clinical composite score (CCS). In addition, there was a significant reduction in 30-day readmissions for HF [60]. Other device-based algorithms such as SmartDelay (Boston Scientific) and SyncAV (Abbott) as well as QuickOpt (Abbott) are also available.

Various metrics exist to guide V-V delay including QLV (measured from the start of the surface QRS to the peak of the R wave on the LV EGM) and RV-LV timing. In the SMART AV trial, both measures were highly correlated ($R^2 = 0.71$), but in a multivariable model, RV-LV emerged as the predictor associated with CRT response and reverse remodeling [61].

SyncAV works by extending the AV delay for 3 beats every 256 beats allowing it to measure the intrinsic AV interval. Fifty milliseconds is then subtracted and this becomes the paced AV interval until the cycle repeats itself. Ventricular pacing can be configured to BiV, LV only or a specific RV-LV delay. As such, this can promote "triple fusion [62]" It has been studied in a real world, propensity matched study comparing SyncAV ON vs. OFF, those who had SyncAV ON had an additional reduction in HFH on top of standard CRT [63].

MSP and MPP

Multi-site pacing (MSP) refers to BiVP from 3 leads—usually 2 LV and 1 RV but may also be 2 RV + 1 LV configuration. In contrast, multi-point pacing (MPP) is pacing from more than one pole of a quadripolar lead. The rationale is to decrease LV activation time which then should lead to improved contractility and clinical outcomes.

Animal models have shown improved dP/dt and some observational studies have shown improvements in hemodynamics, LVEF and functional capacity with MSP and MPP [64, 65]. The MPP study, a trial that randomized 381 patients 3 months after CRT implant, showed that MPP was non-inferior to BiVP when using a clinical composite score [66]. SMART MSP enrolled CRT non-responders (NR) 6 months post-CRT implant and found that 51.3% of prior NR were now responders via a CCS [67]. A subsequent study called MORE-CRT-MPP looking at 467 non-responders was negative and showed no significant difference in converting NR to responders [68].

While technically MPP is more feasible than MSP, it is not in routine use due to conflicting data as above. However, a post hoc analysis of the MPP study showed that a distance of 30 mm between LV1 and LV2 as well as a delay of at least 5 ms portended a higher response rate suggesting that perhaps the differences in the studies were secondary to programming [66]. Phase II of MORE CRT MPP will address this issue.

LV Endocardial Pacing

Wireless stimulation endocardial CRT (WiSE CRT) is a novel technology by which an endocardial receiver electrode is placed in the LV and then is powered wirelessly by a subcutaneous ultrasound pulse transmitter. The system also includes a standard pacemaker or ICD and the transmitter synchronizes with RV pacing, emits a signal, that then causes LV pacing. The LV electrode is placed via a retrograde aortic approach. The first in-man experience was in 2013 [69].

A meta-analysis involving 5 studies with 175 patients reviewed outcomes with WiSE CRT. In this analysis, WiSE CRT showed statistically significant reductions in QRS duration and LV volumes as well as improvements in LVEF [70].

The technology is not without risk, in the SELECT LV study—3 of 34 patients had serious adverse events (AE) including VF during implant (requiring a prolonged resuscitation), electrode embolization to the L tibial artery and then subsequent development of a femoral artery fistula requiring surgical repair. An additional 8 patients had AE within a month including a stroke, 3 infections, 2 femoral artery pseudoaneurysms, 1 pocket hematoma and 1 death (of the aforementioned VF patient) [71].

ALSYNC included 118 patients who all received LV endocardial pacing with a 3830 Medtronic pacing lead placed via a transseptal puncture. All patients enrolled were either CRT non-responders or had failed CS implants. Overall, both groups improved LVEF, NYHA class and quality of life with reductions in LVESVi. Those with a failed CS implant were more likely to have a CRT super response (LVESVi reduction >30%) compared to prior non-responders [72].

Poor Prognosis in Non-responders

Chung et al. reviewed 5 prospective CRT studies and classified patients as improved, stabilized or worsened at 6 months post-CRT based on LVESVi or CCS. Compared to the group who worsened, those who improved or even stabilized post-CRT on the basis of either metric had a significant reduction in mortality The same held true for annual-adjusted HF hospitalizations [73].

In the ADVANCE CRT registry that looked at 1327 patients at 69 centers, in those who were defined as non-responders, 44% received no interventions to improve their response to CRT. Similar to the Chung paper, the authors found a 3-fold increase in all cause hospitalizations in the non-responder group at 6–12 months. There was also an astounding 5-fold increase in mortality in this group [74].

In summary, there is some benefit to be seen by stabilizing patients with CRT. Those who continue to worsen are at high risk for HF hospitalizations and death and need to be followed closely for the need for advanced therapies [73, 74].

In addition, average US Medicare reimbursement is nearly double in the CRT non-responders ($13,861/patient year vs. $7205 USD/patient year).

In the case of patients who do respond to CRT it is critical that the augmentation of blood pressure and cardiac performance provided by CRT be used as an opportunity to titrate neurohormonal antagonists. Small retrospective studies have demonstrated that CRT facilitates titration of BB and ACEI with simultaneous weaning of diuretics [75].

Atrial Fibrillation

Atrial fibrillation (AF) is exceedingly common in patients with HF and becomes more prevalent with increasing degrees of HF severity. The OPTIME CHF and CONSENSUS studies assessing the utility of milrinone and enalapril respectively in patients with NYHA IV symptoms demonstrated a prevalence of 35–50% [76]. It is therefore not surprising that AF is amongst the most common reasons for loss of BiV pacing by facilitating rapid AV conduction that outpaces programmed AV delays or exceeding the upper tracking limit. For this reason, CRT trials have uniformly excluded patients with AF.

Particularly in patients with AF it is critical to confirm biventricular pacing by ECG as device diagnostics may spuriously report BiV pacing. Kamath et al. demonstrated that 12-lead Holter monitoring in patients with permanent atrial fibrillation frequently revealed inadequate BiV pacing percentages in patients with device diagnostics reporting very high rates of BiV pacing [77]. Approaches to AF in CRT include algorithms to achieve higher BiV pacing rates including ventricular sensed response, conducted AF response, and atrial tracking recovery; intensification of rate control; anti-arrhythmic drug therapy; and ultimately AV nodal ablation. The updated ACC/AHA/HRS guidelines provide a IIa indication for CRT in these patients only if appropriate measures are taken to achieve high rates of BiV pacing (Table 23.1).

Evidence for AVN Ablation and CRT

Ganesan et al. performed a meta-analysis examining the utility of AVN ablation in AF patients combined with CRT. They demonstrated that AVN ablation was associated with significant reductions in all-cause and cardiovascular mortality, as well as improvement in mean NYHA functional class when compared to rate control strategies [78].

Since then, the CERTIFY study, an observational prospective study at 95 European centers, was published compared outcomes in patients with AF who underwent CRT and then underwent AVN ablation vs. rate control. They found long term survival to be similar in sinus rhythm compared to the AF+AVJ ablation and worse survival in the group on rate control alone [79].

Similar results were seen out of Italy in a propensity matched analysis, where patients with HFrEF, a narrow QRS and permanent AF who underwent an AVN ablation and CRT had similar prognosis to those who were in NSR undergoing ICD alone, but significantly lower mortality than those who remained in AF in the control arm [80].

Another pooled analysis of data from 3358 CRT patients enrolled in ADVANCE CRT-D, ADVANCE III and the Italian Clinical Service prospective observational project revealed a reduction in ICD shocks as well as in all cause and HF hospitalizations in the AVN ablation/CRT arm vs. AF+drugs arm [81].

APAF CRT was a RCT that enrolled patients with severe symptomatic AF of more than 6 months duration, narrow QRS (<110 ms) and one HF hospitalization in the preceding year regardless of LVEF and randomized to AVN ablation/CRT vs. rate control with medications. Despite a small sample size, there was an astounding 18% absolute risk reduction in death from any cause in an ITT analysis [82]. Subsequent editorials have called into question the validity of these results given a low fragility index [83] and have called for larger RCT to see if these results can be replicated.

Controversies in CRT

Mechanical Dyssynchrony and Narrow Complex QRS

Currently, only a minority of HF patients meet the QRS criteria for CRT and not all CRT candidates are clinical responders. As such, there are ongoing efforts to identify measures of mechanical dyssynchrony that can assist in better predicting response. Beshai et al. assessed the utility of CRT in 172 patients with narrow QRS complexes but with echocardiographic evidence of mechanical dyssynchrony (defined as opposing-wall delay of ≥65 ms on tissue Doppler imaging or a mechanical dyssynchrony in the septal-to-posterior wall of ≥130 ms) in the ReithinQ trial. They found that while CRT treated patients had a significant improvement in NYHA class there was no significant improvement in quality of life, 6-min walk, LV reverse remodeling, or the primary endpoint of peak VO_2 [84]. The Predictors of Response to CRT (PROSPECT) trial assessed the efficacy of 12 echocardiographic parameters of mechanical dyssynchrony in predicting CRT response in 498 patients as evinced by an improvement in clinical composite score and a ≥15% reduction in the LV end systolic volume at 6 months. In general these parameters demonstrated poor sensitivity and specificity with receiver operating characteristic area under the curves (ROC AUC) for most parameters falling between 0.5 and 0.6 [85].

In contrast to these disappointing results, the Speckle Tracking and Resynchronization (STAR) study assessed the ability of radial, circumferential, transverse, and longitudinal strain evidence of mechanical dyssynchrony (≥130 ms opposing wall delay) to predict improvements in LVEF and adverse long-term events including death, transplant, or left ventricular assist device therapy. Radial and transverse dyssynchrony predicted improved LVEF response. Interestingly, patients undergoing CRT without transverse or radial dyssynchrony had a significantly higher rate of adverse HF endpoints [44]. In the NARROW-CRT study, Muto et al., demonstrated that in patients with ischemic cardiomyopathy, narrow QRS complexes and echocardiographic evidence of mechanical dyssynchrony (≥60 ms difference in septal and lateral time-to-peak systolic velocity), CRT-D resulted in improvements in clinical composite scores and a reduction in the composite endpoint of HF hospitalization, HF death, and spontaneous ventricular fibrillation [48]. While intriguing STAR and NARROW-CRT were small studies and require corroboration in larger scale trials. While data has not yet been published, the largest study to date investigating CRT in patients with narrow QRS complexes, EchoCRT was terminated early due to futility after recruiting over 1000 patients [86]. LESSER EARTH was also terminated early for futility and safety concerns after randomizing 85 patients [87].

Patients with NYHA Class IV HF

The majority of patients in CRT trials of advanced HF patients had NYHA class III symptoms with ambulatory class IV patients representing a small minority. These were truly ambulatory patients with resting HF symptoms and did not include patients requiring inotropic or parenteral vasodilator therapy. Sub-study analysis of 217 ambulatory class IV patients from the COMPANION trial demonstrated that CRTP and CRTD provided substantial reductions in HF hospitalization and all-cause mortality [88]. Subsequent studies have demonstrated improvements in ventricular remodeling and clinical composite scores. Despite these benefits, studies continue to show that 1- and 2-year mortality remain high in these patients at 25% and 38% respectively [89].

Hernandez et al. reviewed 151 patients in 8 studies who were inotrope dependent and received a CRT device. Seven out of the eight studies reported successful inotrope wean. Six studies reported an improvement in NYHA class, 35% to Class II, 43% to Class III with all patients being Class IV at baseline. Twelve-month survival in this high-risk population was 69% including 6 patients who underwent heart transplant. Fifty-three patients had died at 1 year or had undergone LVAD [90].

While CRT should generally not be regarded as a salvage therapy for end-stage ACC/AHA stage D HF patients, it may be appropriate in selected individuals.

CRT in LVAD Patients

While great strides have been made in cardiac resynchronization therapy (CRT) in the last decade, there remains a 1/3 CRT non-response rate, some of these patients will go on to have left ventricular assist devices. Given that they are non-responders, ongoing use of the LV lead only serves to deplete the battery and lead to the need for generator changes which as mentioned above, are associated with significant morbidity.

Hemodynamic studies have not shown any change in cardiac indices or filling pressures comparing CRT to RV pacing post-LVAD [91, 92]. In fact, Chung et al. showed an improvement with RV pacing in daily step count, 6MWT distance and KCCQ-12 score compared to BiV pacing when they studied 30 patients in a crossover fashion. They also noted that significantly fewer patients had NSVT or sustained VT during RV pacing vs. BiV pacing (13% vs. 30%, $p = 0.03$) [93]. In addition, the TRAViATA registry found an increased risk of late RV failure in those with a CRT-D device [94].

A 2021 meta-analysis looking at 7 retrospective studies and 1 RCT showed no differences in mortality and all-cause hospitalizations in the RV vs. BiV pacing groups. In those who had a CRT device and had the CRT ON compared with CRT OFF, there was a lower number of VA and ICD shocks in the CRT ON group but it should be noted that the CRT OFF group was sicker [95]. Chou et al. found that the group who had LV pacing ON had more VA and ES, though it was not a randomized comparison and in this trial, the LV pacing ON group was sicker and there was no protective effect seen of LV pacing [96].

Patients with LVEF > 35%

There are several studies examining the utility of CRT in patients with moderately reduced LV systolic function (LVEF 35–45%). Substudy analysis from the PROSPECT trial including 86 patients with LVEF > 35% demonstrated benefits comparable to patients with more severely depressed EFs in LV end systolic volume and clinical composite score [97]. In the BLOCK-HF trial, Curtis et al. examined the role of CRT vs. RV pacing in 691 patients with advanced atrioventricular block necessitating pacing and an LVEF ≤ 50% with NYHA class I–III symptoms. They demonstrated a 26% reduction in the primary composite endpoint of time to death from any cause, urgent care visit for HF, or a 15% or more increase in LV end-systolic volume index in patients with a mean QRS duration of 122 ms [98]. MIRACLE EF was to assess the utility of CRT-P in those with LVEF 35–50% and LBBB, it was stopped early due to poor enrollment after 13 months [99].

Non LBBB Patients

A study by Kawata et al. used Medicare data from the NCDR looking at patients who had non-LBBB but received CRT-D. In those with RBBB, CRT was not associated with improved outcomes. However, in those with an IVCD and wide QRS > 150 ms, CRT-D reduced mortality at 3 years vs. ICD alone [100].

Similar findings were seen when patient level data from 6264 patients was analyzed from 8 landmark CRT trials (MIRACLE, MIRACLE ICD, MIRACLE ICD II, REVERSE, RAFT, BLOCK HF, COMPANION, MADIT CRT). In patients with a QRS duration >150 ms, both LBBB and IVCD were associated with a lower risk of death or HF hospitalization, but RBBB was not [101].

LBBAP may hold some promise in those with RBBB. In a retrospective, multicenter observational study, 121 patients with RBBB, wide QRS > 120 ms, NYHA II-IV and LVEF < 50% with an indication for pacing or CRT underwent LBBAP. The implant was successful in 88% (107 patients). There was mild QRS narrowing (156 ms to 150 ms) with roughly a third had complete elimination of the RBBB. An improvement in LVEF from 35% to 43% was also seen on echo [102].

Similar results were seen in a recent propensity matched analysis by Tan et al. comparing CSP (either HBP or LBBAP) to BiVP in 96 consecutive patients with non-LBBB patterns (51% were RBBB). Patients who underwent CSP were more likely to have an echo response (LVEF improvement of >10%). In addition, there was a 58% relative risk reduction in the composite of mortality and HF hospitalizations [103].

Summary

CRT has emerged as a critically important therapy for patients with persistent symptoms of systolic HF despite optimal medical therapy. An extensive program of clinical trials has demonstrated substantial benefits in HF morbidity and mortality in appropriately selected patients. Current efforts focus on refining candidate selection to identify patients most likely to respond and perhaps expand candidacy with conduction system pacing to patients who do not meet conventional criteria. More efforts need to be made to identify non-responders as they portend a very high-risk group.

Competing Interests The authors declare no competing interests.

References

1. Jessup M, Brozena S. Heart failure. N Engl J Med. 2003;348(20):2007–18. CrossRef PubMed.
2. Wiggers CJ. The muscle reactions of the mammalian ventricles to artificial surface stimuli. Am J Phys. 1925;73:346–78.
3. Askenazi J, Alexander JH, Koenigsberg DI, Belic N, Lesch M. Alteration of left ventricular performance by left bundle branch block simulated with atrioventricular sequential pacing. Am J Cardiol. 1984;53(1):99–104. CrossRef PubMed.
4. Burkhoff D, Oikawa RY, Sagawa K. Influence of pacing site on canine left ventricular contraction. Am J Phys. 1986;251(2 Pt 2):H428–35.
5. Zile MR, Blaustein AS, Shimizu G, Gaasch WH. Right ventricular pacing reduces the rate of left ventricular relaxation and filling. J Am Coll Cardiol. 1987;10(3):702–9. CrossRef PubMed.
6. Gottipaty V, Krelis S, Lu F. Vesnarinone study analysis (abstract 847–4). J Am Coll Cardiol. 1999;33(2):145.
7. Lattuca JJ, Cohen TJ, Mower MM. Biventricular pacing to improve cardiac hemodynamics. Clin Rev. 1990;38:882.
8. Cazeau S, Ritter P, Bakdach S, Lazarus A, Limousin M, Henao L, et al. Four chamber pacing in dilated cardiomyopathy. Pacing Clin Electrophysiol. 1994;17(11 Pt 2):1974–9. CrossRef PubMed.
9. Nelson GS, Berger RD, Fetics BJ, Talbot M, Spinelli JC, Hare JM, et al. Left ventricular or biventricular pacing improves cardiac function at diminished energy cost in patients with dilated cardiomyopathy and left bundle-branch block. Circulation. 2000;102(25):3053–9. CrossRef PubMed.
10. Thackray S, Easthaugh J, Freemantle N, Cleland JGF. The effectiveness and relative effectiveness of intravenous inotropic drugs acting through the adrenergic pathway in patients with heart failure—a meta-regression analysis. Eur J Heart Fail. 2002;4(4):515–29. CrossRef PubMed.
11. Kass DA. Pathobiology of cardiac dyssynchrony and resynchronization. Heart Rhythm. 2009;6(11):1660–5. CrossRef PubMed PubMedCentral.
12. Haddad H, Dwivedi G, Haddad T, Abo-Shasha R, McArdle B, Wells RG, et al. The effect of CRT therapy on RV function in patients with severe LV dysfunction: a Matched Control Study. J Am Coll Cardiol. 2013;61(10_S):e649.
13. Auricchio A, Stellbrink C, Sack S, Block M, Jü V, Bakker P, et al. Long-term clinical effect of hemodynamically optimized cardiac resynchronization therapy in patients with heart failure and ventricular conduction delay. J Am Coll Cardiol. 2002;39(12):2026–33. CrossRef PubMed.
14. Cazeau S, Leclercq C, Lavergne T, Walker S, Varma C, Linde C, et al. Effects of multisite biventricular pacing in patients with heart failure and intraventricular conduction delay. N Engl J Med. 2001;344(12):873–80. CrossRef PubMed.
15. Abraham WT, Fisher WG, Smith AL, Delurgio DB, Leon AR, Loh E, et al. Cardiac resynchronization in chronic heart failure. N Engl J Med. 2002;346(24):1845–53. CrossRef PubMed.
16. Young JB, Abraham WT, Smith AL, Leon AR, Lieberman R, Wilkoff B, Canby RC, Schroeder JS, Liem LB, Hall S, Wheelan K, Multicenter InSync ICD Randomized Clinical Evaluation (MIRACLE ICD) Trial Investigators. Combined cardiac resynchronization and implantable cardioversion defibrillation in advanced chronic heart failure: the miracle icd trial. JAMA. 2003;289(20):2685–94.
17. McAlister Fa EJHN, et al. Cardiac resynchronization therapy for patients with left ventricular systolic dysfunction: a systematic review. JAMA. 2007;297(22):2502–14. CrossRef PubMed.
18. Bristow MR, Saxon LA, Boehmer J, Krueger S, Kass DA, De Marco T, et al. Cardiac-resynchronization therapy with or without an implantable defibrillator in advanced chronic heart failure. New Engl J Med. 2004;350(21):2140–50. CrossRef PubMed.
19. Cleland JGF, Daubert J-C, Erdmann E, Freemantle N, Gras D, Kappenberger L, et al. The effect of cardiac resynchronization on morbidity and mortality in heart failure. N Engl J Med. 2005;352(15):1539–49. CrossRef PubMed.
20. Cleland JGF, Daubert J-C, Erdmann E, Freemantle N, Gras D, Kappenberger L, et al. Longer-term effects of cardiac resynchronization therapy on mortality in heart failure [the CArdiac REsynchronization-Heart

Failure (CARE-HF) trial extension phase]. Eur Heart J. 2006;27(16):1928–32. CrossRef PubMed.
21. Abraham WT, Young JB, León AR, Adler S, Bank AJ, Hall SA, et al. Effects of cardiac resynchronization on disease progression in patients with left ventricular systolic dysfunction, an indication for an implantable cardioverter-defibrillator, and mildly symptomatic chronic heart failure. Circulation. 2004;110(18):2864–8. CrossRef PubMed.
22. Linde C, Abraham WT, Gold MR, St. John Sutton M, Ghio S, Daubert C. Randomized trial of cardiac resynchronization in mildly symptomatic heart failure patients and in asymptomatic patients with left ventricular dysfunction and previous heart failure symptoms. J Am Coll Cardiol. 2008;52(23):1834–43. CrossRef PubMed.
23. Tang ASL, Wells GA, Talajic M, Arnold MO, Sheldon R, Connolly S, et al. Cardiac-resynchronization therapy for mild-to-moderate heart failure. N Engl J Med. 2010;363(25):2385–95. CrossRef PubMed.
24. Moss AJ, Hall WJ, Cannom DS, Klein H, Brown MW, Daubert JP, et al. Cardiac-resynchronization therapy for the prevention of heart-failure events. N Engl J Med. 2009;361(14):1329–38. CrossRef PubMed.
25. Santangeli P, Di Biase L, Pelargonio G, Dello Russo A, Casella M, Bartoletti S, et al. Cardiac resynchronization therapy in patients with mild heart failure: a systematic review and meta-analysis. J Interv Card Electrophysiol. 2011;32(2):125–35. CrossRef PubMed.
26. Stevenson WG, Hernandez AF, Carson PE, Fang JC, Katz SD, Spertus JA, et al. Indications for cardiac resynchronization therapy: 2011 update from the Heart Failure Society of America Guideline Committee. J Card Fail. 2012;18(2):94–106. CrossRef PubMed.
27. Randolph TC, Hellkamp AS, Zeitler EP, Fonarow GC, Hernandez AF, Thomas KL, et al. Utilization of cardiac resynchronization therapy in eligible patients hospitalized for heart failure and its association with patient outcomes. Am Heart J. 2017;189:48–58.
28. Mullens W, Aurichhio A, Martens P, Witte K, Cowie MR, et al. Optimized implementation of cardiac resynchronization therapy: a call for action for referral and optimization of care: a joint position statement from the Heart Failure Association (HFA), European Heart Rhythm Association (EHRA), and European Association of Cardiovascular Imaging (EACVI) of the European Society of Cardiology. Eur J Heart Fail. 2020;22(12):2349–69.
29. Deshmukh P, Casavant DA, Romanyshyn M, Andersen K. Permanent, direct His-bundle pacing: a novel approach to cardiac pacing in patients with normal His-Purkinje activation. Circulation. 2000;101(8):869–77.
30. Beer D, Sharma PS, Subzposh FA, Naperkowski A, Pietrasik GM, Durr B, et al. Clinical outcomes of selective versus nonselective his bundle pacing. JACC Clin Electrophysiol. 2019;5(7):766–74.
31. Qi J, Jia X, Wang Z. His bundle pacing for cardiac resynchronization therapy: a systematic literature review and meta-analysis. J Interv Card Electrophysiol. 2020;59(2):463–70.
32. Huang W, Su L, Wu S, Xu L, Xiao F, Zhou X, Ellenbogen KA, et al. A novel pacing strategy with low and stable output: pacing the left bundle branch immediately beyond the conduction block. Can J Cardiol. 2017;33:1736.e1–3.
33. Parlavecchio A, Vetta G, Caminiti R, Coluccia G, Magnocavallo M, Ajello M, et al. Left bundle branch pacing versus biventricular pacing for cardiac resynchronization therapy: a systematic review and meta-analysis. Pacing Clin Electrophysiol. 2023;46(5):432–9.
34. Wang Y, Zhu H, Hou X, Wang Z, Zou F, Qian Z, et al. Randomized trial of left bundle branch vs biventricular pacing for cardiac resynchronization therapy. J Am Coll Cardiol. 2022;80(13):1205–16.
35. Chung MK, Patton KK, Lau CP, Dal Forno ARJ, Al-Khatib SM, Arora V, et al. 2023 HRS/APHRS/LAHRS guideline on cardiac physiologic pacing for the avoidance and mitigation of heart failure. J Arrhythm. 2023;39(5):681–756.
36. Heist EK, Fan D, Mela T, Arzola-Castaner D, Reddy VY, Mansour M, et al. Radiographic left ventricular–right ventricular interlead distance predicts the acute hemodynamic response to cardiac resynchronization therapy. Am J Cardiol. 2005;96(5):685–90. CrossRef PubMed.
37. Koplan BA, Kaplan AJ, Weiner S, Jones PW, Seth M, Christman SA. Heart failure decompensation and all-cause mortality in relation to percent biventricular pacing in patients with heart failure. J Am Coll Cardiol. 2009;53(4):355–60. CrossRef PubMed.
38. Dimaano VLJ, Abraham TP. The role of echocardiography and tissue doppler imaging in optimal cardiac resynchronization therapy. In: Abraham WT, Baliga RR, editors. Cardiac resynchronization therapy in heart failure. Philadelphia: Lippincott Williams & Wilkins; 2010. p. 59–75.
39. Ellenbogen KA, Gold MR, Meyer TE, Fernndez Lozano I, Mittal S, Waggoner AD, et al. Primary results from the smartdelay determined av optimization: a comparison to other av delay methods used in cardiac resynchronization therapy (SMART-AV) Trial: a randomized trial comparing empirical, echocardiography-guided, and algorithmic atrioventricular delay programming in cardiac resynchronization therapy. Circulation. 2010;122(25):2660–8. CrossRef PubMed.
40. Boriani G, Gardini B, Diemberger I, Bacchi Reggiani ML, Biffi M, Martignani C, et al. Meta-analysis of randomized controlled trials evaluating left ventricular vs. biventricular pacing in heart failure: effect on all-cause mortality and hospitalizations. Eur J Heart Fail. 2012;14(6):652–60. CrossRef PubMed.

41. León AR, Abraham WT, Curtis AB, Daubert JP, Fisher WG, Gurley J, et al. Safety of transvenous cardiac resynchronization system implantation in patients with chronic heart failure: combined results of over 2,000 patients from a multicenter study program. J Am Coll Cardiol. 2005;46(12):2348–56. CrossRef PubMed.
42. Fornwalt BK, Sprague WW, BeDell P, Suever JD, Gerritse B, Merlino JD, et al. Agreement is poor among current criteria used to define response to cardiac resynchronization therapy. Circulation. 2010;121(18):1985–91. CrossRef PubMed PubMedCentral.
43. Hsu JC, Solomon SD, Bourgoun M, McNitt S, Goldenberg I, Klein H, et al. Predictors of super-response to cardiac resynchronization therapy and associated improvement in clinical outcome: the MADIT-CRT (Multicenter Automatic Defibrillator Implantation Trial With Cardiac Resynchronization Therapy) Study. J Am Coll Cardiol. 2012;59(25):2366–73. CrossRef PubMed.
44. Tanaka H, Nesser H-J, Buck T, Oyenuga O, RA J, et al. Dyssynchrony by speckle-tracking echocardiography and response to cardiac resynchronization therapy: results of the Speckle Tracking and Resynchronization (STAR) study. Eur Heart J. 2010;31(14):1690–700. CrossRef PubMed PubMedCentral.
45. Stefan L, Sedláček K, Černá D, Krýže L, Vančura V, Marek T, et al. Small left atrium and mild mitral regurgitation predict super-response to cardiac resynchronization therapy. Europace. 2012;14(11):1608–14. CrossRef PubMed.
46. Stefan L, Sedláček K, Černá D, Krýže L, Vančura V, Marek T, Kautzner J. Small left atrium and mild mitral regurgitation predict super-response to cardiac resynchronization therapy. Europace. 2012;14(11):1608–14. CrossRef PubMed.
47. Sade LE, Özin B, Atar I, et al. Right ventricular function is a determinant of long-term survival after cardiac resynchronization therapy. J Am Soc Echocardiogr. 2013;26(7):706–13. CrossRef PubMed.
48. Muto C, Solimene F, Gallo P, Nastasi M, La Rosa C, Calvanese R, et al. A randomized study of CRT-D versus dual-chamber ICD in ischemic cardiomyopathy with narrow QRS: the NARROW-CRT Study. Circ Arrhythm Electrophysiol. 2013;6:538.
49. Jansen AHM, Bracke F, JM v D, KH P, JC P, van den Bosch HCM, et al. The influence of myocardial scar and dyssynchrony on reverse remodeling in cardiac resynchronization therapy. Eur J Echocardiogr. 2008;9(4):483–8. PubMed.
50. Hummel JP, Lindner JR, Belcik JT, Ferguson JD, Mangrum JM, Bergin JD, et al. Extent of myocardial viability predicts response to biventricular pacing in ischemic cardiomyopathy. Heart Rhythm. 2005;2(11):1211–7. CrossRef PubMed.
51. Dong Y-X, Powell BD, Asirvatham SJ, Friedman PA, Rea RF, Webster TL, et al. Left ventricular lead position for cardiac resynchronization: a comprehensive cinegraphic, echocardiographic, clinical, and survival analysis. Europace. 2012;14(8):1139–47. CrossRef PubMed
52. Dupont M, Rickard J, Baranowski B, Varma N, Dresing T, Gabi A, et al. Differential response to cardiac resynchronization therapy and clinical outcomes according to QRS morphology and QRS duration. J Am Coll Cardiol. 2012;60(7):592–8. CrossRef PubMed.
53. Mullens W, Grimm RA, Verga T, Dresing T, Starling RC, Wilkoff BL, et al. Insights from a cardiac resynchronization optimization clinic as part of a heart failure disease management program. J Am Coll Cardiol. 2009;53(9):765–73. CrossRef PubMed.
54. Gorodeski E, Magnelli-Reyes C, Moennich LA, Grimaldi A, Rickard J. Cardiac resynchronization therapy-heart failure (CRT-HF) clinic: a novel model of care. PLoS One. 2019;14(9):e0222610.
55. Hayes DL, Boehmer JP, Day JD, Gilliam FR III, Heidenreich PA, Seth M, et al. Cardiac resynchronization therapy and the relationship of percent biventricular pacing to symptoms and survival. Heart Rhythm. 2011;8(9):1469–75.
56. Koplan BA, Kaplan AJ, Weiner S, Jones PW, Seth M, Christman SA. Heart failure decompensation and all-cause mortality in relation to percent biventricular pacing in patients with heart failure: is a goal of 100% biventricular pacing necessary? J Am Coll Cardiol. 2009;53(4):355–60.
57. Ruwald MH, Mittal S, Ruwald AC, Aktas MK, Daubert JP, McNitt S, et al. Association between frequency of atrial and ventricular ectopic beats and biventricular pacing percentage and outcomes in patients with cardiac resynchronization therapy. J Am Coll Cardiol. 2014;64(10):971–81.
58. Van den Bruck JH, Middeldorp M, Sultan A, Scheurlen C, Seuthe K, Wormann J, et al. Impact of ventricular arrhythmia management on suboptimal biventricular pacing in cardiac resynchronization therapy. J Interv Card Electrophysiol. 2023;66(2):353–61.
59. Lakkireddy D, Di Biase L, Ryschon K, Biria M, Swarup V, Reddy YM, et al. Radiofrequency ablation of premature ventricular ectopy improves the efficacy of cardiac resynchronization therapy in nonresponders. J Am Coll Cardiol. 2012;60(16):1531–9.
60. Starling RC, Krum H, Bril S, Tsintzos SI, Rogers T, Hudnall JH, Martin DO. Impact of a novel adaptive optimization algorithm on 30-day readmissions: evidence from the adaptive CRT trial. JACC Heart Fail. 2015;3(7):565–72.
61. Field ME, Yu N, Wold N, Gold MR. Comparison of measures of ventricular delay on cardiac resynchronization therapy response. Heart Rhythm. 2020;17(4):615–20.

62. Varma N. Programming algorithms for cardiac resynchronization therapy. Card Electrophysiol Clin. 2022;14(2):243–52.
63. Varma N, Hu Y, Connolly AT, Thibault B, Singh B, Mont L, Nabutovsky Y, Zareba W. Gain in real-world cardiac resynchronization therapy efficacy with SyncAV dynamic optimization: heart failure hospitalizations and costs. Heart Rhythm. 2021;18(9):1577–85.
64. Thibault B, Mondesert B, Cadrin-Tourigny J, Dubuc M, Macle L, Khairy P. Benefits of multisite/multipoint pacing to improve cardiac resynchronization therapy response. Card Electrophysiol Clin. 2019;11(1):99–114.
65. Jain SK, Saba S. Multisite left ventricular pacing in cardiac resynchronization therapy. Card Electrophysiol Clin. 2022;14(2):253–61.
66. Niazi I, Baker J II, Corbisiero R, Love C, Martin D, Sheppard R, et al. Safety and efficacy of multipoint pacing in cardiac resynchronization therapy: the multipoint pacing trial. JACC Clin Electrophysiol. 2017;3(13):1510–8.
67. Saba S, Nair D, Ellis CR, Ciuffo A, Cox M, Gupta N, et al. Usefulness of multisite ventricular pacing in nonresponders to cardiac resynchronization therapy. Am J Cardiol. 2022;164:86–92.
68. Leclercq C, Burri H, Curnis A, Delnoy PP, Rinaldi CA, Sperzel J, et al. Cardiac resynchronization therapy non-responder to responder conversion rate in the MORE-CRT MPP trial. Europace. 2023;25(10):euad294.
69. Hanley A, Heist EK. Left ventricular endocardial pacing/leadless pacing. Card Electrophysiol Clin. 2019;11(1):155–64.
70. Cang J, Liu Y, Zhu D, Liu S, Shen J, Miao H, Zhou Q, Chen L. WiSE CRT is beneficial for heart failure patients as a rescue therapy: evidence from a meta-analysis. Front Cardiovasc Med. 2022;9:823797.
71. Reddy VY, Miller MA, Neuzil P, Sogaard P, Butter C, Seifert M, et al. Cardiac resynchronization therapy with wireless left ventricular endocardial pacing: the SELECT-LV study. J Am Coll Cardiol. 2017;69(17):2119–29.
72. Biffi M, Defaye P, Jais P, Ruffa F, Leclercq C, Gras D, et al. Benefits of left ventricular endocardial pacing comparing failed implants and prior non-responders to conventional cardiac resynchronization therapy: a subanalysis from the ALSYNC study. Int J Cardiol. 2018;259:88–93.
73. Chung ES, Gold MR, Abraham WT, Young JB, Linde C, Anderson C, et al. The importance of early evaluation after cardiac resynchronization therapy to redefine response: pooled individual patient analysis from 5 prospective studies. Heart Rhythm. 2022;19(4):595–603.
74. Varma N, Boehmer J, Bhargava K, Yoo D, Leonelli F, Costanzo M, et al. Evaluation, management, and outcomes of patients poorly responsive to cardiac resynchronization device therapy. J Am Coll Cardiol. 2019;74(21):2588–603.
75. Aranda JM, Woo GW, Schofield RS, Handberg EM, Hill JA, Curtis AB, et al. Management of heart failure after cardiac resynchronization therapy. J Am Coll Cardiol. 2005;46(12):2193–8. CrossRef PubMed.
76. Savelieva I, John CA. Atrial fibrillation and heart failure: natural history and pharmacological treatment. Europace. 2004;5:5–19. CrossRef.
77. Kamath GS, Cotiga D, Koneru JN, Arshad A, Pierce W, Aziz EF, et al. The utility of 12-lead holter monitoring in patients with permanent atrial fibrillation for the identification of nonresponders after cardiac resynchronization therapy. J Am Coll Cardiol. 2009;53(12):1050–5. CrossRef PubMed.
78. Ganesan AN, Brooks AG, Roberts-Thomson KC, Lau DH, Kalman JM, Sanders P. Role of av nodal ablation in cardiac resynchronization in patients with coexistent atrial fibrillation and heart failure. J Am Coll Cardiol. 2012;59(8):719–26. CrossRef PubMed.
79. Gasparini M, Leclercq C, Lunati M, Landolina M, Auricchio A, Santini M, et al. Cardiac resynchronization therapy in patients with atrial fibrillation: the CERTIFY study (Cardiac Resynchronization Therapy in Atrial Fibrillation Patients Multinational Registry). JACC Heart Fail. 2013;1(6):500–7.
80. Palmisano P, Ziacchi M, Ammendola E, Dell'Era G, Guerra F, Donateo P, et al. Impact of atrioventricular junction ablation and CRT-D on long-term mortality in patients with left ventricular dysfunction, permanent, refractory atrial fibrillation, and narrow QRS: results of a propensity-matched analysis. J Cardiovasc Electrophysiol. 2022;33(11):2288–96.
81. Gasparini M, Kloppe A, Lunati M, Anselme F, Landolina M, Martinez-Ferrer JB, et al. Atrioventricular junction ablation in patients with atrial fibrillation treated with cardiac resynchronization therapy: positive impact on ventricular arrhythmias, implantable cardioverter-defibrillator therapies and hospitalizations. Eur J Heart Fail. 2018;20(10):1472–81.
82. Brignole M, Pentimalli F, Palmisano P, Landolina M, Quartieri F, Occhetta E, et al. AV junction ablation and cardiac resynchronization for patients with permanent atrial fibrillation and narrow QRS: the APAF-CRT mortality trial. Eur Heart J. 2021;42(46):4731–9.
83. Kaur H, McIntyre WF, Belley-Cote EP. Ablate and pace for patients with atrial fibrillation: a fragile option? Eur Heart J. 2022;43(22):2160.
84. Beshai JF, Grimm RA, Nagueh SF, Baker JH, Beau SL, Greenberg SM, et al. Cardiac-resynchronization therapy in heart failure with narrow qrs complexes. N Engl J Med. 2007;357(24):2461–71. CrossRef PubMed.
85. Chung ES, Leon AR, Tavazzi L, Sun J-P, Nihoyannopoulos P, Merlino J, et al. Results of the predictors of response to CRT (PROSPECT) trial. Circulation. 2008;117(20):2608–16. CrossRef PubMed.

86. NCT00683696: Echocardiography Guided Resynchronization Therapy (EchoCRT) 2013. Available from: http://clinicaltrials.gov/ct2/show/study/NCT00683696?show_locs=Y.
87. Thibault B, Harel F, Ducharme A, White M, Ellenbogen KA, Frasure-Smith N, et al. Cardiac resynchronization therapy in patients with heart failure and a QRS complex <120 milliseconds: the evaluation of Resynchronization Therapy for Heart Failure (LESSER-EARTH) trial. Circulation. 2013;127(8):873–81.
88. Lindenfeld J, Feldman AM, Saxon L, Boehmer J, Carson P, Ghali JK, et al. Effects of cardiac resynchronization therapy with or without a defibrillator on survival and hospitalizations in patients with New York Heart Association class IV heart failure. Circulation. 2007;115(2):204–12. CrossRef PubMed.
89. van Bommel RJ, van Rijnsoever E, Borleffs CJW, Delgado V, Marsan NA, Bertini M, et al. Effect of cardiac resynchronization therapy in patients with New York Heart Association functional class IV heart failure. Am J Cardiol. 2010;106(8):1146–51. CrossRef PubMed.
90. Hernandez GA, Blumer V, Arcay L, Monge J, Viles-Gonzalez JF, Lindenfeld J, et al. Cardiac resynchronization therapy in inotrope-dependent heart failure patients: a systematic review and meta-analysis. JACC Heart Fail. 2018;6(9):734–42.
91. Tomashitis B, Baicu CF, Butschek RA, Jackson GR, Winterfield J, Tedford RJ, et al. Acute hemodynamic effects of cardiac resynchronization therapy versus alternative pacing strategies in patients with left ventricular assist devices. J Am Heart Assoc. 2021;10(6):e018127.
92. Cotarlan V, Johnson F, Goerbig-Campbell J, Ligh-McGroary K, Inampudi C, Franzwa J, et al. Usefulness of cardiac resynchronization therapy in patients with continuous flow left ventricular assist devices. Am J Cardiol. 2019;123(1):93–9.
93. Chung BB, Grinstein JS, Imamura T, Kruse E, Nguyen AB, Narang N, et al. Biventricular pacing versus right ventricular pacing in patients supported with LVAD. JACC Clin Electrophysiol. 2021;7(8):1003–9.
94. Darden D, Ammirati E, Brambatti M, Lin A, Hsu JC, Shah P, et al. Cardiovascular implantable electronic device therapy in patients with left ventricular assist devices: insights from TRAViATA. Int J Cardiol. 2021;340:26–33.
95. Shah K, Karpe V, Turagam MK, Shah M, Natale A, Gopinathannair R, et al. Cardiac resynchronization therapy in continuous flow left ventricular assist device recipients: a systematic review and meta-analysis from ELECTRAM Investigators. J Atr Fibrill. 2020;13(4):2441.
96. Chou A, Larson J, Deshmukh A, Cascino TM, Ghannam M, Latchamsetty R, et al. Association between biventricular pacing and incidence of ventricular arrhythmias in the early post-operative period after left ventricular assist device implantation. J Cardiovasc Electrophysiol. 2022;33(5):1024–31.
97. Chung ES, Katra RP, Ghio S, Bax J, Gerritse B, Hilpisch K, et al. Cardiac resynchronization therapy may benefit patients with left ventricular ejection fraction >35%: a PROSPECT trial substudy. Eur J Heart Fail. 2010;12(6):581–7. CrossRef PubMed.
98. Curtis AB, Worley SJ, Adamson PB, Chung ES, Niazi I, Sherfesee L, et al. Biventricular pacing for atrioventricular block and systolic dysfunction. N Engl J Med. 2013;368(17):1585–93.
99. Linde C, Curtis AB, Fonarow GC, Lee K, Little W, Tang A, et al. Cardiac resynchronization therapy in chronic heart failure with moderately reduced left ventricular ejection fraction: lessons from the Multicenter InSync Randomized Clinical Evaluation MIRACLE EF study. Int J Cardiol. 2016;202:349–55.
100. Kawata H, Bao H, Curtis JP, Minges KE, Mitiku T, Birgersdotter-Green U, et al. Cardiac resynchronization defibrillator therapy for nonspecific intraventricular conduction delay versus right bundle branch block. J Am Coll Cardiol. 2019;73(24):3082–99.
101. Friedman DJ, Al-Khatib SM, Dalgaard F, Fudim M, Abraham WT, Cleland JGF, et al. Cardiac resynchronization therapy improves outcomes in patients with intraventricular conduction delay but not right bundle branch block: a patient-level meta-analysis of randomized controlled trials. Circulation. 2023;147(10):812–23.
102. Vijayaraman P, Cano O, Ponnusamy SS, Molina-Lerma M, Chan JYS, Padala S, et al. Left bundle branch area pacing in patients with heart failure and right bundle branch block: results from International LBBAP Collaborative-Study Group. Heart Rhythm O2. 2022;3(4):358–67.
103. Tan ESJ, Soh R, Lee JY, Boey E, de Leon J, Chan SP, et al. Conduction system versus biventricular pacing in heart failure with non-left bundle branch block. J Cardiovasc Electrophysiol. 2023;34(4):976–83.

Revascularization and Heart Failure

24

Vakhtang Tchantchaleishvili
and John W. C. Entwistle III

Abbreviations

AWESOME	Angina With Extremely Serious Operative Mortality Evaluation
CABG	Coronary artery bypass grafting
CASS	Coronary Artery Surgery Study
CCS	Canadian Cardiovascular Society
CHF	Congestive heart failure
DES	Drug-eluting stent
DSE	Dobutamine stress echocardiography
HEART	Heart Failure Revascularization Trial
IABP	Intra-aortic balloon pump
IMA	Internal mammary artery
LAD	Left anterior descending
LVAD	Left ventricular assist device
LVEDVI	Left ventricular end diastolic volume index
LVESVI	Left ventricular end systolic volume index
LVEF	Left ventricular ejection fraction
MRI	Magnetic resonance imaging
NYHA	New York Heart Association
OMM	Optimal medical management
PARR-2	PET and Recovery Following Revascularization
PAsP	Pulmonary artery systolic pressure
PCI	Percutaneous coronary intervention
PET	Positron emission tomography
REHEAT	REvascularization in Ischemic HEart Failure Trial
SPECT	Single-photon emission computed tomography
STICH	Surgical Treatment for Ischemic Heart Failure
SVR	Surgical ventricular reconstruction

Introduction

Management of patients with important myocardial dysfunction and concomitant coronary artery disease can be challenging. There is a dearth of data from randomized studies to help guide the decision-making process, and the available data can be confusing due to small sample sizes, inconsistent definitions, lack of rigorous criteria for study enrollment and the retrospective nature of many studies. The increase in public reporting of surgical and interventional cardiologic results may potentially lead to pressure to deny high-risk patients appropriate therapy if there is unclear evidence for benefit, especially if there is a sense

V. Tchantchaleishvili · J. W. C. Entwistle III (✉)
Division of Cardiothoracic Surgery, Department of Surgery, Thomas Jefferson University Hospital, Philadelphia, PA, USA
e-mail: vakhtang.tchantchaleishvili@jefferson.edu; john.entwistle@jefferson.edu

H. J. Eisen (ed.), *Heart Failure I*, https://doi.org/10.1007/978-3-032-12626-9_24

that the risk-stratification system will not adequately account for the risk factors. A clear understanding of the available data can help ensure that patients receive appropriate revascularization when there is a reasonable chance for improved survival or symptom abatement.

For the typical patient with ischemic cardiomyopathy, the decision to proceed with revascularization is relatively easy based on the patient's symptoms and coronary anatomy as there are large studies or guidelines to support that decision. Occasionally, an assessment of myocardial viability may be useful in guiding treatment. However, some patients need additional evaluation as there are findings that lead to a very high operative mortality or suggest less opportunity for favorable long-term outcome with revascularization, and patients with those factors should only receive revascularization with caution. An understanding of the available data can help simplify the decision-making process.

The key factor in directing patient care should always be improvement of the patient's condition, whether that be fewer symptoms, fewer hospitalizations or better survival. Revascularization in ischemic cardiomyopathy can be achieved in many patients with relatively low surgical risk. While it is clear that some patients represent high surgical risk, most patients with ischemic cardiomyopathy are at high risk for medical management as well. In order to make the choice between high-risk surgery and high-risk medical management, it is important to understand the outcomes of both therapies and to try to select that which is best for the individual patient.

Major Trials and Studies

Randomized Controlled Trials

CASS Trial

The CASS Trial randomized 780 patients with coronary artery disease to treatment with either CABG or medical therapy. It excluded those with significant angina, left ventricular ejection fraction (LVEF) <35%, or stenosis of the left main artery. Of those that had an LVEF between 35 and 49%, survival in the surgical group was better than the medical group at 7 years (84% vs. 70%) [1]. However, the benefit in survival was only seen in those with triple-vessel disease, compared to those with single- or double-vessel disease. There was no operative mortality in the surgical group, and the survival curves began to separate at 2 years. This represented the first randomized evidence of the benefit of CABG in low LVEF over medical management, albeit with a medical regimen that is out of date by today's standards.

Veterans Study

In the 1970s, a large trial was conducted in 13 hospitals in the Veterans Administration system [2], where 686 patients with stable angina were randomized to medical management or CABG surgery. About half of those patients were diagnosed with impaired ventricular function (LVEF of less than 50% or contraction grade >2). In those patients, CABG surgery was associated with improved survival compared to medical management at 7 years, but not at 11 years. However, medical management consisted primarily of nitrates and beta blockers, and IMA usage appears to have been uncommon, limiting the potential long-term benefit of CABG.

STICH

The STICH Trial was an NIH-funded study designed to answer two basic questions. The main focus of the study was to determine if patients who were candidates for CABG and had a large area of anterior akinesia or dyskinesia were better treated with CABG alone or CABG plus surgical ventricular reconstruction (SVR) (Hypothesis 2). This portion of the study was highly criticized for deviations from its protocol involving patient enrollment and management. The other question was whether patients with a reduced LVEF and coronary artery disease were better treated with optimal medical management (OMM) or OMM plus CABG (Hypothesis 1). There were 1212 patients with an LVEF ≤35% randomized in the Hypothesis 1 arm of the trial [3]. Patients with ≥50% stenosis of the left main (LM), or with Canadian Cardiovascular Society

(CCS) Class III or IV angina were excluded from the trial as these patients were felt to be best served with surgical therapy. While the overall death rate at 56 months was similar (41% medical vs 36% CABG), the rate of cardiovascular death was less in the CABG group (33% medical vs 28% CABG, $p = 0.05$), and the CABG group had a lower combined outcome of death from any cause or readmission for cardiovascular cause. One concern with the study was the high cross-over rate such that 17% of the patients assigned to OMM alone received CABG and 9% of the patients randomized to CABG were treated medically. The study was designed to assess therapy on an intent-to-treat basis, so the large number of cross-over patients may have contributed to the apparently equivalent results. When analyzed in an as-treated manner, there was a survival advantage for surgery that was also present when cross-over patients were excluded.

Subsequently, 10-year data from the STICH Trial [4] demonstrated a lower overall mortality in the group randomized to CABG (58.9%) compared to medical management alone (66.1%), and the effect of CABG on improvement in survival was greatest in younger patients [5]. Median survival was 18 months longer in the CABG group. CABG patients also performed better in relation to a lower rate of cardiovascular death, or lower rate of the combined outcome of death from any cause or rehospitalization for cardiovascular causes. Despite the favorable results demonstrated with CABG at nearly 10 years, the limitations that were present originally persist with respect to the high rate of cross-over patients, The mortality rate for CABG remained lower than for medical management alone when examined in an as-treated manner or when only looking at per-protocol patients. One important message from this trial is that ischemic cardiomyopathy carries a high mortality regardless of treatment strategy with 62.5% of the patients dead at nearly 10 years. As CABG surgery generally shows superiority over percutaneous coronary intervention (PCI) when looking at long-term results, the STICH Trial confirmed that CABG becomes superior to medical management in patients with coronary disease and a severely depressed LVEF when long-term results are used. Thus, for those patients where long-term survival after CABG is a realistic possibility, the long-term STICH data show that CABG is the preferred treatment option.

Another issue with the STICH trial is that only about 50% of the cohort underwent any sort of viability testing before randomization, limiting the ability to do effective subgroup analysis. An attempt to analyze the effects of viability on outcome [6] showed that unadjusted mortality with revascularization was lower in patients with viable myocardium, but this difference was not present after adjustment for baseline variables. In addition, there did not appear to be a survival benefit for surgical patients over their medical counterparts regardless of viability on an intent-to-treat basis. However, this study also had several problems with viability testing, most notably the potentially non-random manner in which viability tests were ordered such that patients with a preoperative viability study may have been significantly different from those without such a test. The preoperative variables published in the two STICH reports [3, 6] contain sufficiently different data sets making comparison of the groups difficult, but it appears that the patients who underwent preoperative viability testing had more heart failure symptoms than those who did not, suggesting that a selection bias did occur. In addition, amongst the patients studied, the viable and non-viable patient groups had several key differences in baseline characteristics, such as EF, left ventricular end diastolic volume index (LVEDVI) and left ventricular end systolic volume index (LVESVI). In the presence of these confounding variables, viability may not be an independent risk factor for poor outcome, but may still be a marker of risk. In the cohort of patients undergoing SVR in addition to revascularization (Hypothesis 2), the degree of volume reduction was judged by many critics to be inadequate, possibly explaining the conclusion of the study that there was not additional benefit in SVR over revascularization alone. Since SVR is felt by many to be useful in the treatment of patients with heart failure symptoms due to a large anterior akinetic area following myocardial infarction, the criteria for patient enrollment in this study were questioned as there were many patients whose ischemic symptoms were greater than their heart failure symptoms and patients were included who did not have evidence of prior myocardial infarction but were subject to anterior volume reduction operations.

HEART

The HEART Trial [7] was designed to help determine the optimal management of patients with a low LVEF and coronary artery disease in the absence of angina. It was established as a trial of patients with an LVEF ≤35% with demonstrated viability who were randomized to either conservative management or angiography followed by either percutaneous coronary intervention (PCI) or CABG as judged appropriate. While there was no difference in outcome between the conservative and invasive management strategies, the study was underpowered as there were only 138 patients enrolled due to slow recruitment of patients and subsequent withdrawal of funding leading to premature closure of the trial. Although this study was unsuccessful in answering its intended question, it raises the issue that patients with ischemic cardiomyopathy and heart failure symptoms may be equally served with revascularization or conservative management. However, a study powered appropriately to answer this question is still needed.

REVIVED

The Revascularization for Ischemic Ventricular Dysfunction (REVIVED) trial looked at the outcomes of patients with LV dysfunction who were randomized to PCI versus medical management. Enrollment criteria included an LVEF of 35% or less, with extensive CAD amenable to PCI, and viability [8]. While there was a trend to better quality of life at 12 months, this disappeared by 24 months. There was no difference in LVEF at 12 months. There was no difference in the combined end-point of death or rehospitalization for heart failure.

As the HEART Trial was terminated prematurely due to lack to funding and the CASS trial and Veterans Study occurred at time when medical care is not representative of today, the 10-year data from the STICH Trial represents the only RCT data on CABG in patients with a low LVEF receiving more modern medical management. While this study demonstrated a survival benefit with CABG over medical management, several observational studies have been conducted to try to better understand the complexities involved.

Observational Studies

CASS Registry

The CASS Registry [9] used a large cohort of non-randomized patients who did not meet the entry criteria for the CASS trial and were followed for outcomes. In the subgroup with an LVEF ≤35%, there were 420 patients treated medically and 231 treated with coronary artery bypass grafting (CABG). There were several different baseline characteristics, and 30% of the CABG patients underwent myocardial plication or resection for aneurysm as well. After controlling for preoperative variables, patients who underwent surgery had better outcomes than their medically treated counterparts, with the greatest benefit seen in patients with an LVEF <25%. In that group, 5-year survival after CABG was 63% versus 43% in medically-managed patients. Patients who presented with angina had greater symptomatic improvement with surgery (30.2% vs 9.8%) while only 6.4% of surgical patients and 5.8% of medical patients presenting with heart failure symptoms were free of limitation. While survival for patients with angina was much better with surgery, those whose primary symptom was dyspnea or fatigue had a 3-year mortality of 45.2% in both groups. Although this study was non-randomized, it represented a large patient population that was closely followed and provided the basis for the treatment of patients with ischemic cardiomyopathy for many years. It helped define the mantra that patients with ischemic cardiomyopathy and angina should undergo revascularization or, alternatively, demonstrated that clinicians were able to successfully use undefined patient characteristics to select therapies for their patients. However, like the CASS Trial, the results are from a time when medical management differs greatly from today.

Duke Databank

The Duke Cardiovascular Disease Databank is a large clinical dataset of patients treated at Duke University Hospital that started enrolling patients in 1969. It includes data on over 200,000 patients and has been a source of information on a variety of cardiovascular problems. In a report of 1391 patients with ischemic cardiomyopathy and heart failure symptoms with an LVEF <40% and New York Heart Association (NYHA) Class II–IV congestive heart failure (CHF), O'Conner et al. [10] looked at outcomes in patients treated medically and compared them to patients treated surgically between 1969 and 1994. There were many differences in the baseline characteristics between the medical and surgical groups. After adjustment for these differences, short-term and long-term outcomes were analyzed. For short-term survival, medical management was superior for single vessel disease. There was no difference for two-vessel disease, and a trend to favor surgery for triple vessel disease. However, all groups were best served with surgery for survival greater than 30 days as this allowed the impact of up-front surgical risk to diminish. Surgery was favored regardless of age, EF, NYHA Class or angina status. Velazquez et al. [11] applied the STICH enrollment criteria to the Duke Databank to compare medical and surgical management in ischemic cardiomyopathy. Patients with LM >50%, CCS Class III–IV, acute myocardial infarction or those treated with PCI were excluded. A total of 763 patients were included, 624 who had received medical treatment and 139 who underwent CABG. After applying propensity analysis methods, there was a survival benefit that favored surgical management through 10 years. While these two studies are from a single institution and are retrospective in nature, they are some of the largest studies that are available to help guide management in these patients.

Meta-Analyses

While randomized controlled trials (RCTs) are generally considered superior to other types of studies, and observational studies are prone to selection bias in patient treatment, the relative lack of sufficiently powered RCTs and observational studies in this area has left a void that many have attempted to fill using other study designs, with variable results. Several meta-analyses have studied the question of revascularization in low LVEF, and some have looked specifically at the type of revascularization to answer questions that were not completely answered in the RCTs or observational studies.

Meta-analyses allow one to find trends in data that otherwise would require larger studies than the ones published by combining datasets to achieve such larger sample sizes. However, a major limitation with this study design is that they are only as good as the quality of data that was synthesized. While systematic review / meta-analysis of homogeneous randomized controlled trials is considered level 1a evidence, the area of revascularization in ischemic cardiomyopathy has been limited with relatively few observational studies on this topic. As such, the meta-analyses tend to use many of the same studies as each other and vary on which studies are selected, how the data are managed and how the individual studies are weighted.

In general, studies have shown that there is an improvement with revascularization compared to medical management in patients with reduced LVEF. Davoudi et al. found that there was an improvement in mortality in patients with a low LVEF who underwent revascularization (PCI or CABG) compared to those treated with medical management [12]. However, Orlandini only found a survival advantage in patients who demonstrated viability, but not when only the randomized studies were examined [13]. One explanation for this lack of significance is that two of the four randomized studies included patients who had experienced an acute myocardial infarction which is a very different patient population than those with chronic ischemic cardiomyopathy.

CABG has been shown to be superior to medical management in terms of mortality [14, 15], myocardial infarction [14] and repeat revascularization [14]. PCI was shown to have a lower rate of mortality in a pairwise analysis against medical management, but not in a network meta-analysis when comparing all treatment modalities simultaneously [14].

From the available data, it is clear that revascularization provides superior outcome to medical management in patients with ischemic cardiomyopathy, which is the basis for the Class 1 indication for CABG in these patients by the American College of Cardiology and the American Heart Association [16]. CABG appears to provide a better result in terms of survival than PCI, but in patients who are not candidates for CABG, refuse CABG, or have a lesser burden of disease, PCI may be better than medical management in terms of survival.

Patient Selection

LM and Angina

The decision to revascularize a patient with ischemic cardiomyopathy needs to be based on patient symptoms, myocardial assessment and clinical judgment. Often, the decision to offer revascularization is relatively easy such as in patients with stenosis of the left main artery or significant angina and is supported by published guidelines. Significant left main stenosis is considered an indication for CABG with or without symptoms [16]. As such, these patients have been excluded from randomized trials of medical versus surgical therapy in ischemic cardiomyopathy. In the absence of other factors that would significantly elevate the risk of intervention, patients with LM stenosis ≥50% should undergo revascularization regardless of the LVEF. Similarly, significant angina despite medical therapy is considered an indication for revascularization in the presence of double- or triple-vessel disease, or significant stenosis of the proximal left anterior descending (LAD) [16], even in the presence of a diminished LVEF. In the presence of compelling coronary anatomy and significant angina (CCS Class III or IV), especially in the absence of significant heart failure symptoms, additional assessment is usually not necessary before proceeding with revascularization as the operative mortality is relatively low, symptomatic improvement is good and the results with revascularization are considerably better than with medical management.

Viability

There is consensus that revascularization is appropriate when there is myocardial viability in the area of intended revascularization such that the procedure can either restore flow to jeopardized myocardium or prevent future ischemic events. Angina may be used as a marker of viability [17, 18], although there is not perfect correlation between symptoms and viability as assessed noninvasively. While prior guidelines [19] recommend assessment of myocardial ischemia and viability in patients with ischemic cardiomyopathy who may be candidates for revascularization in the absence of angina, the STICH Trial showed no correlation between the presence or absence of viability on survival, and there was no interaction between the presence of viability and the benefit derived from CABG over medical management alone [20]. However, the lack of standardization of viability testing protocols in the STICH Trial may have obscured any benefit the testing may have provided [16]. As such, the 2021 ACC/AHA/SCAI Guideline for Coronary Artery Revascularization make no recommendation for the use of viability testing in ischemic cardiomyopathy [16].

Viability can be assessed by several means. Dobutamine stress echocardiography (DSE), single-photon emission computed tomography (SPECT), positron emission tomography (PET) and magnetic resonance imaging (MRI) are the most commonly utilized methods. They work by assessing cellular integrity, metabolic function, microcirculation or contractile reserve. Each has strengths and weaknesses, but there is no apparent difference in clinical outcome based on the test chosen [21, 22]. Ideally, viability testing would accurately determine how much of the dysfunctional myocardium may recover function with restoration of blood flow and how much is scar and is incapable of functional recovery.

Myocardial stunning is defined as myocardium that has normal blood flow but is dysfunctional due to an acute event. Stunned myocardium has the potential to recover full function in the absence of additional injury. In the setting of ischemic cardiomyopathy, myocardium may be adequately perfused at rest but under-perfused during stress, creating stunning due to repeated episodes of ischemia. As this process continues, the stunned segments may progress to become hibernating myocardium. Hibernating myocardium is dysfunctional myocardium that has down-regulated its pattern of genetic expression in response to chronic inadequate blood flow, and has the potential for full recovery with the resumption of normal perfusion. The critical distinction between stunned and hibernating myocardium is that stunned myocardium usually recovers function within 3 months whereas hibernating myocardium may take longer to recover [23].

Transmural scar is a full thickness myocardial injury that is permanent, while non-transmural scar represents an area of non-viable tissue (often subendocardium) with viable myocardium making up the rest of the thickness of the ventricular wall. While an area of non-transmural myocardium may appear viable on some studies due to perfusion of the adjacent viable tissue, the scar may limit the ability of this muscle to produce a contractile segment.

In a given patient, the ination of viability is generally based on the presence of dysfunctional but viable myocardium in sufficient amount to be clinically significant with the understanding that enough myocardium needs to be salvageable with revascularization for the patient to gain a survival or symptom advantage over medically treated patients. Quantification of viability is often made first by assessing the number of dysfunctional myocardial segments that are viable by one of the accepted methods. The percentage of dysfunctional segments in patients with ischemic cardiomyopathy varies significantly. Three studies labeled 25% [24], 69% [23] and 46% [25] of the studied segments dysfunctional, and 37% [24], 45% [23] and 81% [25] of those segments were viable in the same studies, respectively, with the remaining dysfunctional segments representing scar. Often, once the viable segments have been identified, the myocardium of patients as a whole is then labeled as a dichotomous state of "viable" or "non-viable" depending upon the percentage of dysfunctional segments in a given patient that are viable, rather than on a continuum of viability. Typically, a patient with approximately 25% of dysfunctional segments identified as viable is considered to have myocardial viability. Percentages of patients with ischemic cardiomyopathy who have viability vary greatly from 27% to 81% [6, 17, 21, 24, 26, 27], with much of the variability likely due to patient selection rather than the method used to ascertain viability.

An early report of the use of PET scanning to determine the influence of viability on outcomes in ischemic cardiomyopathy included 93 patients referred for PET scans at a central facility [28] who were treated at their local hospitals. There were 50 patients who were treated medically and 43 who underwent CABG in this multi-center retrospective study. Predictors of survival included CHF class, history of prior MI and mismatch on the PET scan. Interestingly, the authors defined mismatch as >5% of the ventricle showing mismatch between perfusion and glucose metabolism, in contrast to most other studies where viability is usually defined as ≥25% of the myocardium with perfused but dysfunctional segments. In this study of unmatched patients, those with PET mismatch had better survival (75% vs. 30% at 4 years) and more improvement in CHF and angina symptoms than their medical counterparts. In patients without mismatch, there was a non-significant improvement in survival if the patient had severe angina but no difference if there were no mismatch and minimal angina. Patients with a low LVEF and severe angina had better survival than their medical counterparts regardless of the presence of viability, confirming that this group of patients does not need to be studied for viability prior to operation. In terms of symptomatic improvement, there was mild improvement in CHF symptoms in medically treated patients. Surgical patients had improved angina class, and an improvement in heart failure class that was more apparent in patients with PET mismatch. Those without mismatch but with severe angina had a trend towards better outcomes with revascularization. Amongst medically-treated patients, those with mismatch had poorer survival than those without (30% vs. 52%). The study demonstrated that patients with viable myocardium should be considered for revascularization regardless of symptoms and it confirmed that patients with angina should undergo revascularization without regard to viability.

Bax et al. [29] evaluated 68 patients with preoperative DSE followed by revascularization by CABG ($n = 60$) or angioplasty ($n = 8$). Sixty two patients had radionuclide ventriculography before and 3 months after revascularization. Viability was associated with better postoperative outcomes. Viable patients had improvement in EF, NYHA Class and CCS Class, while non-viable patients as a whole showed improvement only in CCS. While there was improvement in NYHA Class in 21% of the individuals without viability, this was not seen in the non-viable group as a whole. There was also a higher event rate in patients with non-viable myocardium when defined as a combined outcome of cardiac death, MI and readmission for CHF. The viability of the myocardium also influenced the recovery of myocardium. On follow-up examination, there was improvement in 27% of the dysfunctional segments of myocardium. Improvement occurred in 90% of the viable segments compared to 25% of the non-viable segments. The improvement in contraction of non-viable segments demonstrates either lack of reproducibility of test methods or difficulty in determining viability by non-invasive means, and it suggests that the presence or absence of viability alone, at least by radionuclide study, cannot be used to predict outcome.

A similar lack of perfect correlation between viability and recovery was reported by Mandegar et al. [30]. In 85 patients with ischemic cardiomyopathy who were deemed viable by DSE, 17.6% of the patients did not show an improvement in LVEF after CABG despite an improvement seen on DSE at the time of initial evaluation. The average improvement in LVEF was 9.9%, and patients with a higher LVESV had a lower likelihood of LVEF recovery, in contrast to other data that showed no correlation between ventricular size and LVEF improvement [29]. The number of viable segments on DSE correlated with outcome. Patients with 6 or more viable segments out of a possible 16 segments had a favorable outcome regardless of the LVESV, but LVESV played an important role in determining outcome in patients with <6 viable segments. In other words, the extent of remodeling becomes an independent predictor of outcome in patients with limited myocardial viability.

In the multicenter PARR-2 trial, 430 patients with ischemic cardiomyopathy were randomized to standard therapy or to have a preoperative PET scan to help guide therapy [31]. The hypothesis was that the information gained from a PET scan in addition to standard of care studies would influence patient management and improve survival. This study demonstrated a trend towards reduction of cardiac events with PET-guided therapy but no difference in the primary outcome of death, MI or cardiac rehospitalization at 1 year. Abraham et al. [32] reported a post hoc analysis of the PARR-2 patients who received care at the University of Ottawa Heart Institute, termed the Ottawa-FIVE study. This was done because the authors from Ottawa had enrolled the majority of the PARR-2 patients and they felt that their results may have differed from those of the other centers, many of which did not have PET scanning on site and may have felt less confident in using PET results to make important patient management decisions. The Ottawa-FIVE PET-assisted subgroup had fewer patients (19%) reach the composite endpoint compared to standard care (41%) despite 78% of the latter group undergoing non-PET viability testing based on standard clinical criteria. The difference in outcome could not be explained solely on the incidence of revascularization since the percentage of patients who underwent revascularization was the same in the PET-assisted and standard care groups. Further, while the Ottawa-FIVE PET-assisted group had better outcomes than the non-Ottawa PARR-2 patients, the Ottawa standard care group fared worse than their PARR-2 counterparts. It appears that the Ottawa-FIVE group, taken as a whole, did about as well as the non-Ottawa PARR-2 patients. Therefore, while there is a suggestion that preoperative PET scanning may be useful in determining the treatment plan for patients with ischemic cardiomyopathy even if they have undergone viability assessment by other means, the data is not clear on this issue. This was also seen in another study where PET was used to guide revascularization decisions [33]. The standard care group had a higher operative mortality and lower long-term survival than those who underwent PET-guided revascularization, but the survival in the patients excluded from CABG due to the PET scan results was so poor that the survival in the overall group was roughly similar between PET-guided therapy and non-PET-guided therapy. Thus, the benefit to PET scanning may be in withholding surgery from those who will do poorly with either treatment rather than increasing overall patient survival. In contrast to PARR-2, a single-center study looking at viability as assessed by PET scanning showed no correlation between percentage of hibernating myocardium or myocardial glucose uptake and improvement in LVEF after revascularization [34].

MRI has the advantage of providing information on cardiac structure, function and viability. Late gadolinium enhancement (LGE) is associated with the presence of myocardial scar, with myocardial segments with larger degrees of LGE representing areas with a greater degree of scar compared to myocardium. In general, segments with less than 50% LGE are considered viable, whereas those with higher degrees of LGE are considered non-viable. Despite the theoretical advantages of MRI, the results have been largely non-predictive. In a HEART sub-study looking at the predictive value of MRI viability, some segments with low LGE showed improved contractile function after revascularization, but the transmural extent of LGE was non-predictive of contractile recovery, as some sections labeled as viable also showed decreased contractile function after revascularization [35]. In a single-center retrospective analysis, an increase in the number of non-viable segments was associated with an increased operative mortality following CABG, but not when patients were analyzed as a dichotomous variable as either viable or non-viable, and anterior wall viability was not predictive of mortality [36].

Viability testing in ischemic cardiomyopathy has limited value when used as a dichotomous variable of "viable" or "non-viable". It is not necessary to determine viability through additional studies in patients with significant angina, as they will do better with revascularization than medical management. It may have use in predicting operative risk and symptomatic improvement in patients with heart failure as a dominant symptom. When performed, viability testing should be used only as one criteria in the decision to perform revascularization, not as an absolute requirement, as some patients without viability will exhibit a reduction in mortality from revascularization [12]. Dichotomizing a continuum invariably weakens the analysis and blurs softer outcomes. Therefore, perhaps viability testing would be best used to direct therapy if viewed on a continuum, where the decision to provide revascularization is made when there is a concordance between segments showing viability with areas of the myocardium that are suitable for revascularization [37]. However, the randomized studies that have been performed did not provide this level of granularity to answer this question.

While no studies have compared the above myocardial viability assessment modalities at a granular level, efforts have been made to pool data from the literature quantitatively. A meta-analysis of 24 prospective trials evaluating myocardial viability using cardiac MRI pooled 698 patients with chronic ventricular dysfunction due to coronary artery disease, and found that delayed enhancement MRI provided the highest sensitivity and negative predictive value (95% and 90%, respectively), whereas stress MRI provided the best specificity and positive predictive value (91% and 93%, respectively) [38]. The authors concluded that integrating these two methods should provide increased accuracy in evaluating patients with chronic LV dysfunction being considered for revascularization. The next best alternative appears to be PET scan (sensitivity 92%, specificity 63%, positive predictive value 74%, negative predictive value 87%), while other myocardial viability assessment methods fall somewhat behind [39].

Mode of Revascularization

Many studies have been conducted to examine the relative benefits and effectiveness of CABG versus PCI in the treatment of patients with coronary artery disease. While the specifics of the studies have varied, they tend to show similar findings: short- and medium-term mortality rates are similar for the two therapies; long-term survival is better with CABG; reintervention rates are higher with PCI; and CABG offers more complete revascularization. Similar results have been seen in patients with ischemic cardiomyopathy. Gioia et al. [40] published a non-randomized multicenter study looking at 220 patients with an LVEF ≤35% who underwent PCI with a drug-eluting stent (DES) or CABG. DES patients had fewer treated vessels (1.3 vs. 3), lower 6-month mortality and a higher reintervention rate. However, CABG patients had better relief from heart failure symptoms. There was no difference in survival or cardiovascular outcomes at 2 years despite only 83% of CABG patients receiving an IMA graft and thienopyridine use for only 3–6 months after DES implantation.

Sedlis et al. [41] reported the results of the Angina With Extremely Serious Operative Mortality Evaluation (AWESOME) trial and registry subgroups with an LVEF <35%. The trial patients (n = 94) were randomized to PCI or CABG to treat medically refractory ischemia, while the registry patients (n = 352) underwent PCI or CABG by either physician or patient choice. While there were some baseline differences in the registry patients that underwent PCI and those that underwent CABG, there was no difference in 36-month survival between the treatment groups. These data suggest that revascularization can be performed with either PCI or CABG with equivalent medium-term outcomes with the caveat that all of the patients had significant angina and patients who were asymptomatic or only had symptoms of heart failure were excluded from the trial.

The Revascularization in Ischemic Heart Failure Trial (REHEAT) [42] was a non-randomized prospective case-controlled comparison of PCI and CABG in 109 patients with an LVEF <40%. There were 55 patients treated with PCI (1.8 vessels treated) and 54 patients who underwent CABG (2.8 bypass grafts). All patients had significant angina, viability by DSE and/or ischemia by a treadmill stress test. Short-term survival was better in patients undergoing PCI. There was no difference in survival at 36 months and better long-term event-free survival rates in CABG patients. Long-term functional status was better in PCI patients by treadmill testing but the NYHA and CCS Classes were similar in both groups and fewer anginal episodes in CABG patients.

The APPROACH Investigators used propensity matching to look at outcomes between CABG and PCI in patients with low LVEF using a large registry. CABG was associated with better survival (hazard ration 1.21 for PCI) and lower rates of revascularization (5.7% vs. 26.7%) out to 15 years [43]. The left internal mammary artery (LIMA) was only used in 91% of the cases, and drug eluting stents (DES) were only available in the last several years of the study.

The CREDO-Kyoto PCI/CABG Registry [44] included 908 patients with 3-vessel or left main stenosis with an LVEF ≤50% who underwent revascularization with CABG or PCI. CABG was associated with a lower risk of all-cause mortality and cardiac mortality at 5 years compared to PCI, in both the groups with LVEF ≤35% and those with an LVEF 35% to 50%.

Several meta-analyses have shown that CABG is better than PCI in terms of mortality [14, 15, 45, 46], myocardial infarction [14, 45, 46] and need for repeat revascularization [14, 45, 46]. Unlike the study that showed no difference, these studies were published later and included a larger number of studies that were included in the meta-analyses.

The quality of the target vessels is an important factor in determining outcomes following surgical revascularization. In a study of 908 patients with ischemic cardiomyopathy undergoing surgical revascularization, target coronary arteries were graded as good, fair or poor based on vessel size and presence of diffuse disease [47]. Predictors of survival (mean 65 months) included good or fair coronary status, viability in the areas grafted and complete revascularization. These were also factors in event-free survival. This study clearly demonstrated that patients with a poor ventricle need complete revascularization, and that the quality of the target vessels is important in making that feasible.

Choosing to treat a patient with ischemic cardiomyopathy with revascularization requires a careful analysis of their symptoms and substrate. While PCI and CABG are both reasonable options in ischemic cardiomyopathy, one may have advantages in a given patient and be the preferred method. It is important to provide complete revascularization when possible. When the patient has a poor ventricle and poor targets, medical management may be the preferred option.

Guidelines on Myocardial Revascularization

Current ACC/AHA recommendations continue to favor revascularization for ischemic cardiomyopathy. However, understanding the evolution of the guidelines may provide the clinician with better insight into the issues involved, and is discussed here.

In 2004, the ACC/AHA guidelines recommended CABG for poor left ventricular function in presence of left main stenosis, left main equivalent, and proximal LAD stenosis with two or three-vessel disease, with class of recommendation I. This was reduced to IIa in absence of the above anatomic patterns, but with presence of significant viable, noncontracting, revascularizable myocardium [48]. Starting in 2011, poor left ventricular function was stratified between mild to moderate (EF 35–50%) and severe (EF <35%). CABG was given class IIa recommendation for LVEF 35–50%, and IIb (of uncertain benefit) for LVEF <35% without significant left main CAD, while indications for PCI were deemed insufficient [49]. The 2012 guidelines, in principle, reiterated the above recommendations for mild to moderate and severe left ventricular dysfunction. However, citing lack of sufficient contemporary data, recommended that the decision of revascularization is best based on "clinical variables, magnitude of LV systolic dysfunction, patient preferences, clinical judgment, and consultation between the interventional cardiologist and the cardiac surgeon"—essentially leaving it open to more individualized decision-making [50]. These recommendations were largely reiterated in 2017 [51]. In 2021, new ACC/AHA guidelines again approached the ischemic cardiomyopathy subset as two groups. For patients with stable ischemic heart disease and appropriate coronary anatomy, CABG was assigned class I indication for LVEF <35% to improve survival, and IIa for LVEF 35–50% to improve survival. Of note, for normal ventricles, both CABG and PCI were given class IIb recommendation for those with stable ischemic heart disease in relation to improving survival [16].

The 2021 guidelines were not endorsed by two of the major cardiothoracic surgical societies, the Society of Thoracic Surgeons, (STS) and the American Association for Thoracic Surgery (AATS), and triggered a strong critique [52]. The main objection to these guidelines focused on the decrease in the class of recommendation for CABG in stable ischemic heart disease with three-vessel coronary disease and mild-to-moderate LV dysfunction from I to IIa in order to improve survival, and giving the equal class of recommendation of IIb to CABG and PCI in patients with three-vessel CAD and normal left ventricular function to improve survival. The critique pointed out that the impact of CABG on survival cannot be ascertained from trials such as ISCHEMIA [53], in which the majority of revascularization procedures performed were PCI and not CABG. Furthermore, ISCHEMIA trial was criticized for making the assumption that PCI and CABG are equivalent revascularization strategies, when in reality PCI and CABG are inherently different revascularization strategies with distinct long-term effects on the coronary blood flow. On the other hand, earlier randomized trials and observational studies (discussed earlier in this chapter) that were considered in the prior ACC/AHA guidelines, were dismissed due to these studies no longer reflecting the advancements made in medical therapy.

Subsequent to this dispute, Mehaffey et al. analyzed the U.S. Centers for Medicare and Medicaid Services database evaluating all beneficiaries with acute coronary syndrome undergoing isolated CABG or multivessel PCI from 2018 through 2020 (a contemporary cohort). Subgroup analysis of patients with preexisting heart failure showed significant reductions in mortality (HR 0.44), myocardial infarction (HR 0.44), reintervention (HR 0.29), and the composite outcome of these three events (HR 0.47) in favor of CABG, compared to PCI [54].

Most recent European guidelines, in general, acknowledge that optimal revascularization strategy for myocardial revascularization in patients with chronic heart failure is not defined, and recommend Heart Team assessment based on patient's clinical status and coronary anatomy, as well as expected completeness of revascularization. Nevertheless, CABG does receive class I recommendation for two-or three-vessel disease with stenosis >50% and severely impaired LV function (LVEF <35%), while PCI has class IIa recommendation for the same indication [55].

In summary, it can be safely stated that revascularization continues to remain the gold standard for ischemic cardiomyopathy and, in general, CABG is preferable over PCI when the anatomy is suitable.

Other Risk Factors

Dyssynchrony

Cardiac resynchronization therapy has emerged as a way to improve cardiac function in patients with left bundle branch block and heart failure symptoms. Mechanical dyssynchrony has been evaluated as a prognostic marker for success after revascularization and must be distinguished from electrical dyssynchrony in that many of these patients with mechanical dyssynchrony have a narrow QRS on the EKG. Mechanical dyssynchrony can be assessed by tissue Doppler, gated PET and SPECT. Penicka et al. [56] reported 215 patients with ischemic cardiomyopathy and an LVEF <40% with NYHA Class I–III CHF symptoms who underwent CABG. All were assessed for viability by SPECT and dyssynchrony by tissue Doppler. The in-hospital mortality was 11.6%. In patients with pre-CABG dyssynchrony ≥119 ms, the operative mortality was 27% compared to 3% in patients without dyssynchrony. The presence of dyssynchrony led to a poor outcome regardless of viability seen on SPECT scan. In addition to use as a preoperative predictor of poor outcome, the presence or absence of dyssynchrony after operation was a marker for long-term outcome. Post-operative dyssynchrony ≥72 ms with 5 or fewer viable segments was associated with a higher rate of late death and rehospitalization compared to patients without dyssynchrony and larger areas of viability. In another study from the same group, 79 patients with a EuroSCORE >10% underwent MRI to assess viability and tissue Doppler to measure dyssynchrony [57]. EuroSCORE underestimated mortality in patients without viability but gave a reasonable assessment of risk in patients with viability. In patients with dyssynchrony ≥105 ms, 30-day mortality was 61% compared to 11% in the absence of dyssynchrony. This study demonstrates the important impact of dyssynchrony in patients who have an elevated operative risk and the inaccuracy of using standard risk models to assess patient risk when dyssynchrony is present. In an observational study that used gated PET to assess dyssynchrony [58], mechanical dyssynchrony was an independent predictor of mortality in patients regardless of whether they were treated with revascularization or medically managed, and patients who underwent CABG had better survival than those treated medically at all levels of dyssynchrony. However, the risk of death with CABG approached that of medical management at the extremes of dyssynchrony. This study suggests that patients with dyssynchrony are better treated with surgery and should be offered operation, albeit at higher risk, unless they have severe dyssynchrony.

These studies demonstrate that a focus on dyssynchrony may allow for better patient selection than by looking at LVEF alone. While assessment of mechanical dyssynchrony is more difficult than EF, there may be no survival advantage with revascularization in patients with severe dyssynchrony, justifying the additional diagnostic study in patients without other clear indications for revascularization.

Left Ventricular Ejection Fraction (LVEF)

There is conflicting evidence assessing whether LVEF is a predictor of outcome following revascularization. Low LVEF has been linked with higher operative mortality [57, 59, 60], but this has not been seen in every study [61]. Long-term survival has been shown to be influenced by preoperative LVEF [33], while others have shown no correlation [59, 61]. Determining the link between LVEF and mortality is complicated by other factors that coexist with low LVEF such as large ventricular volumes or non-viability. These other factors are associated with a poor outcome, making the identification of LVEF as an independent risk factor difficult. While LVEF should be taken into consideration when deciding for or against operation, other factors such as viability, symptoms, LV size and the state of compensation may be more important.

Left Ventricular Size or Volume

One of the greatest predictors of long-term survival in heart failure patients is left ventricular volume. The risk for early death with a severely enlarged heart is significantly higher than with mild LV enlargement. Ventricular volume has also been evaluated as a risk factor for poor outcome following CABG in ischemic cardiomyopathy. Kim et al. [62] reported outcomes in 42 patients with an LVEF $\leq$30% who underwent volume determinations by radionuclide angiography. The decision to operate was based on clinical grounds more than the results of viability testing. The patients were divided into groups based on the LVESVI. Group A had an LVESVI <100 ml/m^2 and Group B >100 ml/m^2. The operative mortality was 5% in both groups, and there was a non-significant improvement in 2-year survival in Group A compared to Group B. More patients in Group A had Class III–IV CHF before operation than in Group B, yet all Group A patients improved to NYHA Class I–II. In contrast, fewer patients in Group B were in Class III–IV CHF before operation because many of these patients would have been referred for heart transplantation rather than CABG. Yet, the Group B patients that did undergo CABG were unlikely to improve to Class I–II CHF. Of the 6 Group B patients with preoperative Class III–IV CHF, only 2 improved to Class I–II and one died after operation. In contrast to the differential effect with heart failure symptoms, both groups experienced decreased angina with CABG. Similar results were seen in 75 patients followed for 8 years after CABG [63] who had preoperative DSE to assess viability. This group was highly selected in that all patients had evidence of viability and those treated with IABP support were excluded. There was 89.3% survival at 8 years. In patients with a LVESVI <100 ml/m^2, there was a 72.1% freedom from CHF symptoms while only 46.9% of patients with an LVESVI >100 ml/m^2 were free from symptoms. There was an improvement in NYHA Class at 4 years, but there was no difference in heart failure symptoms between the preoperative and 8-year time points, suggesting that the symptomatic improvement in CHF is not durable even in patients with preoperative viability.

Bax et al. [64] reported on 79 patients with ischemic cardiomyopathy who underwent preoperative assessment by both PET and SPECT. Viability was present in 49 of the patients. Of the viable patients, 5 died before reassessment at 1 year, 24 had an improvement in LVEF and 20 showed no improvement in EF. In contrast, the non-viable patients had no improvement in LVEF as a group, although 11 of 27 individual patients did show some improvement. The greatest predictor of improvement in LVEF was the LVESV, in that patients with a large ventricle were less likely to show an improvement, these results being similar to that seen by Mandegar et al. [30]. In the article by Bax et al. [64], patients were followed for 3 years. Events were characterized as death, MI and hospital readmission for CHF. The event rate strongly correlated with ventricular size. The event rate in patients with an LVESV ≥130 mL was 37%, in LVESV ≥160 mL was 53% and in LVESV ≥180 mL was 63%. The event rate was 67% in patients with a large LV without viability compared to 5% if the ventricles were small with viability.

Preoperative left ventricular size has been associated with outcome independent of viability or LVEF. In the severely enlarged heart, remodeling may be so severe that the myocardium is essentially end-stage and is not capable of improving despite revascularization. Patients with severely enlarged ventricles may be better treated by means other than revascularization.

Right Ventricular Function

Biventricular dysfunction, as compared to isolated left ventricular dysfunction alone, represents a major operative risk factor that has not received sufficient attention in regards to patient selection for CABG. Pouleur showed that in patients with mean LVEF of 25%, in-hospital mortality rate was significantly higher in patients with right ventricular systolic dysfunction on MRI (18.7% vs 2.7%, $p = 0.004$) [65]. As such, coexisting right ventricular dysfunction should be considered at least a relative contraindication to CABG in ischemic cardiomyopathy. Predicting acute postoperative right ventricular failure has been extensively studied in patients undergoing LVAD placement. In this rather similar patient population, dysfunctional right ventricle has been shown convincingly to be associated with both increased morbidity and mortality after LVAD placement [66]. While such data are lacking on patients undergoing isolated CABG, intuitively it would follow that if right ventricular dysfunction is associated with higher morbidity and mortality even after reestablishing full flow on the left side with an LVAD, it should be at least as bad, if not worse, after CABG where the left ventricular function usually does not improve immediately. To that end, the risk stratification of right ventricular function used for patient evaluation for LVAD could be extrapolated to the coronary revascularization patients, such as PAPI [67] and RVSWI [68], to name a few. If, based on such considerations, postoperative right ventricular failure would be a concern with LVAD placement, then CABG should perhaps be avoided.

Very Poor Prognostic Signs

The overall mortality rate for patients with ischemic cardiomyopathy undergoing operation is in the range of 3–10%, although there have been reports with higher and lower mortality rates. Much of this variability depends upon patient selection. Many studies have noted subgroups of patients that have fared much worse than the other patients. Patients with very poor prognostic signs should probably not undergo revascularization without careful consideration since an operative mortality of 20–30% could easily eliminate any survival advantage that revascularization could otherwise bestow. Table 24.1 [18, 56, 57, 59, 60, 69, 70] lists many of the factors that have been found to put patients at very high operative risk.

Decompensated Patients

While many of the observational studies excluded patients with recent myocardial infarction or worsening heart failure, some have included patients who had more acute presentations. Elefteriades et al. [59] reported on 83 patients with ischemic cardiomyopathy (EF ≤ 30%) who underwent CABG. While the overall mortality rate was 8.4%, it was 22.7% in patients who were admitted to the ICU immediately before operation due to cardiogenic shock compared to 3.3% in those who were stable prior to operation.

Table 24.1 Factors that indicate very high operative risk [18, 56, 57, 59, 60, 69, 70]

Risk factor	Mortality associated	Mortality without	References
Dyssynchrony by tissue Doppler ≥119 ms >105 ms with EuroSCORE >10	 27% 61%	 3% 11%	 Penicka et al. [56] Maruskova et al. [57]
Cardiogenic shock	22.7%	3.3%	Elefteriades et al. [59]
Elevated filling pressures LVEDP ≥23 mmHg LVEDP ≥20 mmHg	 20% 3× increase	 2.7%	 Bouchart et al. [69] Pocar et al. [70]
Emergent operation	25% 38.9%	n/a n/a	Bouchart et al. [69] Fedoruk et al. [18]
Pulmonary artery pressure (systolic) >70	25%	n/a	Hovnanian et al. [60]

Emergency operation was also cited as a risk factor for perioperative death by others [18, 47, 61, 69]. In the study by Bouchart et al. [69], 49 of 141 patients with an LVEF ≤25% had a transmural infarction within 30 days of operation and 37 patients underwent operation within 24 h of catheterization due to clinical need. The operative mortality was 25% in those patients requiring operation within 12 h of catheterization. Pocar et al. [70] studied 45 patients with significant heart failure (NYHA Class III–IV) who had undergone preoperative PET scanning prior to elective CABG. While these patients were clinically stable, the preoperative hemodynamics demonstrated a degree of decompensation in many of them. An LVEDP ≥25 mmHg was associated with a threefold increase in the risk of death and an LVEDP ≥20 mmHg was associated with an increased need for IABP support. None of the patients with an LVEDP ≥25 mmHg improved to NYHA Class I. A high operative mortality was also seen by Bouchart et al. [69] where patients with an LVEDP ≥23 mmHg had a mortality of 20% compared to 2.7% without this risk factor. One theory is that an elevated LVEDP inhibits diastolic flow of the subendocardium and this is responsible for the poor results seen with an elevated LVEDP. Thus, patients who are unstable should be stabilized and optimized if possible before undergoing revascularization. Alternatively, high LVEDP may be a marker for more advanced cardiac injury, decompensation or remodeling, and should prompt consideration for other therapies such as mechanical circulatory support. Some have advocated for the use of temporary MCS in this patient population [71]. As this is a newer technology, there has not been enough time for sufficient data to accumulate on its concomitant use with CABG. However, there are substantial perceived advantages. While IABP reduces afterload and augments coronary perfusion, the improvement in systemic perfusion is often insufficient in most patients with post-cardiotomy shock. On the other hand, while ECMO can provide full systemic circulatory support, it comes at a price of increased LV afterload resulting in myocardial distension and ischemia, as well as pulmonary venous congestion. As such, temporary MCS with a device that directly unloads the left ventricle in the setting of post-cardiotomy shock may normalize systemic perfusion while decreasing the work load on the left ventricle. In patients with EF < 35% and high risk features for developing postoperative cardiogenic shock, one group has reported routine expedited formal LVAD backup process, and placement of a right axillary 10 mm graft at the beginning of CABG for use in Impella insertion if needed. The Impella insertion rate is between 15% and 30% of these patients [71].

Other High Risk Patients

Elevated pulmonary artery pressure has also been indicted as a significant risk factor in patients undergoing revascularization. Hovnanian et al. [60] reported on 244 patients with an LVEF ≤35% who had viability by thallium scanning. In-hospital mortality was 3.7%, but was 25% in those patients with a pulmonary artery systolic pressure (PAsP) >70 mmHg. However, 17% of the patients had a mitral valve intervention as well as CABG, making it more difficult to apply these data to patients with coronary disease alone. Selim Isbir et al. [72] also reported a negative survival effect with an elevated pulmonary artery pressure by multivariable analysis, but no recommended cutoff was provided above which the risk rises, and pulmonary artery catheters were not placed preoperatively on a routine basis.

NYHA

Many of the patients with ischemic cardiomyopathy have symptoms of CHF. Those with important angina in addition to heart failure symptoms have good survival and symptom relief with revascularization. However, patients with predominantly Class IV CHF symptoms are at higher operative risk [47, 60, 69], have lower long-term survival [60, 61, 69] and have less resolution of their symptoms [63]. It may be difficult to opt for revascularization in a patient with no angina and Class IV heart failure symptoms, especially when the operative mortality can reach 29% [69], but these same patients are also at high risk for death with medical management alone. Choosing the patient with stable Class IV heart failure symptoms for revascularization and directing the decompensated patients towards medical management, heart transplantation or ventricular assist device therapy may minimize the operative risk and maximize outcomes.

Patient Optimization

The best results are clearly seen in patients who can undergo elective operation and those with compensated symptoms. Appropriate patient selection is the single greatest factor in achieving low operative mortality. In terms of conduct of the operation, myocardial protection is critical to limit additional ischemic damage. Complete revascularization is important in all patients, especially those with ischemic cardiomyopathy [47]. Perioperative management with an intra-aortic balloon pump (IABP) has been shown to be beneficial [72]. The operation also needs to be conducted in a time-efficient manner as longer cross-clamp and bypass times have been associated with lower survival [72]. Choice of conduit may not be as important in ischemic cardiomyopathy as it is with a normal ventricle. Selim Isbir et al. [72] used the left internal mammary artery (IMA) in only 50.4% of patients and found no correlation between IMA use and outcome out to 4 years. Even though there is evidence that some patients without ischemic cardiomyopathy may benefit from the use of bilateral IMA grafts, it was not better than the use of single IMAs in patients with an LVEF <30%, although there was slightly better outcome with bilateral IMAs seen in patients with an LVEF ≥30% [73]. While these results may be influenced by patient selection in that patients with lower risk may have received bilateral IMAs, these results probably reflect the relative dominance of the cardiomyopathy in determining long-term outcomes rather than the details of the revascularization.

Results

Angina/CHF

One of the main reasons to perform revascularization is to improve symptoms. Angina is present in a significant number of patients with ischemic cardiomyopathy. Revascularization leads to significant improvement in angina score [24, 59], even in the absence of viability [29]. As angina usually signifies the presence of viability, its improvement without demonstrated viability probably represents a limitation in the assessment techniques. The improvement in CHF seems less robust, but improvement can occur [24, 59], although not in the absence of viability [29]. Unfortunately, the improvement in CHF symptoms may not be durable [63]. The improvement in angina and CHF is independent from any change in LVEF [74]. Patients with ischemic cardiomyopathy who are referred for revascularization can expect improvement in angina symptoms, but should only expect improvement in CHF symptoms if there is myocardial viability present.

LVEF/Volumes

LVEF is a marker for mortality in patients with heart failure. Studies have shown an improvement in LVEF following revascularization [42, 69], although some have only shown improvement in patients with viability [20, 29, 30, 63, 64] or no improvement at all [35]. However, when seen, the improvements in LVEF are generally modest. In CABG patients the mean improvement was 4.4 percentage points [75]. Small, equivalent changes were observed in patients undergoing PCI or CABG [42], CABG or medical management [20] or PCI or medical management [8]. In general, there is no consistent improvement in LVEF in patients with nonviable myocardium [29, 64]. Some have shown that recovery of LVEF is dependent upon LVESV [24, 30], with larger ventricles showing less likelihood for recovery of EF. Finally, the status of the coronary arteries to be revascularized plays a role in the recovery of ventricular function. LVEF improved in patients with good or fair coronary arteries but did not change in patients with poor target vessels [47].

While revascularization may improve LVEF, it is not clear that this improvement correlates with better outcome. In a study of 104 patients with ischemic cardiomyopathy and LVEF ≤30% [74] with preoperative and postoperative assessment of EF, only 68 of the patients demonstrated an improvement in LVEF of ≥5% above baseline. In this group, the LVEF increased from 24% to 39%. In contrast, the remaining patients showed no significant improvement (<5%). Despite this difference in response to revascularization, survival was the same in both groups. In addition, both groups had equivalent improvements in angina and heart failure symptoms. Thus, the improvement in LVEF may make clinicians feel better about performing revascularization, but is probably not a clinically important marker of outcome. The STICH Trial showed no correlation between the changes in LVEF and survival [20] suggesting that any potential mortality benefits of CABG in ischemic cardiomyopathy may not be due to changes in the EF, but preservation of viable myocardium with revascularization [37].

Similar to EF, ventricular dimensions may improve with revascularization. Bouchart et al. [69] reported a decrease in LVEDVI in patients with ischemic cardiomyopathy who underwent revascularization but these changes were not seen by others [42]. Even if the ventricular dimensions improve with revascularization, there is no evidence that this will lead to a clinically relevant improvement in outcome.

Survival

Based on the few randomized and several nonrandomized comparison studies, it is clear that select patients do much better with revascularization than with medical management alone. Many studies have shown good results in patients undergoing revascularization but lack a comparison group, making it difficult to make a definitive statement of benefit. In one large meta-analysis of 4119 patients from 26 studies, 5-year survival was an impressive 73.4% in patients undergoing on-pump revascularization [75]. This compares favorably to medical management which has been associated with an annual mortality rate of 16% in patients with viability and 6.2% in those who were non-viable [21]. Several authors have identified groups of patients who are at high risk for death following surgical revascularization. These patients may be the most difficult to manage, as they likely also have poor outcome with medical management alone. While they may have a high operative mortality, it may be superior to their results with medical management, but may not be high enough to be cost-effective or worth it for the patient and their family. Until better data is available to determine the relative effectiveness of revascularization and medical management in these high-risk patients, other options should be considered.

Other Options

Surgical Ventricular Reconstruction (SVR)

Yoon et al. reported their results in 1468 patients with an LVEF <30%. Patients were either treated with CABG, CABG with mitral valve repair or replacement, CABG with SVR or listing for transplantation. Viability testing was performed in only about 20% of the patients. The treatment plan was based on the clinical situation. In their retrospective analysis, they determined that most patients would have benefited most with either CABG or listing for transplantation, despite the 18% mortality seen on the waiting list in this cohort. The authors believe that mitral repair in ischemic cardiomyopathy provides few benefits to most patients. The addition of mitral repair to CABG in patients with 3+ or 4+ mitral regurgitation has been shown to produce no survival benefit and no long-term relief from significant heart failure over CABG alone [76]. Left ventricular reconstruction is, at best, useful in a limited number of patients with ischemic cardiomyopathy as it works best in the setting of an anterior-septal infarct. Although the STICH Trial has cast some doubt about its use in a larger patient population, other data document marked symptomatic improvement and survival benefit when compared with historic controls [77, 78]. A recent meta-analysis of 7685 patients undergoing surgical ventricular reconstruction, that excluded patients from the STICH trial, showed significant improvements in mean pooled values of LVEF (29.9–40.9%), LVESD (49.9–45 mm), LVEDD (63.8–58.23 mm), LVESVI (83.9–46.8 mL/m^2), LVEDVI (119.9–79.6 mL/m^2), and NYHA class (3–1.8). Concomitant CABG was undertaken in 92%. The 30-day mortality was 4% while late mortality was 19% at a mean follow-up of 27.5 months [79].

Durable Left Ventricular Support Device (LVAD)

With current third-generation centrifugal flow LVADs widely available, this should be considered a better option than revascularization for many of these high-risk patients. In the elective setting and good patient selection, LVAD therapy can achieve excellent survival. Recently, Schmitto reported 100% 5-year survival after HeartMate 3 LVAD in the initial 8 consecutive patients from the HeartMate 3™ CE Mark Clinical Trial. Besides 100% survival, no right heart failure, hemolysis, pump thrombosis, mechanical pump malfunction, or neurologic events occurred [80]. While this cohort represented a small number of very carefully selected patients, a broader group of patients from the MOMENTUM trial ($n = 536$) implanted with the HeartMate 3 LVAD achieved 5-year survival of 58.4% [81]. When examining third generation LVADs implanted in the most recent era (2017–2021) in all-comers, 2022 INTERMACS annual report showed 51.9% 5-years survival [82]. Besides median survival exceeding 5 years, heart failure symptoms are greatly improved and the results seem to be durable with more consistent relief of heart failure symptoms in LVAD patients than seen in patients undergoing revascularization. This therapy is particularly suited for many of the patients who are considered high risk for revascularization alone—those with very large ventricles, NYHA Class IV symptoms, low cardiac index, high LVEDP and significant mitral regurgitation. Since LVAD therapy does not rely on the adequacy of LV function, the presence of viability is not a concern. In addition, while presence of significant mitral regurgitation would mandate concomitant mitral valve surgery in addition to CABG and further increase the operative risk, mitral regurgitation does not represent a major concern when instituting LVAD therapy. As such, need for concomitant mitral valve surgery can be considered an additional factor in favor of LVAD over CABG [83]. Recent progress in LVAD technology has led the Centers for Medicare and Medicaid Services (CMS) to revise the national coverage determination (NCD) for artificial hearts and related devices, including LVADs. Patients who meet the following criteria can qualify for short-term or long-term Mechanical Circulatory Support: NYHA Class IV, LVEF <25%, and inotrope dependency or cardiac index <2.2 on optimal medical management [84]. As LVADs continue to improve and their costs are lowered, this treatment modality will likely become therapy of choice for even larger number of patients with ischemic cardiomyopathy and important risk factors for revascularization alone.

Heart Transplantation

Finally, if patients are deemed extraordinarily high risk for CABG with little probability of symptomatic or survival benefit, and biventricular failure precludes LVAD implantation, then transplantation is a reasonable option with excellent results.

Conclusion

Patients with significant stenosis of the left main coronary artery or significant angina should undergo revascularization unless there are compelling reasons to treat them medically. Those with significant angina do not need routine viability testing before operation. When indicated, viability testing can be performed by SPECT, DSE, PET or MRI. Although MRI may offer most versatile approach with highest sensitivity (delayed enhancement MRI) and specificity (stress MRI), due to lack of sufficient evidence the choice of testing method should ultimately be based primarily on local expertise. Patients with viability should not be treated with medical management alone as the magnitude of improvement in survival with surgery is probably greatest in patients with myocardial viability. Angina will often improve after revascularization, regardless of the results of viability testing. Symptoms of heart failure are more likely to improve if there is viability, but this improvement may not be durable as the underlying cardiomyopathy is still present. Very low LVEF should not preclude operation by itself, but may be a marker for higher surgical risk even though the survival benefit with CABG is greatest in this group of patients. LVEF is more likely to improve in patients who exhibit viability, but this may not be clinically relevant. Perioperative support should be considered in high risk patients.

Patients at very high-risk for early mortality should receive revascularization only after careful consideration of other options, and modification of their risk factors if possible. These include patients who have had a recent myocardial infarction, very large ventricles, dyssynchrony as assessed by tissue Doppler, or hemodynamic parameters consistent with cardiogenic shock. These patients should be strongly considered for alternative therapies such as LVAD support or heart transplantation.

References

1. Passamani E, Davis KB, Gillespie MJ, Killip T. A randomized trial of coronary artery bypass surgery. Survival of patients with a low ejection fraction. N Engl J Med. 1985;312(26):1665–71. https://doi.org/10.1056/NEJM198506273122603.
2. Veterans Administration Coronary Artery Bypass Surgery Cooperative Study Group. Eleven-year survival in the Veterans Administration randomized trial of coronary bypass surgery for stable angina. N Engl J Med. 1984;311(21):1333–9. https://doi.org/10.1056/NEJM198411223112102.
3. Velazquez EJ, Lee KL, Deja MA, Jain A, Sopko G, Marchenko A, STICH Investigators, et al. Coronary-artery bypass surgery in patients with left ventricular dysfunction. N Engl J Med. 2011;364(17):1607–16.
4. Velazquez EJ, Lee KL, Jones RH, Al-Khalidi HR, Hill JA, Panza JA, Michler RE, Bonow RO, Doenst T, Petrie MC, Oh JK, She L, Moore VL, Desvigne-Nickens P, Sopko G, Rouleau JL, STICHES Investigators. Coronary-artery bypass surgery in patients with ischemic cardiomyopathy. N Engl J Med. 2016;374(16):1511–20. https://doi.org/10.1056/NEJMoa1602001. Epub 2016 Apr 3
5. Petrie MC, Jhund PS, She L, Adlbrecht C, Doenst T, Panza JA, Hill JA, Lee KL, Rouleau JL, Prior DL,

Ali IS, Maddury J, Golba KS, White HD, Carson P, Chrzanowski L, Romanov A, Miller AB, Velazquez EJ, STICH Trial Investigators. Ten-year outcomes after coronary artery bypass grafting according to age in patients with heart failure and left ventricular systolic dysfunction: an analysis of the extended follow-up of the STICH trial (surgical treatment for ischemic heart failure). Circulation. 2016;134(18):1314–24. https://doi.org/10.1161/CIRCULATIONAHA.116.024800. Epub 2016 Aug 29
6. Bonow RO, Maurer G, Lee KL, Holly TA, Binkley PF, Desvigne-Nickens P, STICH Trial Investigators, et al. Myocardial viability and survival in ischemic left ventricular dysfunction. N Engl J Med. 2011;364(17):1617–25.
7. Cleland JG, Calvert M, Freemantle N, Arrow Y, Ball SG, Bonser RS, et al. The HEART failure revascularisation trial (HEART). Eur J Heart Fail. 2011;13(2):227–33.
8. Perera D, Clayton T, O'Kane PD, Greenwood JP, Weerackody R, Ryan M, Morgan HP, Dodd M, Evans R, Canter R, Arnold S, Dixon LJ, Edwards RJ, De Silva K, Spratt JC, Conway D, Cotton J, McEntegart M, Chiribiri A, Saramago P, Gershlick A, Shah AM, Clark AL, Petrie MC, REVIVED-BCIS2 Investigators. Percutaneous revascularization for ischemic left ventricular dysfunction. N Engl J Med. 2022;387(15):1351–60. https://doi.org/10.1056/NEJMoa2206606. Epub 2022 Aug 27
9. Alderman EL, Fisher LD, Litwin P, Kaiser GC, Myers WO, Maynard C, et al. Results of coronary artery surgery in patients with poor left ventricular function (CASS). Circulation. 1983;68(4):785–95.
10. O'Connor CM, Velazquez EJ, Gardner LH, Smith PK, Newman MF, Landolfo KP, et al. Comparison of coronary artery bypass grafting versus medical therapy on long-term outcome in patients with ischemic cardiomyopathy (a 25-year experience from the Duke Cardiovascular Disease Databank). Am J Cardiol. 2002;90(2):101–7.
11. Velazquez EJ, Williams JB, Yow E, Shaw LK, Lee KL, Phillips HR, et al. Long-term survival of patients with ischemic cardiomyopathy treated by coronary artery bypass grafting versus medical therapy. Ann Thorac Surg. 2012;93(2):523–30.
12. Davoudi F, Miyashita S, Yoo TK, Imahira U, Kimmelstiel C, Huggins GS, Downey BC. Do patients with non-viable myocardium from ischemic cardiomyopathy benefit from revascularization? A systematic review and meta-analysis. Cardiovasc Revasc Med. 2023;47:27–32. https://doi.org/10.1016/j.carrev.2022.08.032. Epub 2022 Aug 28
13. Orlandini A, Castellana N, Pascual A, Botto F, Cecilia Bahit M, Chacon C, Luz Diaz M, Diaz R. Myocardial viability for decision-making concerning revascularization in patients with left ventricular dysfunction and coronary artery disease: a meta-analysis of non-randomized and randomized studies. Int J Cardiol. 2015;182:494–9. https://doi.org/10.1016/j.ijcard.2015.01.025. Epub 2015 Jan 7
14. Gaudino M, Hameed I, Khan FM, Tam DY, Rahouma M, Yongle R, Naik A, Di Franco A, Demetres M, Petrie MC, Jolicoeur EM, Girardi LN, Fremes SE. Treatment strategies in ischaemic left ventricular dysfunction: a network meta-analysis. Eur J Cardiothorac Surg. 2020:ezaa319. https://doi.org/10.1093/ejcts/ezaa319. Epub ahead of print
15. Wolff G, Dimitroulis D, Andreotti F, Kołodziejczak M, Jung C, Scicchitano P, Devito F, Zito A, Occhipinti M, Castiglioni B, Calveri G, Maisano F, Ciccone MM, De Servi S, Navarese EP. Survival benefits of invasive versus conservative strategies in heart failure in patients with reduced ejection fraction and coronary artery disease: a meta-analysis. Circ Heart Fail. 2017;10(1):e003255. https://doi.org/10.1161/CIRCHEARTFAILURE.116.003255.
16. Lawton JS, Tamis-Holland JE, Bangalore S, Bates ER, Beckie TM, Bischoff JM, Bittl JA, Cohen MG, DiMaio JM, Don CW, Fremes SE. 2021 ACC/AHA/SCAI guideline for coronary artery revascularization: executive summary: a report of the American College of Cardiology/American Heart Association Joint Committee on Clinical Practice Guidelines. Circulation. 2022;145(3):e4–17.
17. Auerbach MA, Schöder H, Hoh C, Gambhir SS, Yaghoubi S, Sayre JW, et al. Prevalence of myocardial viability as detected by positron emission tomography in patients with ischemic cardiomyopathy. Circulation. 1999;99(22):2921–6.
18. Fedoruk LM, Tribble CG, Kern JA, Peeler BB, Kron IL. Predicting operative mortality after surgery for ischemic cardiomyopathy. Ann Thorac Surg. 2007;83(6):2029–35.
19. Hunt SA, Abraham WT, Chin MH, Feldman AM, Francis GS, Ganiats TG, et al. American College of Cardiology Foundation; American Heart Association. 2009 Focused update incorporated into the ACC/AHA 2005 Guidelines for the Diagnosis and Management of Heart Failure in Adults A Report of the American College of Cardiology Foundation/American Heart Association Task Force on Practice Guidelines Developed in Collaboration With the International Society for Heart and Lung Transplantation. J Am Coll Cardiol. 2009;53(15):e1–e90. Erratum in: J Am Coll Cardiol. 2009;54(25):2464
20. Panza JA, Ellis AM, Al-Khalidi HR, Holly TA, Berman DS, Oh JK, Pohost GM, Sopko G, Chrzanowski L, Mark DB, Kukulski T, Favaloro LE, Maurer G, Farsky PS, Tan RS, Asch FM, Velazquez EJ, Rouleau JL, Lee KL, Bonow RO. Myocardial viability and long-term outcomes in ischemic cardiomyopathy. N Engl J Med. 2019;381(8):739–48. https://doi.org/10.1056/NEJMoa1807365.
21. Allman KC, Shaw LJ, Hachamovitch R, Udelson JE. Myocardial viability testing and impact of revascularization on prognosis in patients with coronary artery disease and left ventricular dysfunction: a meta-analysis. J Am Coll Cardiol. 2002;39(7):1151–8.
22. Lin LC, Ho YL, Wu CC, Chen MF, Liau CS, Su CT, et al. Comparison of simultaneous dobutamine echo-

cardiography and thallium-201 stress-reinjection single-photon emission computed tomography in predicting improvement of chronic myocardial dysfunction after revascularization. Am J Cardiol. 2000;86(3):293–8.
23. Bax JJ, Visser FC, Poldermans D, Elhendy A, Cornel JH, Boersma E, et al. Time course of functional recovery of stunned and hibernating segments after surgical revascularization. Circulation. 2001;104(12 Suppl 1):I314–8.
24. Schinkel AF, Poldermans D, Rizzello V, Vanoverschelde JL, Elhendy A, Boersma E, et al. Why do patients with ischemic cardiomyopathy and a substantial amount of viable myocardium not always recover in function after revascularization? J Thorac Cardiovasc Surg. 2004;127(2):385–90.
25. Hernandez-Pampaloni M, Bax JJ, Morita K, Dutka DP, Camici PG. Incidence of stunned, hibernating and scarred myocardium in ischaemic cardiomyopathy. Eur J Nucl Med Mol Imaging. 2005;32(3):314–21.
26. Schinkel AF, Bax JJ, Boersma E, Elhendy A, Roelandt JR, Poldermans D. How many patients with ischemic cardiomyopathy exhibit viable myocardium? Am J Cardiol. 2001;88(5):561–4.
27. Rizzello V, Poldermans D, Schinkel AF, Biagini E, Boersma E, Elhendy A, et al. Long term prognostic value of myocardial viability and ischaemia during dobutamine stress echocardiography in patients with ischaemic cardiomyopathy undergoing coronary revascularisation. Heart. 2006;92(2):239–44.
28. Di Carli MF, Maddahi J, Rokhsar S, Schelbert HR, Bianco-Batlles D, Brunken RC, et al. Long-term survival of patients with coronary artery disease and left ventricular dysfunction: implications for the role of myocardial viability assessment in management decisions. J Thorac Cardiovasc Surg. 1998;116(6):997–1004.
29. Bax JJ, Poldermans D, Elhendy A, Cornel JH, Boersma E, Rambaldi R, et al. Improvement of left ventricular ejection fraction, heart failure symptoms and prognosis after revascularization in patients with chronic coronary artery disease and viable myocardium detected by dobutamine stress echocardiography. J Am Coll Cardiol. 1999;34(1):163–9.
30. Mandegar MH, Yousefnia MA, Roshanali F, Rayatzadeh H, Alaeddini F. Interaction between two predictors of functional outcome after revascularization in ischemic cardiomyopathy: left ventricular volume and amount of viable myocardium. J Thorac Cardiovasc Surg. 2008;136(4):930–6.
31. Beanlands RS, Nichol G, Huszti E, Humen D, Racine N, Freeman M, PARR-2 Investigators, et al. F-18-fluorodeoxyglucose positron emission tomography imaging-assisted management of patients with severe left ventricular dysfunction and suspected coronary disease: a randomized, controlled trial (PARR-2). J Am Coll Cardiol. 2007;50(20):2002–12.
32. Abraham A, Nichol G, Williams KA, Guo A, deKemp RA, Garrard L, PARR 2 Investigators, et al. 18F-FDG PET imaging of myocardial viability in an experienced center with access to 18F-FDG and integration with clinical management teams: the Ottawa-FIVE substudy of the PARR 2 trial. J Nucl Med. 2010;51(4):567–74.
33. Boehm J, Haas F, Bauernschmitt R, Wagenpfeil S, Voss B, Schwaiger M, et al. Impact of preoperative positron emission tomography in patients with severely impaired LV-function undergoing surgical revascularization. Int J Card Imaging. 2010;26(4):423–32.
34. Luong TV, Ebbehoj A, Kjaerulff MLG, Nielsen R, Nielsen PH, Christiansen EH, Tolbod LP, Søndergaard E, Gormsen LC. Clinical use of cardiac 18 F-FDG viability PET: a retrospective study of 44 patients undergoing post-test revascularization. Int J Cardiovasc Imaging. 2022;38(11):2447–58. https://doi.org/10.1007/s10554-022-02661-5. Epub 2022 Jun 23
35. McDiarmid AK, Loh H, Nikitin N, Cleland JG, Ball SG, Greenwood JP, Plein S, Sparrow P. Predictive power of late gadolinium enhancement for myocardial recovery in chronic ischaemic heart failure: a HEART sub-study. ESC Heart Fail. 2014;1(2):146–53. https://doi.org/10.1002/ehf2.12019. Epub 2015 Jan 13
36. Yap J, Lim FY, Gao F, Wang SZ, Low SCS, Le TT, Tan RS. Effect of myocardial viability assessed by cardiac magnetic resonance on survival in patients with severe left ventricular dysfunction. Circ Rep. 2020;2(6):306–13. https://doi.org/10.1253/circrep.CR-19-0126.
37. Panza JA, Chrzanowski L, Bonow RO. Myocardial viability assessment before surgical revascularization in ischemic cardiomyopathy: JACC review topic of the week. J Am Coll Cardiol. 2021;78(10):1068–77. https://doi.org/10.1016/j.jacc.2021.07.004.
38. Romero J, Xue X, Gonzalez W, Garcia MJ. CMR imaging assessing viability in patients with chronic ventricular dysfunction due to coronary artery disease: a meta-analysis of prospective trials. JACC Cardiovasc Imaging. 2012;5(5):494–508.
39. Schinkel AF, Bax JJ, Poldermans D, Elhendy A, Ferrari R, Rahimtoola SH. Hibernating myocardium: diagnosis and patient outcomes. Curr Probl Cardiol. 2007;32(7):375–410.
40. Gioia G, Matthai W, Gillin K, Dralle J, Benassi A, Gioia MF, et al. Revascularization in severe left ventricular dysfunction: outcome comparison of drug-eluting stent implantation versus coronary artery by-pass grafting. Catheter Cardiovasc Interv. 2007;70(1):26–33.
41. Sedlis SP, Ramanathan KB, Morrison DA, Sethi G, Sacks J, Henderson W, Department of Veterans Affairs Cooperative Study #385, Angina With Extremely Serious Operative Mortality Evaluation (AWESOME) Investigators. Outcome of percutaneous coronary intervention versus coronary bypass grafting for patients with low left ventricular ejection fractions, unstable angina pectoris, and risk factors for adverse outcomes with bypass (the AWESOME Randomized Trial and Registry). Am J Cardiol. 2004;94(1):118–20.

42. Buszman P, Szkróbka I, Gruszka A, Parma R, Tendera Z, Leśko B, et al. Comparison of effectiveness of coronary artery bypass grafting versus percutaneous coronary intervention in patients with ischemic cardiomyopathy. Am J Cardiol. 2007;99(1):36–41.
43. Nagendran J, Norris CM, Graham MM, Ross DB, Macarthur RG, Kieser TM, Maitland AM, Southern D, Meyer SR, APPROACH Investigators. Coronary revascularization for patients with severe left ventricular dysfunction. Ann Thorac Surg. 2013;96(6):2038–44. https://doi.org/10.1016/j.athoracsur.2013.06.052. Epub 2013 Aug 20
44. Marui A, Kimura T, Nishiwaki N, Mitsudo K, Komiya T, Hanyu M, Shiomi H, Tanaka S, Sakata R, CREDO-Kyoto PCI/CABG Registry Cohort-2 Investigators. Comparison of five-year outcomes of coronary artery bypass grafting versus percutaneous coronary intervention in patients with left ventricular ejection fractions≤50% versus >50% (from the CREDO-Kyoto PCI/CABG registry Cohort-2). Am J Cardiol. 2014;114(7):988–96. https://doi.org/10.1016/j.amjcard.2014.07.007. Epub 2014 Jul 16
45. Cui K, Zhang D, Lyu S, Song X, Yuan F, Xu F, Zhang M. Meta-analysis comparing percutaneous coronary revascularization using drug-eluting stent versus coronary artery bypass grafting in patients with left ventricular systolic dysfunction. Am J Cardiol. 2018;122(10):1670–6. https://doi.org/10.1016/j.amjcard.2018.08.002. Epub 2018 Aug 20
46. Zhang D, Lyu S, Song X, Yuan F, Xu F, Zhang M, Zhang M. Coronary artery bypass grafting versus percutaneous coronary intervention in patients with left ventricular systolic dysfunction: a meta-analysis. Angiology. 2017;68(1):19–28. https://doi.org/10.1177/0003319716639197. Epub 2016 Apr 10
47. Kleikamp G, Maleszka A, Reiss N, Stüttgen B, Körfer R. Determinants of mid- and long-term results in patients after surgical revascularization for ischemic cardiomyopathy. Ann Thorac Surg. 2003;75(5):1406–12.
48. Eagle KA, Guyton RA, Davidoff R, Edwards FH, Ewy GA, Gardner TJ, American College of Cardiology, American Heart Association Task Force on Practice Guidelines, American Society for Thoracic Surgery and the Society of Thoracic Surgeons, et al. ACC/AHA 2004 guideline update for coronary artery bypass graft surgery: summary article: a report of the American College of Cardiology/American Heart Association Task Force on Practice Guidelines (Committee to Update the 1999 Guidelines for Coronary Artery Bypass Graft Surgery). Circulation. 2004;110(9):1168–76. Erratum in: Circulation. 2005;111(15):2014.
49. Hillis LD, Smith PK, Anderson JL, Bittl JA, Bridges CR, Byrne JG, Cigarroa JE, Disesa VJ, Hiratzka LF, Hutter JAM, Jessen ME, American Association for Thoracic Surgery, Society of Cardiovascular Anesthesiologists, Society of Thoracic Surgeons. 2011 ACCF/AHA guideline for coronary artery bypass graft surgery. A report of the American College of Cardiology Foundation/American Heart Association Task Force on Practice Guidelines. Developed in collaboration with the American Association for thoracic surgery, society of cardiovascular anesthesiologists, and society of thoracic surgeons. J Am Coll Cardiol. 2011;58(24):e123–210.
50. Fihn SD, Gardin JM, Abrams J, Berra K, Blankenship JC, Dallas AP, Douglas PS, Foody JM, Gerber TC, Hinderliter AL, King SB III. ACCF/AHA/ACP/AATS/PCNA/SCAI/STS guideline for the diagnosis and management of patients with stable ischemic heart disease: a report of the American College of Cardiology Foundation/American Heart Association task force on practice guidelines, and the American College of Physicians, American Association for Thoracic Surgery, Preventive Cardiovascular Nurses Association, Society for Cardiovascular Angiography and Interventions, and Society of Thoracic Surgeons. Circulation. 2012;126(25):e354–471.
51. Patel MR, Calhoon JH, Dehmer GJ, Grantham JA, Maddox TM, Maron DJ, Smith PK. ACC/AATS/AHA/ASE/ASNC/SCAI/SCCT/STS 2017 appropriate use criteria for coronary revascularization in patients with stable ischemic heart disease: a report of the American College of Cardiology appropriate use criteria task force, American Association for Thoracic Surgery, American Heart Association, American Society of Echocardiography, American Society of Nuclear Cardiology, Society for Cardiovascular Angiography and Interventions, Society of Cardiovascular Computed Tomography, and Society of Thoracic.... J Am Coll Cardiol. 2017;69(17):2212–41.
52. Sabik JF, Bakaeen FG, Ruel M, Moon MR, Malaisrie SC, Calhoon JH, Girardi LN, Guyton R. The American Association for Thoracic Surgery and the Society of Thoracic Surgeons reasoning for not endorsing the 2021 ACC/AHA/SCAI coronary revascularization guidelines. J Thorac Cardiovasc Surg. 2022;163(4):1362–5.
53. Maron DJ, Hochman JS, Reynolds HR, Bangalore S, O'Brien SM, Boden WE, Chaitman BR, Senior R, López-Sendón J, Alexander KP, Lopes RD. Initial invasive or conservative strategy for stable coronary disease. N Engl J Med. 2020;382(15):1395–407.
54. Mehaffey JH, Hayanga JA, Kawsara M, Sakhuja A, Mascio C, Rankin JS, Badhwar V. Contemporary coronary artery bypass grafting versus multivessel percutaneous coronary intervention. Ann Thorac Surg. 2023;
55. Neumann FJ, Sousa-Uva M, Ahlsson A, Alfonso F, Banning AP, Benedetto U, Byrne RA, Collet JP, Falk V, Head SJ, Jüni P. 2018 ESC/EACTS guidelines on myocardial revascularization. The task force on myocardial revascularization of the European Society of Cardiology (ESC) and European Association for Cardio-Thoracic Surgery (EACTS). Giornale italiano di cardiologia (2006). 2019;20(7-8 Suppl 1):1S–61S.
56. Penicka M, Bartunek J, Lang O, Medilek K, Tousek P, Vanderheyden M, et al. Severe left ventricular dyssynchrony is associated with poor prognosis in patients

with moderate systolic heart failure undergoing coronary artery bypass grafting. J Am Coll Cardiol. 2007;50(14):1315–23.
57. Maruskova M, Gregor P, Bartunek J, Tintera J, Penicka M. Myocardial viability and cardiac dyssynchrony as strong predictors of perioperative mortality in high-risk patients with ischemic cardiomyopathy having coronary artery bypass surgery. J Thorac Cardiovasc Surg. 2009;138(1):62–8.
58. AlJaroudi W, Alraies MC, Hachamovitch R, Jaber WA, Brunken R, Cerqueira MD, et al. Association of left ventricular mechanical dyssynchrony with survival benefit from revascularization: a study of gated positron emission tomography in patients with ischemic LV dysfunction and narrow QRS. Eur J Nucl Med Mol Imaging. 2012;39(10):1581–91.
59. Elefteriades JA, Tolis G Jr, Levi E, Mills LK, Zaret BL. Coronary artery bypass grafting in severe left ventricular dysfunction: excellent survival with improved ejection fraction and functional state. J Am Coll Cardiol. 1993;22(5):1411–7.
60. Hovnanian AL, Matos Soeiro A, Serrano CV, Oliveira SA, Jatene FB, Stolf NA, et al. Surgical myocardial revascularization of patients with ischemic cardiomyopathy and severe left ventricular disfunction. Clinics (Sao Paulo). 2010;65(1):3–8.
61. Trachiotis GD, Weintraub WS, Johnston TS, Jones EL, Guyton RA, Craver JM. Coronary artery bypass grafting in patients with advanced left ventricular dysfunction. Ann Thorac Surg. 1998;66(5):1632–9.
62. Kim RW, Ugurlu BS, Tereb DA, Wackers FJ, Tellides G, Elefteriades JA. Effect of left ventricular volume on results of coronary artery bypass grafting. Am J Cardiol. 2000;86(11):1261–4, A6
63. Soliman Hamad MA, Tan ME, van Straten AH, van Zundert AA, Schönberger JP. Long-term results of coronary artery bypass grafting in patients with left ventricular dysfunction. Ann Thorac Surg. 2008;85(2):488–93.
64. Bax JJ, Schinkel AF, Boersma E, Elhendy A, Rizzello V, Maat A, et al. Extensive left ventricular remodeling does not allow viable myocardium to improve in left ventricular ejection fraction after revascularization and is associated with worse long-term prognosis. Circulation. 2004;110(11 Suppl 1):II18–22.
65. Pouleur AC, Rousseau MF, Ahn SA, Amzulescu M, Demeure F, de Meester C, Vancraeynest D, Pasquet A, Vanoverschelde JL, Gerber BL. Right ventricular systolic dysfunction assessed by cardiac magnetic resonance is a strong predictor of cardiovascular death after coronary bypass grafting. Ann Thorac Surg. 2016;101(6):2176–84.
66. Dang NC, Topkara VK, Mercando M, Kay J, Kruger KH, Aboodi MS, Oz MC, Naka Y. Right heart failure after left ventricular assist device implantation in patients with chronic congestive heart failure. J Heart Lung Transplant. 2006;25(1):1–6.
67. Morine K, Kiernan M, Kapur N, Baumgartner R, Pham D, Denofrio D. Pulmonary artery pulsatility index as a novel marker of right ventricular failure following LVAD surgery. J Card Fail. 2013;19(8):S17.
68. Fukamachi K, McCarthy PM, Smedira NG, Vargo RL, Starling RC, Young JB. Preoperative risk factors for right ventricular failure after implantable left ventricular assist device insertion. Ann Thorac Surg. 1999;68(6):2181–4.
69. Bouchart F, Tabley A, Litzler PY, Haas-Hubscher C, Bessou JP, Soyer R. Myocardial revascularization in patients with severe ischemic left ventricular dysfunction. Long term follow-up in 141 patients. Eur J Cardiothorac Surg. 2001;20(6):1157–62.
70. Pocar M, Moneta A, Grossi A, Donatelli F. Coronary artery bypass for heart failure in ischemic cardiomyopathy: 17-year follow-up. Ann Thorac Surg. 2007;83(2):468–74.
71. Tong MZ, Weiss AJ, Bakaeen F, Soltesz EG. CABG in failing hearts: a how-to-guide to using modern mechanical support as backup. Innovations. 2021;16(3):227–30.
72. Selim Isbir C, Yildirim T, Akgun S, Civelek A, Aksoy N, Oz M, et al. Coronary artery bypass surgery in patients with severe left ventricular dysfunction. Int J Cardiol. 2003;90(2–3):309–16.
73. Galbut DL, Kurlansky PA, Traad EA, Dorman MJ, Zucker M, Ebra G. Bilateral internal thoracic artery grafting improves long-term survival in patients with reduced ejection fraction: a propensity-matched study with 30-year follow-up. J Thorac Cardiovasc Surg. 2012;143(4):844–53.
74. Samady H, Elefteriades JA, Abbott BG, Mattera JA, McPherson CA, Wackers FJ. Failure to improve left ventricular function after coronary revascularization for ischemic cardiomyopathy is not associated with worse outcome. Circulation. 1999;100(12):1298–304.
75. Kunadian V, Zaman A, Qiu W. Revascularization among patients with severe left ventricular dysfunction: a meta-analysis of observational studies. Eur J Heart Fail. 2011;13(7):773–84.
76. Mihaljevic T, Lam BK, Rajeswaran J, Takagaki M, Lauer MS, Gillinov AM, et al. Impact of mitral valve annuloplasty combined with revascularization in patients with functional ischemic mitral regurgitation. J Am Coll Cardiol. 2007;49(22):2191–201.
77. Athanasuleas CL, Buckberg GD, Stanley AW, Siler W, Dor V, DiDonato M, RESTORE Group, et al. Surgical ventricular restoration: the RESTORE Group experience. Heart Fail Rev. 2004;9(4):287–97.
78. Dor V, Civaia F, Alexandrescu C, Sabatier M, Montiglio F. Favorable effects of left ventricular reconstruction in patients excluded from the Surgical Treatments for Ischemic Heart Failure (STICH) trial. J Thorac Cardiovasc Surg. 2011;141(4):905–16. 916.e1–4
79. Ferrell BE, Jimenez DC, Ahmad D, Malkani K, Rosen JL, Gaw G, Plestis KA, Guy TS, Massey HT, Tchantchaleishvili V. Surgical ventricular reconstruction for ischemic cardiomyopathy—a systematic review and meta-analysis of 7,685 patients. Ann Cardiothorac Surg. 2022;11(3):226–38.

80. Schmitto JD, Mariani S, Li T, Dogan G, Hanke JS, Bara C, Pya Y, Zimpfer D, Krabatsch T, Garbade J, Rao V. Five-year outcomes of patients supported with HeartMate 3: a single-centre experience. Eur J Cardiothorac Surg. 2021;59(6):1155–63.
81. Mehra MR, Goldstein DJ, Cleveland JC, Cowger JA, Hall S, Salerno CT, Naka Y, Horstmanshof D, Chuang J, Wang A, Uriel N. Five-year outcomes in patients with fully magnetically levitated vs axial-flow left ventricular assist devices in the MOMENTUM 3 randomized trial. JAMA. 2022;328(12):1233–42.
82. Yuzefpolskaya M, Schroeder SE, Houston BA, Robinson MR, Gosev I, Reyentovich A, Koehl D, Cantor R, Jorde UP, Kirklin JK, Pagani FD. The society of thoracic surgeons Intermacs 2022 annual report: focus on the 2018 heart transplant allocation system. Ann Thorac Surg. 2023;115(2):311–27.
83. Maltais S, Tchantchaleishvili V, Schaff HV, Daly RC, Suri RM, Dearani JA, Topilsky Y, Stulak JM, Joyce LD, Park SJ. Management of severe ischemic cardiomyopathy: left ventricular assist device as destination therapy versus conventional bypass and mitral valve surgery. J Thorac Cardiovasc Surg. 2014;147(4):1246–50.
84. Centers for Medicare and Medicaid Services. Proposed decision memo for artificial hearts and related device, including ventricular assist devices for bridge-to-transplant and destination therapy (CAG-00453N) [Internet]. Available from: https://www.cms.gov/medicare-coverage-database/details/nca-proposed-decision-memo.aspx?NCAId=298. Accessed 8/3/2023.

Valve Repair and Replacement in Congestive Heart Failure

25

Tirth A. Patel, Khulkar Mirzozoda, Salil V. Deo, Soon J. Park, and Nicholas Ruggiero

Mitral Regurgitation

Introduction

The mitral valve consists of two leaflets, two papillary muscles, and multiple chordae, which transmit the command of the papillary muscle to the leaflets. Yet this simple description does not do justice the extremely complex interplay of these structures, which helps to promote a well-functioning competent mitral valve. While degenerative mitral valve disease affects primarily the mitral valve leaflets, mitral regurgitation in congestive heart failure primarily involves the annular and sub-valvar apparatus. Carpentier was the first to introduce a systematic classification of mitral valve disease [1], which is based on the mechanism of mitral regurgitation. Thereafter many labels like "ischemic", "cardiomyopathy induced", "functional" or "non-organic" have been interchangeably used to define this condition. Yet in reality the degree and mechanism of regurgitation changes according to the extent of left ventricular dysfunction [2–5]. As Repogle et al. [5] have described, ischemic mitral regurgitation (IMR) can be divided into the following categories: (a) *Acute MR*: This can be due to myocardial infarction and associated papillary muscle ischemia or ventricular dysfunction. (b) *MR due to end-stage Ischemic cardiomyopathy* & (c) *Chronic MR*: Ischemic heart disease with changes in the regional wall motion leading to chronic mitral regurgitation. Another group of patients who further confuse the overall picture are those with coronary artery disease and associated mitral valve prolapse or myxomatous mitral valve disease [6]. In an attempt to provide some clarity to the situation, it is prudent to separate these patients into two main entities: Ischemic mitral regurgitation (IMR) and Functional mitral regurgitation (FMR) [7].

Ischemic Mitral Regurgitation

The basis for IMR is a localized change in the ventricular geometry. McGee et al. have demonstrated increase incidence of IMR with inferior as compared to anterior wall ischemia [8]. A similar finding was detected by echocardiographic analysis of segmental leaflet anatomy [9]. There are subtle differences in mitral pathology depending upon the location of the infarction. Three-dimensional echocardiography has demonstrated that anterior infarction is associated with more

T. A. Patel (✉) · K. Mirzozoda · N. Ruggiero
Division of Cardiology, Thomas Jefferson University Hospital, Philadelphia, PA, USA
e-mail: tirth.patel@jefferson.edu; khulkar.mirzozoda@jefferson.edu; nicholas.ruggiero@jefferson.edu

S. V. Deo · S. J. Park
Division of Cardiac Surgery, University Hospitals, Case Western Reserve University, Cleveland, OH, USA
e-mail: svd14@case.edu; soon.park@uhhospitals.org

H. J. Eisen (ed.), *Heart Failure I*, https://doi.org/10.1007/978-3-032-12626-9_25

depressed left ventricular function, annular dilatation in the antero-posterior axis and annular flattening [10–12]. Inferior infarction has a higher tendency to cause early IMR, likely due to greater dis co-ordination of the papillary muscles [13, 14]. Greater leaflet tension with resultantly more MR occurs when the papillary muscles are displaced in a postero-lateral and apical direction [15]. This phenomenon is more likely with inferior rather than anterior infarction. Dis-synchrony among left ventricular myocardium especially at the area of papillary muscle insertion is an important contributory factor for IMR [16].

Annular dilatation is associated with IMR too, but unlike FMR it is not the primary cause of regurgitation. In fact patients with acute IMR may have significant regurgitation due to a disturbed ventriculo-annular relationship without much annular dilatation.

Functional Mitral Regurgitation

FMR should be reserved for patients with depressed left ventricular function and dilated cardiomyopathy, whether it is ischemic or idiopathic. Studies have demonstrated that leaflet tethering due to alteration in left ventricular global geometry is the primary etiology of FMR [17–20]. Animal models have demonstrated that FMR depends on the left ventricle developing a globular shape [19]. Annular dilatation, which takes place predominantly in a septo-posterior direction, has been found to be an important factor for the production of FMR, with limited regurgitation in patients with minimal increase in annular size [21]. A geometrical change in the left ventricle, promotes increase in the inter-papillary distance, resulting in restricted leaflet motion and a reduction in the coaptation area [22].

Thus IMR and FMR are the two end-points of the entire spectrum of mitral regurgitation associated with congestive heart failure. In the real world, patients may present with a variable combination of both conditions (Fig. 25.1) [7].

Dynamic Nature of Mitral Regurgitation

IMR/FMR is also very dynamic in nature with variation in severity over time and level of activity. Inotropes will increase the dp/dt promoting more closing of the valve and reducing MR [23, 24]. Conditions (anesthesia, diuretic therapy) leading to a reduction in preload and left ventricular diastolic size will reduce MR [25]. Lancellotti et al. have demonstrated the importance of exercise echocardiography as a tool in unmasking MR in patients with congestive heart failure [26, 27]. A change in the effective regurgitant orifice area (EROA) is due to a systolic expansion of the mitral annulus; leading to increase in cooptation distance, increase in the tenting area (area between the mitral annulus and the leaflet cooptation line) and the sphericity index (both end-systolic and end-diastolic) [28]. A sudden increase in MR during daily activities can provoke flash pulmonary edema, acute systolic pulmonary hypertension and electromechanical dys-synchrony promoting further MR [27, 29, 30]. Any discrepancy between symptoms and resting echocardiographic findings should be investigated with exercise testing to unmask latent MR. Exercise induced MR is of great prog-

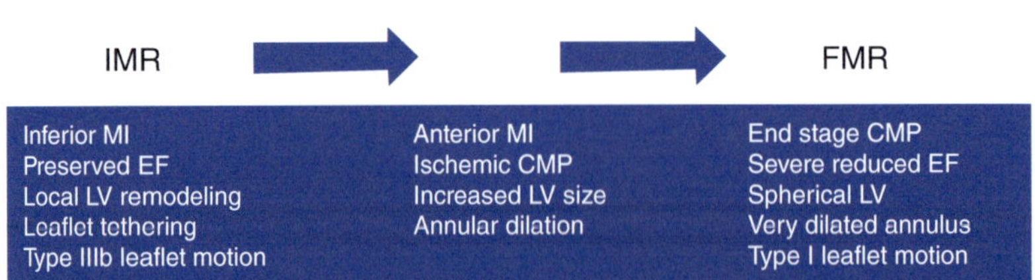

Fig. 25.1 This figure demonstrates the subtle differences in ischemic mitral regurgitation (IMR) and functional mitral regurgitation (FMR). (Reprinted from Timek and Miller [7], © 2011, with permission from Elsevier)

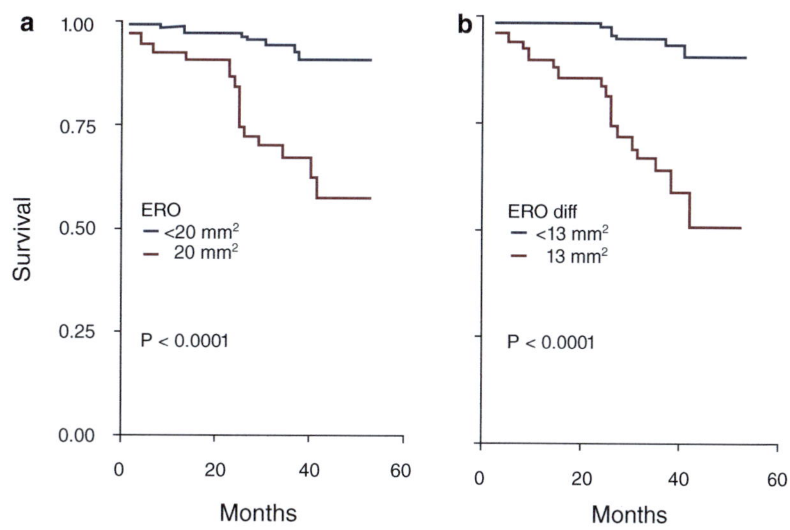

Fig. 25.2 Lancellotti and colleagues demonstrated that survival was significantly different in patients stratified by effective regurgitant orifice (ERO); important cut-off values being ERO ≥20 mm² at rest (**a**) and an increase in ERO ≥13 mm² on exercise (**b**). (Reprinted with permission from Lancellotti et al. [31] by permission of Oxford University Press)

nostic importance in these patients; a change in EROA >13 mm² being a significant predictor of late mortality as demonstrated by Lancelotti and colleagues [31, 32] (Fig. 25.2).

Quantification of Ischemic Mitral Regurgitation/Functional Mitral Regurgitation

The following factors need to be considered for the quantification of IMR/FMR:

(a) Severity of MR; number and direction of the regurgitant jets &.
(b) Degree of LV dilatation, dysfunction and remodeling.

Echocardiography needs to focus on both the mitral valve anatomy as well as the LV geometry: The important factors which need to be considered for evaluating a patient with mitral regurgitation are: LV indices: left ventricular volumes, ejection fraction, sphericity index, the diastolic function and wall motion abnormalities & MV indices: mitral annular dimensions, effective regurgitant orifice area (EROA), co-aptation depth, tenting area and tenting volume on 3-D Echo (Fig. 25.3) [16]. Table 25.1 denotes the measurements obtained with echocardiographic examination of 21 control subjects and 128 patients with left ventricular dysfunction (<50%).

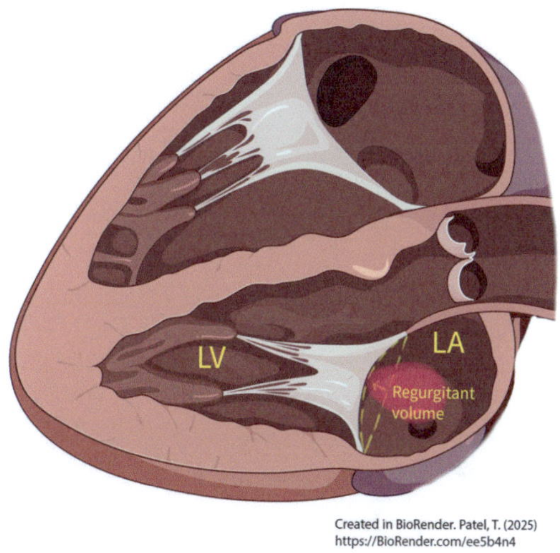

Fig. 25.3 A diagrammatic representation of the co-aptation depth (H), the tenting area (T) and Regurgitant volume; all are important in the quantification of mitral regurgitation. (Reprinted with permission from Agricola et al. [16], by permission of Oxford University Press)

Secondary Changes in Leaflet Structure

Although this is primarily a condition of the left ventricle, the leaflets themselves are far from innocent by-standers in the disease process (Fig. 25.4). While the leaflets may appear grossly normal at surgery, significant biochemical changes have been identified in the leaflets in patients with long-standing cardiomyopathy.

Table 25.1 denotes the measurements obtained with echocardiographic examination of 21 control subjects and 128 patients with left ventricular dysfunction (<50%)

	Comparison with controls			Comparison within LVD					Correlation with ERO	
Variable	Control ($n = 21$)	LVD ($n = 128$)	p	No MR ($n = 21$)	ERO <10 mm^2	ERO 10—<20 mm^2	ERO >20 mm^2	p for trend	r	p
Baseline characteristics										
Age, y	62 ± 10	65 ± 13	0.20	57 ± 16	68 ± 13	65 ± 14	68 ± 11	0.03	0.20	0.02
Sex, % males	57	65	0.50	76	42	70	68	0.56	−0.14	0.12
BSA, m^2	1.9 ± 0.3	1.9 ± 0.2	0.52	2.0 ± 0.2	1.8 ± 0.3	1.9 ± 0.2	1.9 ± 0.2	0.61	−0.04	0.70
SBP, mmHg	134 ± 19	125 ± 21	0.05	126 ± 18	133 ± 21	127 ± 21	116 ± 19	0.003	−0.37	0.0001
CI, L/min^2/m^2	2.9 ± 0.4	2.4 ± 0.5	0.0003	2.7 ± 0.5	2.6 ± 0.5	2.4 ± 0.5	2.3 ± 0.6	0.0005	−0.34	0.0001
Global LV remodeling										
EDVI, ml/m^2	65 ± 10	149 ± 46	<0.0001	115 ± 28	150 ± 34	145 ± 52	169 ± 46	0.0001	0.49	0.0001
ESVI, ml/m^2	24 ± 6	106 ± 43	<0.0001	78 ± 29	108 ± 33	104 ± 51	119 ± 42	0.002	−0.31	0.0005
Systolic L/D	2.5 ± 0.5	1.5 ± 0.2	<0.0001	1.6 ± 0.2	1.4 ± 0.2	1.5 ± 0.2	1.4 ± 0.2	0.012	−0.31	0.0005
Diastolic L/D	1.9 ± 0.2	1.4 ± 0.2	0.0001	1.5 ± 0.2	1.3 ± 0.2	1.4 ± 0.1	1.3 ± 0.2	0.007	−0.29	0.001
EF, %	64 ± 4	31 ± 9	<0.0001	34 ± 10	28 ± 7	30 ± 10	31 ± 9	0.83	−0.09	0.32
ESWS, g/cm^2	158 ± 26	271 ± 67	<0.0001	244 ± 56	284 ± 81	281 ± 65	267 ± 65	0.68	0.13	0.17

Reprinted with permission from Yiu et al. [33] © 2000, with permission from Wolters Kluwer Health, Inc

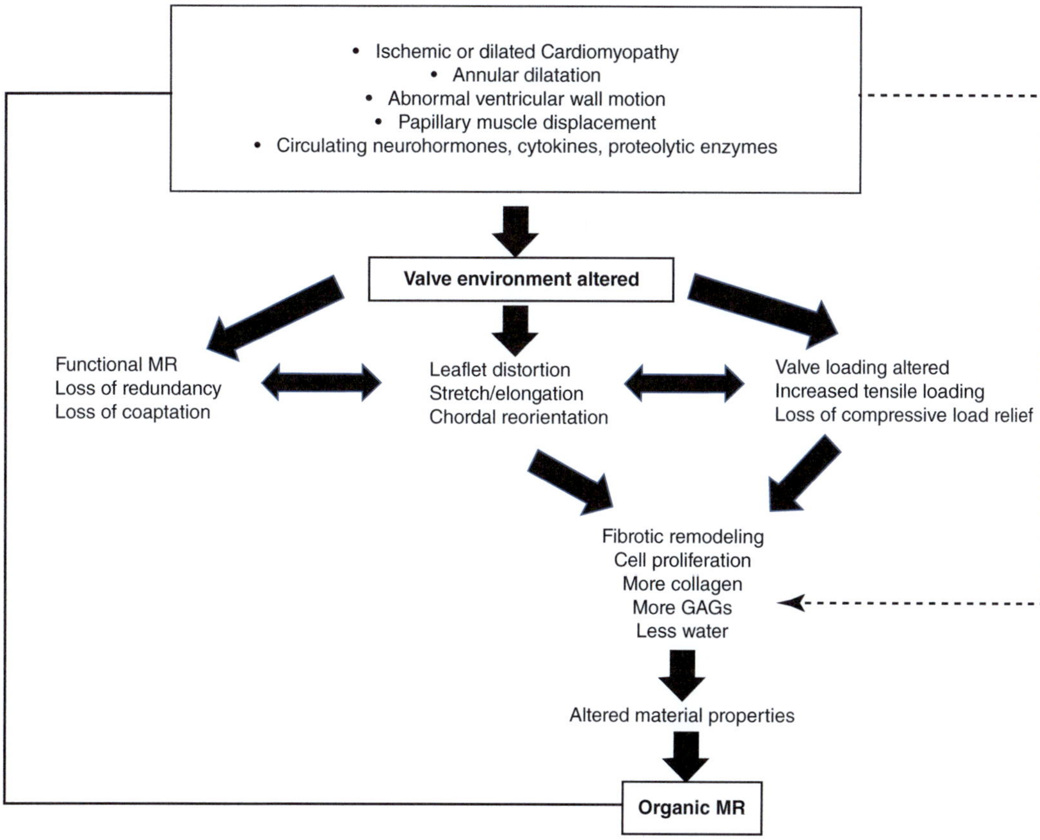

Fig. 25.4 The flowchart by Gravnde-Allen et al. demonstrates changes in leaflet structure and composition in ischemic/functional mitral regurgitation. (Reprinted from Grande-Allen et al. [34], © 2005, with permission from Elsevier)

Grande-Allen and colleagues studied leaflet tissue obtained from recipient hearts explanted at the time of transplantation and tested them with tissue obtained from normal hearts at autopsy. Biochemically these leaflets had a higher cellular count (78% more), higher collagen density (15% more) and lower water content (7% less). These changes made the leaflets thicker and less pliable compared to their normal counterparts. The chordae tendinae also had a smaller cross-sectional area compared to the normal cohort. The leaflets were 28–41% longer than normal [34]. The leaflet length correlated with left atrial diameter, annular diameter while thickness correlated with annular size as well as left ventricular and left atrial dimensions [34].

Importance of Mitral Regurgitation on Survival with Heart Failure

The presence of IMR has a profound influence on survival. In 1988, Hickey et al. demonstrated a 34% increase in mortality for patients with severe IMR compared to those with coronary artery disease and no MR. Even patients with mild IMR had a 4% increase in mortality above baseline [35]. The Survival and Ventricular enlargement study (SAVE) demonstrated that even the presence of mild MR was an independent risk factor for cardiovascular mortality (Relative Risk = 2(1.28–3.04)) during a 3.5 years follow-up period [36]. Grigioni and colleagues compared 194 (IMR+) and 104 (IMR –ve) after matching them for age, gender and ejection fraction over a patient-year period of 817 years [37]. The IMR cohort experienced a much higher long-term mortality (62 +/− 5% vs 39 +/− 6%; $p < 0.001$) at the end of 5 years, with the presence of IMR independently affecting survival on a multi-variate analysis. The mean ejection fraction in this study was in the approximate range of 26–36% for both cohorts (Fig. 25.5).

Trichon et al. evaluated 2057 pts. with symptomatic systolic heart failure undergoing evaluation in the cardiac catheterization laboratory over a 14-year period. While 56% had IMR of any grade, importantly almost half of these patients had moderate/severe IMR. They have demonstrated a 40% survival at 5 years and have demonstrated that the presence of even moderate IMR is a risk factor for early mortality [38]. A study from the University of Michigan in 1421 patients with congestive heart failure (LV ejection fraction <35%) demonstrated 50% survival of 628 +/− 47 days for patients with severe IMR [39]. Importantly almost 50% of the patients in this study had at least moderate MR, which demonstrates the important relationship between left ventricular systolic dysfunction and the presence of MR. Ellis et al. demonstrated an inferior outcomes in patients with IMR undergoing percutaneous intervention, especially in the subset of patients with LVEF <40% [40].

Thus many retrospective studies have demonstrated poorer survival in patients with IMR with approximately 40–50% survival at the end of 3–5 years.

What Degree of Ischemic Mitral Regurgitation Should Be Addressed?

All agree that moderate-severe IMR should be addressed at the time of coronary artery bypass grafting (CABG) [41, 42]. Correcting regurgitation at the time of CABG improves exercise capacity, symptoms and promotes reverse ventricular remodeling [43, 44]. The American College of Cardiology recommends concomitant mitral valve surgery in patients with LVEF <40% with severe symptomatic mitral regurgitation. The committee prefers valve repair; but if that is not possible then replacement should be carried out with chordal preservation [45].

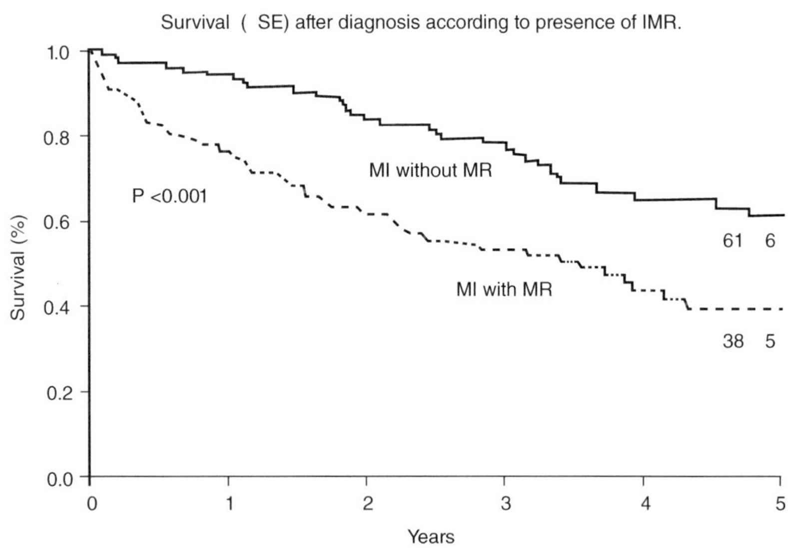

Fig. 25.5 Patients with ischemic MR clearly have a poorer survival as demonstrated by this Kaplan-Meier curve. (Reprinted from Grigioni et al. [37], © 2001, with permission from Wolters Kluwer Health Inc./American Heart Publications)

Results of Repair and Replacement with Ischemic/Functional Mitral Regurgitation

David and colleagues were among the first to demonstrate good results with mitral valve replacement while preserving the subvalvar apparatus [46]. Bolling and Bach were the first to demonstrate successful mitral annuloplasty (MVA) in patients with cardiomyopathy. They were successful in operating on 16 patients (mean ejection fraction 16 +/– 5%) without peri-operative mortality and demonstrated significant improvements in stroke volume, ejection fraction and cardiac output with concomitant reduction in regurgitant volume and fraction [2]. This landmark achievement disputed the theory of the "pop-off" effect of the mitral valve for a failing left ventricle. The Bolling hypothesis is that there is an " annular solution for a ventricular problem… such that reconstruction of the mitral valve annulus` geometric abnormality by an undersized ring restores valvular competency, alleviates excessive ventricular workload, improves ventricular geometry and improves ventricular function". This concept was validated by the Stanford group using animal models [47]. Mihaljevic and colleagues studied patients undergoing CABG + MVA (290) and CABG alone (100) and presented their results in a propensity-matched cohort [48]. A restrictive annuloplasty with the use of both rigid rings (22%) (Carpentier-Edwards Classic Annuloplasty ring, Edward Lifesciences, Irvine, CA), partially flexible posterior annuloplasty bands (63%) (Cosgrove-Edwards Annuloplasty system, Edward Lifesciences, Irvine, CA) and even posterior suture plication with autologous pericardium or Peri-Guard graft (6.9%) (Baxter Healthcare Corp., Deerfield, IL) was performed. Their estimated survival for MVA + CABG (92%, 74% and 39%) and CABG (88%, 75% and 47%) at the end of 1, 5 and 10 years was comparable ($p = 0.3$). In the early period of follow-up, renal insufficiency, severe wall motion abnormalities, and surgery in an earlier time period were the predictors of mortality. For the late constant hazard phase insulin dependent diabetes, renal insufficiency, older age, were significant predictors. The benefit of MVA was in abolishing early post-operative MR. Unfortunately this study failed to demonstrate any incremental clinical benefit of concomitant MVA. In fact they caution that the longer ischemic time needed for MVA could be detrimental in the sick, old patient. They have projected a recurrence of 3 +/ 4 + MR in 9% and 20% in the CABG + MVA cohort at the end of 1 and 5 years respectively. Grossi et al. [42] studied a cohort of 223 patients over two decades, with 152 undergoing MVA (77% ring and 23% suture annuloplasty). As they have found the era of surgery to be an important predictor of outcome, we will concentrate on their results in patients operated after 1988. Analyzing their entire cohort, they report that type of surgery (repair vs replacement), papillary muscle rupture, congestive heart failure and acute MR impair long-term survival. In their contemporary series of patients (surgery after 1988) however, outcome are poorer for mitral valve replacement (hazard Ratio; 0.45(0.22–0.93)) and emergency surgery (hazard ratio 0.19(0.06–0.64)). Using complicated statistical models, they conclude that NYHA functional class and patient selection determine outcome rather than surgical procedure. Impressively almost 82% from the MVA cohort were free of significant MR. They recommend restrictive MVA as the first strategy for patients with an annular pathology, while those with significant leaflet tethering or papillary muscle dysfunction would do better with posterior chordal preservation and MVR. Mayo Clinc recently presented their experience of 431 patients who underwent mitral valve repair/replacement for ischemic MR over a 14 year period [6]. Overall survival for the entire cohort was 82.7%, 55.2% and 24.3% at the end of 1, 5 and 10 years respectively. All patients in the repair cohort underwent either an undersized band or rigid ring annuloplasty. Details of sub-annular apparatus preservation are unfortunately not available in individual patients due to the retrospective nature of the study, although institutional policy is to perform at least posterior chordal preservation. Prior CABG, emergency surgery and age were risk factors for early mortality (<1 year) while age, renal insufficiency and diabetes contributed to the late constant hazard phase. These results are similar to those at the Cleveland Clinic [48]. This underlines the importance of patient factors rather than procedure to late outcome.

Fukuda and colleagues [49] reported results of 126 patients with severe left ventricular dysfunction ($\leq 30\%$), who underwent mitral valve annuloplasty. They found that annuloplasty is not a predictor of improved survival. However they, as well as many others have demonstrated an improved quality of life and functional capacity after mitral valve surgery.

Two important issues regarding repair of ischemic mitral regurgitation are recurrent regurgitation and a more recently introduced concept of exercise induced mitral stenosis. The incidence of recurrent regurgitation after repair is not small. Gilinov et al. have reported a repair failure rate of 9% over a 5-year period [41]. Chan and coworkers have demonstrated a recurrence rate of 23% in their study evaluating 65 patients with mitral valve repair [50].

Exercise induced mitral stenosis is being increasingly reported with patients undergoing restrictive annuloplasty [51]. Magne and coworkers have reported increase in trans-valvular gradients with restrictive annuloplasty leading to pulmonary hypertension and increased clinical symptoms [51]. Some authors have implicated left ventricular dysfunction and pulmonary vascular disease rather Exercise induced mitral stenosis than mitral valve gradients as the cause for pulmonary hypertension after ischemic mitral valve repair [52, 53].

Geometric Rings for Ischemic Mitral Regurgitation

The Geoform™ ring (Edwards Lifesciences, Irvine, CA) has a unique three dimensional shape designed to reduce the anteroposterior diameter and elevate P_2 segment of the leaflet. DeBonis et al. demonstrated survival of 81.1 +/− 6.6% at 3.5 years, while recurrent regurgitation was present in 16%. Significant exercise induced mitral stenosis was not found in any of the survivors. Restricted motion of the posterior leaflet is an important predictor of recurrent regurgitation.

The Carpentier-McCarty-Adams ETLogixring™ is the first ring specifically designed to treat asymmetrical restriction of the posterior leaflet. Initial results are favorable with a low residual grade of regurgitation and improvement in echocardiographic parameters early after surgery [54]. A recent study demonstrates significant reduction ($p < 0.0006$) in the mitral annular diameter, tenting area as well as tenting height after use of the ETLogixring™. They conclude that the ring is useful for selective patients with ischemic mitral regurgitation. While functional mitral stenosis has not been reported with the Geoform™ ring, Martin and colleagues have recently reported their results on 40 patients with the ETLogixring™ [55].

The choice of ring for the repair of ischemic regurgitation is a very complex issue, and an exhaustive discussion regarding this issue is beyond the purview of this article. However while energy and dollars are being spent on devising and marketing new rings, reports are also available demonstrating comparable changes in the geometry of the mitral valve [56].

Percutaneous Techniques to Deal with Mitral Regurgitation

As discussed in the earlier part of the chapter, mortality and morbidity associated with the surgical treatment of mitral regurgitation may be significant. Patients may be denied surgery on the grounds that it is too high risk [57]. Various techniques are present attempting to correct mitral regurgitation in a minimally invasive manner. A detailed discussion of various percutaneous techniques available for secondary mitral regurgitation is provided by Wunderlich and colleagues in their comprehensive review [58]. Percutaneous devices used to treat mitral regurgitation include transcatheter edge-to-edge repair, direct and indirect annuloplasty, transcatheter mitral valve replacement, chordal apparatus, and ventricular restoration.

Transcatheter Edge-to-Edge Repair

The most common percutaneous mitral valve intervention which is approved by the U.S. Food and Drug Administration for both primary/degenerative and secondary MR is the MitraClip™ (Abbott Vascular, Santa Clara, CA). The technique is based on the open surgical technique of Alfieri where the anterior and posterior leaflets are approximated together to create a double mitral orifice. A steerable catheter is utilized to deploy the clip. The approach is antegrade via a trans-septal puncture. In 2009, Feldman and colleagues reported the mid-term results of the EVEREST (Endovascular Valve Edge-to-edge Repair trial) trial, the first randomized controlled single arm study aimed at assessing feasibility of percutaneous mitral valve repair [59]. A total of 107 patients underwent MitraClip™ repair with <1% in-hospital mortality. Overall, 74% had procedural success, defined as residual mitral regurgitation ≤2 + at the end of the procedure. At the end of 1 year, 66% were free of ≥2 + MR, surgery or death. During surgery, repair was still possible in the majority of patients. Although clip embolization was not an issue, partial clip dislodgement occurred in 9%. The EVEREST II trial (NCT 00209274) was undertaken comparing surgical repair and MitraClip™ in a 2:1 randomized manner. The non-inferiority endpoint of the study was met, demonstrating that device therapy was comparable to surgical repair at the end of 1 year of follow-up. In another sub-study of EVEREST II, high-risk patients (STS score >12%) undergoing MitraClip™ repair were compared to similar patients electing for optimal medical therapy. This study demonstrated a significant improvement in clinical symptoms and left ventricular reverse remodeling after 12 months in the device cohort. Based on these results, U.S. Food and Drug Administration, provided the approval for the use of MitraClip™ for primary/degenerative MR in patients with prohibitive surgical risk in 2013. In 2018, Stone and colleagues reported the results of the COAPT (Cardiovascular Outcomes Assessment of the MitraClip™ Percutaneous Therapy), a landmark multi-center, randomized, controlled, parallel-group clinical trial which demonstrated in patients with heart failure and symptomatic moderate to severe or severe secondary mitral regurgitation despite the use of maximally tolerated guideline-directed medical therapy, transcatheter mitral valve repair resulted in a lower rate of heart failure hospitalization and lower all-cause mortality within 24 months of follow-up compared to medical therapy alone [60]. Of the 614 patients in this trial, a total of 302 were assigned to undergo transcatheter mitral valve repair plus medical therapy and 312 were assigned to receive medical therapy alone. The primary end-point of annual rate of all hospitalizations for heart failure within 24 months was significantly lower, 35.8% per patient-year in the device group as compared with 67.9% in the control group. The primary safety end-point, rate of freedom from device-related complications at 12 months was 96.6% for the device group. Of the secondary endpoints, all-cause mortality within 24 months was much lower, 29.1% in the device group as compared with 46.1% in the control group. These results remained significant even after adjustments for differences in guide-line directed medical therapy at baseline. In the secondary analysis of the COAPT trial, Lindman and colleagues demonstrated that while LV reverse remodeling at 6 month was associated with reduced cardiovascular mortality between 6 months and 24 months in both device and control groups, this was not affected by transcatheter mitral valve repair or residual MR severity [61]. A separate secondary analysis of COAPT trial data performed by Pio and colleagues demonstrated a significant improvement in left atrial strain 60.4% in the device group vs 39.6% in the control group at 6 month follow-up [62]. Left atrial strain improvement was significantly associated with reduction of composite outcome of death or heart failure hospitalization between 6 months and 24 months in both device and medical treatment groups. In 2023, Stone and colleagues reported the 5-year follow up of outcomes of the original COAPT trial [63]. A total of 89% of patients in the device group and 85% of patients in the control group completed the five-year follow-up. The annual rate of hospitalization for heart failure was again significantly lower 33.1% per year in the device group compared with 57.2% per year in the control group. Similarly, all-cause mortality at five-year follow-up was significantly lower 57.3% in the device group as compared to 67.2% in the control group. Composite outcome of death or heart failure hospitalization through 5 years was significantly lower 73.6% in the device group as compared to 91.5% in the control group. The majority of the difference in rate of heart failure hospitalizations was within the first 36 months and difference in mortality was within the first 24 months with no significant difference afterwards. Importantly, at 4-year follow-up, rate of stroke or transient ischemic attack was not statistically different, 0.7% in the device group as compared to 0% in the control group [64]. The primary safety end-point, rate of freedom from device-related complications at 5 years remained high at 89.2%. Based on these results, U.S. Food and Drug Administration approved a new indication for MitraClip™ for secondary mitral regurgitation.

PASCAL (Edwards Lifesciences Corp, Irvine, CA) is another U.S. Food and Drug administration transcatheter edge-to-edge repair device based on the Alfieri surgical technique. PASCAL offers broader paddles, central spacer and 3D maneuvering making it more suitable for patients with complex mitral valve anatomy and for those patients requiring more than one MitraClip. In 2023, Zahr and colleagues reported the 1-year outcomes from the CLASP IID (Edwards PASCAL TrAnScatheter Valve RePair System Pivotal Clinical) a randomized controlled trial comparing the outcomes of PASCAL vs MitraClip in patients with significant symptomatic mitral regurgitation with prohibitive surgical risk [65]. A total of 204 patients were randomized to PASCAL and 96 patients were randomized to MitraClip. Noninferiority was met for primary effectiveness (rates of MR $\leq$ 2+ at 6 months) and secondary effectiveness (rates of MR $\leq$ 2+ and MR $\leq$ 1+ at 1-year) and primary safety endpoint (major adverse event at 30-days) for PASCAL. In addition to that, at year 1, there were not statistical differences for key secondary clinical outcomes including all-cause mortality, stroke or heart failure hospitalizations. CLASP IID/IIF (NCT03706833), a prospective, multicenter, randomized, controlled trial to evaluate the safety and effectiveness of PASCAL compared to MitraClip in patients with degenerative mitral regurgitation with prohibitive surgical risk, and in patients with functional mitral regurgitation on guideline directed medical therapy is currently ongoing [66].

The most current 2020 ACC/AHA Valvular Heart disease Guidelines give transcatheter edge-to-edge repair a class 2a recommendation for patients severely symptomatic patients with NYHA class III or IV with primary/degenerative severe mitral regurgitation and high or prohibitive surgical risk, if mitral valve anatomy is favorable for the repair procedure and patient life expectancy is at least 1 year [67]. Similarly, class 2a recommendation is given for transcatheter edge-to-edge repair in patients with chronic severe secondary mitral regurgitation related to LV systolic dysfunction with NYHA Class II-IV symptoms, LVEF of 20% to 50%, LVESD of $\leq$70 mm and PASP $\leq$70 mm Hg with suitable anatomy.

Transcatheter Mitral Valve Replacement

Transcatheter mitral valve replacement is another percutaneous option for treatment of mitral regurgitation in patients with anatomy not suitable for transcatheter edge-to-edge repair. There are many devices currently under clinical investigation for transcatheter mitral valve replacement delivered via transapical or trans-septal approach. SAPIEN 3, SAPIEN 3 Ultra, and SAPIEN 3 Ultra RESILIA Transcatheter Heart Valve System (Edwards Lifesciences Corp, Irvine, CA) are the only systems currently approved by the U.S. Food and Drug Administration for commercial use. In 2023, Guerrero and colleagues reported the final 5-year outcomes of the MITRAL (Mitral Implantation of Transcatheter Valves) trial which was the first prospective trial to evaluate the safety and feasibility of transcatheter heart valves in patients with failed surgical bioprostheses or annuloplasty rings and severe mitral annular calcification treated with mitral valve-in-valve (MViV), valve-in-ring (MViR), or valve-in-mitral annular calcification (ViMAC) [68]. A total of 91 patients were enrolled in the study. Primary endpoints of this analysis included all-cause mortality, clinical effectiveness including NYHA functional class and performance endpoint of mean mitral valve gradient and residual mitral regurgitation. At 5-year follow-up, all-cause mortality was 21.4%, 65.5% and 67.9% in MViV, MViR and ViMAC groups respectively. The percentage of patients in NYHA functional class I or II was 94.7%, 50% and 55.6% in MViV, MViR and ViMAC groups respectively. Mean mitral gradients remained stable at 6.6 ± 2.5 mm Hg, 5.8 ± 0.1 and 6.7 ± 2.5 mm Hg in MViV, MViR and ViMAC groups respectively. Current U.S. Food and Drug Administration approved indications for Edwards SAPIEN 3, SAPIEN 3 Ultra, and SAPIEN 3 Ultra RESILIA Transcatheter Heart Valve System include replacement of native mitral valve with annuloplasty ring in patient with symptomatic heart failure and mitral regurgitation with prohibitive surgical risk and replacement of bioprosthetic mitral valve in patients with symptomatic heart failure and mitral regurgitation who intermediate or greater risk for surgery [69]. While transcatheter mitral valve replacement expands the population of patients eligible for percutaneous mitral valve intervention for mitral regurgitation, it also comes with its own challenges associated with anatomical complexity of the valve such as valve migration and embolization, paravalvular leak and LVOT obstruction [70]. Despite these challenges there is growing evidence for successful use of these devices and further clinical trials are needed to establish long-term clinical safety and effectiveness outcomes [71].

Percutaneous Mitral Annuloplasty

There are two types of percutaneous mitral annuloplasty, direct annuloplasty in which a device is attached directly to the mitral annulus and indirect annuloplasty in which a device is placed into coronary sinus to reduce the size of the mitral valve annulus and thereby improve valve leaflet coaptation [72]. Several different devices are under clinical investigation for percutaneous mitral valve annuloplasty, while several (Cardioband, Mitralign and Carillon) received the Conformité Europééne (CE) mark, none are approved by U.S. Food and Drug Administration for commercial use so far.

In 2019, Messika-Zeitoun and colleagues reported the 1-year outcomes of the transcatheter mitral valve repair for functional mitral regurgitation using the Cardioband (Edwards Lifesciences Corp, Irvine, CA), the most commonly used direct percutaneous mitral valve annuloplasty [73]. A total of 60 patients with moderate or severe secondary mitral regurgitation and high surgical risk underwent placement of Cardioband device. At 1 year follow-up, overall survival, survival free of readmission for heart failure, and survival free of reintervention were 87%, 66%, and 78%, respectively. Mitral regurgitation severity decreased, functional status, exercise capacity and quality of life improved in majority of the patients.

Carillon (Cardiac Dimensions Inc., Kirkland, WA) is the most widely used indirect percutaneous mitral valve annuloplasty device with the most clinical data. The device is made of two self-expanding nitinol anchors placed into proximal coronary sinus and great cardiac vein connected by fixed length nitinol cable. The device has been studied in several clinical trials including AMADEUS, TITAN, TITAN II and REDUCE-FMR. The most recent trial, REDUCE-FMR was a randomized, placebo-controlled, double-blind, proof-of-concept study to evaluate the outcomes of Carillon device on mitral regurgitation severity and left ventricular remodeling [74]. A total of 87 patients were randomized to receive the actual device and 33 patients underwent the sham procedure. The primary endpoint of reduction in mitral regurgitant volume was met with reduction in 7.1 mL/beat in the device group vs increase of 3.3 mL/beat in the control group. There were also statistically significant differences in left ventricular volumes and left ventricular end systolic volumes. The major drawback of the device has been potential for left circumflex artery compression. In the REDUCE-FMR trial, a total of 8 (9%) of patients had to have the device be recaptured due to compression of the left circumflex artery.

Surgical therapy will always remain the gold standard of care for these patients, and the use of alternative therapies needs to be done with an informed discussion with the patient regarding the possibility of recurrent regurgitation. However, open surgical approach is not without significant morbidity and postoperative recovery. A careful balance needs to be achieved between attaining a better clinical endpoint and the patient's quality of life.

To summarize, mitral regurgitation is a predictor of mortality in patients with poor ventricular function. Significant mitral regurgitation (moderate or more) warrants surgical intervention, even more so if done concomitantly with coronary artery surgery. Surgery in the form of a restrictive annuloplasty can be performed with an early mortality of 5–10%. While late survival will not be favorably altered with mitral valve surgery, quality of life and functional capacity is definitely superior. Mitral valve replacement is comparable to repair with regards outcome, especially if performed using the chordal sparing approach. Patient factors like renal dysfunction, age, diabetes, and era of surgery are important predictors of survival. Important concerns with repair like the risk of recurrence and the risk of inducing functional mitral stenosis have to be considered while making the decision to repair or replace the valve.

Percutaneous interventions for mitral valve have now become widespread in their use especially in patient with prohibitive surgical risk. Transcatheter edge-to-edge repair with MitraClip and PASCAL, the most performed procedure, has proven to be a safe and effective technique for patients with either degenerative or functional mitral regurgitation in patients with high surgical risk. While many other techniques and devices are still under clinical investigation, there is growing evidence supporting the use of minimally invasive percutaneous mitral valve interventions in appropriately selected patient populations. As always, heart team approach in decision making process remains the integral part of selecting the most appropriate approach and improving clinical outcomes for the patients.

Tricuspid Regurgitation

Tricuspid valve disease may occur in patients with congestive heart failure. It is primarily due to two mechanisms: (a) Tricuspid regurgitation (TR) develops secondary to pulmonary hypertension and right ventricular dysfunction (b) Primary tricuspid valve disease can occur due to isolated right ventricular dysfunction or more commonly due to pacemaker lead induced damage.

Secondary TR is the most common tricuspid valve pathology associated with congestive heart failure. Right ventricular dysfunction results in a gradual increase in the annular diameter of the tricuspid valve. This enlargement occurs at the anterior aspect of the annulus corresponding to the right ventricular free wall. Its shape changes from a saddle to a more planar dimension [75]. An enlarged annulus leads to improper coaptation of the leaflets and a predominantly central jet of regurgitation. They may suffer from ascites, pedal edema and hepatomegaly, the classical features of right-sided failure. Additionally, they also demonstrate reduced functional capacity, fatigue and dyspnea on exertion.

Dreyfus et al. have demonstrated that TR may fail to resolve after correction of the left sided pathology [76]. The presence of severe TR is also an independent predictor of mortality [39]. Hence severe TR is best corrected surgically at the time of mitral valve surgery (Class I indication) [77]. Data regarding tricuspid valve surgery in isolated TR or TR after prior correction of left sided pathology is less clear (Class IIA indication) [77]. In patients with ischemic/functional mitral regurgitation, TR is a more important issue. Matsunaga et al. demonstrated a 30% prevalence of 2^{+}TR in patients undergoing mitral valve surgery. In spite of adopting a very liberal policy towards surgical correction of the tricuspid valve, almost 2/3rd of the patients developed moderate TR at the end of 3 years [78].

Tricuspid valve repair consists of various procedures like (1) autologous procedures viz. bicuspidalization [79] or De Vega annuloplasty & (2) annuloplasty procedures using rigid or flexible bands/rings. A large series of 790 patients demonstrates the use of four different techniques: DeVega repair, Peri-Guard® pericardial strip annuloplasty, Edwards-Cosgrove flexible band and Carpentier-Edwards semi-rigid ring.

Tricuspid valve replacement can be performed using either a mechanical or bioprosthetic. As a rule, tissue valves are preferred unless specifically contra-indicated for other reasons. Readers are encouraged to pursue the article by Chikwe et al. for a detailed description of the available surgical procedures [80].

Concomitant tricuspid valve surgery with mitral procedures can be done very safely (1–2% early mortality). A comparison of the various available procedures demonstrates more durable results with prosthetic annuloplasty compared to autologous procedures [81].

Results after the surgical repair of isolated tricuspid valve repair are less satisfactory. Severe underlying right ventricular failure has been implicated as an important causative factor. Predictors of poor outcome after isolated tricuspid surgery are poor NYHA functional class, pre-operative hemoglobin and right ventricular end-systolic area [82].

A study reviewing the Mayo Clinic experience with isolated tricuspid valve replacement demonstrated that NYHA class IV and a higher Charlson index were independent predictors for late mortality [83]. The only echocardiographic predictor identified was right index of myocardial performance (RIMP) ratio [83]. Among survivors, almost a quarter needed re-admission for congestive heart failure during the follow-up period. Hence intensive surveillance is important even after surgery to ensure good functional status and quality of life.

The poor results are partly due to a reluctance of surgeons to operate on the tricuspid valve. Analysis of the Society of Thoracic Surgeons cardiac database from 2004 to 2007 demonstrates that tricuspid valve surgery is conducted in very small numbers [84]. Authors at the Mayo clinic demonstrate that surgery can be done with a reasonable outcome if patients are operated before the onset of severe right ventricular failure [83].

Percutaneous Techniques to Deal with Tricuspid Regurgitation

Given unmet clinical need due to high prevalence of tricuspid regurgitation which carries increased risk of mortality combined with reluctance of surgeons to operate on the tricuspid valve given highly variable outcomes [85], there has been a recent emphasis on development minimally invasive, percutaneous tricuspid valve interventions. These interventions can be subdivided into three categories including valve replacement, valve repair (transcatheter edge-to-edge repair, annuloplasty, chordal system) and valve implantation. A detailed discussion of various percutaneous techniques available for tricuspid regurgitation is provided by Seligman and colleagues in their comprehensive review [86].

Transcatheter Edge-to-Edge Repair

Transcatheter edge-to-edge repair using the TriClip™ (Abbott Vascular, Santa Clara, CA) and with PASCAL (Edwards Lifesciences, Irvine, CA) is the most utilized percutaneous tricuspid valve intervention given due to its safety and ease of use. In 2023, Sorajja and colleagues reported the results of the TRILUMINATE Pivotal trial (The Trial to Evaluate Cardiovascular Outcomes in Patients Treated with the Tricuspid Valve Repair System Pivotal), a proscpective, randomized, controlled trial evaluating the outcomes of the transcatheter edge-to-edge repair with TriClip as compared with medical therapy alone [87]. A total of 175 patients were randomized to the device group and 175 were randomized to the medical therapy group. The primary end point was a hierarchical composite including death from any cause or tricuspid-valve surgery, heart failure hospitalization and an improvement in quality of life as measured with the Kansas City Cardiomyopathy Questionnaire at the 1-year follow-up. TriClip was found to be superior to the medical therapy for the primary end-point which was primarily driven by the improvement in quality of life without any significant differences in death from any cause of heart failure hospitalizations. There was a statistically significant reduction in tricuspid regurgitation in the device group, 87% of patients in the device group compared to 4.8% in the medical therapy group had no greater than moderate tricuspid regurgitation at 30-days. The device was also found to be safe with 98.3% of patients in the device group without any major adverse event. Similarly, PASCAL has demonstrated promising results in the first-in-human compassionate use experience in patients with severe tricuspid regurgitation [88]. A total of 28 patients underwent treatment with PASCAL system and 85% achieved TR grade ≤2+ and mortality of 7.1% at 30-day follow-up. The ongoing CLASP II TR trial which is currently ongoing will evaluate the safety and effectiveness of the PASCAL system for patients with severe tricuspid regurgitation deemed to be at intermediate or greater surgical risk compared to medical therapy alone [89].

Transcatheter Valve Replacement

Several different transcatheter valve systems are currently under clinical investigation for tricuspid valve replacement. The system with the most clinical data so far is the EVOQUE System (Edwards Lifesciences, Irvine, CA). The safety and effectiveness of the device was demonstrated in the TRISCEND early feasibility study [90]. Most recently, Hahn and colleagues reported the results of the TRISCEND II Pivotal, a prospective, randomized, controlled trial which evaluated the safety and effectiveness of transcatheter tricuspid-valve replacement using the EVOQUE tricuspid valve-replacement system along with medical therapy to medical therapy alone in for patients with symptomatic, severe tricuspid regurgitation [91]. A total of 267 patients were assigned to the valve replacement group and 133 to medical therapy alone. The hierarchical composite primary outcome was death from any cause, implantation of a right ventricular assist device or heart transplantation, post index tricuspid-valve intervention, hospitalization for heart failure, an improvement of at least 10 points in the score on the Kansas City Cardiomyopathy Questionnaire overall summary, an improvement of at least one New York Heart Association functional class, and an improvement of at least 30 m on the 6-min walk distance. The EVOQUE device group was found to be superior to the medical therapy alone in the hierarchical composite primary outcome which was primarily driven primarily by improvements in symptoms, quality of life, and functional capacity.

Transcatheter Caval Valve Implantation

For patients in whom direct tricuspid valve intervention is not feasible, heterotopic, caval valve implantation has emerged as an additional percutaneous intervention option. TricValve (P&F Products and Features, Wien, Austria) is a bicaval valve system which is implanted into the superior and inferior vena cava to reduce the congestive effects of severe tricuspid regurgitation. Safety and effectiveness of TricValve have been demonstrated in the early feasibility, first-in-human experience studies TRICUS (Safety and Efficacy of the TricValve Transcatheter Bicaval Valves System in the Superior and Inferior Vena Cava in Patients With Severe Tricuspid Regurgitation) and TRICUS EURO studies in patients with severe tricuspid regurgitation with significant caval backflow with prohibitive surgical risk [92]. At 1-year follow-up, improvement in Kansas City Cardiomyopathy Questionnaire score ≥15, improvement to NYHA functional class to I or II, or an increase ≥40 m in the 6-min walk test was observed in 96% of the patients who underwent placement of the TricValve system. Mortality was 6.8% at 1-year follow-up. TRICAV-I and TRICAV-II clinical trials are currently ongoing to evaluate the safety and effectiveness of the TricValve System with optimal medical therapy compared to optimal medical therapy alone in the treatment of patients with severe TR and caval reflux [93].

One of the important aspects to consider with percutaneous tricuspid valve intervention is the afterload that it can impose on the right ventricle and right ventricle-pulmonary artery coupling (RV-PA coupling) which can result from the right ventricular failure. Brener and colleagues demonstrated that RV-PA coupling is a strong, independent predictor of all-cause mortality in patients undergoing transcatheter tricuspid valve repair or replacement [94]. In this study RV-PA coupling ratios for the patients who underwent transcatheter tricuspid valve repair or replacement from the TriValve registry by dividing the tricuspid annular plane systolic excursion (TAPSE) by the PA systolic pressure (PASP) from transthoracic echocardiograms performed before the procedure and 30 days after the procedure. Higher TAPSE/PASP ratio >0.406 was associated with lower risk of all cause mortality compared to lower TAPSE/PASP ratio of ≤0.406.

Transcatheter tricuspid interventions are quickly emerging as safe and effective alternative to surgical repair or medical therapy alone fulfilling the unmet clinical need. Many questions still remain unanswered when it comes to timing, patient selection and optimal strategy selection for which further clinical trials are required.

Aortic Valve Disease

Aortic Regurgitation

Aortic regurgitation produces predominantly a volume overload on the left ventricle. The lesion is well tolerated initially, and symptoms are minimal. However, a left ventricular end-systolic diameter >50 mmHg is associated with increased mortality and is an indication for aortic valve replacement. Guidelines recommend surgery even for asymptomatic patients with left ventricular dysfunction (LVEF <50%), however studies have demonstrated a significant reluctance to conduct surgery in these high-risk patients [77]. The Euro Heart Survey has demonstrated that only 22% with LVEF in the range of 30–50% underwent surgery while only 3% with severe LV dysfunction (LVEF <30%) received operative intervention [95]. A retrospective single center study demonstrated that only a third of the patients with severe AR and LV dysfunction underwent surgery. The pre-operative factors cited for non-intervention were an older age, female gender, presence of diabetes and renal dysfunction, and the need for concomitant procedures. Operative mortality is in the range of 7–10% [96]. Kamath and co-workers have demonstrated that in severe AR patients with severe LV dysfunction, AVR is an independent predictor of improved survival [97]. AVR had significant survival benefit with 1-year, 2-year, and 5-year survival rates of 88%, 82%, and 70%, respectively, compared to 65%, 50%, and 37%, respectively, in the population who did not receive AVR surgery ($p < 0.001$). Patients with severe LV dysfunction (LVEF <35%) and (LVEF <20%) demonstrated a 5-year survival of 70% and 60% respectively. Although survival cannot match the age-matched normal population, we have still demonstrated a benefit for surgical intervention. Propensity matched results have also demonstrated the advantage of surgical therapy [96].

A study from the Mayo Clinic demonstrated that preoperative ejection fraction, left ventricular end-systolic dimension, indexed end-systolic dimension, end-diastolic dimension, and indexed end-diastolic dimension were univariate predictors of late ejection fraction. In a multivariate model, the only predictor of late normal ejection fraction was a higher preoperative ejection fraction (odds ratio, 2.85; $p < 0.001$) [98].

Thankfully, regression in left ventricular dimensions has been demonstrated after aortic valve replacement. Bonow et al. monitored changes in left ventricular dimensions and ejection fraction after aortic valve replacement in 61 patients [99]. They utilized echocardiography and radionuclide scanning to assess them over a 7-year period. Between preoperative and early postoperative studies, left ventricular end-diastolic dimension decreased (from 75 ± 6 to 56 ± 9 mm, $p < 0.001$), peak systolic wall stress decreased (from 247 ± 50 to 163 ± 42 dynes), and ejection fraction increased (from 43 ± 9% to 51 ± 16%, $p < 0.001$). However, patients without early increase in the ejection fraction failed to demonstrate any improvement long-term. They further demonstrate a significant improvement in ejection fraction even in patients with severe LV dysfunction [96].

Hence, aortic valve replacement is beneficial even in patients with advanced left ventricular dysfunction. Compared to medical therapy, benefit in terms of quality of life and functional capacity is observed after surgery. Associated preoperative factors and a higher operative mortality rate must be considered when considering surgical intervention in patients with severe aortic regurgitation and left ventricular dysfunction.

Aortic valve replacement is one of the most common adult cardiac procedures performed in the USA. Patients with a poor ejection fraction typically develop a subset of aortic stenosis (AS): a low gradient, low flow (LF-LG) severe AS.

Definition

LF-LG severe AS is defined as a combination of an EOA ≤1.0 cm^2 (or EOA index <0.6 cm^2/m^2) with a low mean trans-valvular gradient (less than 40 mmHg). Low flow means either a cardiac index <3 l/m^2/min or an ejection fraction (less than 40% or 35%).

Pseudo-Severe Aortic Stenosis

Patients with primarily left ventricular dysfunction may have a small aortic valve area with low trans-valvular gradient due to their sub-normal stroke volume. The small effective orifice area of the aortic valve in these patients is secondary to incomplete opening during systole.

This stratification has a significant clinical consequence as aortic valve replacement fails to improve the symptomatology in the latter cohort and may be detrimental.

Role of Dobutamine Stress Echocardiography

Dobutamine stress echocardiography [100] is implemented as a confirmatory test for assessing LF-LG AS. While true aortic stenosis will present with a significant increase in gradient (mean transvalvular gradient >40 mmHg) with minimally increase flow and aortic valve orifice area (change <0.3 cm^2, valve area <1 cms^2) pseudo-severe aortic stenosis will demonstrate an increased flow without much change in the gradient [77]. The European Committee for guidelines on valvular heart disease recommends this test for all patients with LF-LG AS. Apart from being a diagnostic test, the increase in ejection fraction helps to assess contractile reserve of the left ventricle, an important prognostic indicator [101]. Contractile reserve is defined as an increase in ejection fraction >20% with dobutamine infusion compared to the baseline [102].

Momin et al. studied the changes in stroke volume, left ventricular ejection fraction, aortic valve area and mean pressure gradient in patients with and without contractile reserve on DSE. Patients with an intact contractile reserve demonstrated an increase in stroke volume (33%), LVEF (12%), aortic valve area (0.1 cm^2) and MPG (47%). Those devoid of contractile reserve demonstrated minimal increase in values on Dobutamine stress echocardiography.

TOPAS Study

The TOPAS (Truly or Pseudo-Severe Aortic Stenosis) is a prospective study conducted to improve the accuracy of differentiating true from pseudo-aortic stenosis. While authors agree that DSE is a reliable test, stenotic indices obtained from the DSE depend upon the magnitude of flow increase achieved. Blais and co-workers have developed a new stenotic index, the EOA_{proj} which determines the orifice area at a standardized flow rate of 250 ml/s, a constant which they have derived using hydraulic models in the laboratory. Hence they have presented their equation as: $EOA_{proj} = EOA_{rest} + VC*(250\text{-}Q_{rest})$. The authors have further indexed this obtained value to the patient's body surface area to derive the indexed projected EOA. Using a cut-off of ≤0.55 cm²/m², the sensitivity of this score increased from 93% to 100% (Fig. 25.6) [103].

While these investigations are useful to the surgeon for risk stratification, clinical assessment and evaluation of risk factors are essential to implement the correct strategy suited to the individual patient. However, optimal medical therapy has proved inferior to surgical AVR irrespective of contractile flow reserve. Five-year mortality with conservative therapy can be as high as 87%. Hence many authors recommend valve replacement for patients with LF LG aortic stenosis [101, 103]. Trans-cutaneous aortic valve implantation is emerging as an exciting option for these high-risk patients.

Results of Conventional AVR

Peri-operative Mortality

Overall peri-operative mortality in this cohort remains high; in the range of 9–22% [101, 104–107]. Cardiogenic shock (79%), sepsis (9%), stroke (3%) and respiratory failure were reported as important causes of death in a multicentric study from Europe [107]. Univariate analysis of this large cohort of patients demonstrated that a higher EuroSCORE, poorer NYHA functional class, coronary artery disease, and longer surgical duration were important predictors of early mortality. Monin et al. [101] have demonstrated that operative risk is significantly higher for patients with a mean pressure gradient (MPG) <20 mmHg (44% vs 11%; $p = 0.0006$). Multivariate analysis from this cohort defined absence of contractile reserve (Odds ratio 10.9; 95% confidence interval 2.6–43.3; $p = 0.001$) and MPG <20 mmHg (Odds ratio 4.7; 95% confidence interval 1.1–21; $p = 0.04$) as predictors of peri-operative mortality. Coronary artery disease and prior myocardial infarction are also important in risk stratification [108]. Importantly, levy et al. [107] have demonstrated that surgical outcomes are better in the present era (2000–2005) (a 10% reduction in mortality; $p = 0.04$) in spite of more emergency cases being conducted (a 9% increase; $p = 0.04$).

While a risk stratification scores selectively devised for this patient population is not yet available, the use of the EuroSCORE or the STS risk score tailored to the individual patient's condition is the best tool to make an informed decision [109, 110]. As described earlier, DSE and contractile reserve are important prognosticators in patient outcome.

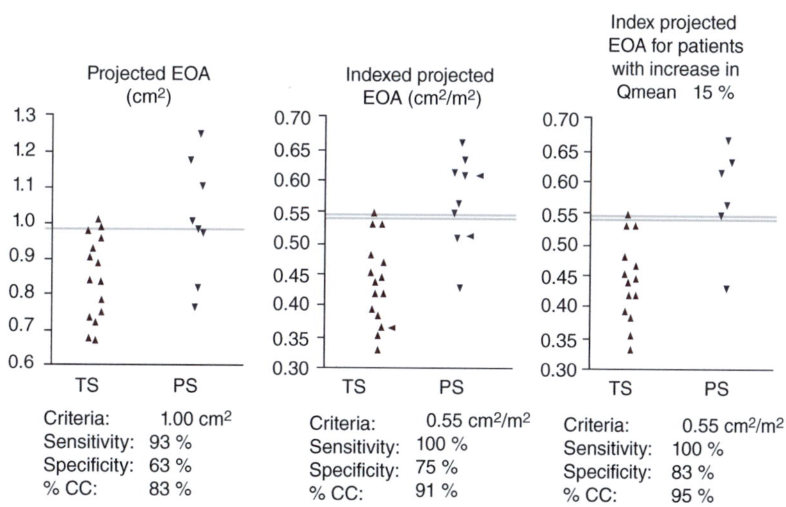

Fig. 25.6 The technique of indexed projected effective orifice area is a reliable test to differentiate true and pseudo-severe aortic stenosis. The panels D-F demonstrate the change of this parameter in patients with true (red triangles) and pseudo-severe (blue triangles) aortic stenosis. (Reprinted with permission Blais et al. [103]. © 2006, with permission from Wolters Kluwer Health Inc)

Functional Capacity After Aortic Valve Replacement

Multiple authors have demonstrated improved functional status after aortic valve replacement [101, 104, 105] While significantly more improvement was found in patients with a contractile reserve >20% on DSE, even patients with no reserve did better after aortic valve replacement [101]. The TOPAS study assessed the Duke Activity Score index (DASI) scores and distance covered in the standard 6-min walk test (6 MW) both before and after AVR. They were able to demonstrate a significant increase in both parameters (DASI and 6 MW) in the AVR cohort (ΔDASI: +5.9 ± 3.3 and Δ6 MW: +66 ± 27) while patients maintained with optimal medical therapy actually demonstrated a decline in function at the end of 1 year of follow-up (ΔDASI: −5.5 ± 2.6 and Δ6 MW: −9 ± 22) [111].

Predictors of Long-Term Survival

A multi-centric study has demonstrated an overall 5-year survival of 49 ± 4% after aortic valve replacement [107]. They have demonstrated a significant difference in survival stratified by ejection fraction (less and more than 20%; $p = 0.005$), multivessel coronary disease ($p = 0.002$) and EuroScore (less and more than 10; $p = 0.0001$). Recent European guidelines for valvular heart disease state that the EuroSCORE may overestimate mortality with the Society of Thoracic Surgeons risk calculator being a more accurate predictor in high-risk patients with severe aortic stenosis [63].

Results in patients with no contractile reserve: (Fig. 25.7).

Tribouilloy et al. [104] conducted a prospective multi-centric study of 81 patients with LF-LG aortic stenosis without contractile reserve. While their operative mortality was relatively high (22%), they demonstrated a significant improvement in 5 year survival in surgically treated patients compared to OMM (54 ± 7% vs 13 ± 7%; $p = 0.001$). Propensity matching demonstrated that an ejection fraction <20% and coronary artery disease were independent predictors of mortality. Hospital survivors demonstrated a 5-year survival of 69 ± 5%.

Thus, they demonstrated that aortic valve replacement was beneficial even in patients without functional reserve, albeit at the cost of a higher operatively mortality.

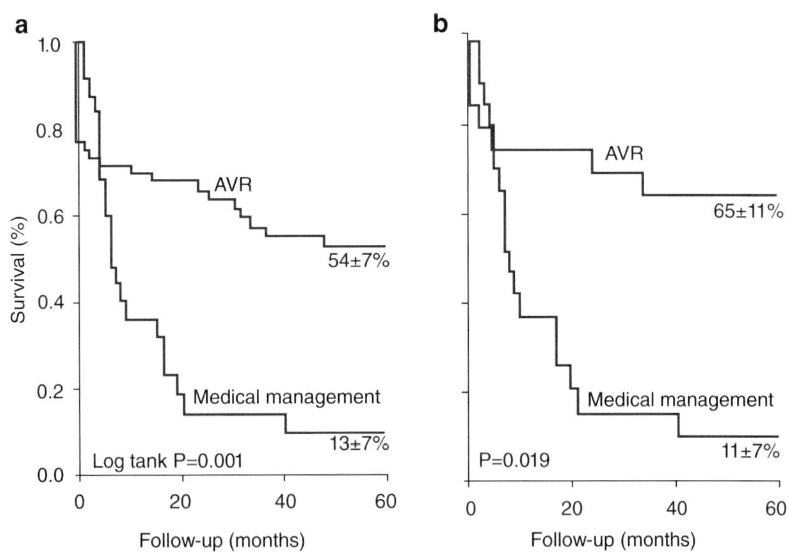

Fig. 25.7 This Kaplan-Meier curve compares survival with aortic valve replacement (AVR) or optimal medical therapy in patients without contractile reserve on Dobutamine Stress Echocardiograph. As depicted, results are significantly superior with AVR; in the entire cohort (**a**) as well a propensity matched sub-group (**b**). (Reprinted with permission from Tribouilloy et al. [104])

Results with Optimal Medical Therapy in Patients with LF-LG Aortic Stenosis

Studies are unanimous in concluding that optimal medical therapy is associated with very poor outcome in these patients. Both survival and functional class are very poor in patients managed non-surgically. Thus, in spite of the high early mortality, surgical aortic valve replacement provides the patient with the best odds for a longer and better quality of life.

Role of TAVI in Patients with LF-LG Severe Aortic Stenosis

Fraccaro et al. [112] have presented their data using Edwards SAPIEN / SAPIEN XT™ as well as then Medtronic CoreValve™ in patients with left ventricular dysfunction. They studied 384 patients undergoing transcutaneous aortic valve implantation (TAVI); 50 patients had LVEF <35% (Group A) while the remaining 334 (Group B) had normal left ventricular function. Patients ($n = 50$) with left ventricular function <35% had a much higher logistic EuroSCORE™, STS®score, higher degree of renal dysfunction and poorer NYHA functional class. While in-hospital mortality was higher in Group A (14%) compared to Group B (4%) ($p = 0.004$), among hospital survivors' cardiovascular mortality was comparable at the end of 1 year (10% in Group A and 6% in Group B; $p = 0.434$). In the group A cohort, ejection fraction increased from a baseline of 27.7 ± 6% to 46.6 ± 13.7% at the end of 1 year ($p < 0.0001$). The Authors conclude that further studies are needed to define the role of TAVI in patients with LF-LG severe aortic stenosis but recommend that left ventricular dysfunction should not be a contraindication for performing TAVI. They further make a recommendation for TAVI without pre-dilatation, as this avoids the need for rapid ventricular pacing which may be very deleterious in these sick patients (Fig. 25.8) [113].

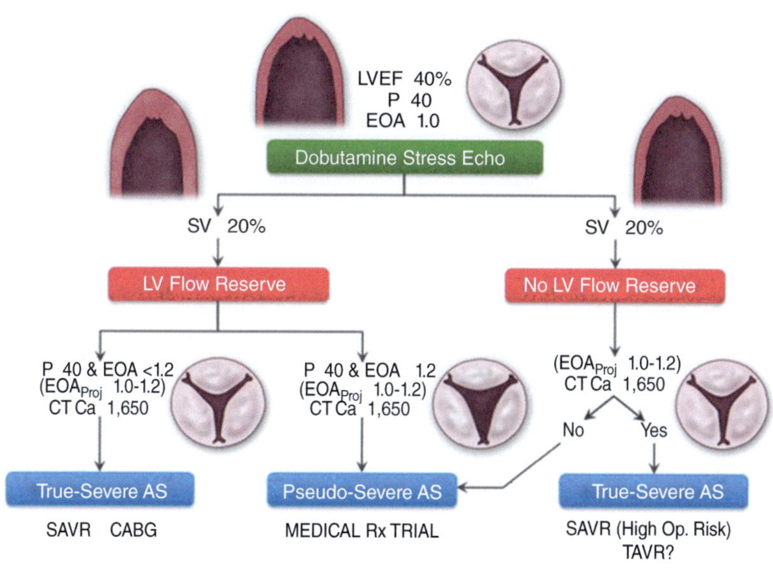

Fig. 25.8 Drs. Pibarot and Dumesnil have outlined this protocol for the management of patients with low-flow low-gradient severe aortic stenosis with a reduced ejection fraction. Abbreviations: EOA effective orifice area (in square centimeters), EOAProj projected EOA at normal flow rate (in square centimeters); P mean transvalvular gradient (in mmHg), CT Ca calcium score (in Agatston Unit) on Computerized tomography, SV stroke volume, Op operative, SAVR surgical aortic valve replacement, TAVR transcatheter aortic valve replacement. (Reprinted and adapted from Pibarot and Dumesnil [113], © 2012, with permission from Elsevier)

Conclusion

The treatment of patients with low flow low gradient aortic stenosis requires a coordinated approach between the cardiologist and surgeon. Dobutamine stress echocardiography is an important tool to separate true aortic stenosis from pseudo-aortic stenosis, a stratification having important clinical and therapeutic consequences. In spite of the higher operative mortality of surgical aortic valve replacement, this therapy provides better long-term survival and quality of life in the majority of survivors. Trans-cutaneous aortic valve implantation presents an exciting option in these patients; although left ventricular dysfunction should not be a contraindication for this procedure, the exact risk-benefit equation is still unknown.

Transcutaneous Aortic Valve Replacement

Surgical aortic valve replacement (SAVR) has been seen as the gold standard for the treatment of critical aortic stenosis for very long time. Recently, Transcutaneous aortic valve implantation (TAVI) has emerged as the gold standard therapy for managing critical aortic stenosis, particularly in patients at high or prohibitive surgical risk. Since Alain Cribier developed TAVI in 2002, it has undergone significant advancements.

TAVI has now been used in patients with high, intermediate, and low-risk patients with severe aortic stenosis as supported in trials like PARTNER 2A and SURTAVI. Both trials showed favorable outcomes in intermediate-risk patients [114, 115]. Newer generations of transcatheter valves have improved features like the ability to reposition, decreased paravalvular leak, and performance improvement [116, 117]. Procedure is less invasive and very frequently performed under local anesthesia under conscious sedation when performed via transfemoral access, which has reduced procedure time, length of stay in the hospital, and procedure-related complications [118, 119]. Pre-procedure planning has improved with advances in imaging techniques. The integration of artificial intelligence and multidetector computed tomography has improved the accuracy of valve sizing and positioning accuracy. It has also helped to reduce complications like paravalvular regurgitation and vascular injury [114, 120]. As providers have become more experienced with procedure and device technology, complication rates have decreased.

These advancements have collectively transformed TAVI into a routine and highly effective treatment for aortic stenosis in many patients.

Overview of Current Devices

Presently two devices are widely being used: The Edwards SAPIEN trans-catheter heart valve (Edwards Lifesciences, Irvine, CA) and the Medtronic CoreValve™ (Medtronic Corp, Minneapolis, MN, USA). The SAPIEN valve is designed from bovine pericardium, like the Edwards PERIMOUNT® valve. It is treated with the same THERMAFIX™ anti-calcification process implemented for all other valves. The Edwards SAPIEN valve is available in 23- and 26-mm sizes. These valves are recommended for annuli in the range of 18–22 mm and 21–25 mm respectively. The Edwards system has been designed for a trans-femoral or a trans-apical approach and is available in two sheath sizes (25Fr and 28Fr). While the trans-femoral delivery system contains a RETROFLEX 3™ delivery system, the trans-apical valve is placed on the ASCENDRA introducer system™.

Since its introduction, the Edwards SAPIEN valve has undergone several modifications to improve procedural outcomes and patient safety. The original SAPIEN valve was the first balloon-expandable transcatheter heart valve used in the pivotal PARTNER trials. It demonstrated efficacy in patients who were inoperable or at high surgical risk [121]. The SAPIEN XT valve was developed to address some of the limitations of the original SAPIEN valve. It has a lower profile and a cobalt-chromium frame, which improves deliverability and reduces vascular complications. The PARTNER II trial showed that the SAPIEN XT was non-inferior to surgical aortic valve replacement in high-risk patients [122]. The SAPIEN 3 valve introduced significant advancements, including an outer sealing skirt to minimize paravalvular regurgitation. It also featured an improved delivery system for more accurate placement. Clinical studies have shown that the SAPIEN 3 valve is associated with lower rates of paravalvular regurgitation and procedural complications than its predecessors [123, 124]. The SAPIEN 3 Ultra is the latest iteration. It further refines the design with sealing skirt and delivery system enhancements. These improvements aim to reduce paravalvular leaks further and simplify the implantation process [125].

The Medtronic CORE-VALVE™ is available in three sizes 26, 29 and 31 mm. The AccuTrak® delivery system is designed to provide a controlled environment of valve delivery without the need for rapid ventricular pacing during deployment. This valve has been designed for delivery via three routes: trans-femoral, direct trans-aortic and via the subclavian artery. Unlike the SAPIEN® valve, which is placed intra-annularly, the CORE-VALVE™ is a supra-annular seating valve with a much longer leaflet coaptation zone. This design has been provided to equitably distribute strain along the valve. The frame is provided with 8 mm gaps, which allow adequate coronary ostial perfusion and instrumentation. The CORE-VALVE™ delivery system is much smaller than the SAPIEN® at 18Fr size irrespective of valve size.

The Medtronic CoreValve system has also undergone significant changes since its introduction. The original CoreValve was a self-expanding valve made of a nitinol frame with a porcine pericardial tissue valve. It was designed to be deployed via a transfemoral approach and provided good hemodynamic performance but had issues with paravalvular leak and the need for permanent pacemaker implantation [126]. The Evolut R introduced a recapturable and repositionable feature, allowing for more precise placement. It also had a lower profile delivery system (14 Fr equivalent), which expanded the patient population eligible for transfemoral TAVR. This iteration showed improved outcomes regarding valve positioning and reduced paravalvular leak [127, 128]. The Evolut PRO added an outer pericardial wrap to the valve to further reduce the paravalvular leak. This design change resulted in lower rates of significant aortic regurgitation while maintaining excellent hemodynamic performance. However, it required a larger sheath size (16 Fr) than the Evolut R [129, 130]. The Evolut PRO+ maintained the features of the Evolut PRO but included enhancements to the delivery system and valve design to improve ease of use and further reduce complications. It continued to show excellent clinical outcomes with low rates of paravalvular leaks and comparable safety profiles [131]. Evolut FX is the latest iteration, which included technical enhancements to improve valve positioning, orientation, and vascular access. These improvements aim to enhance procedural success and reduce periprocedural complications, maintaining the trend of better clinical outcomes and valve performance [132].

Randomized Trials

The first US implant occurred as part of the REVIVAL I study in March 2005. This trial was designed to compare outcomes between TAVI with balloon aortic valvuloplasty. After technical problems due to antegrade implantation, modifications to design were made and the REVIVAL II was introduced, the first patient being enrolled in December 2005. This trial was designed to include only a trans-femoral approach, with 55 patients being enrolled.

The PARTNER (Placement of AoRticTraNscathetER Valves; Clinicaltrials.gov Identifier: NCT0053084) trial was the first prospective, multi-centric, pivotal, randomized controlled trial conducted to determine the efficacy of TAVI. The PARTNER A study consists of two cohorts: (A) a comparison of TAVI (either trans-femoral or transapical) using the SAPIEN® and SAVR in patients who are deemed high risk. (B) a comparison of trans-femoral TAVI and optimal medical management (OMM) in patients considered inoperable.

The PARTNER IA consisted of 699 high-risk patients with critical calcific aortic stenosis undergoing either transfemoral (TF) or transapical (TA) aortic valve replacement. The study was powered to achieve a statistical significance for all-cause mortality at the 1 year (non-inferiority). After including 492 and 207 patients in the TF and TA cohorts respectively, patients were assigned to TAVI or surgical aortic valve replacement with 1:1 randomization [133, 134].

The PARTNER IB study consisted of 358 patients considered too high risk for conventional surgery, but eligible for transfemoral TAVI. They were randomized equally between TF-TAVI and standard therapy, defined as Balloon aortic valvotomy (78.2%), medial therapy alone (7.9%), aortic valve replacement (6.1%) apical-aortic conduits (3.3%) or TAVI outside the USA (2.2%).

The PARTNER committee recently presented 2-year outcomes of the PARTNER IA study [135]. The PARTNER IA study met its non-inferiority endpoint demonstrating that TAVI has comparable outcomes to SAVR. The PARTNER IA study met its non-inferiority endpoint demonstrating that TAVI has comparable outcomes to SAVR. At the end of 2 years, all-cause mortality was comparable in both SAVR and TAVI cohorts at 35% and 33.9% respectively ($p = 0.78$). Bleeding complications were significantly higher in the SAVR cohort (29.5% vs 19%; $p = 0.002$) while stroke/TIA were more common in the TAVI cohort (11.2% vs 6.5%; $p = 0.05$). Vascular complications were present in 11.6% of TAVI patients, majority of them were related to the trans-femoral approach. Pacemaker requirement, dialysis, and endocarditis were comparable in both cohorts. Predictors of mortality for the TAVI cohort were a smaller body mass index (Hazard ratio 0.93(0.90, 0.97)), higher mean gradient (Hazard ratio 0.82(0.72, 0.94)), creatinine at baseline (Hazard ratio 1.06 (1.00, 1.13)) and prior vascular surgery or stent (Hazard ratio 1.85(1.10, 3.39)). The study demonstrated a satisfactory decline in the mean gradient and increase in the aortic valve area after TAVI during the 2-year follow-up.

The main concerns raised with TAVI were the occurrence of neurological events post-procedure and the presence of residual peri-prosthetic regurgitation. A separate article focusing on neurological events in this PARTNER IA study, demonstrated that there are two distinct hazard phases associated with adverse CNS events. While the initial phase was driven by the procedure (hazard function 2.21 + 0.68) the late phase was predominantly influenced by patient-related factors (like history of prior stroke and NYHA class) [136].

PARTNER investigators have found paravalvular regurgitation to be an important predictor of mortality. The presence of paravalvular leak (mild–severe) increased the odds of mortality twofold (1.43–3.10) over an estimated 3-year period ($p < 0.01$; log-rank test). The valve cover index, defined as 100* [(valve prosthesis diameter-annulus diameter)/valve prosthesis diameter] was lower in patients with paravalvular leak, demonstrating that valve under sizing was an important causative factor [137]. Colli et al. have introduced a calcification score, which allows prediction of post-procedure para- and overall aortic regurgitation [138].

The PARTNER IB cohort results demonstrate significant advantage of TAVI over OMM. TAVI reduced the occurrence of all-cause mortality and re-hospitalizations by 29.1% at the end of 1 year. The major concern was a higher incidence of stroke (5% vs 1.1%; $p = 0.06$) and major vascular complications (16.2% vs 1.1%; $p < 0.001$) in the TAVI; important to note that as part of the study design all patients in the TAVI arm underwent a trans-femoral approach. A significant improvement in functional status was present in the TAVI cohort compared to the OMM group.

Data is also available from several registries which look at results of TAVI in the "real world". They all report a procedural success rate ranging from 88% to more than 95%. The lowest reported 1-year morality is 6.7% while 30.7% is the highest [132].

The Medtronic Core Valve® US pivotal trial was published in May 2014. It compared TAVR using a self-expanding transcatheter aortic-valve bio prosthesis with SAVR in patients with severe aortic stenosis at increased surgical risk. The study included 795 patients who were randomly assigned to either TAVR or SAVR, with the primary endpoint being the death rate from any cause at 1 year. The results showed a significantly lower death rate in the TAVR group compared to the surgical group (14.2% vs. 19.1%), with an absolute risk reduction of 4.9 percentage points ($P < 0.001$ for noninferiority; $P = 0.04$ for superiority). Additionally, TAVR was non-inferior to SAVR regarding echocardiographic indexes, functional status, and quality of life. Exploratory analyses indicated a reduction in major adverse cardiovascular and cerebrovascular events and no increase in stroke risk [139].

PARTNER 2 trial compared transcatheter and surgical aortic valve replacement in intermediate-risk patients. It was published in April 2016. Authors of the study randomized 2032 intermediate-risk patients with severe aortic stenosis to undergo either TAVR or SAVR. The primary endpoint was the rate of death from any cause or disabling stroke at 2 years. Patients were enrolled from 57 centers *across USA and Canada*, with 76.3% in the transfemoral-access cohort and 23.7% in the transthoracic-access cohort. The results indicated that the rate of death from any cause or disabling stroke was similar between the TAVR and SAVR groups, with Kaplan-Meier event rates of 19.3% in the TAVR group and 21.1% in the SAVR group (hazard ratio, 0.89; 95% CI, 0.73–1.09; $P = 0.25$). In the transfemoral-access cohort, TAVR resulted in a lower rate of death or disabling stroke compared to SAVR (hazard ratio, 0.79; 95% CI, 0.62–1.00; $P = 0.05$), whereas outcomes were similar in the transthoracic-access cohort. TAVR was associated with lower rates of acute kidney injury, severe bleeding, and new-onset atrial fibrillation, while SAVR had fewer major vascular complications and less paravalvular aortic regurgitation. These findings support the use of TAVR as a non-inferior alternative to SAVR in intermediate-risk patients with severe aortic stenosis [140].

In SURTAVI, investigators assessed clinical outcomes in intermediate-risk patients with severe, symptomatic aortic stenosis by comparing TAVR using a self-expanding prosthesis with SAVR. This trial was performed in multiple centers across USA, Netherland and Denmark. The primary endpoint was a composite of death from any cause or disabling stroke at 24 months. Bayesian analytical methods were employed to evaluate the noninferiority of TAVR compared to SAVR. A total of 2032 patients were randomly assigned to either TAVR or SAVR at 57 centers. Patients were divided into two cohorts based on clinical and imaging findings: 76.3% were in the transfemoral-access cohort, and 23.7% were in the transthoracic-access cohort. The primary hypothesis was that TAVR would not be inferior to SAVR. The results indicated that the rate of death from any cause or disabling stroke was similar between the TAVR and SAVR groups, with Kaplan-Meier event rates of 19.3% in the TAVR group and 21.1% in the SAVR group (hazard ratio, 0.89; 95% CI, 0.73–1.09; $P = 0.25$). In the transfemoral-access cohort, TAVR resulted in a lower rate of death or disabling stroke compared to SAVR (hazard ratio, 0.79; 95% CI, 0.62–1.00; $P = 0.05$), while outcomes were similar in the transthoracic-access cohort. TAVR was associated with larger aortic-valve areas and lower rates of acute kidney injury, severe bleeding, and new-onset atrial fibrillation. In contrast, SAVR had fewer major vascular complications and less paravalvular aortic regurgitation [141].

The most recent clinical trial assessing TAVR in asymptomatic patients with severe aortic stenosis is the EARLY TAVR trial. This trial compared early TAVR using a balloon-expandable valve with clinical surveillance in 901 patients. The primary endpoint was a composite of death, stroke, or unplanned hospitalization for cardiovascular causes at 24 months. The results demonstrated that early TAVR significantly reduced the incidence of the primary endpoint compared to clinical surveillance (26.8% vs. 45.3%; hazard ratio, 0.50; 95% CI, 0.40–0.63; $P < 0.001$). Mortality occurred in 8.4% of patients assigned to transcatheter aortic valve replacement (TAVR) and in 9.2% of those assigned to clinical surveillance. Stroke rates were 4.2% in the TAVR group and 6.7% in the clinical surveillance group. Unplanned hospitalization for cardiovascular causes occurred in 20.9%of the TAVR group and 41.7% of the clinical surveillance group. During a median follow-up of 3.8 years, 87.0% of patients in the clinical surveillance group underwent aortic-valve replacement. There were no significant differences in procedure-related adverse events between patients in the TAVR group and those in the clinical surveillance group who eventually underwent aortic-valve replacement [142].

Ongoing studies are evaluating the long-term durability of TAVI valves, which is crucial as the procedure is increasingly used in younger, lower-risk populations [143].

Valve in Valve

The **valve-in-valve (ViV) procedure** treats failed bioprosthetic valves by implanting a new transcatheter heart valve within the existing bioprosthetic valve. This approach is particularly beneficial for patients at high surgical risk who have previously undergone surgical aortic valve replacement (SAVR) or transcatheter aortic valve replacement (TAVR) and now present with structural valve deterioration or other valve dysfunctions [144, 145].

In the context of transcatheter aortic valve replacement (TAVR) for asymptomatic patients with severe aortic stenosis, the ViV procedure is relevant as it provides a less invasive reintervention option if the initial TAVR valve deteriorates over time. The American College of Cardiology and the American Heart Association guidelines indicate that a second TAVR within the first prosthesis (ViV TAVR) is likely possible if significant valve deterioration occurs [144]. This is particularly important for younger patients or those with longer life expectancies, as it offers a feasible solution for managing valve durability concerns [146].

Economic Aspects of TAVI

A detailed cost-analysis of the PARTNER study revealed that procedural cost for transapical arm of TAVI ($90,000 ± 40,000) was higher than conventional aortic valve replacement ($80,000 ± 47,000). The cost of a transfemoral and conventional AVR were comparable. However, total expenditure at the end of 1 year in both cohorts was comparable [147]. While TF-TAVI resulted in improved quality of life (QOL) as well as cost benefit, patients undergoing TA-TAVI and conventional AVR had similar procedural cost and QOL scores. Thus, they conclude that at present TF-TAVI is economically beneficial to surgical AVR.

2021 ESC/EACTS Guidelines for the Management of Aortic Stenosis

Aortic stenosis is heterogenous condition and selection of the most appropriate mode of intervention should be carefully considered by the Heart Team for all patients, accounting for individual age and estimated life expectancy, comorbidities (including frailty and overall quality of life, section 3), anatomical and procedural characteristics (Tables 25.2 and 25.3), the relative risks of SAVR and TAVI and their long-term outcomes, prosthetic heart valve durability, feasibility of transfemoral TAVI, and local experience and outcome data. These factors should be discussed with the patient and their family to allow informed treatment choice [148].

Table 25.2 An outline of the present recommendations for TAVI in the management of symptomatic aortic stenosis [148]

Recommendations in symptomatic aortic stenosis	Class	Level
Intervention is recommended in symptomatic patients with severe, high-gradient aortic stenosis [mean gradient ≥40 mmHg, peak velocity ≥4.0 m/s, and valve area ≤1.0 cm^2 (or ≤0.6 cm^2/m^2)]	I	B
Intervention is recommended in symptomatic patients with severe low-flow (SVi ≤35 mL/m^2), low-gradient (<40 mmHg) aortic stenosis with reduced ejection fraction (<50%), and evidence of flow (contractile) reserve.	I	B
Intervention should be considered in symptomatic patients with low-flow, low-gradient (<40 mmHg) aortic stenosis with normal ejection fraction after careful confirmation that the aortic stenosis is severed	IIa	C
Intervention should be considered in symptomatic patients with low-flow, low-gradient severe aortic stenosis and reduced ejection fraction without flow (contractile) reserve, particularly when CCT calcium scoring confirms severe aortic stenosis.	IIa	C
Intervention is not recommended in patients with severe comorbidities when the intervention is unlikely to improve quality of life or prolong survival >1 year.	III	C

Table 25.3 A list of absolute and relative contra-indications for TAVI in the management of severe calcific aortic valve stenosis

Absolute contraindications
Absence of a 'heart team' and no cardiac surgery on the site
Appropriateness of TAVI, as an alternative to AVR, not confirmed by a 'heart team'
Clinical
Estimated life expectancy <1 year
Improvement of quality of life by TAVI unlikely because of comorbidities
Severe primary associated disease of other values with major contribution to the patient's symptoms, that can be treated only by surgery
Anatomical
Inadequate annulus size (<18 mm, >29 mm)
Thrombus in the left ventricle
Active endocarditis
Elevated risk of coronary ostium obstruction (asymmetric valve calcification, short distance between annulus and coronary ostium, small aortic sinuses)
Plaques with mobile thrombi in the ascending aorta, or arch
For transfemoral/subclavian approach: inadequate vascular access (vessel size, calcification, tortuosity)
Relative contraindication
Bicuspid or non-calcification
Untreated coronary artery disease requiring revascularization
Hemodynamic instability
LVEF <20%
For transapical approach: severe pulmonary disease, LV apex not accessible

Acknowledgements We would like to thank Dr. Ishan K Shah for his help in the preparation of the manuscript. We also thank Ms. Melody Roller for assisting us to obtain copyright permission for the reproduced figures in this chapter.

Disclosure We do not have any disclosure related to this article.

References

1. Carpentier A. Cardiac valve surgery—the "French correction". J Thorac Cardiovasc Surg. 1983;86(3):323–37.
2. Bolling SF, Deeb GM, Brunsting LA, Bach DS. Early outcome of mitral valve reconstruction in patients with end-stage cardiomyopathy. J Thorac Cardiovasc Surg. 1995;109(4):676–82; discussion 682–73.
3. Bach DS, Bolling SF. Early improvement in congestive heart failure after correction of secondary mitral regurgitation in end-stage cardiomyopathy. Am Heart J. 1995;129(6):1165–70.
4. Calafiore AM, Gallina S, Di Mauro M, et al. Mitral valve procedure in dilated cardiomyopathy: repair or replacement? Ann Thorac Surg. 2001;71(4):1146–52; discussion 1152–43
5. Replogle RL, Campbell CD. Surgery for mitral regurgitation associated with ischemic heart disease. Results and strategies. Circulation. 1989;9(6 Pt 2):I122–5.
6. Maltais S, Schaff HV, Daly RC, et al. Mitral regurgitation surgery in patients with ischemic cardiomyopathy and ischemic mitral regurgitation: factors that influence survival. J Thorac Cardiovasc Surg. 2011;142(5):995–1001.

7. Timek TA, Miller DC. Another multidisciplinary look at ischemic mitral regurgitation. Semin Thorac Cardiovasc Surg. 2011;23(3):220–31.
8. McGee EC, Gillinov AM, Blackstone EH, et al. Recurrent mitral regurgitation after annuloplasty for functional ischemic mitral regurgitation. J Thorac Cardiovasc Surg. 2004;128(6):916–24.
9. Bin J, Zhibin C, Weidong R, et al. Assessment of mitral annulus (p3 segment) asymmetric deformity in myocardial infarction with ischemic regurgitation by real time three-dimensional echocardiography. Echocardiography. 2012;29(1):42–50.
10. Watanabe N, Ogasawara Y, Yamaura Y, et al. Geometric differences of the mitral valve tenting between anterior and inferior myocardial infarction with significant ischemic mitral regurgitation: quantitation by novel software system with transthoracic real-time three-dimensional echocardiography. J Am Soc Echocardiogr. 2006;19(1):71–5.
11. Watanabe N, Ogasawara Y, Yamaura Y, et al. Mitral annulus flattens in ischemic mitral regurgitation: geometric differences between inferior and anterior myocardial infarction: a real-time 3-dimensional echocardiographic study. Circulation. 2005;112(9 Suppl):I458–62.
12. Watanabe N, Ogasawara Y, Yamaura Y, et al. Geometric deformity of the mitral annulus in patients with ischemic mitral regurgitation: a real-time three-dimensional echocardiographic study. J Heart Valve Dis. 2005;14(4):447–52.
13. Gorman 3rd JH, Jackson BM, Gorman RC, et al. Papillary muscle discoordination rather than increased annular area facilitates mitral regurgitation after acute posterior myocardial infarction. Circulation. 1997;96(9 Suppl):II-124–7.
14. Gorman 3rd JH, Gorman RC, Jackson BM, et al. Distortions of the mitral valve in acute ischemic mitral regurgitation. Ann Thorac Surg. 1997;64(4):1026–31.
15. He S, Fontaine AA, Schwammenthal E, et al. Integrated mechanism for functional mitral regurgitation: leaflet restriction versus coapting force: in vitro studies. Circulation. 1997;96(6):1826–34.
16. Agricola E, Oppizzi M, Pisani M, et al. Ischemic mitral regurgitation: mechanisms and echocardiographic classification. Eur Heart J Cardiovasc Imaging. 2008;9(2):207–21.
17. Di Salvo TG, Acker MA, William Dec G, Byrne JG. Mitral valve surgery in advanced heart failure. J Am Coll Cardiol. 2010;55(4):271–82.
18. Kono T, Sabbah HN, Rosman H, et al. Left ventricular shape is the primary determinant of functional mitral regurgitation in heart failure. J Am Coll Cardiol. 1992;20(7):1594–8.
19. Sabbah HN, Kono T, Rosman H, et al. Left ventricular shape: a factor in the etiology of functional mitral regurgitation in heart failure. Am Heart J. 1992;23(4):961–6.
20. Kono T, Sabbah HN, Stein PD, et al. Left ventricular shape as a determinant of functional mitral regurgitation in patients with severe heart failure secondary to either coronary artery disease or idiopathic dilated cardiomyopathy. Am J Cardiol. 1991;68(4):355–9.
21. Boltwood CM, Tei C, Wong M, Shah PM. Quantitative echocardiography of the mitral complex in dilated cardiomyopathy: the mechanism of functional mitral regurgitation. Circulation. 1983;68(3):498–508.
22. Sadeghpour A, Abtahi F, Kiavar M, et al. Echocardiographic evaluation of mitral geometry in functional mitral regurgitation. J Cardiothorac Surg. 2008;3:54.
23. Keren G, Katz S, Strom J, et al. Dynamic mitral regurgitation. An important determinant of the hemodynamic response to load alterations and inotropic therapy in severe heart failure. Circulation. 1989;80(2):306–13.
24. Lancellotti P, Magne J. Stress testing for the evaluation of patients with mitral regurgitation. Curr Opin Cardiol. 2012;27(5):492–8.
25. Bach DS, Deeb GM, Bolling SF. Accuracy of intraoperative transesophageal echocardiography for estimating the severity of functional mitral regurgitation. Am J Cardiol. 1995;76(7):508–12.
26. Lancellotti P, Lebrun F, Pierard LA. Determinants of exercise-induced changes in mitral regurgitation in patients with coronary artery disease and left ventricular dysfunction. J Am Coll Cardiol. 2003;42(11):1921–8.
27. Lebrun F, Lancellotti P, Pierard LA. Quantitation of functional mitral regurgitation during bicycle exercise in patients with heart failure. J Am Coll Cardiol. 2001;38(6):1685–92.
28. Giga V, Ostojic M, Vujisic-Tesic B, et al. Exercise-induced changes in mitral regurgitation in patients with prior myocardial infarction and left ventricular dysfunction: relation to mitral deformation and left ventricular function and shape. Eur Heart J. 2005;26(18):1860–5.
29. Pierard LA, Lancellotti P. The role of ischemic mitral regurgitation in the pathogenesis of acute pulmonary edema. N Engl J Med. 2004;351(16):1627–34.
30. Lancellotti P, Melon P, Sakalihasan N, et al. Effect of cardiac resynchronization therapy on functional mitral regurgitation in heart failure. Am J Cardiol. 2004;94(11):1462–5.
31. Lancellotti P, Gerard PL, Pierard LA. Long-term outcome of patients with heart failure and dynamic functional mitral regurgitation. Eur Heart J. 2005;26(15):1528–32.
32. Lancellotti P, Troisfontaines P, Toussaint AC, Pierard LA. Prognostic importance of exercise-induced changes in mitral regurgitation in patients with chronic ischemic left ventricular dysfunction. Circulation. 2003;108(14):1713–7.
33. Yiu SF, Enriguqez-Sarano M, Tribouilloy C, et al. Determinants of the degree of functional mitral regurgitation in patients with systolic left ventricular dysfunction: a quantitative clinical study. Circulation. 2000;102(12):1400–6.

34. Grande-Allen KJ, Borowski AG, Troughton RW, et al. Apparently normal mitral valves in patients with heart failure demonstrate biochemical and structural derangements: an extracellular matrix and echocardiographic study. J Am Coll Cardiol. 2005;45(1):54–61.
35. Hickey MS, Smith LR, Muhlbaier LH, et al. Current prognosis of ischemic mitral regurgitation. Implications for future management. Circulation. 1988;78(3 Pt 2):I51–9.
36. Lamas GA, Mitchell GF, Flaker GC, et al. Clinical significance of mitral regurgitation after acute myocardial infarction survival and ventricular enlargement investigators. Circulation. 1997;96(3):827–33.
37. Grigioni F, Enriquez-Sarano M, Zehr KJ, et al. Ischemic mitral regurgitation: long-term outcome and prognostic implications with quantitative doppler assessment. Circulation. 2001;103(13):1759–64.
38. Trichon BH, Felker GM, Shaw LK, et al. Relation of frequency and severity of mitral regurgitation to survival among patients with left ventricular systolic dysfunction and heart failure. Am J Cardiol. 2003;91(5):538–43.
39. Koelling TM, Aaronson KD, Cody RJ, et al. Prognostic significance of mitral regurgitation and tricuspid regurgitation in patients with left ventricular systolic dysfunction. Am Heart J. 2002;144(3):524–9.
40. Ellis SG, Whitlow PL, Raymond RE, Schneider JP. Impact of mitral regurgitation on long-term survival after percutaneous coronary intervention. Am J Cardiol. 2002;89(3):315–8.
41. Gillinov AM, Wierup PN, Blackstone EH, et al. Is repair preferable to replacement for ischemic mitral regurgitation? J Thorac Cardiovasc Surg. 2001;122(6):1125–41.
42. Grossi EA, Goldberg JD, LaPietra A, et al. Ischemic mitral valve reconstruction and replacement: comparison of long-term survival and complications. J Thorac Cardiovasc Surg. 2001;122(6):1107–24.
43. Bax JJ, Braun J, Somer ST, et al. Restrictive annuloplasty and coronary revascularization in ischemic mitral regurgitation results in reverse left ventricular remodeling. Circulation. 2004;110(11 Suppl 1):II103–8.
44. Geidel S, Lass M, Schneider C, et al. Downsizing of the mitral valve and coronary revascularization in severe ischemic mitral regurgitation results in reverse left ventricular and left atrial remodeling. Eur J Cardiothorac Surg. 2005;27(6):1011–6.
45. Bonow RO, Carabello BA, Chatterjee K, et al. 2008 focused update incorporated into the ACC/AHA 2006 guidelines for the management of patients with valvular heart disease: a report of the American College of Cardiology/American Heart Association Task Force on Practice Guidelines (Writing Committee to revise the 1998 guidelines for the management of patients with valvular heart disease). Endorsed by the Society of Cardiovascular Anesthesiologists, Society for Cardiovascular Angiography and Interventions, and Society of Thoracic Surgeons. J Am Coll Cardiol. 2008;52(13):e1–142.
46. David TE, Uden DE, Strauss HD. The importance of the mitral apparatus in left ventricular function after correction of mitral regurgitation. Circulation. 1983;68(3 Pt 2):II76–82.
47. Tibayan FA, Rodriguez F, Langer F, et al. Undersized mitral annuloplasty alters left ventricular shape during acute ischemic mitral regurgitation. Circulation. 2004;110(11 Suppl 1):II98–102.
48. Mihaljevic T, Lam BK, Rajeswaran J, et al. Impact of mitral valve annuloplasty combined with revascularization in patients with functional ischemic mitral regurgitation. J Am Coll Cardiol. 2007;49(22):2191–201.
49. Fukuda S, Gillinov AM, Song JM, et al. Echocardiographic insights into atrial and ventricular mechanisms of functional tricuspid regurgitation. Am Heart J. 2006;152(6):1208–14.
50. Chan V, Ruel M, Mesana TG. Mitral valve replacement is a viable alternative to mitral valve repair for ischemic mitral regurgitation: a case-matched study. Ann Thorac Surg. 2011;92(4):1358–65; discussion 1365–56.
51. Magne J, Senechal M, Mathieu P, et al. Restrictive annuloplasty for ischemic mitral regurgitation may induce functional mitral stenosis. J Am Coll Cardiol. 2008;51(17):1692–701.
52. Kainuma S, Taniguchi K, Toda K, et al. Pulmonary hypertension predicts adverse cardiac events after restrictive mitral annuloplasty for severe functional mitral regurgitation. J Thorac Cardiovasc Surg. 2011;142(4):783–92.
53. Kainuma S, Taniguchi K, Daimon T, et al. Does stringent restrictive annuloplasty for functional mitral regurgitation cause functional mitral stenosis and pulmonary hypertension? Circulation. 2011;124(11 Suppl):S97–106.
54. Daimon M, Fukuda S, Adams DH, et al. Mitral valve repair with Carpentier-McCarthy-Adams IMR ETlogix annuloplasty ring for ischemic mitral regurgitation: early echocardiographic results from a multi-center study. Circulation. 2006;114(1 Suppl):I588–93.
55. Martin CE, Castano M, Gomez-Plana J, et al. Mitral stenosis after IMR ETlogix ring annuloplasty for ischemic regurgitation. Asian Cardiovasc Thorac Ann. 2012;20(5):534–8.
56. Wong VM, Wenk JF, Zhang Z, et al. The effect of mitral annuloplasty shape in ischemic mitral regurgitation: a finite element simulation. Ann Thorac Surg. 2012;93(3):776–82.
57. Mirabel M, Iung B, Baron G, et al. What are the characteristics of patients with severe, symptomatic, mitral regurgitation who are denied surgery? Eur Heart J. 2007;28(11):1358–65.
58. Wunderlich NC, Shechter A, Swaans MJ, et al. Current percutaneous approaches to treat mitral valve regurgitation. Curr Treat Options Cardio Med. 2023;25:793–817.

59. Feldman T, Kar S, Rinaldi M, et al. Percutaneous mitral repair with the MitraClip system: safety and midterm durability in the initial EVEREST (Endovascular Valve Edge-to-Edge REpair Study) cohort. J Am Coll Cardiol. 2009;54(8):686–94.
60. Stone GW, Lindenfeld JA, et al. For the COAPT investigators transcatheter mitral-valve repair in patients with heart failure. N Engl J Med. 2018;379:2307–18. https://doi.org/10.1056/NEJMoa1806640.
61. Lindman B, Asch F, Grayburn P, et al. Ventricular remodeling and outcomes after mitral transcatheter edge-to-edge repair in heart failure: the COAPT trial. J Am Coll Cardiol Intv. 2023;16(10):1160–72. https://doi.org/10.1016/j.jcin.2023.02.031.
62. Pio S, Medvedofsky D, Delgado V, et al. Left atrial improvement in patients with secondary mitral regurgitation and heart failure: the COAPT trial. J Am Coll Cardiol Img. 2024;17(9):1015–27. https://doi.org/10.1016/j.jcmg.2024.03.016.
63. Stone GW, Abraham WT, Lindenfeld JA, et al. Five-year follow-up after transcatheter repair of secondary mitral regurgitation. N Engl J Med. 2023;388:2037–48. https://doi.org/10.1056/NEJMoa2300213.
64. Vincent F, Redfors B, Kotinkaduwa L, et al. Cerebrovascular events after transcatheter edge-to-edge repair and guideline-directed medical therapy in the COAPT trial. J Am Coll Cardiol Intv. 2023;16(12):1448–59. https://doi.org/10.1016/j.jcin.2023.03.023.
65. Zahr F, Smith RL, Gillam LD, Chadderdon S, Makkar R, et al. One-year outcomes from the CLASP IID randomized trial for degenerative mitral regurgitation. JACC Cardiovasc Interv. 2023;S1936-8798(23):01358–4. https://doi.org/10.1016/j.jcin.2023.10.002. Epub ahead of print
66. Edwards PASCAL CLASP IID/IIF Pivotal Clinical Trial (CLASP IID/IIF). https://clinicaltrials.gov/study/NCT03706833
67. Otto CM, Nishimura RA, et al. ACC/AHA guideline for the management of patients with valvular heart disease: a report of the American College of Cardiology/American Heart Association Joint Committee on Clinical Practice Guidelines. Circulation. 2020;143(5):e35–71. https://doi.org/10.1161/CIR.0000000000000923.
68. Guerrero ME, Eleid MF, Wang DD, Pursnani A, Kodali SK, George I, Palacios I, Russell H, Makkar RR, Kar S, Satler LF, Rajagopal V, Dangas G, Tang GHL, McCabe JM, Whisenant BK, Fang K, Balan P, Smalling R, Kaptzan T, Lewis B, Douglas PS, Hahn RT, Thaden J, Oh JK, Leon M, O'Neill W, Rihal C. 5-year prospective evaluation of mitral valve-in-valve, valve-in-ring, and valve-in-MAC outcomes: MITRAL trial final results. JACC Cardiovasc Interv. 2023;16(18):2211–27. https://doi.org/10.1016/j.jcin.2023.06.041.
69. Edwards SAPIEN 3, Edwards SAPIEN 3 Ultra, and Edwards SAPIEN 3 Ultra RESILIA Transcatheter Heart Valve Edwards Commander Delivery System. https://www.accessdata.fda.gov/cdrh_docs/pdf14/P140031S162C.pdf
70. Alperi A, Granada J, Bernier M, et al. Current status and future prospects of transcatheter mitral valve replacement: JACC state-of-the-art review. JACC. 2021;77(24):3058–78. https://doi.org/10.1016/j.jacc.2021.04.051.
71. Hensey M, Brown R, Lal S, et al. Transcatheter mitral valve replacement: an update on current techniques, technologies, and future directions. J Am Coll Cardiol Intv. 2021;14(5):489–500. https://doi.org/10.1016/j.jcin.2020.12.038.
72. Khatib D, Neuburger PJ, Pan S, Rong LQ. Transcatheter mitral valve interventions for mitral regurgitation: a review of mitral annuloplasty, valve replacement, and chordal repair devices. J Cardiothorac Vasc Anesth. 2022;36(10):3887–903. https://doi.org/10.1053/j.jvca.2022.05.005. Epub 2022 May 8
73. Messika-Zeitoun D, Nickenig G, Latib A, Kuck K-H, Baldus S, Schueler R, La Canna G, Agricola E, Kreidel F, Huntgeburth M, Zuber M, Verta P, Grayburn P, Vahanian A, Maisano F. Transcatheter mitral valve repair for functional mitral regurgitation using the Cardioband system: 1 year outcomes. Eur Heart J. 2019;40(5):466–72. https://doi.org/10.1093/eurheartj/ehy424.
74. Witte K, Lipiecki J, Siminiak T, et al. The REDUCE FMR trial: a randomized sham-controlled study of percutaneous mitral annuloplasty in functional mitral regurgitation. J Am Coll Cardiol HF. 2019;7(11):945–55. https://doi.org/10.1016/j.jchf.2019.06.011.
75. Pinney SP. The role of tricuspid valve repair and replacement in right heart failure. Curr Opin Cardiol. 2012;27(3):288–95.
76. Dreyfus GD, Corbi PJ, Chan KM, Bahrami T. Secondary tricuspid regurgitation or dilatation: which should be the criteria for surgical repair? Ann Thorac Surg. 2005;79(1):127–32.
77. Vahanian A, Alfieri O, Andreotti F, et al. Guidelines on the management of valvular heart disease (version 2012): the joint task force on the management of valvular heart disease of the European Society of Cardiology (ESC) and the European Association for Cardio-Thoracic Surgery (EACTS). Eur J Cardiothorac Surg. 2012;42(4):S1–44.
78. Matsunaga A, Duran CM. Progression of tricuspid regurgitation after repaired functional ischemic mitral regurgitation. Circulation. 2005;112(9 Suppl):I453–7.
79. Deloche A, Guerinon J, Fabiani JN, et al. Anatomical study of rheumatic tricuspid valve diseases: application to the study of various valvuloplasties. Ann Chir Thorac Cardiovasc. 1973;12(4):343–9.
80. Chikwe J, Anyanwu AC. Surgical strategies for functional tricuspid regurgitation. Semin Thorac Cardiovasc Surg. 2010;22(1):90–6.

81. McCarthy PM, Bhudia SK, Rajeswaran J, et al. Tricuspid valve repair: durability and risk factors for failure. J Thorac Cardiovasc Surg. 2004;127(3):674–85.
82. Kim YJ, Kwon DA, Kim HK, et al. Determinants of surgical outcome in patients with isolated tricuspid regurgitation. Circulation. 2009;120(17):1672–8.
83. Topilsky Y, Khanna AD, Oh JK, et al. Preoperative factors associated with adverse outcome after tricuspid valve replacement. Circulation. 2011;123(18):1929–39.
84. Rogers JH, Bolling SF. The tricuspid valve: current perspective and evolving management of tricuspid regurgitation. Circulation. 2009;119(20):2718–25.
85. Sarano ME, Zeitoun DM, Topilsky Y, Tribouilloy C, Benfari G, Michelena H. Tricuspid regurgitation is a public health crisis. Prog Cardiovasc Dis. 2019;62(6):447–51. https://doi.org/10.1016/j.pcad.2019.10.009.
86. Seligman H, et al. The current landscape of transcatheter tricuspid valve intervention. J Soc Cardiovasc Angiogr Interv. 2023;2(6):101201.
87. Sorajja P, Whisenant B, Hamid N, Naik H, Makkar R, Tadros P, Price MJ, Singh G, Fam N, Kar S, Schwartz JG, Mehta S, Bae R, Sekaran N, Warner T, Makar M, Zorn G, Spinner EM, Trusty PM, Benza R, Jorde U, McCarthy P, Thourani V, Tang GHL, Hahn RT, Adams DH, TRILUMINATE Pivotal Investigators. Transcatheter repair for patients with tricuspid regurgitation. N Engl J Med. 2023;388(20):1833–42. https://doi.org/10.1056/NEJMoa2300525. Epub 2023 Mar 4
88. Fam NP, Braun D, von Bardeleben RS, Nabauer M, Ruf T, Connelly KA, Ho E, Thiele H, Lurz P, Weber M, Nickenig G, Narang A, Davidson CJ, Hausleiter J. Compassionate use of the PASCAL transcatheter valve repair system for severe tricuspid regurgitation: a multicenter, observational, first-in-human experience. JACC Cardiovasc Interv. 2019;12(24):2488–95. https://doi.org/10.1016/j.jcin.2019.09.046.
89. Edwards PASCAL Transcatheter Valve Repair System Pivotal Clinical Trial (CLASP II TR) ClinicalTrials.gov ID NCT04097145. https://clinicaltrials.gov/study/NCT04097145
90. Kodali S, Hahn RT, George I, Davidson CJ, Narang A, Zahr F, Chadderdon S, Smith R, Grayburn PA, O'Neill WW, Wang DD, Herrmann H, Silvestry F, Elmariah S, Inglessis I, Passeri J, Lim DS, Salerno M, Makar M, Mack MJ, Leon MB, Makkar R, TRISCEND Investigators. Transfemoral tricuspid valve replacement in patients with tricuspid tegurgitation: TRISCEND study 30-day results. JACC Cardiovasc Interv. 2022;15(5):471–80. https://doi.org/10.1016/j.jcin.2022.01.016.
91. Hahn RT, Makkar R, Thourani VH, Makar M, Sharma RP, Haeffele C, Davidson CJ, Narang A, O'Neill B, Lee J, Yadav P, Zahr F, Chadderdon S, Eleid M, Pislaru S, Smith R, Szerlip M, Whisenant B, Sekaran NK, Garcia S, Stewart-Dehner T, Thiele H, Kipperman R, Koulogiannis K, Lim DS, Fowler D, Kapadia S, Harb SC, Grayburn PA, Sannino A, Mack MJ, Leon MB, Lurz P, Kodali SK, TRISCEND II Trial Investigators. Transcatheter valve replacement in severe tricuspid regurgitation. N Engl J Med. 2025;392(2):115–26. https://doi.org/10.1056/NEJMoa2401918. Epub 2024 Oct 30
92. Blasco-Turrión S, Briedis K, Estévez-Loureiro R, et al. Bicaval TricValve implantation in patients with severe symptomatic tricuspid regurgitation: 1-year follow-up outcomes. J Am Coll Cardiol Intv. 2024;17(1):60–72. https://doi.org/10.1016/j.jcin.2023.10.043.
93. Sugiura A, Tanaka T, Kavsur R, Öztürk C, Vogelhuber J, Silaschi M, Weber M, Zimmer S, Nickenig G. Tricuspid regurgitation: innovation, current landscape, and future perspective of transcatheter tricuspid valve interventions. J Cardiol. 2025., ISSN 0914-5087,; https://doi.org/10.1016/j.jjcc.2025.03.009.
94. Brener MI, Lurz P, Hausleiter J, Rodés-Cabau J, et al. Right ventricular-pulmonary arterial coupling and afterload reserve in patients undergoing transcatheter tricuspid valve repair. J Am Coll Cardiol. 2022;79(5):448–61., ISSN 0735-1097. https://doi.org/10.1016/j.jacc.2021.11.031.
95. Iung B, Baron G, Butchart EG, et al. A prospective survey of patients with valvular heart disease in Europe: the Euro Heart Survey on valvular heart disease. Eur Heart J. 2003;24(13):1231–43.
96. Chaliki HP, Mohty D, Avierinos JF, et al. Outcomes after aortic valve replacement in patients with severe aortic regurgitation and markedly reduced left ventricular function. Circulation. 2002;106(21):2687–93.
97. Kamath AR, Varadarajan P, Turk R, et al. Survival in patients with severe aortic regurgitation and severe left ventricular dysfunction is improved by aortic valve replacement: results from a cohort of 166 patients with an ejection fraction < or =35%. Circulation. 2009;120(11 Suppl):S134–8.
98. Brown ML, Schaff HV, Suri RM, et al. Indexed left ventricular dimensions best predict survival after aortic valve replacement in patients with aortic valve regurgitation. Ann Thorac Surg. 2009;87(4):1170–5; discussion 1175–76.
99. Bonow RO, Dodd JT, Maron BJ, O'Gara PT, White GG, McIntosh CL, et al. Long-term serial changes in left ventricular function and reversal of ventricular dilatation after valvereplacement for chronic aortic regurgitation. Circulation. 1988;78(5 Pt 1):1108–20.
100. deFilippi CR, Willett DL, Brickner ME, et al. Usefulness of dobutamine echocardiography in distinguishing severe from nonsevere valvular aortic stenosis in patients with depressed left ventricular function and low transvalvular gradients. Am J Cardiol. 1995;75(2):191–4.
101. Monin JL, Quere JP, Monchi M, et al. Low-gradient aortic stenosis: operative risk stratification and predictors for long-term outcome: a multicenter study

using dobutamine stress hemodynamics. Circulation. 2003;108(3):319–24.
102. Monin JL, Monchi M, Gest V, et al. Aortic stenosis with severe left ventricular dysfunction and low transvalvular pressure gradients: risk stratification by low-dose dobutamine echocardiography. J Am Coll Cardiol. 2001;37(8):2101–7.
103. Blais C, Burwash IG, Mundigler G, et al. Projected valve area at normal flow rate improves the assessment of stenosis severity in patients with low-flow, low-gradient aortic stenosis: the multicenter TOPAS (Truly or Pseudo-Severe Aortic Stenosis) study. Circulation. 2006;113(5):711–21.
104. Tribouilloy C, Levy F, Rusinaru D, et al. Outcome after aortic valve replacement for low-flow/low-gradient aortic stenosis without contractile reserve on dobutamine stress echocardiography. J Am Coll Cardiol. 2009;53(20):1865–73.
105. Connolly HM, Oh JK, Schaff HV, et al. Severe aortic stenosis with low transvalvular gradient and severe left ventricular dysfunction: result of aortic valve replacement in 52 patients. Circulation. 2000;101(16):1940–6.
106. Pai RG, Varadarajan P, Razzouk A. Survival benefit of aortic valve replacement in patients with severe aortic stenosis with low ejection fraction and low gradient with normal ejection fraction. Ann Thorac Surg. 2008;86(6):1781–9.
107. Levy F, Laurent M, Monin JL, et al. Aortic valve replacement for low-flow/low-gradient aortic stenosis operative risk stratification and long-term outcome: a European multicenter study. J Am Coll Cardiol. 2008;51(15):1466–72.
108. Powell DE, Tunick PA, Rosenzweig BP, et al. Aortic valve replacement in patients with aortic stenosis and severe left ventricular dysfunction. Arch Intern Med. 2000;160(9):1337–41.
109. Malfatto G, Branzi G, Giglio A, et al. Diastolic dysfunction and abnormal exercise ventilation predict adverse outcome in elderly patients with chronic systolic heart failure. Eur J Prev Cardiol. 2012;19(3):396–403.
110. Gardin JM, Leifer ES, Kitzman DW, et al. Usefulness of doppler echocardiographic left ventricular diastolic function and peak exercise oxygen consumption to predict cardiovascular outcomes in patients with systolic heart failure (from HF-ACTION). Am J Cardiol. 2012;110(6):862–9.
111. Clavel MA, Fuchs C, Burwash IG, et al. Predictors of outcomes in low-flow, low-gradient aortic stenosis: results of the multicenter TOPAS study. Circulation. 2008;118:S234–42.
112. Fraccaro C, Al-Lamee R, Tarantini G, et al. Transcatheter aortic valve implantation in patients with severe left ventricular dysfunction: immediate and mid-term results, a multicenter study. Circ Cardiovasc Interv. 2012;5(2):253–60.
113. Pibarot P, Dumesnil JG. Low-flow, low-gradient aortic stenosis with normal and depressed left ventricular ejection fraction. J Am Coll Cardiol. 2012;60(19):1845–53.
114. Cahill TJ, Chen M, Hayashida K, Latib A, Modine T, Piazza N, Redwood S, Søndergaard L, Prendergast BD. Transcatheter aortic valve implantation: current status and future perspectives. Eur Heart J. 2018;39(28):2625–34. https://doi.org/10.1093/eurheartj/ehy244.
115. Postolache A, Sperlongano S, Lancellotti P. TAVI after more than 20 years. J Clin Med. 2023;12(17):5645. https://doi.org/10.3390/jcm12175645.
116. Avvedimento M, Tang GHL. Transcatheter aortic valve replacement (TAVR): recent updates. Prog Cardiovasc Dis. 2021;69:73–83. https://doi.org/10.1016/j.pcad.2021.11.003. Epub 2021 Nov 17
117. Bourantas CV, Modolo R, Baumbach A, et al. The evolution of device technology in transcatheter aortic valve implantation. EuroIntervention. 2019;14(18):e1826–33. https://doi.org/10.4244/EIJ-D-18-01048.
118. Barbe T, Levesque T, Durand E, et al. Transcatheter aortic valve implantation: the road to a minimalist "stent-like" procedure. Arch Cardiovasc Dis. 2022;115(4):196–205. https://doi.org/10.1016/j.acvd.2022.03.004. Epub 2022 Apr 29
119. Tagliari AP, Taramasso M. New practices in transcatheter aortic valve implantation: how I do it in 2023. J Clin Med. 2023;12(4):1342. https://doi.org/10.3390/jcm12041342.
120. Mas-Peiro S, Fichtlscherer S, Walther C, Vasa-Nicotera M. Current issues in transcatheter aortic valve replacement. J Thorac Dis. 2020;12(4):1665–80. https://doi.org/10.21037/jtd.2020.01.10.
121. Minha S, Waksman R. Evaluation of the Edwards Lifesciences SAPIEN transcatheter heart valve. Expert Rev Med Devices. 2014;11(6):553–62. https://doi.org/10.1586/17434440.2014.947272. Epub 2014 Aug 9
122. Webb JG, Doshi D, Mack MJ, et al. A randomized evaluation of the SAPIEN XT transcatheter heart valve system in patients with aortic stenosis who are not candidates for surgery. JACC Cardiovasc Interv. 2015;8(14):1797–806. https://doi.org/10.1016/j.jcin.2015.08.017.
123. Schymik G, Wendler O, Hengstenberg C, et al. SOURCE 3 and SOURCE XT Investigators. Outcomes of transfemoral balloon expandable transcatheter aortic valve implantation: comparison of two subsequent valve generations. Catheter Cardiovasc Interv. 2020;96(4):930–9. https://doi.org/10.1002/ccd.28621. Epub 2019 Dec 3
124. Amat-Santos IJ, Dahou A, Webb J, et al. Comparison of hemodynamic performance of the balloon-expandable SAPIEN 3 versus SAPIEN XT transcatheter valve. Am J Cardiol. 2014;114(7):1075–82. https://doi.org/10.1016/j.amjcard.2014.07.019. Epub 2014 Jul 17

125. Solomonica A, Choudhury T, Bagur R. Newer-generation of Edwards transcatheter aortic valve systems: SAPIEN 3, Centera, and SAPIEN 3 Ultra. Expert Rev Med Devices. 2019;16(2):81–7. https://doi.org/10.1080/17434440.2019.1555465. Epub 2018 Dec 10
126. Grube E, Buellesfeld L, Mueller R, Sauren B, et al. Progress and current status of percutaneous aortic valve replacement: results of three device generations of the CoreValve Revalving system. Circ Cardiovasc Interv. 2008;1(3):167–75. https://doi.org/10.1161/CIRCINTERVENTIONS.108.819839.
127. Piazza N, Martucci G, Lachapelle K, et al. First-in-human experience with the Medtronic CoreValve Evolut R. EuroIntervention. 2014;9(11):1260–3. https://doi.org/10.4244/EIJV9I11A215.
128. Manoharan G, Walton AS, Brecker SJ, et al. Treatment of symptomatic severe aortic stenosis with a novel resheathable supra-annular self-expanding transcatheter aortic valve system. JACC Cardiovasc Interv. 2015;8(10):1359–67. https://doi.org/10.1016/j.jcin.2015.05.015.
129. Hellhammer K, Piayda K, Afzal S, et al. The latest evolution of the medtronic CoreValve system in the era of transcatheter aortic valve replacement: matched comparison of the Evolut PRO and Evolut R. JACC Cardiovasc Interv. 2018;11(22):2314–22. https://doi.org/10.1016/j.jcin.2018.07.023.
130. Forrest JK, Kaple RK, Tang GHL, et al. Three generations of self-expanding transcatheter aortic valves: a report from the STS/ACC TVT registry. JACC Cardiovasc Interv. 2020;13(2):170–9. https://doi.org/10.1016/j.jcin.2019.08.035.
131. Bhogal S, Rogers T, Merdler I, et al. Evolut PRO/PRO+ versus Evolut R system for transcatheter aortic valve replacement. Int J Cardiol. 2023;389:131196. https://doi.org/10.1016/j.ijcard.2023.131196. Epub 2023 Jul 19
132. Panagides V, Mesnier J, Nuche J, Delarochellière R, et al. From the Evolut Pro to the Evolut FX self-expanding transcatheter aortic valve replacement systems: current status and future perspectives. Expert Rev Med Devices. 2022;19(7):561–9. https://doi.org/10.1080/17434440.2022.2113386. Epub 2022 Aug 25
133. Leon MB, Smith CR, Mack M, et al. Transcatheter aortic-valve implantation for aortic stenosis in patients who cannot undergo surgery. N Engl J Med. 2010;363:1597–607.
134. Smith CR, Leon MB, Mack MJ, et al. Transcatheter versus surgical aortic-valve replacement in high-risk patients. N Engl J Med. 2011;364:2187–98.
135. Kodali SK, Williams MR, Smith CR, et al. Two-year outcomes after transcatheter or surgical aortic-valve replacement. N Engl J Med. 2012;366:1686–95.
136. Miller DC, Blackstone EH, Mack MJ, et al. Transcatheter (TAVR) versus surgical (AVR) aortic valve replacement: occurrence, hazard, risk factors, and consequences of neurologic events in the PARTNER trial. J Thorac Cardiovasc Surg. 2012;143(4):832–843.e13.
137. Detaint D, Lepage L, Himbert D, et al. Determinants of significant paravalvular regurgitation after transcatheter aortic valve: implantation impact of device and annulus discongruence. JACC Cardiovasc Interv. 2009;2(9):821–7.
138. Colli A, D'Amico R, Kempfert J, et al. Transesophageal echocardiographic scoring for transcatheter aortic valve implantation: impact of aortic cusp calcification on postoperative aortic regurgitation. J Thorac Cardiovasc Surg. 2011;142(5):1229–35.
139. Adams DH, Popma JJ, Reardon MJ, et al. Transcatheter aortic-valve replacement with a self-expanding prosthesis. N Engl J Med. 2014;370(19):1790–8. https://doi.org/10.1056/NEJMoa1400590. Epub 2014 Mar 29
140. Leon MB, Smith CR, Mack MJ, et al. Transcatheter or surgical aortic-valve replacement in intermediate-risk patients. N Engl J Med. 2016;374(17):1609–20. https://doi.org/10.1056/NEJMoa1514616. Epub 2016 Apr 2
141. Reardon MJ, Van Mieghem NM, Popma JJ, et al. Surgical or transcatheter aortic-valve replacement in intermediate-risk patients. N Engl J Med. 2017;376(14):1321–31. https://doi.org/10.1056/NEJMoa1700456. Epub 2017 Mar 17
142. Généreux P, Schwartz A, Oldemeyer JB, et al. Transcatheter aortic-valve replacement for asymptomatic severe aortic stenosis. N Engl J Med. 2025;392(3):217–27. https://doi.org/10.1056/NEJMoa2405880.
143. Rahhab Z, El Faquir N, Tchetche D, et al. Expanding the indications for transcatheter aortic valve implantation. Nat Rev Cardiol. 2020;17(2):75–84. https://doi.org/10.1038/s41569-019-0254-6.
144. Writing Committee Members, Otto CM, Nishimura RA, et al. 2020 ACC/AHA guideline for the management of patients with valvular heart disease: a report of the American College of Cardiology/American Heart Association Joint Committee on Clinical Practice Guidelines [published correction appears in J Am Coll Cardiol. 2021;77(4):509. 10.1016/j.jacc.2020.12.040.] [published correction appears in J Am Coll Cardiol. 2021;77(9):1275. 10.1016/j.jacc.2021.02.007.] [published correction appears in J Am Coll Cardiol. 2023;82(9):969. 10.1016/j.jacc.2023.07.010.] [published correction appears in J Am Coll Cardiol. 2024;84(18):1772. 10.1016/j.jacc.2024.09.025.]. J Am Coll Cardiol. 2021;77(4):e25–e197. https://doi.org/10.1016/j.jacc.2020.11.018.
145. Groginski T, Mansour A, Kamal D, Saad M. Transcatheter aortic valve replacement for failed surgical or transcatheter bioprosthetic valves: a comprehensive review. J Clin Med. 2024;13(5):1297. Published 2024 Feb 25. https://doi.org/10.3390/jcm13051297.

146. Beerkens FJ, Tang GHL, Kini AS, et al. Transcatheter aortic valve replacement beyond severe aortic stenosis: JACC state-of-the-art review. J Am Coll Cardiol. 2025;85(9):944–64. https://doi.org/10.1016/j.jacc.2024.11.051.
147. Reynolds MR, Magnuson EA, Lei Y, et al. Cost-effectiveness of transcatheter aortic valve replacement compared with surgical aortic valve replacement in high-risk patients with severe aortic stenosis: results of the PARTNER (Placement of Aortic Transcatheter Valves) trial (Cohort A). J Am Coll Cardiol. 2012;60(25):2683–92.
148. Vahanian A, Praz F, Milojevic M, et al. 2021 ESC/EACTS Guidelines for the management of valvular heart disease. EuroIntervention. 2022;17(14):e1126–96. https://doi.org/10.4244/EIJ-E-21-00009.
149. Vahanian A, Alfieri O, Andreotti F, et al. Guidelines on the management of valvular heart disease (version 2012): the joint task force on the management of valvular heart disease of the European Society of Cardiology (ESC) and the European Association for Cardio-Thoracic Surgery (EACTS). Eur J Cardiothorac Surg. 2012;33(19):2451–96.

Index

H. J. Eisen (ed.), *Heart Failure I*, https://doi.org/10.1007/978-3-032-12626-9

E

F

T

U

V

W

MIX
Papier aus verantwortungsvollen Quellen
Paper from responsible sources
FSC® C105338

If you have any concerns about our products,
you can contact us on
ProductSafety@springernature.com

In case Publisher is established outside the EU,
the EU authorized representative is:
Springer Nature Customer Service Center GmbH
Europaplatz 3, 69115 Heidelberg, Germany

Printed by Libri Plureos GmbH
in Hamburg, Germany